Medicine in a Day: Revision Notes

For Medical Exams, Finals, UKMLA and Foundation Years

Medicine in a Day: Revision Notes

For Medical Exams, Finals, UKMLA and Foundation Years

BERENICE AGUIRREZABALA ARMBRUSTER, MB ChB, BSc

Foundation Year Doctor
University Hospitals Coventry & Warwickshire NHS Foundation Trust
Coventry, UK

HANNAH PUNTER, MB ChB, MA, MSci

Foundation Year Doctor
University Hospitals Bristol and Weston NHS Foundation Trust
Bristol, UK

GREGORY PETER OXENHAM, MB ChB, BA

Junior ED Registrar
Palmerston North Hospital
MidCentral DHB, NZ

HOLLIE BLABER, MB ChB, BSc

Foundation Year Doctor
Milton Keynes University Hospital
Buckinghamshire, UK

MARCUS DRAKE, MA, DM, FRCS (Urol)

Academic Lead, Final Year
Bristol Medical School
Bristol, UK

For your complete, downloadable eBook version, see inside front cover for access details.

ELSEVIER

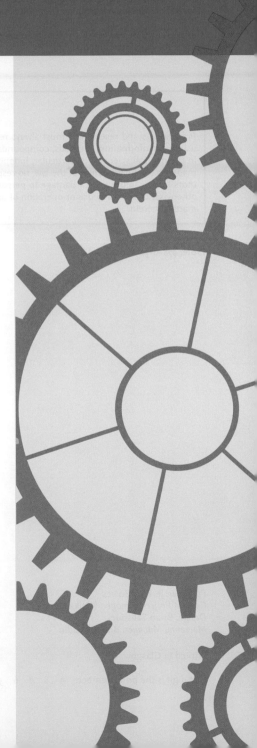

Notices

ISBN: 978-0-323-87098-6

Publisher: Jeremy Bowes
Content Project Manager: Kritika Kaushik
Design: Brian Salisbury
Marketing Manager: Belinda Tudin

Printed in Glasgow, UK

Last digit is the print number: 9 8 7 6 5 4 3 2 1

CONTENTS

I am delighted to write a foreword to this handy book, which aims to summarise 'medical practice' for junior doctors. Whilst no-one would advise practicing medicine without extensive background reading and experience, there are many situations where a concise summary to revise a clinical topic is invaluable. This book is the perfect text for those situations.

The book covers clinical conditions, complications, and common presentations, with considerations of equality and inclusion embedded throughout. It has been led by former medical students (now qualified doctors) from the University of Bristol. Amazingly, Berenice, Hannah and Greg managed to do this whilst studying for exams and then practicing as full-time

junior doctors in a pandemic. At the same time Hollie produced her beautiful illustrations. They have been supported by a large number of authors and experts to ensure that the key knowledge is included.

I am so impressed by the output - it just shows that with vision, determination, good team working and the right support, amazing achievements become possible. I commend this book to anyone trying to pass exams or survive as a junior doctor, and hope that you enjoy reading it as much as I have.

Jane Norman
Dean, Faculty of Health Sciences
University of Bristol

PREFACE

In *Medicine in a Day*, you will find the core knowledge a junior doctor needs, presented succinctly to facilitate rapid scrutiny. We aim the book at people who have previously been taught the subjects, but want a rapid refresher to remind them of the fundamentals. Once you are practising, this will be useful when you start a job in a new specialty, or need to deal with an issue that you have not seen for a while. And of course, for exams, this is a one-stop resource for that final burst of fact-cramming. The content covers the syllabus of the UK Medical Licensing Assessment, and will be sufficient for most other medical finals exams.

We have named the book "Medicine in a Day", but we admit that to cover all this in only 24 hours would be rather tough. We wish to express our utmost respect to any determined individual who manages the challenge. Many people may prefer to take a week, for a less demanding revision experience.

We have endeavoured to illustrate conditions with extensive representation of all skin tones. To help achieve this, we partnered with Don't Forget the Bubbles (DFTB) Skin Deep (https://dftbskindeep.com/about/), which provides an open-access bank of high-quality photographs of medical conditions in a range of skin tones for use by both healthcare professionals and the public.

We are sincerely grateful to the large number of people who have made this project possible. In particular, we would like to extend our immense gratitude to Professor Sanjay Gandhi, Dr Jacob Whitworth, Dr Simranjeet Kaur and their Radiology departments for provision of the radiological images. Dr Hollie Blaber has demonstrated incredible talent with her illustrations, which we believe greatly enrich the book. Working with everyone has been a privilege, and we thank all involved.

Please accept our best wishes for the success of your revision for Finals and other exams, and subsequent medical careers.

Berenice, Hannah, Greg, Hollie and Marcus

CONTRIBUTORS

The editor(s) would like to acknowledge and offer grateful thanks for the input of all contributors, without whom this edition would not have been possible.

Dr Viren Ahluwalia, MB ChB, BSc, MRCP

Dr Rebecca Allam, MB BS, BSc, MRCP

Dr Berenice Aguirrezabala Armbruster, MB ChB, BSc

Dr Oliver Arnold, MB ChB, BSc

Dr Denize Atan, BM BCh, PhD, MA, MRCP, FRCOphth

Dr Georgina Beckley, MB BS, BSc, FRCP

Dr Tom Bird, MB ChB, MSc, MRCP FRCR

Mr Matthew Boissaud-Cooke, MB ChB, BMedSc, MRCS

Dr Thomas Brankin-Frisby, MB ChB, BSc

Dr Chiara Bucciarelli-Ducci, MD, PhD, FRCP, FESC, FACC

Dr Yvonne Chang, MD, MRCP, FHEA

Professor Emma Clark, MB BS, PhD, FRCP

Dr Laura Cochran, MB BS, MA, MRCP (Pall Med)

Dr Ellie Crook, MRCP

Dr Joanne Davies, MB ChB, BA, MRCPsych

Professor Marcus Drake, DM, MA, FRCS (Urol)

Dr Judith Fox, MB BS, DPhil, MA, MSc

Professor Sanjay Gandhi, MB BS, MD, FRCR, FHEA

Dr Peter Goodrem, FRCP (Resp)

Dr Charlotte Hayden, MB ChB, BSc, MRCP

Miss Cherrie Ho, MB ChB, MSc, MRCS

Dr Paddy Horner, MB BS, MD, FRCP

Dr Ben Howes, MB ChB, FRCA

Dr Nagarjun Konda, MB ChB, BSc

Dr Angeliki Kosti, MB BS, BSc, MRCS

Miss Chrissie Laban, MD, FRCS

Dr Mark Lam, MB ChB, BDS

Mrs Claire Langton-Hewer, BM BCh, MA, FRCS (ORL-HNS)

Mr James Li, MB BChir, MRCS

Dr Jason Louis, MB ChB, FRCSEd, FRCEM

Dr Dan Magnus, BM BS, MSc, BMedSci, MRCPCH

Dr Dominic Mahoney, MB ChB, BSc

Dr Frankie Mayes, MB ChB, BSc

Dr Viola Mendonca, MB ChB, BSc

Professor Richard Morris, PhD, BSc

Dr Osamuyimen Omoragbon, MB ChB, BSc

Dr Gregory Oxenham, MB ChB, BA

Dr Dolcie Paxton, MB ChB, BSc

Dr Ruth Perkins, MB ChB, BSc

Dr Hannah Punter, MB ChB, MA, MSci

Mr Jonathan Rees, PhD, MSc, FRCS, FHEA

Dr Alexander Royston, MB ChB, MSc, BA

Dr Luke Rutter, MB ChB

Dr Jane Sansom, MB ChB, FRCP

Professor Simon Satchell, MB BS, PhD, MRCP

Dr Sanchita Sen, MB BS, FRCOG

Mr Karanjit Mangat, FRCS (Tr & Orth)

Dr Matthew Smith, BM BS, BSc, MRCP

Dr Nicola Taylor, MRCPsych

Dr Jonathan
Tyrrell-Price, FRCP

Dr Dillon Vyas,
MB ChB, MSc

Professor Michael
Whitehouse, PhD, MSc,
FRCS (Tr & Orth),
FHEA

Dr James Wiggins,
MB ChB, BMedSc

Dr Phil Wild,
MB BChir, MA

Dr Julia Wolf, MB BCh,
MRCP

Dr Jeffrey Wu, MB ChB,
BA, BSc

ACKNOWLEDGEMENTS

To our friends and family for their love and support, and for believing in us.

Especially to Berenice's mum, without whom this would not have been possible, to Toby, for his magnificent mnemonics, to our co-editors for their never-ending enthusiasm, motivation and guidance and to

Mark, for reliable provision of cups of tea! Plus, to Yotam Ottolenghi, as Greg loves your cookbooks.

To all those who contributed to this book – we are so proud of all of you.

And finally… To all those who dream to become the best doctor; WE WISH YOU THE VERY BEST!

HOW TO USE THIS BOOK

Medicine in a Day: Revision Notes for Medical Exams, Finals, UKMLA and Foundation Years covers all conditions stated by the UKMLA plus more! We included things that we thought are essential for your medical training.

Please note the following:

Buzzwords: We have mentioned the most common risk factors and presentations. However, more may be present.

Investigations: Any test marked with an asterisk (e.g. *CT*) means it is the gold standard test. Baseline bloods include FBC (full blood count), U&Es (urea and electrolytes), LFTs (liver function tests), CRP (C-reactive protein), and clotting. Pre-operative bloods may include baseline bloods + group and save +/− cross-match.

Differentials. We have mentioned some common differentials to consider and/or differentials not to miss. However, more differentials may be considered

Management: Antibiotics mentioned in this book are based on the British National Formulary (BNF) recommendations (UK) and/or the National Institute for Health and Care Excellence (NICE) guidelines (UK). However, always check local guidelines and keep up to date with new recommendations. Management guidelines may be updated over time. Therefore, also ensure you keep up to date with them.

For your revision, and to ensure you cover everything for your exams, you can either tick all boxes of the table of contents by UKMLA condition (see Table 1) or tick all the boxes in the table of contents by specialty (see Table 2).

TABLE 1 UKMLA Conditions and Where to Find Them

Conditions	Chapter	Page	Revised?
Acid-base abnormality	Chapter 20: Renal Medicine and Chemical Pathology in an Hour	516	
Acne vulgaris	Chapter 5: Dermatology in an Hour	112	
Acoustic neuroma	Chapter 6: ENT and Ophthalmology in an Hour	138	
Acute bronchitis	Chapter 21: Respiratory Medicine in an Hour	542	
Acute cholangitis	Chapter 9: General Surgery in an Hour	226	
Acute coronary syndromes	Chapter 3: Cardiology and ECGs in an Hour	46	
Acute glaucoma	Chapter 6: ENT and Ophthalmology in an Hour	162	
Acute kidney injury	Chapter 20: Renal Medicine and Chemical Pathology in an Hour	502	
Acute pancreatitis	Chapter 9: General Surgery in an Hour	227	
Acute stress reaction	Chapter 18: Psychiatry in an Hour	443	
Addison's disease	Chapter 8: Endocrinology in an Hour	205	
Adverse drug effects	Prescribing appendix	Prescribing appendix	
Alcoholic hepatitis	Chapter 1: Anaesthetics and Critical Care in an Hour Chapter 10: Gastroenterology in an Hour	19, 250	
Allergic disorder	Chapter 5: Dermatology in an Hour Chapter 7: Emergency Medicine in an Hour	111, 175	
Anaemia	Chapter 11: Haematology in an Hour	263	
Anal fissure	Chapter 9: General Surgery in an Hour	235	
Anaphylaxis	Chapter 7: Emergency Medicine in an Hour	175	
Aneurysms, ischaemic limb and occlusions	Chapter 2: Breast and Vascular Surgery in an Hour	32	

TABLE 1　UKMLA Conditions and Where to Find Them—cont'd

Conditions	Chapter	Page	Revised?
Ankylosing spondylitis	Chapter 22: Rheumatology in an Hour	553	
Anxiety disorder: generalised	Chapter 18: Psychiatry in an Hour	442	
Anxiety disorder: post-traumatic stress disorder	Chapter 18: Psychiatry in an Hour	443	
Anxiety, phobias, OCD	Chapter 18: Psychiatry in an Hour	442	
Aortic aneurysm	Chapter 2: Breast and Vascular Surgery in an Hour	35	
Aortic dissection	Chapter 2: Breast and Vascular Surgery in an Hour	36	
Aortic valve disease	Chapter 3: Cardiology and ECGs in an Hour	55	
Appendicitis	Chapter 9: General Surgery in an Hour	228	
Arrhythmias	Chapter 3: Cardiology and ECGs in an Hour	61	
Arterial thrombosis	Chapter 2: Breast and Vascular Surgery in an Hour	32	
Arterial ulcers	Chapter 2: Breast and Vascular Surgery in an Hour	30	
Asbestos-related lung disease	Chapter 21: Respiratory Medicine in an Hour	541	
Ascites	Chapter 10: Gastroenterology in an Hour	251	
Asthma	Chapter 16: Paediatrics in an Hour Chapter 21: Respiratory Medicine in an Hour	399, 535	
Asthma COPD overlap syndrome	Chapter 21: Respiratory Medicine in an Hour	540	
Atopic dermatitis and eczema	Chapter 5: Dermatology in an Hour	105	
Atrophic vaginitis	Chapter 15: Obstetrics, Gynaecology and Sexual Health in an Hour	375	
Attention deficit hyperactivity disorder	Chapter 18: Psychiatry in an Hour	448	
Autism spectrum disorder	Chapter 18: Psychiatry in an Hour	448	
Bacterial vaginosis	Chapter 15: Obstetrics, Gynaecology and Sexual Health in an Hour	383	
Basal cell carcinoma	Chapter 5: Dermatology in an Hour	115	
Bell's palsy	Chapter 13: Neurology in an Hour	311	
Benign eyelid disorders	Chapter 6: ENT and Ophthalmology in an Hour	167	
Benign paroxysmal positional vertigo	Chapter 6: ENT and Ophthalmology in an Hour	136	
Benign prostatic hyperplasia	Chapter 24: Urology in an Hour	607	
Biliary atresia	Chapter 16: Paediatrics in an Hour	403	
Bipolar affective disorder	Chapter 18: Psychiatry in an Hour	439	
Bladder cancer	Chapter 24: Urology in an Hour	617	
Blepharitis	Chapter 6: ENT and Ophthalmology in an Hour	167	
Brain abscess	Chapter 14: Neurosurgery in an Hour	344	
Brain metastases	Chapter 14: Neurosurgery in an Hour Chapter 17: Palliative Care and Oncology in an Hour	345, 428	
Breast abscess/ mastitis	Chapter 2: Breast and Vascular Surgery in an Hour	26	
Breast cancer	Chapter 2: Breast and Vascular Surgery in an Hour	27	
Breast cysts	Chapter 2: Breast and Vascular Surgery in an Hour	25	
Bronchiectasis	Chapter 21: Respiratory Medicine in an Hour	537	
Bronchiolitis	Chapter 16: Paediatrics in an Hour	399	

continued

TABLE 1   UKMLA Conditions and Where to Find Them—cont'd

Conditions	Chapter	Page	Revised?
Depression	Chapter 18: Psychiatry in an Hour	438	
Developmental delay	Chapter 16: Paediatrics in an Hour	390	
Diabetes in pregnancy (gestational and pre-existing)	Chapter 15: Obstetrics, Gynaecology and Sexual Health in an Hour	361	
Diabetes insipidus	Chapter 8: Endocrinology in an Hour	201	
Diabetes mellitus type 1 and 2	Chapter 8: Endocrinology in an Hour	212	
Diabetic eye disease	Chapter 6: ENT and Ophthalmology in an Hour	152	
Diabetic ketoacidosis	Chapter 7: Emergency Medicine in an Hour	183	
Diabetic nephropathy	Chapter 20: Renal Medicine and Chemical Pathology in an Hour	510	
Diabetic neuropathy	Chapter 13: Neurology in an Hour	320	
Disease prevention/screening	Integrated throughout relevant chapter	N/A	
Disseminated intravascular coagulation	Chapter 11: Haematology in an Hour	271	
Diverticular disease	Chapter 9: General Surgery in an Hour	228	
Down's syndrome	Chapter 16: Paediatrics in an Hour	412	
Drug overdose	Chapter 7: Emergency Medicine in an Hour	187	
Eating disorders	Chapter 18: Psychiatry in an Hour	447	
Ectopic pregnancy	Chapter 15: Obstetrics, Gynaecology and Sexual Health in an Hour	373	
Encephalitis	Chapter 13: Neurology in an Hour	312	
Endometrial cancer	Chapter 15: Obstetrics, Gynaecology and Sexual Health in an Hour	379	
Endometriosis	Chapter 15: Obstetrics, Gynaecology and Sexual Health in an Hour	374	
Epididymitis and orchitis	Chapter 24: Urology in an Hour	610	
Epiglottitis	Chapter 6: ENT and Ophthalmology in an Hour	142	
Epilepsy	Chapter 13: Neurology in an Hour	306	
Epistaxis	Chapter 6: ENT and Ophthalmology in an Hour	140	
Essential or secondary hypertension	Chapter 3: Cardiology and ECGs in an Hour	42	
Essential tremor	Chapter 13: Neurology in an Hour	317	
Extradural haemorrhage	Chapter 14: Neurosurgery in an Hour	344	
Febrile convulsion	Chapter 16: Paediatrics in an Hour	412	
Fibroadenoma	Chapter 2: Breast and Vascular Surgery in an Hour	26	
Fibroids	Chapter 15: Obstetrics, Gynaecology and Sexual Health in an Hour	375	
Fibromyalgia	Chapter 22: Rheumatology in an Hour	560	
Fibrotic lung disease	Chapter 21: Respiratory medicine in an Hour	540	
Folliculitis	Chapter 12: Infectious Diseases in an Hour	297	
Gallstones and biliary colic	Chapter 9: General Surgery in an Hour	225	
Gangrene	Chapter 12: Infectious Diseases in an Hour	297	
Gastric cancer	Chapter 9: General Surgery in an Hour	219	
Gastrointestinal perforation	Chapter 9: General Surgery in an Hour	237	

continued

TABLE 1   UKMLA Conditions and Where to Find Them—cont'd

Conditions	Chapter	Page	Revised?
Gastro-oesophageal reflux disease	Chapter 10: Gastroenterology in an Hour Chapter 16: Paediatrics in an Hour	244, 403	
Gonorrhoea	Chapter 15: Obstetrics, Gynaecology and Sexual Health in an Hour	382	
Haemochromatosis	Chapter 10: Gastroenterology in an Hour	252	
Haemoglobinopathies	Chapter 11: Haematology in an Hour	269	
Haemophilia	Chapter 11: Haematology in an Hour	274	
Haemorrhoids	Chapter 9: General Surgery in an Hour	235	
Head lice	Chapter 12: Infectious Diseases in an Hour	297	
Henoch-Schonlein purpura	Chapter 22: Rheumatology in an Hour	564	
Hepatitis	Chapter 10: Gastroenterology in an Hour	247	
Hernias	Chapter 9: General Surgery in an Hour	236	
Herpes simplex virus	Chapter 5: Dermatology in an Hour Chapter 15: Obstetrics, Gynaecology and Sexual Health in an Hour	102. 384	
Hiatus hernia	Chapter 9: General Surgery in an Hour	220	
Hospital acquired infections	Chapter 12: Infectious Diseases in an Hour Chapter 21: Respiratory medicine in an Hour	293 (C.diff), 543 (HAP)	
Human immunodeficiency virus	Chapter 15: Obstetrics, Gynaecology and Sexual Health in an Hour	384	
Human papilloma virus infection	Chapter 15: Obstetrics, Gynaecology and Sexual Health in an Hour	378, 383	
Hypercalcaemia of malignancy	Chapter 17: Palliative Care and Oncology in an Hour	429	
Hyperlipidemia	Chapter 3: Cardiology and ECGs in an Hour	43	
Hyperosmolar hyperglycaemic state	Chapter 7: Emergency Medicine in an Hour	184	
Hyperparathyroidism	Chapter 8: Endocrinology in an Hour	209	
Hyperthermia and hypothermia	Chapter 7: Emergency Medicine in an Hour	187	
Hypoglycaemia	Chapter 7: Emergency Medicine in an Hour	183	
Hypoparathyroidism	Chapter 8: Endocrinology in an Hour	211	
Hyposplenism/splenectomy	Chapter 11: Haematology in an Hour	281	
Hypothyroidism	Chapter 8: Endocrinology in an Hour	203	
Idiopathic arthritis	Chapter 22: Rheumatology in an Hour	566	
Impetigo	Chapter 5: Dermatology in an Hour	101	
Infectious colitis	Chapter 12: Infectious Diseases in an Hour	290	
Infectious diarrhoea	Chapter 12: Infectious Diseases in an Hour	292	
Infectious mononucleosis	Chapter 12: Infectious Diseases in an Hour	297	
Infective endocarditis	Chapter 3: Cardiology and ECGs in an Hour	51	
Infective keratitis	Chapter 6: ENT and Ophthalmology in an Hour	160	
Inflammatory bowel disease	Chapter 10: Gastroenterology in an Hour	255	
Influenza	Chapter 12: Infectious Diseases in an Hour	296	
Intestinal ischaemia	Chapter 2: Breast and Vascular Surgery in an Hour Chapter 9: General Surgery in an Hour	38, 238	

TABLE 1   UKMLA Conditions and Where to Find Them—cont'd

continued

TABLE 1   UKMLA Conditions and Where to Find Them—cont'd

Conditions	Chapter	Page	Revised?
Non-accidental injury	Chapter 16: Paediatrics in an Hour	417	
Notifiable diseases	Chapter 12: Infectious Diseases in an Hour	288	
Obesity	Chapter 16: Paediatrics in an Hour	392	
Obesity and pregnancy	Chapter 15: Obstetrics, Gynaecology and Sexual Health in an Hour	358	
Obstructive sleep apnoea	Chapter 6: ENT and Ophthalmology in an Hour	142	
Occupational lung disease	Chapter 21: Respiratory Medicine in an Hour	541	
Oesophageal cancer	Chapter 9: General Surgery in an Hour	219	
Optic neuritis	Chapter 6: ENT and Ophthalmology in an Hour	160	
Osteoarthritis	Chapter 23: Trauma and orthopaedics in an Hour	589	
Osteomalacia	Chapter 22: Rheumatology in an Hour	560	
Osteomyelitis	Chapter 23: Trauma and Orthopaedics in an Hour	587	
Osteoporosis	Chapter 22: Rheumatology in an Hour	558	
Otitis externa	Chapter 6: ENT and Ophthalmology in an Hour	133	
Otitis media	Chapter 6: ENT and Ophthalmology in an Hour	134	
Ovarian cancer	Chapter 15: Obstetrics, Gynaecology and Sexual Health in an Hour	380	
Pancreatic cancer	Chapter 9: General Surgery in an Hour	224	
Pancytopenia	Chapter 11: Haematology in an Hour	262	
Parkinson's disease	Chapter 13: Neurology in an Hour	316	
Pathological fracture	Chapter 23: Trauma and Orthopaedics in an Hour	572	
Patient on anti-coagulant therapy	Chapter 11: Haematology in an Hour Prescribing Appendix	262 Prescribing Appendix	
Patient on anti-platelet therapy	Prescribing Appendix	Prescribing Appendix	
Pelvic inflammatory disease	Chapter 15: Obstetrics, Gynaecology and Sexual Health in an Hour	382	
Peptic ulcer disease and gastritis	Chapter 10: Gastroenterology in an Hour	245	
Perianal abscesses and fistulae	Chapter 9: General Surgery in an Hour	236	
Pericardial disease	Chapter 3: Cardiology and ECGs in an Hour	53	
Periorbital and orbital cellulitis	Chapter 6: ENT and Ophthalmology in an Hour	163	
Peripheral nerve injuries/palsies	Chapter 6: ENT and Ophthalmology in an Hour Chapter 23: Trauma and Orthopaedics in an Hour	148, 570	
Peripheral vascular disease	Ch2: Breast and Vascular Surgery in an Hour	32	
Peritonitis	Chapter 9: General Surgery in an Hour	237	
Personality disorder	Chapter 18: Psychiatry in an Hour	445	
Pituitary tumours	Chapter 8: Endocrinology in an Hour Chapter 14: Neurosurgery in an Hour	206, 345	
Placenta praevia	Chapter 15: Obstetrics, Gynaecology and Sexual Health in an Hour	364	
Placental abruption	Chapter 15: Obstetrics, Gynaecology and Sexual Health in an Hour	365	
Pneumonia	Chapter 21: Respiratory medicine in an Hour	542	
Pneumothorax	Chapter 7: Emergency Medicine in an Hour	175	

TABLE 1 UKMLA Conditions and Where to Find Them—cont'd

Conditions	Chapter	Page	Revised?
Polycythaemia	Chapter 11: Haematology in an Hour	280	
Polymyalgia rheumatica	Chapter 22: Rheumatology in an Hour	560	
Postpartum haemorrhage	Chapter 15: Obstetrics, Gynaecology and Sexual Health in an Hour	369	
Pre-eclampsia, gestational hypertension	Chapter 15: Obstetrics, Gynaecology and Sexual Health in an Hour	363	
Pressure sores	Chapter 2: Breast and Vascular Surgery in an Hour	30	
Prostate cancer	Chapter 24: Urology in an Hour	619	
Psoriasis	Chapter 5: Dermatology in an Hour	109	
Pulmonary embolism	Chapter 7: Emergency Medicine in an Hour	177	
Pulmonary hypertension	Chapter 21: Respiratory Medicine in an Hour	546	
Pyloric stenosis	Chapter 16: Paediatrics in an Hour	405	
Radiculopathies	Chapter 14: Neurosurgery in an Hour	351	
Raised intracranial pressure	Chapter 14: Neurosurgery in an Hour	335	
Reactive arthritis	Chapter 22: Rheumatology in an Hour	552	
Respiratory arrest	Chapter 1: Anaesthetics and Critical Care	10	
Respiratory failure	Chapter 1: Anaesthetics and Critical Care	10	
Retinal detachment	Chapter 6: ENT and Ophthalmology in an Hour	160	
Rheumatoid arthritis	Chapter 22: Rheumatology in an Hour	549	
Rhinosinusitis	Chapter 6: ENT and Ophthalmology in an Hour	140	
Right heart valve disease	Chapter 3: Cardiology and ECGs in an Hour	58	
Rubella	Chapter 16: Paediatrics in an Hour	414	
Sarcoidosis	Chapter 21: Respiratory Medicine in an Hour	540	
Scabies	Chapter 5: Dermatology in an Hour	105	
Schizophrenia	Chapter 18: Psychiatry in an Hour	441	
Scleritis	Chapter 6: ENT and Ophthalmology in an Hour	162	
Self-harm	Chapter 18: Psychiatry in an Hour	446	
Sepsis	Chapter 7: Emergency Medicine in an Hour	179	
Septic arthritis	Chapter 23: Trauma and Orthopaedics in an Hour	588	
Sickle cell disease	Chapter 11: Haematology in an Hour	269	
Somatisation	Chapter 18: Psychiatry in an Hour	444	
Spinal cord compression	Chapter 14: Neurosurgery in an Hour	351, 430	
	Chapter 17: Palliative Care and Oncology in an Hour		
Spinal cord injury	Chapter 14: Neurosurgery in an Hour	352	
Spinal fracture	Chapter 14: Neurosurgery in an Hour	346	
Squamous cell carcinoma	Chapter 5: Dermatology in an Hour	118	
Stroke	Chapter 13: Neurology in an Hour	308	
Subarachnoid haemorrhage	Chapter 14: Neurosurgery in an Hour	337	
Subdural haemorrhage	Chapter 14: Neurosurgery in an Hour	340	
Substance use disorder	Chapter 18: Psychiatry in an Hour	447	
Surgical site infection	Prescribing Appendix	Prescribing Appendix	
Syphilis	Chapter 15: Obstetrics, Gynaecology and Sexual Health in an Hour	383	
Systemic lupus erythematosus	Chapter 22: Rheumatology in an Hour	554	

continued

TABLE 2 Specialties Covered in This Book

Medicine	Revised?
Chapter 3: Cardiology and ECGs in an Hour	
Chapter 5: Dermatology in an Hour	
Chapter 8: Endocrinology in an Hour	
Chapter 10: Gastroenterology in an Hour	
Chapter 11: Haematology in an Hour	
Chapter 12: Infectious Diseases in an Hour	
Chapter 13: Neurology in an Hour	
Chapter 16: Paediatrics in an Hour	
Chapter 17: Palliative Care and Oncology in an Hour	
Chapter 18: Psychiatry in an Hour	
Chapter 20: Renal Medicine and Chemical Pathology in an Hour	
Chapter 21: Respiratory Medicine in an Hour	
Chapter 22: Rheumatology in an Hour	

Surgery	Revised?
Chapter 2: Breast Surgery and Vascular Surgery in an Hour	
Chapter 6: Ear, Nose and Throat and Ophthalmology in an Hour	
Chapter 9: General Surgery in an Hour	
Chapter 14: Neurosurgery in an Hour	
Chapter 15: Obstetrics and Gynaecology and Sexual Health in an Hour	
Chapter 23: Trauma and Orthopaedics in an Hour	
Chapter 24: Urology in an Hour	

Anaesthetics, Critical Care and Emergency Medicine	Revised?
Chapter 1: Anaesthetics and Critical Care in an Hour	
Chapter 7: Emergency Medicine in an Hour	

Other	Revised?
Chapter 4: Clinical Epidemiology in an Hour	
Chapter 19: Radiology in an Hour	
Prescribing Appendix	

ABBREVIATIONS

Abbreviation	Term
2WW	Two-week-wait
5-FU	5-fluorouracil
AA	Amyloid A protein
AAA	Abdominal aortic aneurysm
AAT	Alpha-1-antitrypsin
ABG	Arterial blood gas
ABPA	Allergic bronchopulmonary aspergillosis
ABPI	Ankle brachial pressure index
ABR	Auditory brainstem response
ABX	Antibiotics
ACE	Angiotensin converting enzyme
ACE-i	Angiotensin-converting-enzyme inhibitor
ACHe	Acetylcholinesterase
ACL	Anterior cruciate ligament
ACOS	Asthma COPD overlap syndrome
ACR	albumin: creatinine ratio
ACS	Acute coronary syndrome
ACTH	Adrenocorticotropic hormone
ADAMTS13	A disintegrin and metalloproteinase with thrombospondin motif 13
ADEM	Acute disseminated encephalomyelitis
ADH	Anti-diuretic hormone
ADHD	Attention deficit hyperactivity disorder
ADL	Activities of daily living
AF	Atrial fibrillation
AFP	Alpha fetoprotein
AIDS	Acquired immunodeficiency syndrome
AIN	Acute interstitial nephritis
AK	Actinic keratosis
AKI	Acute kidney injury
AL	Amyloid light chain
ALI	Acute limb ischaemia
A-LKM	Anti-liver kidney microsomal antibody
ALL	Acute lymphoblastic leukaemia
ALP	Alkaline phosphatase
ALS	Advanced life support
ALT	Alanine aminotransferase
AMA	Anti-mitochondrial antibody
AMD	Age-related macular degeneration
AMHP	Approved mental health professional
AMI	Acute mesenteric ischaemia

AML	Acute myeloid leukaemia
AN	Anorexia nervosa
ANA	Antinuclear antibody
ANCA	Antineutrophil cytoplasmic antibody
Anti-CCP	Anti-cyclic citrullinated peptide antibody
Anti-dsDNA	Anti-double stranded DNA antibody
Anti-GBM	Anti-glomerular basement membrane
Anti-HBc IgG	IgG antibodies against Hep B core antigen
Anti-HBc IgM	IgM antibodies against Hep B core antigen
Anti-HBs	Antibodies against Hep B surface antigen
Anti-HCV	Antibodies against Hepatitis C virus
Anti-HEV IgM	IgM antibodies against Hepatitis E
Anti-SRP	Anti-signal recognition particle antibody
Anti-TNF	Anti-tumour necrosis factor
Anti-TTG	Anti-tissue transglutaminase antibody
AOM	Acute otitis media
AP	Anterior-posterior
APD	Automated peritoneal dialysis
APH	Antepartum haemorrhage
APLS	Antiphospholipid syndrome
APTT	Activated partial thromboplastin time
AR	Aortic regurgitation
ARB	Angiotension II receptor blocker
ARDS	Acute respiratory distress syndrome
ARLD	Alcohol-related liver disease
AS	Aortic stenosis
ASA	American Society of Anesthesiologists
ASD	Autistic spectrum disorder or Atrial septal defect
ASDH	Acute subdural haemorrhage
ASMA	Anti-smooth muscle antibody
AST	Aspartate aminotransferase
ATLS	Advanced trauma and life support
ATN	Acute tubular necrosis
AV	Atrioventricular or arterio-venous
AVM	Arterio-venous malformation or atrioventricular malformations
AVN	Avascular necrosis
AVNRT	Atrioventricular nodal re-entrant tachycardia
AVPU	Alert, Voice, Pain, Unresponsive
AVR	Aortic valve replacement
AVRT	Atrioventricular re-entrant tachycardia
AVSD	Atrioventricular defect
AXR	Abdominal x-ray
BAL	Bronchoalveolar lavage
BASDAI	Bath Ankylosing Spondylitis Disease Activity Index
BCC	Basal cell carcinoma
BCG	Bacillus Calmette-Guérin
BDI-II	Beck's Depression Inventory 2

BE	Base excess
β-HCG	β-Human chorionic gonadotrophin
BiPAP	Bi-level positive airway pressure
BMD	Bone mineral density
BMI	Body mass index
BNP	B-type natriuretic peptide
BOO	Bladder outlet obstruction
BP	Blood pressure
BPAD	Bipolar affective disorder
BPE	Benign prostatic enlargement
BPPV	Benign paroxysmal positional vertigo
BSO	Bilateral salpingo-oophorectomy
BT	Breslow thickness
BTS	British Thoracic Society
BV	Bacterial vaginosis
BVM	Bag valve mask
Ca	Calcium
Ca125	Cancer antigen 125
Ca15-3	Cancer antigen 15-3
Ca19-9	Cancer antigen 19-9
CABG	Coronary artery bypass graft
CAD	Coronary artery disease
CAH	Congenital adrenal hyperplasia
CAM	Confusion assessment method
CAP	Community-acquired pneumonia
CAPD	Continuous ambulatory peritoneal dialysis
CAR-T cell	Chimeric antigen receptor T-cell
CAUTI	Catheter-associated urinary tract infection
CBG	Capillary blood glucose
CBP	Clinic blood pressure
CBT	Cognitive behavioural therapy
CCB	Calcium channel blocker
CCF	Congestive cardiac failure
CEA	Carcinoembryonic antigen
CF	Cystic fibrosis
CFTR	Cystic fibrosis transmembrane conductance regulator
CFU	Colony-forming units
CI	Confidence interval
CIDP	Chronic inflammatory demyelinating polyneuropathy
CIN	Cervical intraepithelial neoplasia
CIS	Carcinoma in situ
CIWA	Clinical Institute Withdrawal Assessment for Alcohol
CJD	Creutzfeldt-Jakob disease
CK	Creatinine kinase
CKD	Chronic kidney disease
CLL	Chronic lymphocytic leukaemia
CMC	Carpo-metacarpal

CMI	Chronic mesenteric ischaemia
CML	Chronic myeloid leukaemia
CMV	Cytomegalovirus
CN	Cranial nerve
CNS	Central nervous system
CO	Cardiac output
COCP	Combined oral contraceptive pill
COL17	Collagen type 17
COPD	Chronic obstructive pulmonary disease
COX-II	Cyclooxygenase-2
CP	Costophrenic
CPAP	Continuous positive airway pressure
CPR	Cardiopulmonary resuscitation
CrCl	Creatinine clearance
CRH	Corticotrophin-releasing hormone
CRP	C-reactive protein
CRPP	Closed reduction and percutaneous pinning
CRRT	Continuous renal replacement therapies
CSDH	Chronic subdural haemorrhage
CSF	Cerebrospinal fluid
CSH	Carotid sinus hypersensitivity
CSOM	Chronic suppurative otitis media
CSU	Catheter stream urine
CSW	Cerebral salt wasting
CT TAP	CT thorax, abdomen pelvis
CT	Computed tomography
CTG	Cardiotocograph
CTPA	Computed tomography pulmonary angiogram
CV	Cardiovascular
CVC	Central venous catheter
CVD	Cardiovascular disease
CVP	Central venous pressure
CVS	Cardiovascular system
CXR	Chest X-ray
DAA	Direct-acting antiviral
DAS	Disease Activity Score
Db HL	Decibels hearing loss
DBP	Diastolic blood pressure
DBT	Dialectical behavioural therapy
DCIS	Ductal carcinoma in situ
DDH	Developmental dysplasia of the hip
DEXA	Dual-energy x-ray absorptiometry
DFNB1	Non-syndromic hearing loss and deafness
DHS	Dynamic hip screw
DI	Diabetes insipidus
DIC	Disseminated intravascular coagulation
DIPs	Distal interphalangeal joints

DKA	Diabetic ketoacidosis
DKD	Diabetic kidney disease
DM	Diabetes mellitus
DMARD	Disease-modifying anti-rheumatic drug
DMSA	Dimercapto succinic acid
DOAC	Direct oral anticoagulant
DRE	Digital rectal exam
DS DNA	Double-stranded DNA
DSD	Disorders of sexual development
DSM	Diagnostic and Statistical Manual of Mental Disorders
DVLA	Driver and Vehicle Licensing Agency
DVT	Deep vein thrombosis
DWI	Diffusion weighted imaging
EAC	External auditory canal
EBV	Epstein-Barr virus
ECG	Electrocardiogram
ECMO	Extra-corporeal membrane oxygenation
ECRB	Extensor carpi radialis brevis
ECRL	Extensor carpi radialis longus
ECT	Electroconvulsive therapy
ECU	Extensor carpi ulnaris
ECV	External cephalic version
ED	Extensor digitorum
EDH	Extra dural haemorrhage
EDM	Extensor digiti minimi
EDS	Ehlers-Danlos syndrome
EDV	End diastolic volume
EEG	Electroencephalogram
EF	Ejection fraction
eGFR	Estimated glomerular filtration rate
EGPA	Eosinophilic granulomatosis with polyangiitis
EIA	Enzyme immunoassay
ELF	Enhanced liver fibrosis
ELISA	Enzyme-linked immunosorbent assay
EM	Erythema multiforme
EMB	Endomyocardial biopsy
EMDR	Eye movement desensitization and reprocessing
EMG	Electromyogram
EN	Erythema nodosum
ENaC	Epithelial sodium channel
EPAP	End positive airway pressure
EPO	Erythropoietin
ER	Oestrogen receptor
ERCP	Endoscopic retrograde cholangiopancreatography
ERG	Electroretinogram
ERP	Exposure and response prevention
ERPC	Evacuation of retained products of conception

ESM	Ejection systolic murmur
ESR	Erythrocyte sedimentation rate
ESRF	End-stage renal failure
ESV	End systolic volume
ESWL	Extracorporeal shockwave lithotripsy
ET	Essential thrombocythaemia or endotracheal
ETT	Endotracheal tube
FAMMM	Familial atypical multiple mole melanoma syndrome
FAP	Familial adenomatous polyposis
FB	Foreign body
FBC	Full blood count
FBS	Fetal blood sampling
FDG PET	Fluorodeoxyglucose positron emission tomography
FEMg	Fractional excretion of magnesium
FeNO	Fractional exhaled nitric oxide
FEV1	Forced expiratory volume in 1 second
FFP	Fresh frozen plasma
FGM	Female genital mutilation
FH	Familial hypercholesterolaemia
FIB-4	Fibrosis-4
FiO_2	Fraction inspired O_2
FIT	Faecal immunochemical test
FMD	Fibromuscular dysplasia
FNAC	Fine needle aspiration cytology
FNE	Flexible nasoendoscopy
FOOSH	Fall on an outstretched hand
FRC	Functional residual capacity
FSGS	Focal segmental glomerulosclerosis
FSH	Follicle-stimulating hormone
FTD	Frontotemporal dementia
FTU	Fingertip units
FVC	Forced vital capacity
G6PD	Glucose-6-phosphate dehydrogenase
GAD	Generalised anxiety disorder
GAS	Group A streptococcus
GBM	Glomerular basement membrane
GBS	Guillain-Barre syndrome
GCA	Giant cell arteritis
GCS	Glasgow Coma Score
GCT	Germ cell tumours
GDM	Gestational diabetes mellitus
GGT	Gamma glutamyl transferase
GH	Growth hormone
GHJ	Gleno-humeral joint
GHRH	Growth hormone-releasing hormone
GI	Gastrointestinal
GLP-1	Glucagon-like peptide-1

GnRH	Gonadotrophin-releasing hormone
GORD	Gastro-oesophageal reflux disease
GPA	Granulomatosis with polyangiitis
GTN	Glyceryl trinitrate
GU	Genitourinary
H	Hydrogen
H_2RA	Histamine 2 receptor antagonist
HACEK	*Haemophilus species, Aggregatibacter actinomycetemcomitans, Cardiobacterium hominis, Eikenella corrodens,* and *Kingella kingae*
HADS	Hospital anxiety and depression scale
HAP	Hospital-acquired pneumonia
HAS	Human albumin solution
HAV	Hepatitis A virus
Hb	Haemoglobin
HbCO	Carboxyhaemoglobin
HBeAg	Hepatitis B envelope antigen
HBsAg	Hep B surface antigen
HBV	Hepatitis B virus
HCC	Hepatocellular carcinoma
HCO_3	Bicarbonate
HCV	Hepatitis C virus
HDL-C	High-density lipoprotein cholesterol
HDV	Hepatitis D virus
Hep B	Hepatitis B
Hep C	Hepatitis C
HER2	Human epidermal growth receptor 2
HEV	Hepatitis E virus
HF	Heart failure
HFpEF	Heart failure with preserved ejection fraction
HFrEF	Heart failure with reduced ejection fraction
HHS	Hyperosmolar hyperglycaemic state
HHT	Hereditary haemorrhagic telangiectasia
HHV	Human herpes virus
HHV6	Human herpes virus 6
HIT	Heparin-induced thrombocytopenia
HIV	Human immunodeficiency virus
HL	Hodgkin lymphoma
HNPCC	Hereditary non-polyposis colorectal cancer
HOCM	Hypertrophic obstructive cardiomyopathy
HP	Hypersensitivity pneumonitis
HPB	Hepatobiliary
HPL	Human placental lactogen
HPLC	High-performance liquid chromatography
HPV	Human papilloma virus
HR	Heart rate
HRS	Hepato-renal syndrome
HRT	Hormone replacement therapy

HSP	Henoch-Schönlein purpura
HSV	Herpes simplex virus
HTN	Hypertension
HUS	Haemolytic uraemic syndrome
IA	Invasive aspergillosis
IABP	Intra-aortic balloon pump
IBD	Inflammatory bowel disease
IBS	Irritable bowel syndrome
IC	Intermittent claudication
ICD	Implantable cardioverter defibrillator
ICD-10	International statistical classification and disease and related health problems
ICER	Incremental cost-effectiveness ratio
ICP	Intracranial pressure
ICS	Inhaled corticosteroid
ICU	Intensive care unit
IE	Infective endocarditis
IECOPD	Infective exacerbation of COPD
IFG	Impaired fasting glucose
IgA	Immunoglobulin A
IGF1	Insulin-like growth factor 1
IGF2	Insulin-like growth factor 2
IGT	Impaired glucose tolerance
IHD	Ischaemic heart disease or intermittent haemodialysis
IIEF	International Index for Erectile Function
IJV	Internal jugular vein
IL	Interleukin
ILD	Interstitial lung disease
IM	Intramuscular
IMB	Intermenstrual bleeding
INR	International normalised ratio
IO	Intraosseous
IPAP	Inspiratory positive airway pressure
IPD/PD	Idiopathic Parkinson's disease
IPPV	Intermittent positive pressure ventilation
IRDS	Infant respiratory distress syndrome
IRT	Immunoreactive trypsinogen
ISUP	International Society of Urological Pathology
ITP	Immune thrombocytopenic purpura
IUD	Intrauterine device
IUGR	Intrauterine growth restriction
IUS	Intrauterine system
IV	Intravenous
IVC	Inferior vena cava
IVDU	Intravenous drug usage
IVI	Intravenous infusion
IVIG	Intravenous immunoglobulins
JPS	Juvenile polyposis syndrome

JVP	Jugular venous pressure
K	Potassium
KCl	Potassium chloride
KUB	Kidney-ureter-bladder
LABA	Long-acting beta 2 agonist
LACS	Lacunar stroke
LAD	Left anterior descending (artery)
LAFB	Left anterior fascicle block
LARC	Long-acting reversible contraception
LBBB	Left bundle branch block
LBO	Large bowel obstruction
LC-1	Liver cytosolic-1
LCIS	Lobular carcinoma in situ
LCL	Lateral collateral ligament
LDH	Lactate dehydrogenase
LDL-C	Low-density lipoprotein cholesterol
LEMS	Lambert-Eaton myasthenic syndrome
LFTs	Liver function tests
LGA	Large for gestational age
LH	Lutenising hormone
LHRH	Luteinising hormone-releasing hormone
LLETZ	Large loop excision of the transformation zone
LLL	Left lower lobe
LLQ	Left lower quadrant
LLZ	Left lower zone
LMA	Laryngeal mask airway
LMN	Lower motor neurone
LMWH	Low-molecular weight heparin
LP	Lumbar puncture
LPFB	Left posterior fascicle block
LRTI	Lower respiratory tract infection
LSCS	Lower segment caesarean section
LTOT	Long-term oxygen therapy
LTRA	Leukotriene receptor antagonist
LUL	Left upper lobe
LUQ	Left upper quadrant
LUTS	Lower urinary tract symptoms
LV	Left ventricle
LVEF	Left ventricular ejection fraction
LVF	Left ventricular failure
LVH	Left ventricular hypertrophy
M, C & S	Microbiology, culture and sensitivities
M2	Mitral valve closure (2nd heart sound)
MAOIs	Monoamine oxidase inhibitors
MART	Maintenance and reliever therapy
MBL	Monoclonal B lymphocytosis

MCA	Middle cerebral artery
MCD	Minimal change disease
MCHC	Mean cell haemoglobin concentration
MCL	Medial collateral ligament
MCPJ	Metacarpal-phalangeal joint
MCUG	Micturating cystourethrogram
MCV	Mean cell volume
MDRTB	Multidrug-resistant tuberculosis
MDS	Myelodysplastic syndrome
MDT	Multidisciplinary team
ME	Myalgic encephalomyelitis
MELD	Model of end-stage liver disease
MEN	Multiple endocrine neoplasia
MEq	Milliequivalents
Mg	Magnesium
MG	Myasthenia gravis
MGRS	Monoclonal gammopathy of renal significance
MGUS	Monoclonal gammopathy of undetermined significance
MHA	Mental Health Act
MI	Myocardial infarction
MM	Multiple myeloma
MMF	Mycophenolate mofetil
MMR	Measles, mumps and rubella
MN	Membranous nephropathy
MND	Motor neurone disease
MOA	Mechanism of action
MODY	Maturity-onset diabetes of the young
MOsm	Milliosmoles
MR	Mitral regurgitation
MRCP	Magnetic resonance cholangiopancreatography
MRI	Magnetic resonance imaging
MRS	Modified Rankin Score
MRSA	Methicillin-resistant *Staphylococcus aureus*
MS	Mitral stenosis or multiple sclerosis
MSA	Multi-system atrophy
MSK	Musculoskeletal
MSM	Men who have sex with men
MSU	Midstream urine
MTC	Major trauma center
MTP	Metatarsophalangeal joint
MUS	Medically unexplained symptoms
MV	Minute ventilations or mitral valve
MVT	Mesenteric venous thrombosis
Na	Sodium
NAAT	Nucleic acid amplification test
NAC	N-acetyl cysteine
NAFLD	Non-alcoholic fatty liver disease
NAI	Non-accidental injury

NASH	Non-alcoholic steatohepatitis
NASS	National Ankylosing Spondylitis Society
NASSA	Noradrenergic and specific serotonin antidepressant
NBM	Nil by mouth
Neb	Nebuliser
NF	Necrotising fasciitis
NFS	NAFLD Fibrosis Score
NFT1	Neurofibromatosis type 1
NFT2	Neurofibromatosis type 2
NG	Nasogastric
NGCT	Non-germ cell tumours
NGS	Next generation sequencing
NGT	Nasogastric tube
NHL	Non-Hodgkin lymphoma
NIHSS	National Institutes of Health Stroke Severity
NIV	Non-invasive ventilation
NMJ	Neuromuscular junction
NMO	Neuromyelitis optica
NNT	Number needed to treat
NOF	Neck of femur
NOF#	Neck of femur fracture
NOMI	Non-occlusive mesenteric ischaemia
NPI	Nottingham prognostic index
NPV	Negative predictive value
NSAIDs	Non-steroidal anti-inflammatory drugs
NSCLC	Non-small cell lung cancer
NSGCT	Non-seminomatous germ cell tumours
NSTEMI	Non ST-elevation myocardial infarction
NTD	Neural tube defect
OA	Occiput anterior
OA	Osteoarthritis
OAB	Overactive bladder
OAE	Otoacoustic emissions
OC	Obstetric cholestasis
OCD	Obsessive compulsive disorder
OCP	Oral contraceptive pill
OD	Overdose
OE	Otitis externa
OGD	Oesophagogastroduodenoscopy
OME	Otitis media with effusion
OMP	Outer membrane protein
ORIF	Open reduction and internal fixation
OSA	Obstructive sleep apnoea
OSD	Osgood-Schlatter disease
OT	Occupational therapist
P2	Pulmonary valve closure (2nd heart sound)
PA	Posterior to anterior
$PACO_2$	Partial pressure of carbon dioxide (alveolar)

PaCO$_2$	Partial pressure of carbon dioxide (arterial)
PACS	Partial anterior circulation stroke
PAD	Peripheral artery disease
PAH	Pulmonary arterial hypertension
PAN	Polyarteritis nodosa
P-ANCA	Perinuclear anti-neutrophil cytoplasmic antibodies
PaO$_2$	Partial pressure of oxygen (arterial)
PAO$_2$	Partial pressure of oxygen (alveolar)
PAP	Pulmonary artery pressure
PAPP-A	Pregnancy-associated plasma protein-A
PASI	Psoriasis area and severity index
PBC	Primary biliary cholangitis
PCA	Patient-controlled analgesia
PCD	Primary ciliary dyskinesia
PCI	Percutaneous intervention
PCKD	Polycystic kidney disease
PCL	Posterior cruciate ligament
PCNL	Percutaneous nephrolithotomy
PCOS	Polycystic ovarian syndrome
PCR	Polymerase chain reaction or protein:creatinine ratio
PCSK	Proprotein convertase subtilisin/kexin type 9 (inhibitor)
PD	Peritoneal dialysis
PDA	Patent ductus arteriosus
PDE-5	Phosphodiesterase-5
PE	Pulmonary embolism
PEA	Pulseless electrical activity
PEEP	Positive end-expiratory pressure
PEFR	Peak expiratory flow rate
PEPSE	Post-exposure prophylaxis following sexual exposure
PFMT	Pelvic floor muscle training
PH	Pulmonary hypertension
PHA	Pseudohypoaldosteronism
PHE	Public Health England
PHQ-9	Patient Health Questionnaire-9
PICC	Peripherally inserted central catheter
PICO	Population, intervention, comparator, outcome
PID	Pelvic inflammatory disease
PIMS	Paediatric multisystem inflammatory syndrome
PIPJ	Proximal interphalangeal joint
PJP (or PCP)	*Pneumocystis jiroveci pneumonia (Pneumocystis carinii pneumonia)*
PJS	Peutz-Jeghers syndrome
PMC	Percutaneous mitral balloon commissurotomy
PMR	Polymyalgia rheumatica
PND	Paroxysmal nocturnal dyspnoea
PO	Per os (taken orally)
PO$_4$	Phosphate
POAC	Preoperative Assessment Clinic
POCS	Posterior circulation stroke

POP	Progesterone-only pill
PPH	Postpartum haemorrhage
PPI	Proton pump inhibitor
PPPD	Pylorus preserving pancreaticoduodenectomy
PPROM	Preterm premature rupture of membranes
PPV	Patent processus vaginalis or Positive predictive value
PR	Per rectum or progesterone receptor
PrEP	Pre-exposure prophylaxis
PRIME-MD	Primary Care Evaluation of Mental Disorders
PROM	Premature rupture of membranes
PS	Pulmonary stenosis
PSA	Prostate-specific antigen
PsA	Psoriatic arthritis
PSC	Primary sclerosing cholangitis
PSGN	Post-streptococcal glomerulonephritis
PSM	Pan systolic murmur
PSP	Progressive supranuclear palsy
PTT	Partial thromboplastin time
PT	Physiotherapy or prothrombin time
PTH	Parathyroid hormone
PTL	Preterm labour
PTSD	Post-traumatic stress disorder
PTX	Pneumothorax
PUVA	Psoralen plus ultraviolet A light therapy
PV	Polycythaemia vera
PVC	Premature ventricular contraction
Q	Perfusion
QALY	Quality adjusted life year
QoL	Quality of life
RA	Rheumatoid arthritis
RAPD	Relative afferent pupillary defect
RB	Retinoblastoma
RBBB	Right bundle branch block
RBC	Red blood cell
RCA	Right coronary artery
RCC	Renal cell carcinoma
RCT	Randomised control trial
Rdiff	Risk difference
REM	Rapid eye movement
RF	Risk factors
RHD	Rheumatic heart disease
RHF	Right heart failure
RhF	Rheumatoid factor
RIPE	Rifampicin, isoniazid pyrazinamide and ethambutol
RLL	Right lower lobe
RLQ	Right lower quadrant
ROM	Range of movement
RPF	Retroperitoneal fibrosis

RPGN	Rapidly progressive glomerulonephritis
RPR	Rapid plasmin reagin
RR	Risk ratio or Respiratory rate
RRT	Renal replacement therapy
RSI	Rapid sequence induction
RSV	Respiratory syncytial virus
RTA	Renal tubular acidosis
RUL	Right upper lobe
RUQ	Right upper quadrant
RV	Residual volume
RVF	Right ventricular failure
RVH	Right ventricular hypertrophy
S1	1st heart sound (closure of atrioventricular valves)
S2	2nd heart sound (closure of semilunar valves)
S3	3rd heart sound (additional)
S4	4th heart sound (additional)
SA	Sinoatrial
SAAG	Serum ascites albumin gradient
SABA	Short-acting beta 2 agonist
SAH	Subarachnoid haemorrhage
SALT	Speech and language therapist
SAN	Sinoatrial node
SBO	Small bowel obstruction
SBP	Systolic blood pressure or Spontaneous bacterial peritonitis
SC	Subcutaneous
SCC	Squamous cell carcinoma
SCI	Spinal cord injury
SCID	Severe combined immunodeficiency
SCLC	Small cell lung cancer
SD	Standard deviation
SDH	Subdural haemorrhage
SE	Standard error
SEs	Side effects
SFH	Symphysial fundal height
SGA	Small for gestational age
SGLT-2	Sodium glucose co-transporter-2
SIAD	Syndrome of inappropriate anti-diuresis
SIADH	Syndrome of inappropriate anti-diuretic hormone
SIBO	Small intestinal bacterial overgrowth
SJS	Stevens Johnson syndrome
SLE	Systemic lupus erythematous
SLJD	Sinding-Larsen-Johansson disease
SNRI	Serotonin-norepinephrine reuptake inhibitor
SOB	Shortness of breath
SOBOE	Shortness of breath on exertion
SOL	Space occupying lesion
SSRI	Selective serotonin uptake inhibitor
SSSS	Staphylococcal scalded skin syndrome

STEMI	ST-elevation myocardial infarction
STI	Sexually transmitted infection
STIR	Short tau inversion recovery (MRI sequence)
SUFE	Slipped upper femoral epiphysis
SUI	Stress urinary incontinence
SV	Stroke volume
SVCO	Superior vena cava obstruction
SVR	Systemic vascular resistance
SVT	Supraventricular tachycardia
T1	1st heart sound - caused by tricuspid valve opening
T1DM	Type 1 diabetes mellitus
T1RF	Type 1 respiratory failure
T2	Tricuspid valve closure (2nd heart sound)
T2DM	Type 2 diabetes mellitus
T2RF	Type 2 respiratory failure
T3	Triiodothyronine
T4	Thyroxine
TACS	Total anterior circulation stroke
TAH	Total abdominal hysterectomy
TAVI	Transcatheter aortic valve implantation
TB	Tuberculosis
TBSA	Total body surface area
TCA	Tricyclic antidepressant
TCC	Transitional cell carcinoma
TD	Traveler's diarrhoea
TDS	Ter die sumendum (to be taken three times daily)
TEN	Toxic epidermal necrolysis
TFTs	Thyroid function tests
TG	Triglyceride
TGA	Transposition of the great arteries
TIPSS	Transjugular intrahepatic portosystemic shunt
TLOC	Transient loss of consciousness
TM	Tympanic membrane
TOE	Transoesophageal echocardiogram
TOF	Tetralogy of Fallot
TORCH	*Toxoplasmosis*, Other agents, *Rubella*, *Cytomegalovirus*, and *Herpes simplex*
TPMT	Thiopurine methyl transferase
TPN	Total parenteral nutrition
TPPA	Treponema pallidum particle agglutination
TR	Tricuspid regurgitation
TR-Ab	Thyroid-stimulating hormone receptor antibodies
TRH	Thyrotropin releasing hormone
TRUS	Transrectal ultrasound
TS	Tricuspid stenosis or tuberous sclerosis
TSH	Thyroid stimulating hormone
TTE	Transthoracic echocardiogram
TTN	Transient tachypnoea of the newborn
TTP	Thrombotic thrombocytopaenic purpura

TURBT	Transurethral resection of bladder tumour
TURP	Transurethral resection of prostate
T-VEC	Talimogene laherparepvec
TVUSS	Transvaginal ultrasound scan
TWI	T-wave inversion
TWOC	Trial without catheter
U&Es	Urea and electrolytes
U/O	Urine output
UC	Ulcerative colitis
UFH	Unfractionated heparin
UGI	Upper GI
UI	Urinary incontinence
ULSE	Upper left sternal edge
UMN	Upper motor neuron
UPSI	Unprotected sexual intercourse
URS	Ureteroscopy
URTI	Upper respiratory tract infection
USS	Ultrasound scan
UTI	Urinary tract infection
UVA	Ultraviolet A
V	Ventilation
Va	Alveolar ventilation
VAP	Ventilator-acquired pneumonia
VATS	Video-assisted thoracic surgery
VBG	Venous blood gas
Vd	Dead space volume
VEGF	Vascular endothelial growth factor
VF	Ventricular fibrillation
VGCC	Voltage-gated calcium channel
vHL	von Hippel-Lindau syndrome
VIN	Vulval intraepithelial neoplasia
V/Q	Ventilation: Perfusion
VSD	Ventricular septal defect
VT	Ventricular tachycardia
Vt	Tidal volume
VTE	Venous thromboembolism
VVC	Vulvo-vaginal candidiasis
VWF	Von Willebrand factor
VZV	*Varicella zoster virus*
WBC	White blood cell
WCC	White cell count
WFNS	World Federation of Neurological Surgeons
WHO	World Health Organization
WLE	Wide local excision
WM	Waldenström macroglobulinaemia
ZN	Ziehl–Neelsen

Anaesthetics and Critical Care in an Hour

Gregory Oxenham and Ben Howes

OUTLINE

ANAESTHETICS

EQUIPMENT

IV Cannulae

Large-bore cannulae: Often required in emergency management of hypovolaemia. This means a *green, grey or orange*.

Choose the smallest gauge needed to do the job, e.g., 22G for IV antibiotics. (Table 1.1 and Fig 1.1)

Oxygen Delivery

Variable performance devices: These devices deliver an unreliable fraction of inspired oxygen (FiO_2) because an unpredictable amount of room air is taken in with each breath regardless of which oxygen flow rate you provide. They include:

Bag valve mask: (Fig 1.2)
- **Flow rate:** up to 15 L/min. >90% oxygen achievable with tight seal. Patients can breathe spontaneously or be manually ventilated.
- **Uses:** can be used for ventilation and oxygen delivery perioperatively and in cardiac arrest/ emergencies.

Nasal cannula: (Fig 1.3 A)
- **Flow rate:** up to 4 L/min, variable FiO_2
- **Uses:** long-term oxygen therapy and for patients requiring little supplemental oxygen. Patients can talk/eat normally.

Simple face mask (Hudson mask): (Fig 1.3 B)
- **Flow rate**: 6–10 L/min, FiO_2 25%–60%
- **Uses:** patients requiring oxygen >4 L/min

Venturi mask (similar to a Hudson mask except there is a coloured attachment at the front – the Venturi device):
- **Flow rate:** delivers a fixed FiO_2 between 0.24 and 0.6. Each colour represents a different FiO_2, with specific oxygen flow rates written on them. Works by entraining a predictable mix of air and oxygen based on the shape of the Venturi device. (Table 1.2)
- **Uses**: when more accurate FiO_2 delivery is desirable (e.g., with COPD); however, still suffers from similar room-air entrainment issues mentioned above.

Non-rebreather mask (i.e., reservoir mask): (Fig 1.3C)
- **Flow rate**: 10–15 L/min, FiO_2 30%–80%
- **Uses:** emergencies and high oxygen-demand situations. Don't forget to occlude the one-way valve inside the facemask before use so that the reservoir bag fills up.

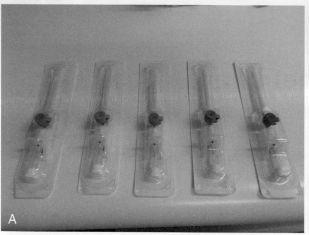
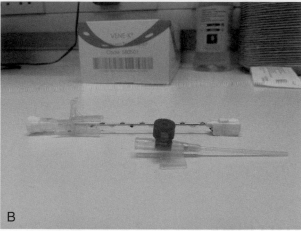

Fig 1.1 (A) Various cannulae. (B) Orange cannula showing intravenous component (*front*) after removal of the needle (*behind*).

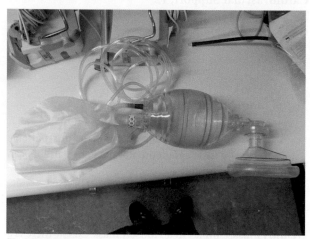

Fig 1.2 Bag Valve Mask. Note oxygen tubing and reservoir bag at one end and patient facemask at the other.

TABLE 1.2	Flow Rate by Venturi Colour	
Colour	O$_2$ Flow Rate (L/min)	FiO$_2$
Blue	2	0.24
White	4	0.28
Orange	6	0.31
Yellow	8	0.35
Red	10	0.40
Green	15	0.60

Airway Adjuncts

Oropharyngeal airway (Fig 1.4):
- **Uses:** supports the airway in patients with reduced consciousness, mainly by moving the tongue anteriorly. Tolerated at a Glasgow Coma Scale (GCS) score of <8. Any gagging or spluttering should prompt removal.
- **Sizing:** incisors to angle of the jaw ('hard to hard').

Nasopharyngeal airway (Fig 1.5):
- **Uses**: patients who cannot open their mouth (status epilepticus, trismus, facial injuries) and in more conscious or awake patients. Avoid in patients with suspected skull-base fractures. Use caution in anticoagulated patients due to the risk of significant epistaxis.
- **Sizing:** nares to tragus of the ear ('soft to soft').

TABLE 1.1	Cannula Size, Length and Flow		
Colour	Size (Gauge)	Length (mm)	Flow (mL/min)
Orange	14G	45	240
Grey	16G	45	180
Green	18G	32	90
Pink	20G	32	60
Blue	22G	25	36

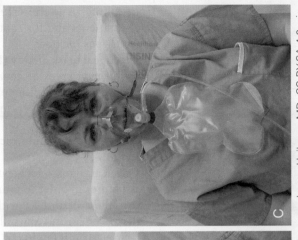

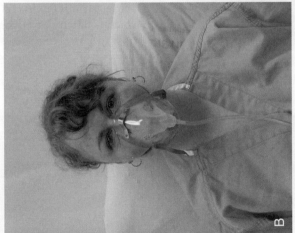

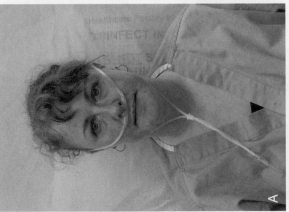

Fig 1.3 (A) Nasal cannula, (B) simple face mask and (C) non-rebreather mask. (Panel A reference: James Heilman, MD, CC BY-SA 4.0, via Wikimedia Commons Panel B reference: James Heilman, MD, CC BY-SA, via Wikimedia Commons); and Panel C reference: James Heilman, MD, CC BY-SA 4.0, via Wikimedia Commons

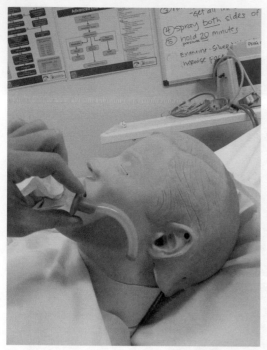

Fig 1.4 Oropharyngeal Airway – Sizing.

Supraglottic airways: In anaesthetised or AVPU-unresponsive patients, these devices can provide a patent airway and moderate protection of the airway from soiling. A useful emergency airway in unconscious patients and for routine day cases/minor surgeries. Types include:

- **Laryngeal mask airway (LMA):** Requires the cuff to be inflated to provide a seal (Fig 1.6).
- **iGel:** Elastomer cuff moulds to the patient's airway, creating a seal. The printed text always faces the crown of the head.

Laryngoscope and endotracheal tube (ETT): (Fig 1.7 and Fig 1.8)

- **Uses:** Laryngoscopes are used to move upper airway structures in order to visualise the larynx and allow placement of an ETT with the cuff resting beneath the vocal cords. Cuff inflation protects the airway from gastric reflux/secretions and generates a seal, which facilitates positive-pressure ventilation.

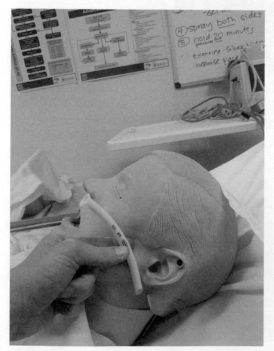

Fig 1.5 Nasopharyngeal Airway - Sizing.

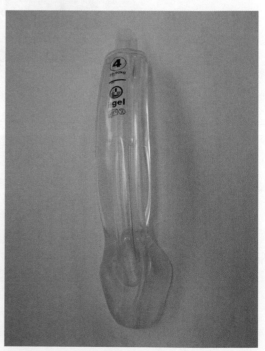

Fig 1.6 iGel Airway. (Reference: i-gel. Qqq1, CC BY-SA 3.0, via Wikimedia Commons.)

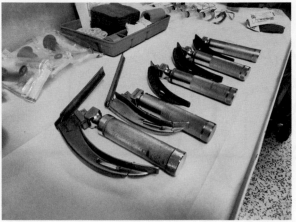

Fig 1.7 Various Laryngoscopes. (Reference: Tom Mallinson, CC BY-SA 4.0, via Wikimedia Commons.)

TABLE 1.3   Nine Independent Risk Factors that Increase Perioperative Risk
i Age
ii Sex
iii Socioeconomic status
iv Aerobic fitness
v *Diagnosed ischaemic heart disease (myocardial infarction and angina)*
vi *Diagnosed heart failure*
vii *Diagnosed ischaemic brain disease (stroke and transient ischaemic attacks)*
viii *Diagnosed kidney failure*
ix *Diagnosed peripheral arterial disease*
Factors in italics each *independently* increase the risk of dying by 1.5x

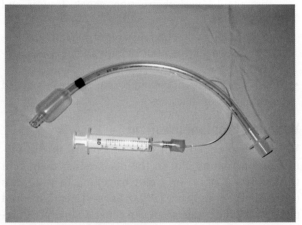

Fig 1.8 Endotracheal Tube with Inflated Cuff. (Reference: bigomar2, CC BY-SA 3.0, via Wikimedia Commons.)

PREOPERATIVE ASSESSMENT

All patients are assessed prior to or on the day of surgery, allowing anaesthetists to discuss the operation, identify risks and confirm that it is still in the patient's best interest to proceed.

A preoperative assessment clinic (POAC) is for patients undergoing elective procedures, especially those who are identified as being high risk.

Perioperative Risk Factors

Patient history, examination, investigations and expert opinions are used to identify perioperative risk factors (see Table 1.3).

Examination

- General condition – frailty, obesity
- Airway assessment – see below
- Pulse – evidence of arrhythmia
- Heart and lungs – identify any new murmurs. If so, should proceed to echocardiogram.
- Relevant anatomy if a regional block is planned

Airway Assessment

History:
- Inherited problems (e.g., Down syndrome, Pierre Robin syndrome)
- Acquired problems (e.g., obesity, radiotherapy, neck fusion)

Examination: factors associated with an increased intubation difficulty:
- **Anatomical features:** small mouth/large tongue/thick neck
- **Mallampati Test (Fig 1.9):**
  - Grade 1 (full visibility of soft palate)
  - Grade 2 (partial visibility of soft palate, but full uvula is still visible)
  - Grade 3 (only base of uvula seen)
  - Grade 4 (soft palate not visible)

Mallampati test

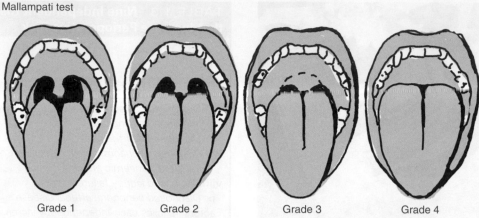

| Grade 1 | Grade 2 | Grade 3 | Grade 4 |

Fig 1.9 Mallampati Test. (Illustrated by Dr Hollie Blaber.)

- **Inability to protrude mandible**
- **Previous difficult intubation**

American Society of Anesthesiologists (ASA) Grade

This is a universal grading system for assessing operative risk.

- **ASA grade 1:** A normal, healthy patient
- **ASA grade 2:** A patient with mild systemic disease
- **ASA grade 3:** A patient with severe systemic disease
- **ASA grade 4:** A patient with severe systemic disease that is a constant threat to life
- **ASA grade 5:** A moribund patient who is not expected to survive without the operation
- **ASA grade 6:** A declared brain-dead patient whose organs are being removed for donor purposes

Aspiration Risk in Adults

Anaesthesia (or unconsciousness resulting from other reasons) obtunds protective airway reflexes, raising the risk of airway soiling. Aspiration of stomach contents has a significant mortality risk. Steps to reduce the risk of aspiration include:

- Intake of water allowed **up to 2 hours** before induction of anaesthesia
- Intake of food (solids, milk and milk-containing drinks) up to **6 hours** before induction of anaesthesia
- Oral medication should be continued with a small volume of water **up to 30 minutes** before induction of anaesthesia

- Consider using proton-pump inhibitors, metoclopramide and anti-acids perioperatively
  - Some factors that **delay emptying** of the stomach are small bowel obstruction, shock, trauma and peritonitis
  - Some factors that **increase regurgitation** are obesity, pregnancy, alcohol/opioids and delayed emptying
- If risk remains high, cricoid pressure may be needed at induction of anaesthesia

Venous Thromboembolism

Venous thromboembolism (VTE) refers to the formation of a blood clot in the deep veins (deep vein thrombosis (DVT)) or a clot travelling to the lungs (pulmonary embolism (PE)). Surgery, trauma and physiological derangement can cause a hypercoagulable state. VTE is a major cause of perioperative morbidity and mortality. See Emergency Medicine for more information and the Prescribing Appendix for common postoperative VTE prophylaxis regimens.

OPERATIVE ANAESTHESIA

World Health Organization (WHO) Surgical Safety Checklist (Fig 1.10)

- Required in all UK operating theatres
- Reduces avoidable surgical complications
- Enhances team work in high-risk environments, reduces human error

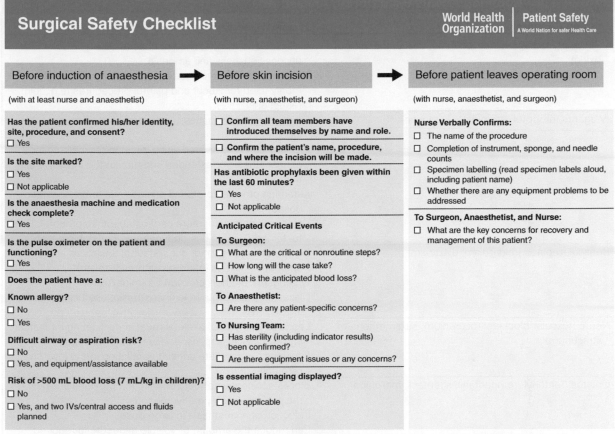

Fig 1.10 World Health Organization Checklist. (Zaydfudim, V. M., Hu, Y., & Adams, R. B. (2021) Principles of preoperative and operative surgery. In C. Townsend (Ed.), *Sabiston textbook of surgery*. Elsevier. (Figure 10.6) Copyright © 2022 Elsevier Inc. All rights reserved.)

The Surgical Stress Response

Surgery is effectively the same as trauma and sets off numerous physiological changes in the body via the endocrine and autonomic nervous systems, with consequent effects on hormone release and metabolism. These include:

- **Increased catecholamines** – cardiovascular changes, catabolism and hyperglycaemia
- **Increased oxygen consumption and tachypnoea**
- **Increased vasopressin** – fluid retention
- **Increased CO_2 production** – acidosis
- **Increased adrenocorticotropic hormone release** – electrolyte disturbances, hyperglycaemia and poor wound healing

- **Neurology** – long-term changes in nociceptive pathways

Pain is a component of the stress response during and after surgery and should be treated accordingly. Blocking nociceptive signals (peripherally or in the CNS) with analgesics or local anaesthetics **reduces this response.**

The Triad of Anaesthesia and Anaesthetic Drugs

The three principal factors involved in providing anaesthesia are:

1. **Autonomic reflex control:** Includes the correction of physiological imbalances caused by the

TABLE 1.4 **Common Agents Used During Anaesthesia**

Common Agents	Principal Uses During Anaesthesia
Volatile inhaled agents (sevoflurane, desflurane, nitrous oxide)	Induction and maintenance of anaesthesia – provoke unconsciousness and amnesia. Nitrous oxide also provides analgesia. Now more commonly used for labour and painful procedures (e.g., joint reductions).
IV agents (propofol, etomidate, ketamine)	Produce unconsciousness and amnesia, common for induction Propofol can be delivered as an infusion for maintenance of anaesthesia or extended sedation in the intensive care unit Ketamine provides profound analgesia at subanaesthetic doses Ketamine/etomidate: more cardiostable than propofol. Useful for induction in haemodynamically unstable patients
Benzodiazepines (midazolam, diazepam)	Preoperative medication for sedation, anxiolysis and amnestic qualities (more so with midazolam) IV sedation for short procedures (midazolam) Diazepam less common in anaesthesia, useful in terminating seizures
Neuromuscular blockers (rocuronium, suxamethonium, atracurium)	Leads to paralysis of skeletal muscle, facilitating intubation and surgical access, especially through the abdomen. Infusions can facilitate difficult ventilation in the intensive care unit
Opiates (fentanyl, remifentanil, alfentanil, morphine)	Blocks nociceptive effects of pain and provides analgesia in the pre/intra/postoperative periods Induction of anaesthesia in large doses Can reduce the amount of volatile anaesthetic required Infusions of alfentanil/remifentanil can provide intraoperative analgesia
Simple analgesia (paracetamol, ibuprofen, diclofenac)	Effective for treating postoperative pain without affecting consciousness

See the Prescribing Appendix

requirements of surgery and anaesthesia (e.g., hypotension caused by vasodilation due to anaesthetic drugs -treated with vasopressor drugs and fluids). It also involves paralysis of muscles for airway management/surgical access.

2. **Unconsciousness:** modifying brain function with drugs, often by unclear mechanisms
3. **Analgesia:** systemically or regionally reducing the nociceptive effects of pain, even in an unconscious patient

Key ideas:
• Neuromuscular blockers have *no analgesic/hypnotic* properties so *must not* be administered to awake patients due to the risk of awareness while paralyzed.
• Drugs are selected to suit the patient and surgery; therefore, no single combination will work for everyone. (Table 1.4)

Pain

Managing pain should be guided by the patient and his or her perception of pain. If a patient has pain, it is important to help them. Pain is commonly either **nociceptive** or **neuropathic**, *but there is often overlap.* While nociceptive pain usually has a physiological role in protecting the body, neuropathic pain is caused by a *dysfunction of* the nervous system and is therefore a maladaptive response.

Pain management technique falls into four categories:
- Pharmacological
- Regional analgesia
- Physical therapy
- Psychological therapy

See Palliative Care for further pain management, including chronic pain, and the Prescribing Appendix for common analgesia strategies.

Local and Regional Anaesthesia

Loss of pain and sensation in an area or region without a loss of consciousness. May be used for interoperative and/or postoperative analgesia, as well as general acute pain management.

Local anaesthesia:
- **Mechanism:** provides a loss of sensation in a small cutaneous area
- **Common uses:** suturing and wound infiltration. Adrenaline can be combined to reduce bleeding (through vasoconstriction).

Regional anaesthesia:
- **Mechanism:** provides analgesia +/- loss of sensation in a nerve/plexus/field distribution
- **Common uses:** fascia iliaca block to help with pain from a Neck of Femur fracture (NOF#). Brachial plexus block to facilitate upper-limb surgery

Neuraxial anaesthesia – a specific form of regional anaesthesia including spinal, epidural:
- **Mechanism:** local anaesthetic agents injected around structures of the CNS
- **Common uses:** surgery below the umbilicus, labour analgesia, caesarean section

These techniques are useful for:
- Smaller, peripheral procedures
- Frail, multimorbid patients in order to avoid general anaesthesia
- *Combined* with a general anaesthetic to improve analgesia
- Awake procedures (such as carotid endarterectomy or craniotomies) to monitor for thromboembolic sequalae or to identify resection margins using intra-operative electroencephalography (EEG) in surgeries for epilepsy

Patient-controlled Analgesia

The anaesthetic team should have developed a postoperative pain plan, which might include regional anaesthesia or patient-controlled analgesia (PCA). Always refer to the specialist pain nurse or anaesthetist if your patient is struggling with postoperative pain. The hospital will have an acute pain guideline which should support any decisions.

Patients often receive IV opioids intraoperatively and immediately postoperatively, with oral/IM routes more commonly seen on the wards. Opioids are sometimes given by the epidural or intrathecal routes, which can be an occult source of opioid toxicity.

A PCA pump is a common and useful postoperative strategy, since patients can request analgesia without delay and can spend more time pain free. In PCA, an opioid is given through an IV cannula from a locked pump with a button attached, so that the patient can press to deliver a bolus, with a lock-out period before another dose can be given (e.g., 1 mg morphine IV + 5-min lockout). Analgesia concentrations with PCA versus intermittent opiate use is represented in Fig 1.11.

| CRITICAL CARE
THE CRITICALLY ILL PATIENT

Critically ill patients are admitted to the ICU for specific organ support, monitoring and enhanced/advanced care. Supporting a failing organ system can prevent a knock-on effect in other organ systems, multiorgan failure and death.

The number of organ systems requiring support at any one time is a simple way of estimating a patient's risk. Regular assessments should be comprehensive and can be remembered as the extended A–E approach. The regular A–E approach learnt in undergraduate training is still essential for assessing sick patients on the wards!
- Airway
- Breathing – **respiratory support**, arterial blood gas (ABG), venous blood gas (VBG)
- Cardiovascular – **circulatory support** (vasopressors/inotropes)
- Disability – **neurological support**, sedation, analgesia
- Electrolytes – replacement and **renal support**
- Fluid balance – part of circulatory support
- Gut, nutrition, blood sugars – **gastrointestinal support**
- Haematology

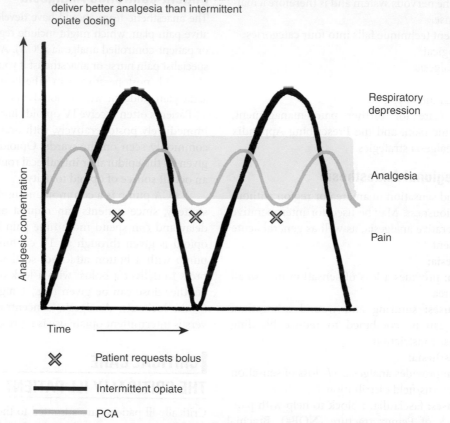

Graph showing how a PCA pump can deliver better analgesia than intermittent opiate dosing

Fig 1.11 Analgesia Concentrations with Patient-Controlled Analgesia versus Intermittent Opiate Use. *PCA, Patient-controlled analgesia. (Illustrated by Dr. Hollie Blaber.)*

TABLE 1.5	Levels of Care	
Level	**Where?**	**What Does it Involve?**
Level 1	Ward-based care	Nursing-to-patient ratio varies
Level 2	High-dependency unit (HDU) care	Nursing-to-patient ratio of 1:2
		Single-organ support (excluding mechanical ventilation)
Level 3	Intensive care unit (ICU) care	Nursing-to-patient ratio of 1:1
		Multiorgan support (or needing mechanical ventilation alone)

- Infection, antibiotics and fevers
- Jugular lines (or other lines) – dates of insertion, which cannulae/catheters/drains/CVCs/arterial lines can we safely remove?
- Kin – are the family updated and can they visit?
  See next sections for specific organ support available and indications.

  Levels of care – used to decide the best place for the patient's care (see Table 1.5).

RESPIRATORY SUPPORT

Respiratory Failure and Arrest

Definition:

- **Respiratory failure:** inability to oxygenate the blood sufficiently to meet the demands of the body. This type of failure is defined by the ABG (see Renal and Chemical Pathology in an Hour) and includes type 1 respiratory failure (T1RF) (primary hypoxia) and type 2 respiratory failure (T2RF) (hypoxia and hypercapnia)

- **Respiratory arrest:** cessation of breathing

Buzzwords:

- **Risk factors:** respiratory conditions (COPD, asthma), cardiovascular conditions (heart failure), neuromuscular conditions (myasthenia gravis, Guillain-Barré syndrome), musculoskeletal conditions (severe kyphoscoliosis, traumatic chest injuries)
- **Presentation:**
  - **T1RF:** hyperventilation, dyspnoea, agitation, tachycardia, cyanosis – *usually a VQ mismatch with an SpO$_2$ <92%*
  - **T2RF:** tachypnoeic or shallow breathing depending on cause, confusion/drowsiness is a late sign – *usually ventilatory failure*
  - **Respiratory arrest:** absence of breathing. Most common cause of cardiac arrest in children. Exhaustion, silent chest and bradycardia are pre-terminal signs
  - Signs of paediatric respiratory distress (see Paediatrics in an Hour)

Investigations:

- ABG (to identify the type of failure): T1RF vs T2RF
- Chest x-ray (CXR) (to identify the cause): consolidation, pleural effusion, pneumothorax – must rule out pneumothorax prior to administering positive-pressure ventilation
- CT imaging (to identify cause): pulmonary embolism, chest trauma, acute respiratory distress syndrome (ARDS)
- Echocardiogram (to identify cause): heart failure, evidence of right heart strain in large PE
- Bedside spirometry: see Guillain-Barré syndrome (see Neurology in an hour)

Differentials: cardiac failure

Management:

- **Oxygen:** escalating support from a nasal cannula to invasive ventilation (see start of chapter for delivery devices). In a hypoxic patient with an unclear cause, give high-flow oxygen first and ask questions later (treatment based on ABG results).
- **T2RF/respiratory arrest:** requires an improvement in *ventilation (i.e., increased minute volume to clear CO$_2$)* and cannot be treated with O$_2$ alone
- **Continuous positive airway pressure (CPAP): (Fig 1.12)**
  - **Indications:** T1RF, left ventricular failure

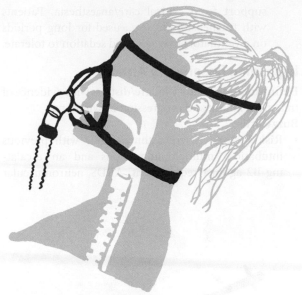

Fig 1.12 Continuous Positive Airway Pressure/Noninvasive Ventilation Mask. Straps help to form a tight seal over the mouth and nose. (Illustrated by Dr Hollie Blaber.)

- **Mechanism:** delivers a constant pressure throughout the respiratory cycle, including at the end of expiration (positive end expiratory pressure (PEEP)). Helps to stent alveoli open and increases the functional residual capacity. FiO$_2$ of 0.21–1.0 is possible
- **Bilevel positive airway pressure (BiPAP),** also known as non-invasive ventilation (NIV)
  - **Indications:** T2RF, hypoventilation
  - **Mechanism:** delivers positive pressure at two levels throughout the respiratory cycle. Gives the patient pressure support whenever they trigger the machine with a breath. Will also trigger if they fail to take a sufficient number of breaths. Improves *ventilation*, reduces PaCO$_2$
- **Inspiratory positive airway pressure (IPAP):** the pressure used to *augment* a regular breath (Fig 1.14)
- **Expiratory positive airway pressure (EPAP):** the pressure maintained at the end of expiration, the same as PEEP (Fig 1.14)
- **Invasive ventilation: (Fig 1.13)**
  - **Indications:** decreased consciousness, airway protection, severe head injury and respiratory failure/arrest
  - **Mechanism:** involves intubation and mechanical ventilation. General anaesthesia is needed, with

support from critical care/anaesthesia. Patients with tracheostomies (e.g., used for long periods on a ventilator) may not need sedation to tolerate.

Impending Respiratory Arrest

Definition: Respiratory failure/distress with evidence of treatment failure and progression of symptoms

Buzzwords:

- **Risk factors:** severe asthma/COPD with previous intubation, multiple admissions and an escalating B2 agonist requirement, ARDS, neuromuscular

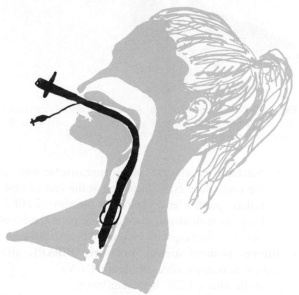

Fig 1.13 Endotracheal Tube In Situ. Note the balloon inflated below the vocal cords, which protects the airway and allows for delivery of positive-pressure ventilation. (Illustrated by Dr Hollie Blaber.)

weakness, traumatic chest injuries, acute heart failure, e.g., large myocardial infarction

- **Presentation:** deteriorating respiratory effort despite best treatment, tripod positioning, unable to complete sentences in one breath, low saturations, rising $PaCO_2$, cyanosis (Fig 1.15 and Fig 1.16), drowsiness, worsening acidosis, Cheyne-Stokes respiratory pattern
  - N.B. Agonal breathing should be treated as respiratory arrest

Investigations and Management:

- *GET HELP*, as above – observation of the patient is most important in diagnosing impending respiratory arrest
- Bag-mask ventilation if patient is in respiratory arrest or RR is <8

CARDIOVASCULAR SUPPORT

Shock

Definition: Circulatory failure with consequent cellular hypoperfusion. Usually associated with a *low blood pressure* and *tachycardia*. There are four types of shock and each is associated with a different underlying pathology. However, in clinical practice they often coexist. The most important points to consider are the most likely causes of shock and the management of shock via basic measures (i.e., fluid resuscitation) whilst getting help:

- Distributive
- Hypovolaemic
- Cardiogenic
- Obstructive

These four types of shock are explained physiologically using variables from Fig 1.17.

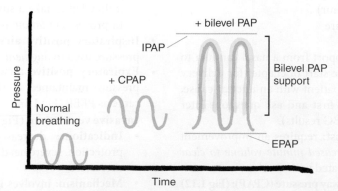

Fig 1.14 Graph Showing Pressure Changes with Continuous Positive Airway Pressure and Bilevel Positive Airway Pressure Compared with Normal Breathing. *CPAP,* Continuous positive airway pressure; *EPAP,* expiratory positive airway pressure; *IPAP,* inspiratory positive airway pressure; *PAP,* positive airway pressure. (Illustrated by Dr Hollie Blaber.)

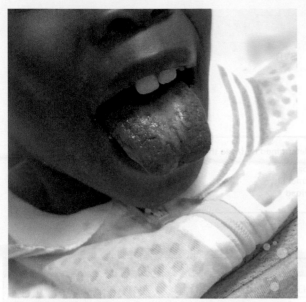

Fig 1.15 Central Cyanosis in Darker Skin. (With permission from Skin Deep.)

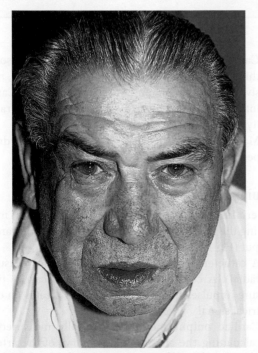

Fig 1.16 Central Cyanosis in Lighter Skin. (With permission from White V.L.C. (2018). Respiratory system. In *Hutchison's Clinical Methods*. Elsevier. Figure 12.1. Copyright © 2018 Elsevier Ltd. All rights reserved.)

Treating the cause: This approach may be distracting. A simpler memory aid for reversible causes of shock/cardiac arrest are the 4 Hs and 4 Ts from life-support training (Table 1.6).

General Management of all Patients in Shock

- **Aim:** to establish normal tissue perfusion, which is evidenced by improved vital signs, production of urine, reducing lactate/normalising pH, an improved GCS score and the clinical impression
- **Fluids:** usually the first drug for circulatory failure. A rise in the blood pressure following a fluid bolus/straight-leg raise indicates fluid responsiveness.
  - Resuscitation: 10 mL/kg crystalloid bolus. Bleeding patients need blood. Repeated boluses in septic shock of up to 30 mL/kg initially
  - Major haemorrhage protocol (see Emergency Medicine in an Hour)
- Major trauma: all need 1g IV tranexamic acid and keeping warm
- Vasopressors (to increase systemic vascular resistance (SVR)): most commonly noradrenaline/vasopressin (in intensive care)
- Inotropes (for cardiogenic shock): most commonly dobutamine (in intensive care)

Distributive shock (Fig 1.18):

- **Presentation:** Patient looks flushed and vasodilated
- **Causes:** sepsis, anaphylaxis, neurogenic (cord injury)
- **Management:** treat cause. Fluid resuscitation +/- vasopressors, adrenaline in anaphylaxis, antibiotics in sepsis
  - Infusion of volumes >30 mL/kg with minimal responsiveness is an indication for vasopressors.

Hypovolaemic shock (Fig 1.19):

- **Presentation:** Patient is cold, peripherally shut down, pale, thirsty and possibly bleeding
- **Causes:** bleeding, fluid loss
- **Management:** treat cause. Blood transfusion, fluid resuscitation, haemostasis, prevent further losses, vasopressors if above measures fail.

Cardiogenic shock (Fig 1.20):

- **Presentation:** Patient looks cold, shut down and dyspnoeic. Poor cardiac function results in venous congestion and pulmonary oedema
- **Causes:** cardiac disease which leads to a reduction in cardiac output (e.g., MI, dysrhythmias, fast atrial fibrillation (AF), acute valve incompetency). Heart unable to pump enough blood to maintain the blood pressure despite peripheral vasoconstriction

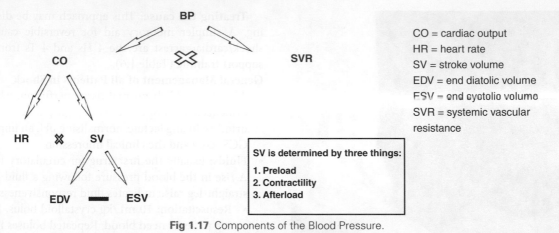

Fig 1.17 Components of the Blood Pressure.

CO = cardiac output
HR = heart rate
SV = stroke volume
EDV = end diatolic volume
ESV = end cystolic volume
SVR = systemic vascular resistance

SV is determined by three things:
1. Preload
2. Contractility
3. Afterload

TABLE 1.6	**The Four Hs and Four Ts**
REVERSIBLE CAUSES OF CARDIAC ARREST	
Hypoxia	Thrombus (coronary/pulmonary embolism)
Hyper/hypokalaemia, hypoglycaemia, acidosis	Tension pneumothorax
Hypovolaemia	Tamponade (cardiac)
Hypothermia	Toxins

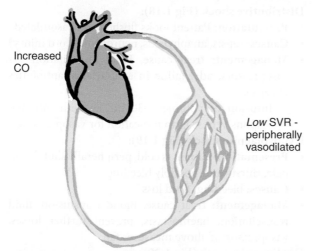

Increased CO

Low SVR - peripherally vasodilated

Fig 1.18 Distributive Shock. *CO*, Cardiac output; *SVR*, systemic vascular resistance. (Illustrated by Dr Hollie Blaber.)

- **Management:** treat cause. Revascularisation, cardioversion, valve repair. Possibly inotropes and intraaortic balloon pump placement

Obstructive shock (Fig 1.21):
- **Presentation:** Patient looks cold, shut down and dyspnoeic. Signs/symptoms of pneumothorax/PE (see Emergency Medicine in an Hour)

- **Causes:** reduction in cardiac output caused by something blocking blood flow out of the heart (e.g., massive PE, tension pneumothorax, tamponade). Can go into shock even with an adequate volume, contractility and SVR
- **Management:** treat cause. Thrombolysis, chest drain, pericardiocentesis

Equipment

Arterial lines: for freely sampling arterial blood, monitoring the heartbeat and BP and estimating the cardiac output (Fig 1.22 and Fig 1.24)
- A catheter is placed in a peripheral artery (usually radial). A continuous column of fluid carries pressure impulses to a transducer which creates an electrical signal.
- Cardiac output monitoring: usually measured by calculating the area under the curve of the arterial waveform. This can be used to assist in diagnosing causes of cardiovascular failure and in monitoring the response to treatment with fluids or vasoactive agents.

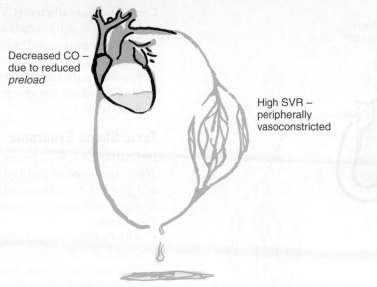

Decreased CO –
due to reduced
preload

High SVR –
peripherally
vasoconstricted

Fig 1.19 Hypovolaemic Shock. *CO*, Cardiac output; *SVR*, systemic vascular resistance. (Illustrated by Dr Hollie Blaber.)

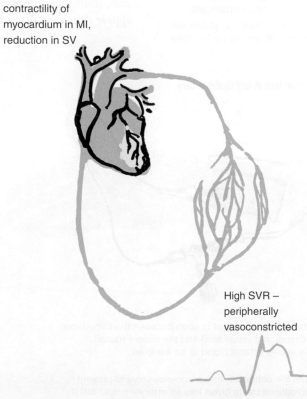

Reduced CO – impaired
contractility of
myocardium in MI,
reduction in SV

High SVR –
peripherally
vasoconstricted

Fig 1.20 Cardiogenic Shock. *CO*, Cardiac output; *MI*, myocardial infarction; *SV*, stroke volume; *SVR*, systemic vascular resistance. (Illustrated by Dr Hollie Blaber.)

Reduced SV in tamponade - impaired diastolic filling, reduced CO

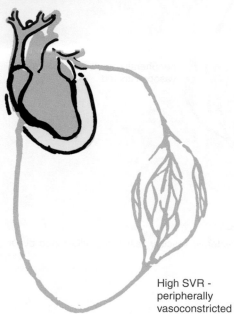

High SVR - peripherally vasoconstricted

Fig 1.21 Obstructive Shock. *CO,* Cardiac output; *SV,* stroke volume; *SVR,* systemic vascular resistance. (Illustrated by Dr Hollie Blaber.)

Central venous catheters (CVCs) (Fig 1.23 and Fig 1.24)

- Delivery of drugs (such as noradrenaline and concentrated potassium), which are dangerous if given peripherally
- Monitoring the central venous pressure (CVP) – trends in this measure can give information about a patient's fluid status

Toxic Shock Syndrome

Definition: A severe, potentially life-threatening syndrome mediated by toxins from *Staphylococcus aureus* and group A *Streptococcus* (GAS), which act as superantigens and cause a disseminated immune reaction.

Buzzwords:

- **Risk factors:** retained foreign body (classically highly absorbent tampons but also nasal packing), wound infection, necrotizing fasciitis. Diabetes and alcohol use disorder increase the risk of severity.
- **Presentation:** prodrome of myalgia, arthralgia, headache; then fever, rash (diffuse erythematous rash that desquamates 1–2 weeks later), hypotension, multiorgan involvement/failure. Patients often appear extremely ill at presentation.

Arterial line in left radial artery.

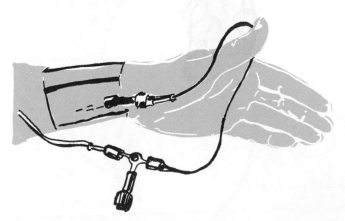

A three-way connector is seen between the transducer (proximal, not visualised) and the patient (distal). This allows arterial blood to be sampled.

Often the connector has a one-way valve to prevent medications being given into an artery – risk of distal necrosis

Fig 1.22 Arterial Line. (Illustrated by Dr Hollie Blaber.)

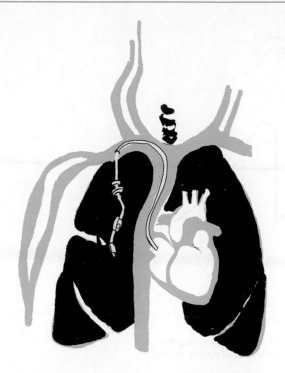

CVC in the right subclavian vein with its tip resting at the entrance to the right heart.
More commonly seen in the internal jugular vein

Fig 1.23 Central Venous Catheter. *CVC,* Central venous catheter. (Illustrated by Dr Hollie Blaber.)

Investigations:
- **Source identification:** pelvic examination in women who use tampons, physical examination for fasciitis, CT imaging of the abdomen/pelvis, imaging of suspected sites of infection – may find retained foreign body
- **Bloods/VBG:** as for sepsis (see relevant section)
- **Cultures of blood, urine, wound, throat swab:** to identify microorganisms

Differentials: sepsis, scarlet fever, Kawasaki's disease, necrotizing fasciitis, erythema multiforme

Management:
- **Aims:** to remove source, treat infection, halt toxin production
- Finding the source and removing it is the most important step, otherwise management is similar to that of sepsis
- Penicillin with activity against *S. aureus* and GAS and Clindamycin. Vancomycin if MRSA is suspected
- Surgical debridement of necrotizing infection/abscesses
- Management of multiorgan failure with referral to ICU if appropriate

NEUROLOGICAL SUPPORT
Assessment
AVPU (Alert, Voice, Pain, Unresponsive) (Table 1.7)
- Used as a fast way to assess alertness
- **A score of 'P' roughly correlates to a GCS score of <8,** which usually means the patient is unable to protect their own airway and may need an adjunctive or secure airway

Glasgow Coma Scale (GCS) (Table 1.8, Fig 1.25, Fig 1.26)
- A GCS score of 15 [E4 V5 M6] is a normal response. A GCS score of 3 is the lowest possible score
- Most suitable for grading progression following a head injury

Sedation and Analgesia
- **Uses:** facilitate treatment, intubation, status epilepticus if other treatments fail
- **Common drugs:** paracetamol/weak opioids (see the Prescribing Appendix), opioids (morphine, alfentanil), benzodiazepines (midazolam), propofol, haloperidol, alpha-2 agonists (clonidine, dexmedetomidine). Many combinations are possible, although the *most likely* combination you will see in a critically unwell and ventilated adult patient is *propofol and alfentanil*

Being in the ICU is distressing and carries a considerable risk of posttraumatic stress disorder. Good sedation and analgesia can help patients recover *psychologically* from critical illness.
- Patients may be sedated to facilitate treatment or to protect them from hurting themselves
- Anxiolysis: Anxiety can lead to a stress response and hyperventilation, which may be deleterious in the critically ill patient
- Sedation allows intubated patients to tolerate the ETT and to dampen the gag/cough reflex
- Status epilepticus: if other treatments have failed, ICU treatment includes sedation with continuous EEG monitoring
- Many patients will have a degree of pain with their illness, especially in the postoperative period after major surgeries

Disordered Consciousness
Definition: an acute change in consciousness resulting in loss of orientation, reactivity or wakefulness not otherwise explained by a preexisting neurodegenerative

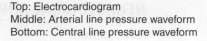

Top: Electrocardiogram
Middle: Arterial line pressure waveform
Bottom: Central line pressure waveform

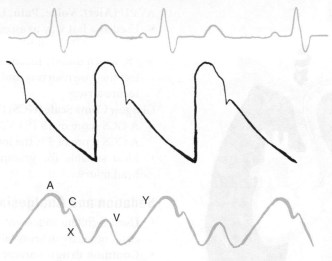

A: Atrial contraction
C: Tricuspid bulging during systole
X: Atrial relaxation

V: Atrial filling during systole
Y: Tricuspid opens, diastole

Fig 1.24 Comparison of Central Venous Catheter/Arterial Pressure Waveforms with an Electrogram for Reference. (Illustrated by Dr Hollie Blaber.)

TABLE 1.7	**AVPU Scoring**
Alert (A)	Fully awake and responsive
Voice (V)	Response to verbal stimulus
Pain (P)	Response to pain stimulus
Unresponsive (U)	No response to verbal or painful stimulus

condition. This definition includes delirium (see Neurology in an Hour), as well as broader differentials.

Buzzwords:

- **Risk factors:** any critical illness, preexisting dementia, frailty, previous overdose (OD), alcohol dependence, epilepsy, diabetes, depression
- **Presentation:** confusion, delirium, seizures, reduced GCS, apnoea, cranial nerve (CN) palsies, fixed dilated pupils, coma, obstructed airway

Investigations: Should not delay initial management (A to E). Guided by differential but likely to include:

- **Blood gas**
- **Bloods:** confusion screen (see Neurology in an Hour)
- **Neuroimaging:** to assess for structural causes
- **Lumbar puncture (if concerns of CNS infection):** see Infectious Diseases in an Hour
- **EEG/visual evoked potentials:** specialist to assess underlying brain activity in persistent coma

Differentials (mnemonic MIST P):

- **Metabolic:** hypo/hyperglycaemia, acidosis, hypercalcaemia, hypo/hypernatraemia, hypercapnia, hypoxia, hepatic encephalopathy, uraemia, myxoedema coma
- **Infective:** CNS infections, sepsis
- **Structural:** head injury, stroke, subarachnoid haemorrhage, cerebral oedema, seizure, hydrocephalus, space-occupying lesion, hypovolaemia
- **Toxins:** OD/intoxication, withdrawal, drug side effects
- **Psychiatric:** catatonia and akinetic mutism

TABLE 1.8   Glasgow Coma Scale Scoring

	Eyes (opening)	Verbal Response	Motor Response
6			Obeys commands
5		Oriented	Localizes to pain
4	Spontaneously	Confused	Withdraws from pain
3	To voice	Inappropriate words	Abnormal flexion (decorticate rigidity)
2	To pain	Incomprehensible sounds	Abnormal extension (decerebrate rigidity)
1	No response	No response	No response

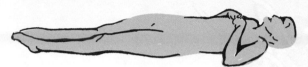

Fig 1.25 Decorticate Positioning (M3). (Illustrated by Dr Hollie Blaber.)

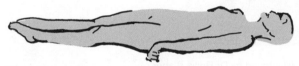

Fig 1.26 Decerebrate Positioning (M2). (Illustrated by Dr Hollie Blaber.)

Management:
- **Aims:** to keep the patient *safe* and *treat reversible causes*
- Get help if unresponsive or in need of a secure airway
- Secure C-spine in cases of trauma
- Head injury – normocapnia and nurse head up
- Treat underlying cause – see differentials and relevant chapters

GASTROINTESTINAL SUPPORT

Enteral nutrition: (Fig 1.27) nutrition into the GI tract. Enteral nutrition is the preferred method over total parenteral nutrition (TPN) because it is less risky and protects the gut's mucosal defences. Options include:
- Nasogastric/nasojejunal tube
- Gastrostomy
- Jejunostomy

- **TPN:** nutrition into a large vein via a central line. Suitable if the enteral route is not an option, e.g., major abdominal resections, bowel obstruction

Acute Liver Failure

Definition: failure of the liver to perform its functions (see list below). Results in the development of encephalopathy and coagulopathy (INR>1.5)
- Synthetic function, e.g., production of albumin and coagulation proteins
- Detoxification of ammonia
- Blood sugar control
- Metabolism of lactate

There are three main patterns:
- **Acute** – within 26 weeks in a previously healthy liver
- **Chronic** – usually with a *background* of cirrhosis (irreversible liver damage)
- **Acute on chronic** – when someone with known liver disease develops acute features of failure

Buzzwords:
- **Risk factors:** cirrhosis (alcohol dependence, intravenous drug use, nonalcoholic steatohepatitis, autoimmune liver disease, hepatitis (alcoholic, viral, ischaemic) (see Gastroenterology in an Hour), drugs (paracetamol), infection (leptospirosis), Budd-Chiari syndrome
- **Presentation:** stigmata of liver disease, encephalopathy, jaundice, bleeding, asterixis, coma. May lead to a syndrome of *multiorgan dysfunction*

Investigations: Should not delay initial management (A to E)
- **Temperature:** Decreases in liver failure
- **Blood gas:** ↑lactate (as it is metabolised in liver), ↓pH, ↓glucose

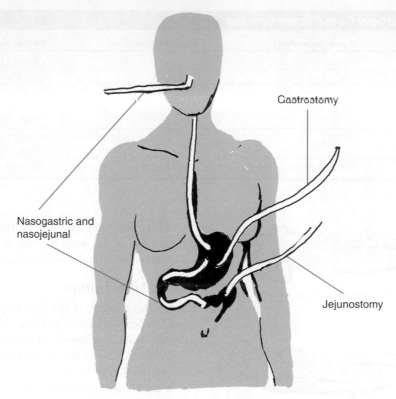

Fig 1.27 Routes for Enteral Nutrition. (Illustrated by Dr Hollie Blaber.)

- **Blood:** FBC (↓platelets), LFTs (deranged enzymes, ↑bilirubin, ↓albumin), clotting (INR>1.5, ↑aPTT), paracetamol levels, viral serology
- **Ascitic tap** (if ascites)
- **Doppler US of portal vein/hepatic vein:** if suspected Budd-Chiari

Differentials: sepsis, disseminated intravascular coagulation, spontaneous bacterial peritonitis, hypoglycaemia, upper GI bleed

Management:

- **Aim:** to treat the underlying cause
- **Organ support as required:**
  - **Respiratory:** intubation and ventilation if unable to protect airway (encephalopathy, haematemesis)
  - **Cardiovascular:** replace fluid loss +/− vasoactive agents for BP. Albumin fluid resuscitation if significant ascites/paracentesis. Fluid balance

- **Gastrointestinal:** regular lactulose (constipation makes encephalopathy worse). Avoid medications with hepatic metabolism. Rifaximin can reduce ammonia absorption. Nutritional support + folate/thiamine replacement. NAC if paracetamol overdose
- **Renal:** Hepato-renal syndrome has a high mortality, monitor for this + renal replacement therapy
- **Metabolic:** avoid hypoglycaemia with IV glucose
- **Haematology:** deranged clotting, bleeding may require FFP/platelet transfusion, IV vitamin K, +/− endoscopy
- **Social:** prophylaxis for alcohol withdrawal
- **Transplant:** indicated for acute liver failure (King's College Criteria), cirrhosis of any cause and some hepatocellular carcinomas

Prognosis: worse if grade III/IV encephalopathy, age >40 years, albumin <30 g/L, drug-induced liver failure

THE ONE-LINE ROUND-UP!

Here are some key words to help you remember each condition/concept

Condition/Concept	One-line Description
Cannulae	Orange, grey, green = large bore
Oxygen delivery	Bag valve mask in respiratory arrest
Aspiration risk	Water 2 hrs, food 6 hrs
Surgical stress response	Same as trauma
Chronic pain	>12 weeks pain, usually neuropathic
Respiratory failure/arrest	Usually T1RF > T2RF > respiratory arrest
Impending respiratory arrest	Beware rising $PaCO_2$ in asthma
Shock	Hypovolaemic, obstructive, distributive, cardiogenic
Toxic shock syndrome	Retained FB leading to critical illness
Disordered consciousness	MIST – differentials are wide
Acute liver failure	Encephalopathy, bleeding and jaundice

READING LIST: ANAESTHETICS AND CRITICAL CARE IN AN HOUR

Anaesthetics
Equipment
Al-Shaikh, B., & Stacey, S. (2019). *Essentials of equipment in anaesthesia, critical care and perioperative medicine.* Elsevier.

Wilkinson, I.B., Raine, T., Wiles, K., Goodhart, A., Hall, C. & O'Neill, H. *Oxford handbook of clinical medicine* (10th ed.). Oxford University Press.

HEE e-LFH. (2020). *Anaesthesia eLA, core training, face masks and oxygen delivery devices.* http://portal.e-lfh.org.uk. [Accessed 21 August 2020].

HEE e-LFH. (2020). *Anaesthesia eLA, core training, standards of monitoring during anaesthesia and recovery.* http://portal.e-lfh.org.uk. [Accessed 25 August 2020].

Perioperative Assessment
AAGBI. (2010). *AAGBI safety guideline. Pre-operative assessment and patient preparation.* http://www.rcoa.ac.uk. [Accessed 18 August 2020].

Artime, C., & Hagberg, C. (2020). Airway management in the adult. In M. A. Gropper, L. I. Eriksson, L. A. Fleisher, J. P. Wienter-Kronish, & K. Leslie (Eds.), *Miller's anaesthesia* (9th ed.). Elsevier.

HEE, e-LFH. (2020). *Anaesthesia eLA, core training, preoperative assessment and management.* http://portal.e-lfh.org.uk. [Accessed 21 August 2020].

HEE, e-LFH. (2020). *Anaesthesia eLA, core training, the purpose of preoperative visiting.* http://portal.e-lfh.org.uk. [Accessed 21 August 2020].

Operative Anaesthesia and Pain
Flood, P., & Shafer, S. (2015). Inhaled anesthetics. In R. Stoelting, P. Flood, J. P. Rathmell, & S. L. Shafer (Eds.), *Stoelting's pharmacology and physiology in anesthetic practice* (5th ed.) (pp. 98–159). Wolters Kluwer.

Rathmell, J., & Rosow, C. (2015). Intravenous sedatives and hypnotics. In R. Stoelting, P. Flood, J. P. Rathmell, & S. L. Shafer (Eds.), *Stoelting's pharmacology and physiology in anesthetic practice* (5th ed.) (pp. 160–203). Wolters Kluwer.

Gomersall, C., Joynt, G., Cheng, C., Yap, F., Lam, P., Torrance, J., Ramsay, S., Boots, R., Graham, C., Freebairn, R., Shivakumar, I., Holley, A., Udy, A. and Loew, C. (2020). *Basic assessment and support in intensive care (course manual).* Shatin, Hong Kong: Department of Anaesthesia & Intensive Care, The Chinese University of Hong Kong.

HEE, e-LFH. (2020). *Anaesthesia eLA, core training, aims of anaesthesia.* http://portal.e-lfh.org.uk. [Accessed 21 August 2020].

World Health Organization. (2009). *WHO guidelines for safe surgery.* http://who.int/teams/integrated-health-services/patient-safety/research/safe-surgery. [Accessed 20 November 2020].

Al-Shaikh, B., & Stacey, S. (2019). *Essentials of equipment in anaesthesia, critical care and perioperative medicine.* Elsevier.

HEE, e-LFH. (2020). *Anaesthesia eLA, core training, administration Techniques – IV PCA.* http://portal.e-lfh.org.uk. [Accessed 20 November 2020].

Shirley, P. (2005). Would you explain what the level 3 or level 2/3 ICU is? What is the difference between ICU and HDU? *BMJ, 330,* s184.

HEE, e-LFH. (2020). *Anaesthesia eLA, core training, a structured approach to the critically ill patient.* http://portal.e-lfh.org.uk. [Accessed 26 August 2020].

Critical Care
The Critically Ill Patient
Shirley, P. (2005). Would you explain what the level 3 or level 2/3 ICU is? What is the difference between ICU and HDU? *BMJ, 330,* s184.

HEE, e-LFH. (2020). *Anaesthesia eLA, core training, A structured approach to the critically ill patient.* http://portal.e-lfh.org.uk. [Accessed 26 August 2020].

Respiratory Support

British Thoracic Society Standards of Care Committee. (2002). Non-invasive ventilation in acute respiratory failure. *Thorax, 57*, 192–211.

Elsevier Point of Care. (2019). *Clinical overview: Asthma in adults.*

Gomersall, C., Joynt, G., Cheng, C., Yap, F., Lam, R., Torrance, J., Ramsay, S., Boots, R., Graham, C., Freebairn, R., Shivakumar, I., Holley, A., Udy, A. and Loew, C. (2020). *Basic assessment and support in intensive care (course manual).* Shatin, Hong Kong: Department of Anaesthesia & Intensive Care, The Chinese University of Hong Kong.

HEE e-LFH. (2020). *Anaesthesia eLA, core training, acute asthma.* http://portal.e-lfh.org.uk. [Accessed 18 November 2020].

Cardiovascular Support

Vahdatpour, C., Collins, D., & Goldberg, S. (2019). Cardiogenic shock. *Journal of the American Heart Association, 8*, 8.

Prescott, C., & Ruff, S. (2021). The shocked patient. *Medicine, 49*, 88–92.

Gomersall, C., Joynt, et al. (2020). *Basic assessment and support in intensive care (course manual).* Shatin, Hong Kong: Department of Anaesthesia & Intensive Care, The Chinese University of Hong Kong.

HEE, e-LFH. (2020). *Anaesthesia eLA, core training, the shocked patient.* http://portal.e-lfh.org.uk. [Accessed 18 November 2020].

Elsevier Point of Care. (2018). *Clinical overview: Toxic shock syndrome.* https://www.clinicalkey.com/#!/content/clinical_overview/67-s2.0-8106cf2d-7991-4c0f-a2a2-97821ea3d2cf.

Rapose, A. (2021). Toxic shock syndrome. In R. D. Kellerman, & D. Rakel (Eds.), *Conn's current therapy 2021* (pp. 666–668). Elsevier.

Neurological Support

BMJ Best Practice. (2021). *Assessment of delirium.* https://bestpractice.bmj.com/topics/en-gb/241.

British Geriatrics Society Clinical Guidelines. (2020). *End of life care in frailty: Delirium.* https://www.bgs.org.uk/resources/end-of-life-care-in-frailty-delirium. [Accessed February 2021].

HEE e-LFH. (2020). *Anaesthesia eLA, core training, the patient with disordered consciousness.* http://portal.e-lfh.org.uk. [Accessed 20 November 2020].

HEE e-LFH. (2020). *Anaesthesia eLA, core training, investigation of coma.* http://portal.e-lfh.org.uk. [Accessed 20 November 2020].

Gastrointestinal Support

Nanchal, R., et al. (2020). Guidelines for the management of adult acute and acute-on-chronic liver failure in the ICU: Cardiovascular, endocrine, hematologic, pulmonary and renal considerations: Executive summary. *Critical Care Medicine, 48*, 415–419.

HEE e-LFH. (2020). *Anaesthesia eLA, core training, the patient with acute liver failure.* http://portal.e-lfh.org.uk. [Accessed 19 November 2020].

Wilkinson, I. B., Raine, T., Wiles, K., Goodhart, A., Hall, C., & O'Neill, H. (2018). Liver failure. *Oxford handbook of clinical medicine* (10th ed.). Oxford University Press.

2

Breast Surgery and Vascular Surgery in an Hour

Hannah Punter, Chrissie Laban; Nagarjun Konda, Thomas Brankin-Frisby and Angeliki Kosti

OUTLINE

BREAST SURGERY

BREAST ANATOMY AND GENETIC RISK FACTORS

Breast Anatomy

Definition: a modified sweat gland covered by skin and subcutaneous tissue comprised of mammary glands and connective tissue (see Fig 2.1A,B). Mammary glands consist of ducts and secretory lobules converging at the nipple. Lymphatic drainage is to the axillary lymph nodes (75%), parasternal lymph nodes (20%) and posterior intercostal lymph nodes (5%).

Genetic Risk Factors

The genes, **BRCA1** and **BRCA2,** have been identified to significantly increase the risk of developing breast and ovarian cancers (see Table 2.1) and account for 5% of all breast cancers.
Key facts:
- Tumour-suppressor genes

- Autosomal-dominant inheritance
- Genetic testing is available
- More common in patients with young presentations

Genetic testing should be carried out if there is:
- First-degree female relative with breast cancer at **<40 years**
- First-degree **male** relative with breast cancer
- First-degree relative with **bilateral breast cancer**
- **Multiple** first or second-degree relatives with breast cancer

BREAST CARE

Breast Care in General Practice

Referral guidelines: General practitioners (GPs) should refer a patient to a one-stop breast clinic with less than a **2-week wait** if:
- Patient is >30 years of age with an unexplained breast or axillary lump
- Patient is >50 years of age with a breast lump, nipple retraction, bloody nipple discharge or other concerning features

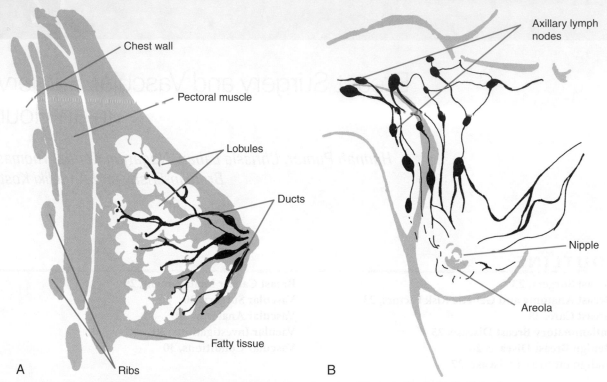

Fig 2.1 (A) Breast anatomy. (B) Breast lymph nodes. (Illustrated by Dr Hollie Blaber.)

TABLE 2.1   **Genetic Risk Factors for Breast and Ovarian Cancer**

	Breast Cancer Risk	Ovarian Cancer Risk
Baseline	12%	1.3%
BRCA1	72%	44%
BRCA2	69%	17%

- Patient has skin changes suggestive of cancer

Nonurgent referral if <30 years of age with a breast lump

All referrals should ask about:

- **Symptoms**: lump, nipple retraction, nipple discharge, skin changes, mastalgia, change in size or shape of breast
- **Systemic features of malignancy:** weight loss, fatigue, shortness of breath, back pain, jaundice
- **Risk factors:** oestrogen exposure, personal history, screening history, family history, radiation, breast feeding, smoking, alcohol, BRCA1, BRCA2

- **Oestrogen exposure**: combined oral contraception pill (COCP), early menarche, late menopause, nulliparity, obesity, polycystic ovary syndrome, hormone replacement therapy (HRT)

Breast Care in Hospitals

Screening program: All women aged **47–73** years are invited every **3 years** for a mammogram. If any problem is detected, they are referred to a one-stop breast clinic.

One-stop breast clinic: All patients requiring further investigation following screening or seeing their GP are referred to a one-stop breast clinic (see Fig 2.2), and a triple assessment is carried out to guide further management. This assessment combines a detailed history and examination followed by a number of investigations (see Table 2.2).

Following the triple assessment, a score (see Table 2.3) is calculated based on three components:

- Examination (P)
- Imaging (U) via ultrasound scan (USS) or (M) for mammogram
- Histology (B) or cytology (C)

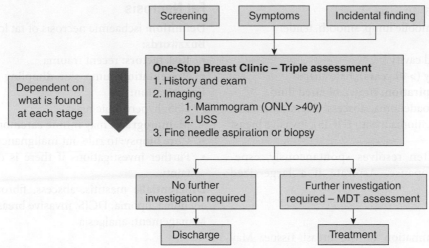

Fig 2.2 One-stop Breast Clinic. *MDT*, Multidisciplinary team; *USS*, ultrasound scan. (Illustrated by Dr Hannah Punter.)

TABLE 2.2   Investigations Performed During a Patient Assessment at a One-stop Breast Clinic

Investigation	Description	Buzzwords for Concerning Features
Examination	Inspection and palpation of both breasts and axillary lymph nodes.	Fixed lump; craggy, rubbery lymph node; peau d'orange; skin dimpling; nipple retraction
Ultrasound scan	High-frequency sound waves useful for highly glandular tissue (<40 years)	Alternate hypo-hyperechogenic lines, deep lesion, incompressible
Mammogram	Two-view x-rays of the breasts. Difficult if breast tissue is very glandular (>40 years)	Calcifications, mass, asymmetry, distortion of underlying tissue
Fine-needle aspiration cytology	Needle inserted into a hypoechogenic lesion identified at imaging for cytology	Malignant cells seen on fine-needle aspiration cytology (C5)
Core biopsy	Tissue samples of the mass is sent to histology. Sample is graded, and immunohistochemistry is performed to assess: • Oestrogen receptor (ER) status • Progesterone receptor (PR) status • Human epidermal growth receptor 2 (HER2) status	Loss of basement membrane, dysplasia, poorly differentiated, **triple negative** (ER, PR and HER2 negative). Grade 1, 2 or 3. Invasive ductal, lobular, papillary or medullary carcinoma

TABLE 2.3   Scoring of the Triple Assessment

No.	Description
1	Normal
2	Benign
3	Suspicious, likely benign
4	Suspicious, likely malignancy
5	Malignancy

For example, a P4, M4, B5 score indicates that the mass looked suspicious and likely malignant on the examination and mammography, with histology confirming malignancy.

INFLAMMATORY BREAST DISEASE

Cyst

Definition: epithelial-lined, fluid-filled cavity
Buzzwords:

- **Risk factors:** 35–50 years of age
- **Presentation:** mobile lump, smooth, tender

Investigations:

- **USS:** fluid-filled cavity
- **Mammography (>40 years):** halo shape
- **Fine-needle aspiration:** straw-coloured fluid

Differentials: fibroadenoma, abscess, ductal adenoma, lipoma, ductal carcinoma in situ (DCIS), invasive breast cancer

Management: often resolves spontaneously, especially after menopause. Aspirate if a large-sized cyst

Mastitis

Definition: inflammation of the breast tissue. May occur whilst breast feeding (lactational) or otherwise (nonlactational).

Buzzwords:

- **Risk factors:** breast feeding, smoking, duct ectasia, *Staphylococcus aureus*
- **Presentation:** cracked nipples, swelling, tender, erythema, induration

Investigations:

- **Blood (if systemically unwell):** ↑white cell count, ↑CRP, positive blood cultures

Differentials: abscess, fat necrosis

Management:

1. Analgesia
2. Antibiotics: flucloxacillin orally (PO) for 5 days (clindamycin if allergic to penicillin)
3. Continue breast feeding (if applicable)

Breast Abscess

Definition: painful collection of pus in the breast tissue.

Buzzwords:

- **Risk factors:** breast feeding, smoking, mastitis
- **Presentation:** fluctuant, erythema, fever, mass

Investigations:

- **USS:** hypoechoic collection with an echogenic capsule

Differentials: mastitis, cyst, fat necrosis, fibroadenoma, ductal adenoma, lipoma, DCIS, invasive breast cancer

Management:

1. Fine-needle aspiration of pus and send for microscopy, culture and sensitivities (MC+S)
2. Antibiotics: co-amoxiclav PO for 5 days
3. Incision and drainage if no improvement
4. Regular clinical follow-up

Fat Necrosis

Definition: ischaemic necrosis of fat lobules

Buzzwords:

- **Risk factors:** recent trauma
- **Presentation:** lump, skin dimpling

Investigation:

- **USS:** hyperechoic mass
- **Mammogram:** may mimic carcinoma
- **Core biopsy:** to rule out malignancy
- Further investigations if there is diagnostic uncertainty

Differentials: mastitis, abscess, fibroadenoma, ductal adenoma, lipoma, DCIS, invasive breast cancer

Management: analgesia

BENIGN BREAST DISEASE

A collection of conditions that are not malignant. Patients are often assessed at a one-stop breast clinic to distinguish from malignant breast disease.

Fibrocystic Change

Definition: increased nodularity of breast tissue in response to hormonal changes

Buzzwords:

- **Risk factors:** 30–50 years of age
- **Presentation:** multiple diffuse lumps, size fluctuation, cyclical mastalgia

Investigation:

- **USS/mammogram:** no concerning features
- FNAC and biopsy rarely carried out

Differentials: fibroadenoma, ductal adenoma, lipoma, DCIS, invasive breast cancer

Management: analgesia and a well-fitted bra

Fibroadenoma

Definition: benign, mobile tumour in the breast lobules ('the breast mouse')

Buzzwords:

- **Risk factors:** COCP, pregnancy, HRT
- **Presentation:** mobile, smooth, painless lump

Investigations:

- **USS (<40 years)** or **mammogram (>40 years):** well circumscribed
- **Biopsy:** only if >2.5 cm, enlarging in size or atypical features

Differentials: fibrocystic change, ductal adenoma, lipoma, DCIS, invasive breast cancer

Management: surgical excision if >3 cm, diagnostic uncertainty, very painful or increasing in size

Ductal Adenoma

Definition: benign glandular tumour
Buzzwords:
- **Risk factors:** >50 years of age
- **Presentation:** lump, painless, nodular

Investigations:
- **USS** (<40 years) or **mammogram** (>40 years): may mimic malignancy
- **Biopsy:** often required to distinguish from malignancy

Differentials: fibroadenoma, lipoma, DCIS, invasive breast cancer
Management: conservative management or surgical excision if diagnostic uncertainty.

Lipoma

Definition: Benign adipose tumour
Buzzwords:
- **Risk factors:** N/A
- **Presentation:** soft, mobile lump

Investigations:
- **Mammogram:** radiolucent, no calcification
- **Biopsy:** ONLY required if enlarging

Differentials: fibroadenoma, ductal adenoma, DCIS, invasive breast cancer
Management: refer to sarcoma team and arrange for MRI if >5 cm in size.

Papilloma

Definition: benign intraductal breast lesion
Buzzwords:
- **Risk factors:** 40–50 years of age
- **Presentation:** lump, subareolar, bloody or clear nipple discharge

Investigations:
- **USS (<40 years):** dilated duct
- **Mammogram (>40 years):** ductal calcifications
- **Biopsy:** often required to exclude malignancy

Differentials: ductal ectasia, fibroadenoma, ductal adenoma, lipoma, DCIS, invasive breast cancer
Management: excision – either a microdochectomy or a major duct excision.

Ductal Ectasia

Definition: dilated, calcified ducts

Buzzwords:
- **Risk factors:** increasing age, perimenopausal
- **Presentation:** green discharge, lump, nipple retraction

Investigations:
- **Mammogram:** calcified ducts
- **Biopsy:** multiple plasma cells

Differentials: papilloma, ductal adenoma, Paget's disease of the nipple, DCIS, invasive breast cancer
Management: duct excision if malignancy concern or persistent discharge

Phyllodes

Definition: rare fibroepithelial tumour that can be benign or malignant.
Buzzwords:
- **Risk factors:** increasing age
- **Presentation:** rapid growth, large mass

Investigations:
- **Core biopsy** shows leaf-like projections

Differentials: fibrocystic change, fibroadenoma, ductal adenoma, DCIS, invasive breast cancer
Management:
1. Wide local excision with clear margins
2. Mastectomy if large

MALIGNANT BREAST DISEASE

Epidemiology:
- Represents 15% of all new cancer cases in the United Kingdom
- Risk of cancer increases with increasing age

Key definitions:
- **In situ:** contained within the basement membrane (see Fig 2.3A)
- **Invasive:** not contained within the basement membrane (see Fig 2.3B)

Ductal Carcinoma In Situ

Definition: malignancy of ductal tissue contained within the basement membrane
Buzzwords:
- **Risk factors:** family history, increased oestrogen exposure, increasing age, alcohol, obesity
- **Presentation:** breast screening

Investigations:
- **Mammogram:** microcalcifications
- **Biopsy:** histological confirmation

Differentials: fibrocystic change, fibroadenoma, ductal adenoma, lipoma, invasive breast cancer
Management: wire-guided, wide local excision, as often nonpalpable

Lobular Carcinoma In Situ (LCIS)

Definition: malignancy of the secretory lobules contained within the basement membrane
Buzzwords:
- **Risk factors:** family history, increased oestrogen exposure, increasing age, alcohol, obesity
- **Presentation:** asymptomatic, incidental

Investigations: usually an incidental finding on biopsy
Differentials: DCIS, invasive breast cancer
Management:
1. Yearly mammogram for 5 years due to an increased risk of invasive disease
2. Excision advised if pleiomorphic LCIS – treat as DCIS

Invasive Breast Cancer

Definition: malignancy of the ductal tissue no longer contained by the basement membrane.
Types:
- Invasive ductal carcinoma (80%)
- Invasive lobular carcinoma (10%)
- Medullary

- Diffuse
Buzzwords:
- **Risk factors:** family history, unopposed oestrogen, increasing age, alcohol, obesity
- **Presentation:** skin dimpling, craggy mass, immobile, nipple retraction, nipple discharge

Investigations:
- **USS:** alternate hypo-hyperechogenic lines, deep lesion, incompressible
- **Mammogram:** calcifications, mass, asymmetry, spiculated distortion of breast tissue
- **Biopsy:** for grading and hormone receptor status
- **Staging CT** (if more than four axillary lymph nodes): TNM staging
- **MRI** (if lobular carcinoma or inconsistency in breast imaging): high-resolution imaging
- **Genetic testing (if triple negative or strongly positive family history):** BRCA1 or BRCA2

Differentials: fibrocystic change, fibroadenoma, ductal adenoma, DCIS, Paget's disease of the nipple
Management: dependent on histology and staging but may include:
1. **Surgical excision:** wide local excision or mastectomy
2. **Sentinel lymph node biopsy:** radioactive and patent blue dye is injected into the areolar area, and the first axillary lymph nodes it drains into are removed

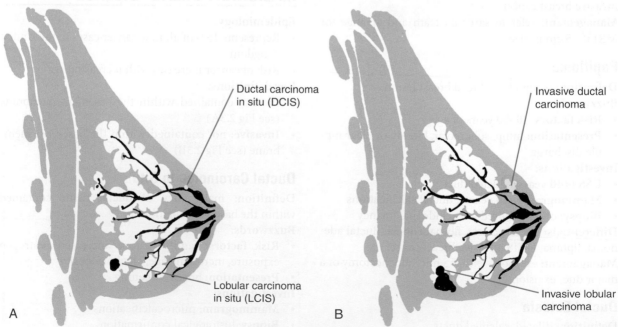

Ductal carcinoma in situ (DCIS)

Lobular carcinoma in situ (LCIS)

A

Invasive ductal carcinoma

Invasive lobular carcinoma

B

Fig 2.3 (A) In Situ Carcinoma. (B) Invasive Carcinoma. (Illustrated by Dr Hollie Blaber).

for further analysis to determine if the tumour has spread to the lymphatic system.

3. **Adjuvant therapy:** chemotherapy, herceptin, radiotherapy, ibandronate and endocrine therapy
4. **Breast reconstruction:** immediate or delayed

Paget's Disease

Definition: Epidermal involvement by malignant ductal carcinoma (Fig 2.4).

Buzzwords:

- **Risk factors:** family history, unopposed oestrogen, increasing age, alcohol, obesity
- **Presentation:** itching, redness, ulceration of nipple, bloody nipple discharge

Investigations:

- **Mammogram:** microcalcifications
- **Nipple biopsy:** histological confirmation
- **MRI:** evidence of invasive breast disease

Differentials: papilloma, ductal adenoma, DCIS, invasive breast cancer

Management: central wide local excision or mastectomy. Adjuvant therapy.

BREAST CANCER MANAGEMENT

At a multi-disciplinary team (MDT) meeting, the following is assessed:

- Size and grade of tumour

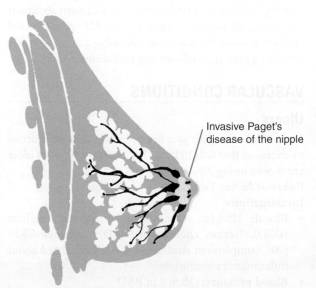

Fig 2.4 Invasive Paget's Disease of the Nipple. (Illustrated by Dr Hollie Blaber.)

- Immunohistochemistry – ER-, PR- and HER2-receptor status
- CT staging (for TNM staging see Palliative Care and Oncology in an Hour)
- Proliferative markers – Ki67

The treatment plan will depend on the factors above and also the patient's functional status and age.

Treatment principles:

- Most cases will be treated surgically followed by adjuvant therapy.
- A wide local excision should be followed by radiotherapy.
- Mastectomy may NOT require adjuvant radiotherapy.
- Axillary node dissection may be required if there is evidence of spread to the lymph nodes.
- If ER positive, adjuvant therapy with tamoxifen (premenopausal) or aromatase inhibitors (postmenopausal) for 5–10 years following surgery is recommended.
- If HER2 positive, adjuvant treatment with Herceptin (trastuzumab) should be offered.
- Breast reconstruction may be offered immediately or delayed.
- Prognosis may be calculated using the Nottingham Prognostic Index.
- If cancer is advanced or recurrent, treatment should focus on the quality of life (see Palliative Care and Oncology in an Hour).
- Treatment side effects should be considered and discussed with the patient (see Table 2.4).
- For side effects of chemotherapy, radiotherapy and immunotherapy, see Palliative Care and Oncology in an Hour.

TABLE 2.4 Breast Cancer Treatments and Side Effects	
Treatment	**Side Effects**
Lymph node dissection	Unilateral lymphoedema Numbness in arm and chest wall
Tamoxifen (anti-oestrogen)	Thrombosis, menopausal symptoms, small increased risk of endometrial cancer
Aromatase inhibitors (anastrozole, letrozole, exemestane)	Menopausal symptoms, joint pain
Trastuzumab=herceptin (monoclonal antibody that targets HER2)	Cardiac toxicity, breathlessness, nausea and vomiting, neutropenia

TABLE 2.5   Nodal Status and Involvement

Nodal Status	Nodes Involved
1	0 nodes
2	1–4 nodes
3	>4 nodes

Nottingham Prognostic index (NPI): made up of three components:

- Size – diameter of the lesion (cm)
- Nodal status (Table 2.5)
- Grade

NPI calculation: (size × 0.2) + nodal status + grade

NPI interpretation: see Table 2.6

THE ONE-LINE ROUND-UP!

Here are some key words to help you remember each condition/concept.

Condition/Concept	One-line Description
Cyst	Halo shape
Mastitis	Breast feeding
Breast abscess	Erythematous and fluctuant
Fat necrosis	Recent trauma
Fibrocystic change	Lumpy breasts
Fibroadenoma	Breast mouse
Papilloma	Subareolar lump
Ductal ectasia	Green discharge
Phyllodes	Leaf-like projections
Malignant breast disease	Immobile, craggy
ER positive	Tamoxifen
HER2 positive	Herceptin
Triple negative	BRCA testing
Paget's disease	Ulceration of nipple
Screening	47–73 years of age

VASCULAR SURGERY

VASCULAR ANATOMY

For a recap on vascular anatomy please see Fig 2.5, Fig 2.6 and Fig 2.7.

VASCULAR INVESTIGATIONS

Ankle-Brachial Pressure Index (ABPI): The ABPI measures the ratio of the systolic blood pressure at the level of the ankle to the systolic blood pressure at the

TABLE 2.6   Nottingham Prognostic Index Score and 5-year Survival

Nottingham Prognostic Index Score	5-year Survival
2–2.4	93%
2.5–3.4	85%
3.5–5.4	70%
>5.4	50%

level of the arm to assess the peripheral arterial perfusion. The specific cutoff values (see Table 2.7) vary according to different guidelines; therefore, the overall clinical picture is more important than the exact ABPI result.

Duplex ultrasonography: A noninvasive imaging technique that combines traditional ultrasonography with Doppler ultrasonography to produce a coloured image to detect blood flow and greyscale to correlate with the surrounding tissues. Blood flow can be characterised by the direction, speed and turbulence. Duplex ultrasonography can be used to detect a deep vein thrombosis (DVT), peripheral arterial disease (PAD) and venous insufficiency by evaluating the degree of vascular stenosis, irregularities in blood flow and occlusion of blood vessels.

CT angiography (CTA): A radiological technique to visualise arterial and venous vessels using IV contrast (see Fig 2.8). It is primarily used to detect stenosis, aneurysms and dissections. Scans can be 3D reconstructed and are commonly used for operative planning. CTA involves a high dose of ionising radiation.

VASCULAR CONDITIONS

Ulcers

Definition: An ulcer is a break in the skin or mucous membranes that fails to heal. The different types of ulcer are shown in Fig 2.9.

Buzzwords: See Table 2.8

Investigations:

- **Blood:** HbA1c >48mmol/mol (diabetes mellitus (DM)), ↑serum cholesterol (PAD); consider CRP/ESR, complement studies/ANCA if concerned about inflammatory conditions
- **Blood pressure:** Often ↑ in PAD
- **ABPI:** ≤0.9 in PAD

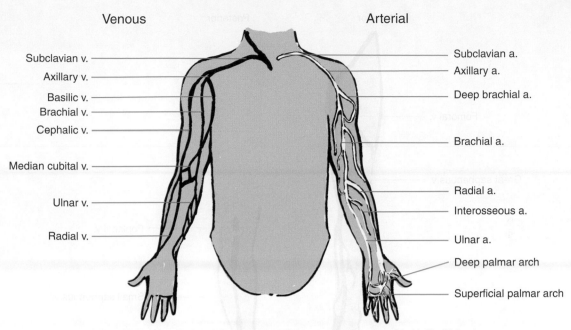

Fig 2.5 Upper-limb Arterial and Venous Systems. (Illustrated by Dr Hollie Blaber.)

Venous

- Subclavian v.
- Axillary v.
- Basilic v.
- Brachial v.
- Cephalic v.
- Median cubital v.
- Ulnar v.
- Radial v.

Arterial

- Subclavian a.
- Axillary a.
- Deep brachial a.
- Brachial a.
- Radial a.
- Interosseous a.
- Ulnar a.
- Deep palmar arch
- Superficial palmar arch

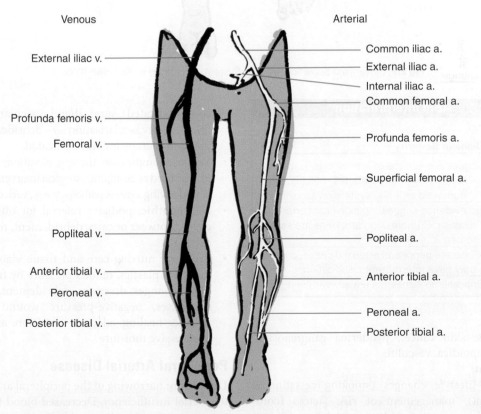

Fig 2.6 Lower-limb Deep Arterial and Venous Systems. (Illustrated by Dr Hollie Blaber.)

Venous

- External iliac v.
- Profunda femoris v.
- Femoral v.
- Popliteal v.
- Anterior tibial v.
- Peroneal v.
- Posterior tibial v.

Arterial

- Common iliac a.
- External iliac a.
- Internal iliac a.
- Common femoral a.
- Profunda femoris a.
- Superficial femoral a.
- Popliteal a.
- Anterior tibial a.
- Peroneal a.
- Posterior tibial a.

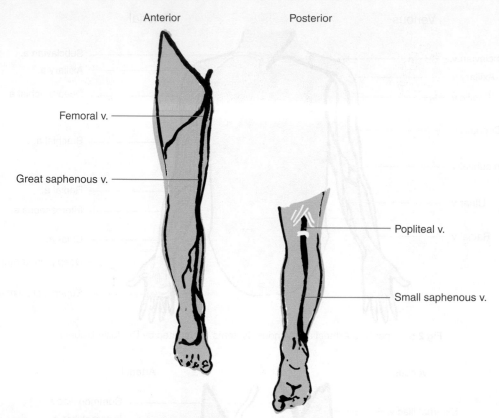

Fig 2.7 Lower-limb Superficial Venous System. (Illustrated by Dr Hollie Blaber.)

TABLE 2.7	ABPI interpretation
Resting ABPI	**Disease Severity**
>1.3	Suggests presence of arterial calcification – commonly due to diabetes mellitus, rheumatoid arthritis, systemic vasculitis
0.8–1.3	No evidence suggesting significant arterial disease. Compression stockings are safe to use
0.5–0.8	Moderate peripheral arterial disease, patient may have intermittent claudication
<0.5	Critical limb ischaemia usually with rest pain

Differentials: skin cancer, pyoderma gangrenosum, necrobiosis lipoidica, vasculitis

Management:

- **Arterial**: lifestyle changes (smoking cessation is paramount), management of risk factors (commence lifelong statin and antiplatelet use if not contraindicated), surgical/endovascular intervention (plan for revascularisation +/- debridement). Compression therapy is contraindicated.
- **Venous**: compression therapy, elevation, pentoxifylline may be used as an adjunct, surgical intervention for repair of underlying venous pathology, e.g., varicose veins
- **Neuropathic**: podiatry referral for offloading, specialist footwear or casts, debridement, regular wound dressings
- **Pressure**: nursing care and tissue viability involvement +/- plastics. offload pressure by frequent positional changes, dressings, debridement, use of foam mattresses, negative-pressure wound therapy to enhance healing, adequate nutrition, and reduction of excessive moisture

Peripheral Arterial Disease

Definition: narrowing of the peripheral arteries leading to arterial insufficiency. Decreased blood flow can lead to pain, impaired healing and ischaemia. This condition

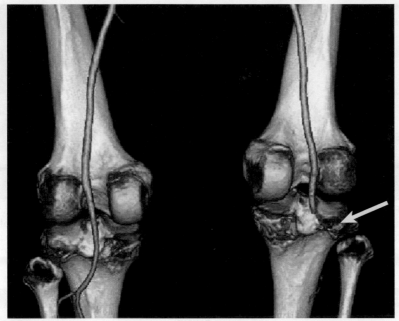

Fig 2.8 Three-Dimensional Reconstruction of a CT Angiogram Showing an Occlusion in the Right Popliteal Artery. (From Godfrey, A. D., Hindi, F., Ettles, C., Pemberton, M., Grewal, P. (2017). Acute thrombotic occlusion of the popliteal artery following knee dislocation: A case report of management, local unit practice, and a review of the literature. *Case Reports in Surgery*, 2017, 5346457.)

TABLE 2.8 Ulcers

	ULCERS			
	Pressure (A)	**Neuropathic (B)**	**Venous (C)**	**Arterial (D)**
Risk Factors	Prolonged bed rest, dementia	Diabetes mellitus, prolonged pressure, microtrauma	Obesity, pregnancy, previous deep vein thrombosis, varicose veins, immobility	Smoking, diabetes, hypertension, peripheral arterial disease, hypercholesterolaemia
Location	Heel, buttocks, bony prominences	Lateral to 5th metatarsal, tips of toes, ball of foot, heel	Gaiter area (between medical malleolus and mid-calf)	Toes and feet, pressure areas, lateral malleolus, tibial areas
Presentation	Deep, often macerated	Deep, calcified rim, insensate	Flat margins and shallow, exudate present, slough at base with granulation tissue	Punched-out lesion, deep, presence of necrotic tissue, painful
Skin Features	Loss of muscle mass, atrophic skin	Dry, cracked skin, calluses	Eczematous, itchy skin, limb oedema, haemosiderin staining	Shiny skin, hair loss, absent or weak pulses, delayed capillary refill, cold peripheries

is caused by atherosclerotic deposits in arteries leading to progressive stenosis. Further categories include:

- **Intermittent claudication (IC):** unable to meet tissue oxygen requirements with exertion
- **Critical limb ischaemia (CLI):** unable to meet tissue oxygen requirements at rest

- **Acute limb ischaemia (ALI):** sudden onset occlusion leading to acute ischaemia

Buzzwords:
- **Risk factors:** smoking, DM, hypertension (HTN), hyperlipidaemia, >40 years of age
- **Presentation:**

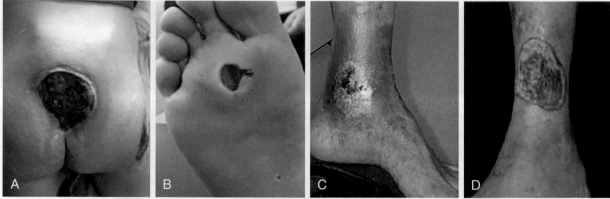

Fig 2.9 (A) Pressure Ulcer, (B) Neuropathic Ulcer, (C) Venous Ulcer, and (D) Arterial Insufficiency Ulcer. (**A,** With permission from Duci, S. B., Arifi, H. M., Selmani, M. E., et al. (2013). Surgical treatment of 55 patients with pressure ulcers at the Department of Plastic and Reconstructive Surgery Kosovo during the period 2000-2010: A retrospective study. Plastic Surgery International, 2013, 129692; **C,** Reprinted with permission from Thomas Jefferson University Clinical Image Database.)

TABLE 2.9   Rutherford Classification of Acute Limb Ischaemia

	SIGNS		DOPPLER SIGNAL	
Category	Sensation Loss	Muscle weakness	Arterial	Venous
I – Viable	None	None	Audible	Audible
IIa – Threatened, marginally	Minimal – toes	None	Inaudible	Audible
IIb – Threatened, immediately	More than toes	Mild–moderate	Inaudible	Audible
III – Irreversible	Profound loss	Paralysis	Inaudible	Inaudible

- **IC:** muscle pain after periods of exercise and exertion, relieved by rest. Commonly affects the calves but may also be felt in the thighs and buttocks and may cause erectile dysfunction. Patients often have absent pulses.
- **CLI:** felt at the extremities (toes) because they are furthest away from the heart and blood supply. Gnawing pain, rest pain, pain worse at night (when lying down, since gravity is not helping blood flow, so relieved by hanging leg out of the bed), absent limb pulses, arterial ulcers and chronic gangrene may be present.
- **ALI:** sudden onset of 6 Ps in order of presentation: pain (constant), pulselessness, pallor (or cyanosis or mottling), perishingly cold, paraesthesia, paralysis (late), fixed mottling (irreversible). See Table 2.9

Investigations:
- **Blood:** ↑serum cholesterol
- **Blood pressure:** ↑
- **ABPI:** ≤0.9 defines PAD

- ***Duplex ultrasonography:** ↑arterial stenosis*

Differentials: spinal stenosis, osteoarthritis, diabetic neuropathy, DVT, chronic compartment syndrome, nocturnal leg cramps, sciatica, metatarsalgia

Management:
- **IC:**
  - Statin and antiplatelet therapy
  - Exercise therapy and aggressive risk factor modification
  - Disease optimisation (HTN, DM)
  - Referral to vascular centre only if improvement is not seen with above therapies after 6 months, if rapid deterioration in walking distance/QoL, if signs and symptoms of CLI or if complex disease
  - Revascularisation: endovascular or surgery as applicable
- **CLI:**
  - URGENT referral to vascular service for investigations and revascularisation +/- debridement
  - Strong analgesia (morphine based)

Types of Aneurysm

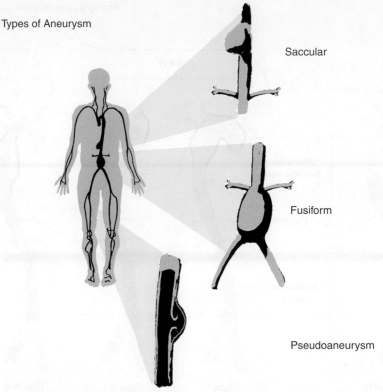

Saccular

Fusiform

Pseudoaneurysm

Fig 2.10 Different Types of Aneurysms. (Illustrated by Dr Hollie Blaber).

- Amputation if revascularisation fails or overwhelming sepsis
- **ALI:** requires emergency intervention
  - Endovascular: percutaneous catheter–directed thrombolysis or percutaneous mechanical thrombus extraction
  - Surgical: thromboembolectomy +/- fasciotomy, endarterectomy or bypass
  - Amputation of unsalvageable limb

Abdominal Aortic Aneurysm (AAA)

Definition: permanent dilation of the abdominal aorta to >3 cm, with more than 90% occurring infrarenally. Dilation is seen in all the layers of the artery (see Fig 2.10). This condition is caused by a loss of elastin and collagen in the adventitia and tunica media, as well as smooth muscle loss.

Buzzwords
- **Risk factors:** male > female, smoking, family history, age >55 years, Marfan syndrome
- **Presentation:** asymptomatic, picked up through national screening program (ultrasound (US) for men aged 65 years old), expansile abdominal mass on palpation
- **Ruptured AAA presentation:** triad of abdominal/back pain, pulsatile abdominal mass and hypotension

Investigations:
- **Abdominal US:** diameter of abdominal aorta >3 cm
- **CTA:** to confirm diagnosis and first choice for operative planning

Differentials: ureteric colic, perforated viscus, diverticulitis, inflammatory bowel disease, ovarian torsion, appendicitis

Management:
- **Surveillance:** asymptomatic and small (3–4.4 cm) = yearly US; medium (4.5–5.4 cm) = repeat US in 3 months; symptomatic or >5.5 cm or an increase in size by >1 cm in 1 year = 2-week-wait referral for repair
- **Reducing rupture risk:** smoking cessation, optimisation of HTN
- **Repair:** open surgical repair or endovascular aneurysm repair (EVAR). Outcomes are similar for both methods for elective, large (AAA >5.5 cm) repairs

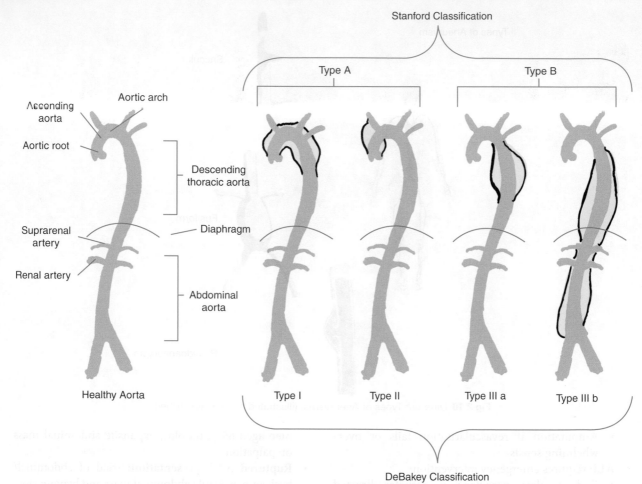

Fig 2.11 Classification of Aortic Dissections: Stanford and DeBakey Classification Systems. (Illustrated by Dr Hollie Blaber).

- **Ruptured AAA:** initial A–E resuscitation followed by immediate surgery. EVAR is preferred to an open repair in those aged over 70 years. High mortality rates

Prognosis: 5-year survival rates after an elective operative repair of an aneurysm are between 60%–75%.

Aortic Dissection

Definition: disruption of the arterial wall intima, leading to a separation of the wall from the lumen of the aorta and providing a false lumen in which blood can accumulate. Classified according to the Stanford and DeBakey classification systems (see Fig 2.11).

Buzzwords:
- **Risk factors:** HTN, smoking, hypercholesterolaemia, bicuspid aortic valve, Marfan syndrome, Ehlers-Danlos syndrome, family history of dissection, male
- **Presentation:** sudden-onset, sharp, tearing chest pain radiating to the retrosternal region; HTN; blood pressure differences between the two upper limbs and a weakened pulse volume. Syncope, hypotension and ischaemic changes are late signs

Investigations:
- **Blood:** group and save/crossmatch in preparation for surgery, electrocardiogram and cardiac enzymes to rule out acute coronary syndromes (ACS), D-dimer for pulmonary embolism (PE)

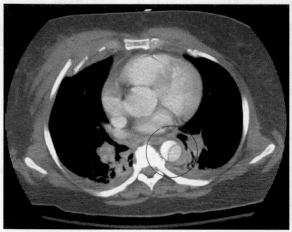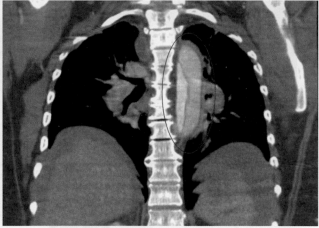

Fig. 2.12 CT Scan Showing an Aortic Dissection (Suspected Stanford Type B) Visualized at the Descending Thoracic Aorta. (From Jason Robert Young, MD, CC BY-SA 4.0 via Wikimedia Commons.)

- **Chest x-ray:** widened mediastinum
- **Transthoracic US:** ↑diameter of aorta
- ***CT thorax:** (see Fig 2.12) *

Differentials: ACS, pericarditis, aortic aneurysm, musculoskeletal pain, PE, cholecystitis

Management:
1. A–E assessment and initial resuscitation
2. IV beta blockade to achieve a heart rate of <60 bpm and a systolic BP of 100–120 mm Hg
3. Analgesia
4. Blood products for impaired end-artery perfusion
5. Surgery: type A (involving the ascending aorta) and complicated type B dissections are usually managed via an open repair. Uncomplicated type B dissections are managed via endovascular stent-graft repair.

Prognosis: Aortic rupture has an 80% mortality rate. The 10-year survival after surgery is around 52%.

Varicose Veins

Definition: Superficial veins that are dilated and tortuous and commonly found in the lower limbs. Varicose veins result from retrograde blood flow in the superficial venous system caused by incompetent valves and hydrostatic pressure caused by gravity. Chronic venous insufficiency can be seen on examination by leg swelling, skin colour and textural changes and venous ulcers.

Buzzwords:
- **Risk factors:** female, older age, family history, increasing parity, previous DVT, obesity

- **Presentation:** leg cramps; fatigue with prolonged standing; visible, bulging, palpable, tortuous superficial veins; may be asymptomatic; spontaneous bleeding; superficial thrombophlebitis

Investigations:
- **Blood:** D-dimer to exclude DVT
- **Duplex US:** reversed flow

Differentials: telangiectasias, cellulitis, superficial thrombophlebitis, DVT

Management:
1. Conservative management: compression stockings (above or below the knee depending on the location of varicosities), increased mobility and leg elevation when resting
2. Refer to secondary care if spontaneous bleeding, thrombophlebitis, skin changes or venous leg ulcers
3. Vascular treatment options include endothermal ablation (radiofrequency or laser), foam sclerotherapy and surgery (ligation or stripping) of vein

Buerger's Disease

Definition: A nonatherosclerotic chronic vasculitic condition that results in inflammation and thrombosis of small- and medium-sized arteries and veins in the distal aspects of the upper and lower limbs in young men who smoke. Also known as thromboangiitis obliterans.

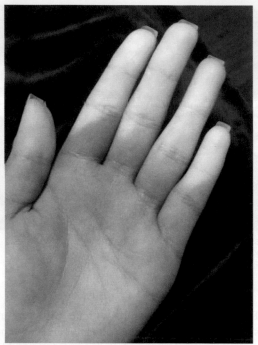

Fig 2.13 Raynaud's Phenomenon. (With permission from MSM98, CC BY-SA 4.0, via Wikimedia Commons.)

Buzzwords:

- **Risk factors:** smoking, Southeast Mediterranean/Middle- and Far-East origins, familial, male, age <40 years
- **Presentation:** claudication and rest pain in extremities, paraesthesia/cyanosis of digits, ulceration/gangrene, loss of digital pulses, Raynaud's phenomenon (see Fig 2.13). It is important to exclude systemic lupus erythematosus (SLE) and scleroderma in these patients

Investigations:

- No specific diagnostic test
- **Blood:** thrombophilia screen, ANA/ESR/dsDNA/anti-centromere Ab to rule out SLE/CREST
- **Duplex US:** embolism/thrombus

Differentials: SLE, scleroderma, PAD, DM, ALI, embolic disease, thrombophilia, CREST syndrome

Management:

1. Smoking cessation
2. Analgesia
3. Calcium-channel blockers (e.g., nifedipine)
4. Oral antibiotics for gangrene
5. Surgical techniques include debridement, revascularisation and lumbar/periarterial sympathectomy

Chronic Mesenteric Ischaemia (CMI)

Definition: a long-standing disease characterised by reduced blood flow to the intestinal region (also referred to as abdominal angina), most commonly due to atherosclerotic changes causing reductions in arterial blood flow

Buzzwords:

- **Risk factors:** smoking, HTN, hypercholesterolaemia, DM, increasing age, female
- **Presentation:** often chronic post-prandial pain (abdominal pain after eating caused by an increased perfusion requirement), weight loss, irregular bowel habits and fear of eating

Investigations:

- **Mesenteric duplex US:** ↓ blood flow
- *CTA: atherosclerotic changes*

Differentials: acute myocardial infarction (MI), gastric/pancreatic/bowel cancer, diverticulitis, gastroesophageal reflux disease (GORD), chronic pancreatitis, chronic pyelonephritis

Management:

1. **If asymptomatic disease:** smoking cessation, statin therapy, antiplatelet therapy, existing disease and risk factor modification
2. **If symptomatic disease:** open surgical repair carries a high risk, so nonsurgical options are preferred (e.g., percutaneous mesenteric angioplasty +/- stenting).

Prognosis: 5-year mortality rate for untreated CMI is close to 100%

Atherosclerosis

Definition: a long-standing disease characterised by hardening and deposition of plaque within the lumen of large- and medium-sized arteries. Over time, it can predispose to MI, PAD, cerebrovascular events and carotid artery stenosis.

Buzzwords:

- **Risk factors:** smoking, hypertension, DM, obesity, diet high in saturated fats, family history, hypercholesterolaemia, stress, alcohol, lack of exercise
- **Presentation:** initially asymptomatic. Over time, this condition may lead to chest pain on exertion (angina) or muscle pain on exertion (IC). Signs include carotid bruits, xanthelasmata, poor peripheral pulses and a reduced ABPI

Investigations: see section on PAD

Management:

- **Conservative and Medical:** see section on PAD
- **Surgical:** coronary artery bypass grafts, endovascular (e.g., stent) or open revascularisation (e.g., bypass graft)

TABLE 2.10	Wells Criteria for Deep Vein Thrombosis				
Criteria				**Criteria**	**Present?**
Active cancer Treatment or palliation within 6 months	No	0		Yes	+1
Bedridden recently > 3 days or major surgery within 12 weeks	No	0		Yes	+1
Calf swelling > 3 cm compared to the other leg Measured 10 cm below tibial tuberosity	No	0		Yes	+1
Collateral (nonvaricose) superficial veins present	No	0		Yes	+1
Entire leg swollen	No	0		Yes	+1
Localized tenderness along the deep venous system	No	0		Yes	+1
Pitting edema, confined to symptomatic leg	No	0		Yes	+1
Paralysis, paresis, or recent plaster immobilization of the lower extremity	No	0		Yes	+1
Previously documeneted DVT	No	0		Yes	+1
Alternative diagnosis to DVT as likely or more likely	No	0		Yes	−2

With permission from Wells' Criteria for DVT. MD+ Calc.

Carotid Artery Stenosis

Definition: progressive narrowing of the carotid arteries caused by a build-up of atherosclerotic plaque. Plaque rupture or carotid occlusion can lead to a cerebrovascular accident.

Buzzwords:

- **Risk factors:** smoking, HTN, DM, obesity, cardiovascular disease, hypercholesterolaemia
- **Presentation:** carotid bruits, focal neurological deficit, transient ischaemic attack (TIA) or stroke

Investigations:

- **Blood:** elevated lipid profile
- **Carotid duplex US:** for visualisation and categorisation of stenosis
- **CT head:** to prove a resolving TIA before considering carotid endarterectomy (CEA)
- ***CTA:** To help delineate anatomy and gather more information prior to consideration of surgery

Management:

- Smoking cessation, alcohol limitation, increased exercise, healthy eating, stress avoidance
- **Asymptomatic:**
  - **With stenosis of <70%:** antiplatelet therapy (aspirin or clopidogrel) and statin
  - **With stenosis of ≥70%:** antiplatelet therapy (aspirin or clopidogrel), statin and consider CEA.
- **Symptomatic** (patients with a resolving TIA or stroke less than 2 weeks ago):
  - **Ipsilateral carotid stenosis of <50%:** antiplatelet therapy (aspirin or clopidogrel) and statin
  - **Ipsilateral carotid stenosis of ≥50%:** antiplatelet therapy (aspirin or clopidogrel), statin and CEA.

- **CEA:** surgical procedure that involves plaque removal from the lumen of the diseased common carotid and internal carotid artery. Complications include an intra/postoperative stroke, MI, pain, swelling, bleeding, infection, mortality, nerve damage to the hypoglossal, glossopharyngeal, recurrent laryngeal and mandibular branches of the facial nerve.

Deep Vein Thrombosis

Definition: a thrombus (blood clot) that has formed in a deep vein, usually in the legs or pelvis, that partially or completely disrupts blood flow:

- **Provoked DVT:** clear cause, e.g., cancer or lower-limb surgery
- **Unprovoked DVT:** no clear cause

Buzzwords:

- **Risk factors:** Hx of DVT, cancer, high BMI, age >60 years, thrombophilia, varicose veins, smoking, recent major surgery, pelvic mass, significant immobility, travel (classically air travel) for >4 h, oestrogen-containing contraception or HRT, dehydration, lower extremity trauma. These feed into Virchow's triad of hypercoagulability, stasis and endothelial injury.
- **Presentation:** unilateral, localised, throbbing pain worse on weight bearing; limb swelling; erythema or warmth; vein distension

Investigations:

- **D-dimer:** raised
- **Venous lower limb US:** reduced venous flow, inability to compress vein with probe

Differentials: cellulitis, ruptured popliteal cysts (Baker's cyst), calf muscle tear/Achilles' tendon tear, lymphoedema, superficial thrombophlebitis.

Management:

1. Calculate a two-level DVT Well's score (see Table 2.10)
   - ≥2 DVT likely: proceed to imaging (first line: whole-leg US) Also refer pregnant women and those up to 6 weeks postpartum for imaging.
   - <2 DVT unlikely: perform D-dimer; if raised, proceed to imaging
2. Thrombus confirmed on imaging:
   - Direct oral anticoagulant (DOAC) (if contraindicated: Low molecular weight heparin (LMWH) followed by warfarin) for 3 months
   - If all anticoagulation is contraindicated, consider an inferior vena cava filter
   - If imaging is delayed by >4 h, give interim anticoagulation
3. Consider graduated compression stockings for distal lower limb DVTs
4. Early ambulation
5. Follow-up:
   - Investigate possible cancer/thrombophilia in patients with an unprovoked DVT
   - If a provoked DVT with a transient provocation factor (e.g., hip replacement), anticoagulation can typically be stopped after 3 months
   - If unprovoked (or provoking factor not transient), reassessment for longer term anticoagulation at 3 months is required

THE ONE-LINE ROUND-UP!

Here are some key words to help you remember each condition/concept.

Condition/Concept	One-line description
Arterial ulcer	Painful, punched out
Venous ulcer	Gaiter area
Neuropathic ulcer	Nonpainful
Pressure ulcer	Bony prominences
PAD	Duplex US is gold standard
AAA	One-off screening program for men at 65 years
Aortic dissection	Marfan/Ehlers-Danlos syndromes can predispose
Varicose veins	Dilated and tortuous superficial veins
Buerger's disease	Smoking cessation halts disease progression
CMI	Postprandial abdominal pain
Atherosclerosis	Arterial plaques
Carotid artery stenosis	Narrowing of carotid arteries
DVT	Raised D-dimer

READING LIST: BREAST SURGERY IN AN HOUR

Breast Anatomy and Genetic Risk Factors

Patient.info. *Anatomy of the breast.* https://patient.info/news-and-features/anatomy-of-the-breast. [Accessed April 2021].

NICE. (2018). *CKS. Breast cancer – managing FH.* https://cks.nice.org.uk/topics/breast-cancer-managing-fh/. [Accessed April 2021].

National Cancer Institute. (2018). *BRCA gene mutations: Cancer risk and genetic testing.* https://www.cancer.gov/about-cancer/causes-prevention/genetics/brca-fact-sheet. [Accessed April 2021].

Breast Care

NICE. (2015). *CKS: Breast cancer – recognition and referral.* https://cks.nice.org.uk/topics/breast-cancer-recognition-referral/. [Accessed April 2021].

NICE. (2017). *CKS: Breast screening.* https://cks.nice.org.uk/topics/breast-screening/. [Accessed April 2021].

NICE. (2014). *CSG1: Improving outcomes in breast cancer.* https://www.nice.org.uk/guidance/csg1. [Accessed April 2021].

Inflammatory Breast Disease

Patient.info. (2016). *Mammary duct ectasia and periductal mastitis.* https://patient.info/doctor/mammary-duct-ectasia-and-periductal-mastitis. [Accessed April 2021].

NICE. (2018). *CKS: Mastitis and breast abscess.* https://cks.nice.org.uk/topics/mastitis-breast-abscess/. [Accessed April 2021].

Patient.info. (2016). *Benign breast disease.* https://patient.info/doctor/benign-breast-disease. [Accessed April 2021].

Benign Breast Disease

Patient.info. (2016). *Benign breast disease.* https://patient.info/doctor/benign-breast-disease. [Accessed April 2021].

Lammie, G. A., & Millis, R. R. (1989). Ductal adenoma of the breast--a review of fifteen cases. *Human Pathology*, 20, 903–908. https://doi.org/10.1016/0046-8177(89)90104-4.

Patient.info. (2017). *Breast lumps.* https://patient.info/womens-health/breast-problems/breast-lumps. [Accessed April 2021].

Malignant Breast Disease

Cancer Research UK. (2017). *Breast cancer statistics.* https://www.cancerresearchuk.org/health-professional/cancer-statistics/statistics-by-cancer-type/breast-cancer#heading-Zero. [Accessed April 2021].

Patient.info. (2016). *Breast cancer.* https://patient.info/doctor/breast-cancer-pro. [Accessed April 2021].

London Cancer Alliance. (2013). *LCA Breast Cancer Clinical Guideline.* http://rmpartners.cancervanguard.nhs.uk/wp-content/uploads/2017/03/lca-breast-cancer-clinical-guidelines-october-2013-updated-march-2016-.pdf. [Accessed April 2021].

NICE. (2018). *NG101: Early and locally advanced breast cancer: diagnosis and management.* https://www.nice.org.uk/guidance/ng101. [Accessed April 2021].

Breast Cancer Management

NICE. (2018). *NG101: Early and locally advanced breast cancer: diagnosis and management.* https://www.nice.org.uk/guidance/ng101. [Accessed April 2021].

Fong, Y., Evans, J., Brook, D., Kenkre, J., Jarvis, P., & Gower-Thomas, K. (2015). The Nottingham Prognostic Index: five- and ten-year data for all-cause survival within a screened population. *Annals of The Royal College of Surgeons of England*, 97, 137–139. https://doi.org/10.1308/003588414X14055925060514.

READING LIST: VASCULAR SURGERY IN AN HOUR

Vascular Investigations

NICE. (2020). *CKS: Interpretation of ABPI.* https://cks.nice.org.uk/topics/leg-ulcer-venous/diagnosis/interpretation-of-abpi/. [Accessed April 2021]. Accessed.

Cheung, M. E., Singh, V., & Firstenberg, M. S. (2020). *Duplex Ultrasound.* StatPearls [Internet]. https://www.ncbi.nlm.nih.gov/books/NBK459266/. [Accessed April 2021].

Kumamaru, K., Hoppel, B., Mather, R., & Rybicki, F. (2010). CT angiography: Current technology and clinical use. *Radiologic Clinics of North America*, 48, 213–235. https://www.ncbi.nlm.nih.gov/pmc/articles/PMC2901244/. [Accessed April 2021].

Vascular Conditions

Ulcers: Arterial, Venous, Neuropathic, Pressure

NICE. (2020). *CKS: Leg ulcer venous.* http://www.cks.nice.org.uk. [Accessed April 2021].

NICE. (2014). *CG179: Pressure ulcers: Prevention and management.* https://www.nice.org.uk/guidance/cg179. [Accessed April 2021]. Accessed.

NICE. (2015). *NG19: Diabetic foot problems: Prevention and management.* https://www.nice.org.uk/guidance/ng19. [Accessed April 2021].

Peripheral Arterial Disease: Acute Limb Ischaemia, Critical Limb Ischaemia and Intermittent Claudication

NICE. (2019). *CKS: Peripheral arterial disease.* https://cks.nice.org.uk/topics/peripheral-arterial-disease/. [Accessed April 2021].

Best Practice, B. M. J. (2020). *Peripheral arterial disease.* https://bestpractice.bmj.com/topics/en-gb/431. [Accessed April 2021].

AAA

NICE. (2020). *NG156: Abdominal aortic aneurysm: diagnosis and management.* https://www.nice.org.uk/guidance/ng156. [Accessed April 2021].

Best Practice, B. M. J. (2020). *Abdominal aortic aneurysm.* https://bestpractice.bmj.com/topics/en-gb/145. [Accessed April 2021].

NHS UK. (2021). *Abdominal aortic aneurysm screening.* https://www.nhs.uk/conditions/abdominal-aortic-aneurysm-screening/. [Accessed April 2021].

Aortic Dissection

Best Practice, B. M. J. (2018). *Aortic dissection.* https://bestpractice.bmj.com/topics/en-gb/445. [Accessed April 2021].

Patient.info. (2020). *Aortic dissection.* https://patient.info/doctor/aortic-dissection. [Accessed April 2021].

Varicose Veins

NICE. (2020). *CKS: Varicose veins.* https://cks.nice.org.uk/topics/varicose-veins/. [Accessed April 2021].

Best Practice, B. M. J. (2020). *Varicose veins.* https://bestpractice.bmj.com/topics/en-gb/630. [Accessed April 2021].

Buerger's Disease

Best Practice, B. M. J. (2018). *Buerger's disease.* https://bestpractice.bmj.com/topics/en-gb/1148?q=Buerger%27s%20disease&c=suggested. [Accessed April 2021].

Patient.info. (2016). *Buerger's disease.* https://patient.info/doctor/buergers-disease-pro. [Accessed April 2021].

Chronic Mesenteric Ischaemia

Best Practice, B. M. J. (2019). *Ischaemic bowel disease.* https://bestpractice.bmj.com/topics/en-gb/818. [Accessed April 2021].

Patient.info. (2019). *Bowel ischaemia.* https://patient.info/doctor/bowel-ischaemia. [Accessed April 2021].

Atherosclerosis

Patient.info. (2016). *Atherosclerosis.* https://patient.info/doctor/atherosclerosis. [Accessed April 2021].

Patient.info. (2014). *Prevention of cardiovascular disease.* https://patient.info/doctor/prevention-of-cardiovascular-disease. [Accessed April 2021].

Carotid Artery Stenosis

Best Practice, B. M. J. (2020). *Carotid artery stenosis.* https://bestpractice.bmj.com/topics/en-gb/1205. [Accessed April 2021].

Patient.info. (2016). *Carotid artery stenosis.* https://patient.info/doctor/carotid-artery-stenosis. [Accessed April 2021].

Deep Vein Thrombosis

Best Practice, B. M. J. (2020). *Deep vein thrombosis.* https://bestpractice.bmj.com/topics/en-gb/70. [Accessed April 2021].

NICE. (2020). *CKS: Deep vein thrombosis.* https://cks.nice.org.uk/topics/deep-vein-thrombosis/. [Accessed April 2021].

3

Cardiology and ECGs in an Hour

Alexander Royston, Oliver Arnold, Chiara Bucciarelli-Ducci and Viren Ahluwalia

BASIC ANATOMY AND KEY CONCEPTS

Surfaces of the Heart

- Anterior (or sternocostal): right ventricle (RV)
- Posterior (or base): left atrium (LA)
- Inferior (or diaphragmatic): left and right ventricles
- Right pulmonary: right atrium (RA)
- Left pulmonary: left ventricle (LV)

Conducting System (See Fig 3.1)

Coronary Vessels and Associated Territories
(See Table 3.1 and Fig 3.2)

Heart Sounds (See Table 3.2)

CARDIOLOGY CONDITIONS

Hypertension

Definition: ambulatory blood pressure monitoring (ABPM) of >135/85 mmHg **and** clinic blood pressure (CBP) of >140/90 mmHg. May be classified as:

- **Primary/essential hypertension** (HTN): no known cause

- **Secondary HTN** (rare): causes include intrinsic renal and renovascular disease, aortic coarctation, endocrine disease (hyperparathyroidism, phaeochromocytoma, Conn's syndrome, Cushing's disease), pre-eclampsia, oral contraceptive pill, drugs

Buzzwords:
- **Risk factors:** family history, age, male, obesity, ethnicity, chronic kidney disease (CKD)
- **Presentation:** usually asymptomatic
  - **Malignant hypertension:** retinal haemorrhage, visual disturbances, headache, dizziness, nausea and vomiting, chest pain and acute kidney injury (AKI)
- **Complications:** stroke risk, erectile dysfunction, hypertensive retinopathy, ischaemic heart disease (IHD) and congestive cardiac failure (CCF), CKD, osteoporosis (see Fig 3.3)

Investigations:
- **ABPM:** diagnostic
- **Risk stratification and end-organ damage:** blood glucose and HbA1c (diabetes mellitus (DM)), cholesterol, albumin-creatinine ratio, renal function, fundoscopy, electrocardiogram (ECG)
- **QRISK3:** an estimate of cardiovascular (CV) event risk over next 10 years

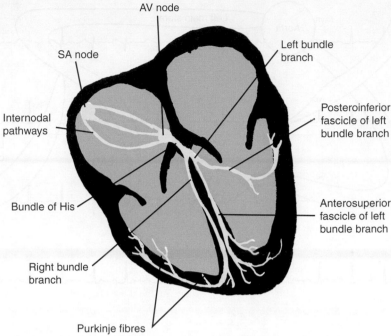

Fig 3.1 Conduction System of the Heart. (Adapted from Andreoli, Kinney & Packa, 1996; Illustrated by Dr Hollie Blaber.)

Management:
- Lifestyle modification to reduce CV risk
- Discuss medical treatment in people with a CBP of >140/90 mmHg if 10-year CV risk is >10% or signs of end-organ damage
- Offer medical treatment to all people with a CBP of >160/100 mmHg
- Targets:
  - CBP of 140/90 mmHg (<80 years), 150/90 mmHg (>80 years)
  - ABPM of 135/85 mmHg (<80 years), 145/85 mmHg (>80 years)
  - DM: 135/85 mmHg, but 130/80 mmHg if comorbid metabolic syndrome/albuminuria
- Antihypertensive choice (see Fig 3.4): drug choice and dose can be titrated relatively rapidly, as 50% of antihypertensive effect is seen after 1 week

Hyperlipidaemia

Definition:
- **Dyslipidaemia**: high levels of low-density lipoprotein cholesterol (LDL-C), low levels of high-density lipoprotein cholesterol (HDL-C), elevated

TABLE 3.1 Coronary Vessels and Associated Territories

Territory	Vessel	Leads
Inferior	Right coronary artery	II, III, aVF
Lateral	Left circumflex	I, aVL, V5–V6
Septal	Left anterior descending (septal branches)	V1–V2
Anterior	Left anterior descending	V3–V4
Anterolateral	Left main stem	I, aVL, V1–V6
Posterior	Right coronary artery	V7, V8, V9 (recip of V1–V3)

triglycerides (TG) and other qualitative lipid abnormalities
- **Hypercholesterolaemia**: high total cholesterol (TC), elevated LDL-C or non-HDL-C. Causes include:
  - **Primary common hypercholesterolaemia** (70% of cases): polygenic, with some inherited component, characterised by ↑LDL-C
  - **Familial hypercholesterolaemia** (FH): monogenic inheritance characterised by very high LDL-C (>7.5 mmol/L)

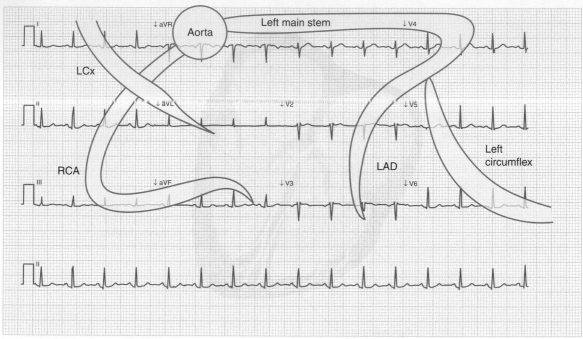

Fig 3.2 Coronary Vessels and Respective Territories. (Adapted from ECG Medical Training on Twitter, 2021; Illustrated by Dr Hollie Blaber.)

TABLE 3.2 Classification of Heart Sounds

Sound	Sounds like	Event/Details	Implication
S1	"lub"	Closure of atrioventricular valves M1 (mitral valve closure) slightly precedes T1 (tricuspid valve closure)	Normal If T1 is very delayed (split S1): suggestive of right bundle branch block
S2	"dub"	A2 (aortic valve closure) and P2 (pulmonary valve closure) A2 precedes P2	Normal Splitting is physiological during inspiration Wide and fixed split: atrial septal defect Wide and variable split: right bundle branch block, pulmonary stenosis, pulmonary hypertension, ventricular septal defect Soft A2: aortic stenosis Loud P2: pulmonary hypertension
S3	"lub-dub-ta"	Protodiastolic gallop Early diastolic, low pitch (not valvular in origin) L-sided: apex, lateral decubitus position R-sided: LLSE	Benign in youth/athletes >40 years of age suggests overload and/or dilated congestive cardiac failure
S4	"ta-lub-dub"	Presystolic/atrial gallop Requires atrial contraction. Absent in atrial fibrillation Immediately before S1, end of diastole Heard apex, left lateral decubitus, breath held	Failing or hypertrophic left ventricle: Systemic hypertension Severe aortic stenosis Hypertrophic cardiomyopathy

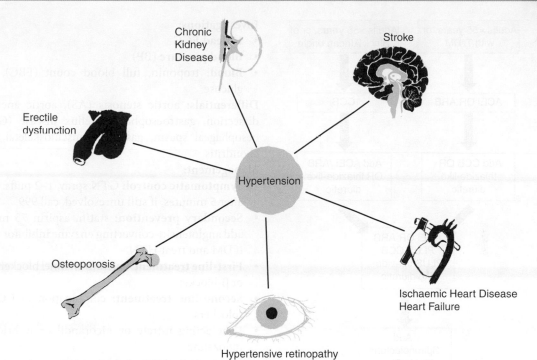

Fig 3.3 Complications of Hypertension. (Illustrated by Dr Hollie Blaber.)

- **Non-familial hypercholesterolaemia**: several genes interact with diet and other risk factors

Buzzwords:
- **Risk factors**: raised BMI, sedentary lifestyle, type 2 diabetes mellitus (T2DM), hypothyroidism, alcohol, family history of early-onset coronary heart disease (CHD) or dyslipidaemia in a first-degree relative (males <55 years, females <65 years), history of CV disease, consumption of saturated fats and trans-fatty acids
  - Secondary hypercholesterolaemia: cholestatic liver disease, Cushing's disease, pancreatitis, thiazides/steroids
- **Presentation**: usually asymptomatic until atherosclerosis is established, arcus cornealis (onset <45 years), xanthelasma (near the inner canthus of the eyelid), tuberous xanthomas (plaques on extensor surfaces of knees, elbow, knuckles; rare), pancreatitis
- **Complications:** major risk factor for atherosclerosis causing CHD, cerebrovascular disease (CVD) and peripheral arterial disease (PAD)

Investigations:
- **Lipid profile** (fasting if necessary): may be artificially deranged in acute illness/immediately post-myocardial infarction (MI). Measurements of TC, LDL-C (estimated or direct), HDL-C and TG
- **Thyroid function tests**: may show hypothyroidism
- Lipoprotein(a)

Differentials: obstructive liver disease, nephrotic syndrome, chronic renal insufficiency

Management:
- Identify familial causes (treat aggressively if found) and treat underlying secondary causes
- Lifestyle modifications: dietary changes, exercise and smoking cessation
- Pharmacological intervention. Aim for an LDL-C <4.0 mmol/L (ideally <3.0). TC:HDL ratio is best predictor of CV risk, aim for <4.5 (6 is high risk)
  - Statin therapy: if QRISK2 >10%, if IHD/peripheral vascular disease history or if DM. Intolerance is significant though often overdiagnosed. Rare but important side effects include myositis – measure CK, if ↑, then stop. Routinely measure liver function tests (LFTs) at 3 months
  - Ezetimibe: cholesterol-absorption inhibitor
  - Fibrates: PPARα antagonists (lower TG)
  - Proprotein convertase subtilisin/kexin type 9 (PCSK9) inhibitor
  - Niacin

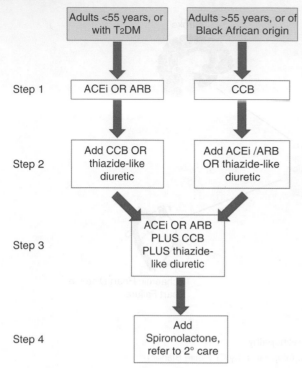

| Step 1 | ACEi OR ARB | CCB |

Adults <55 years, or with T2DM | Adults >55 years, or of Black African origin

Step 1 — ACEi OR ARB / CCB

Step 2 — Add CCB OR thiazide-like diuretic / Add ACEi /ARB OR thiazide-like diuretic

Step 3 — ACEi OR ARB PLUS CCB PLUS thiazide-like diuretic

Step 4 — Add Spironolactone, refer to 2° care

Fig 3.4 Treatment Steps for Hypertension. *ACEi,* Angiotensin-converting enzyme inhibitor; *ARB,* angiotension-receptor blocker; *CCB,* calcium-channel blocker; *T2DM,* type 2 diabetes mellitus (Adapted from National Institute of Health and Care Excellence (NICE). (2019). *NG136: Hypertension in adults: diagnosis and management.)*

Ischaemic Heart Disease (IHD)

Definition: an inability to adequately perfuse the myocardium, caused by atherosclerosis of epicardial branches of the coronary arteries (see Fig 3.5). Stable IHD is differentiated from acute coronary syndromes (ACS) (same disease process) by symptoms being manageable and not rapidly progressive. The term IHD is often used interchangeably with coronary artery disease (CAD).

Buzzwords:
- **Risk factors:**
  - **Modifiable:** HTN, DM, smoking, cholesterol, obesity
  - **Non-modifiable:** age, male, family history (MI <55 years), genetics (hyperlipidaemias)
- **Presentation:** Central crushing or tightness/'heaviness', can radiate to jaw/left arm, triggered by exertion (stable angina), relieved by rest/nitrates, exacerbated by anaemia and tachyarrhythmias

Investigations:
- **12-lead ECG**
- **Blood pressure** (BP)
- **Blood:** troponin, full blood count (FBC), lipids, glucose

Differentials: aortic stenosis (AS), aortic aneurysm/dissection, gastroesophageal reflux disease (GORD), oesophageal spasm, gastritis, musculoskeletal, costochondritis

Management:
- **Symptomatic control:** GTN spray, 1–2 puffs. Repeat after 5 minutes, if still unresolved, call 999.
- **Secondary prevention:** statin, aspirin 75 mg, also add angiotensin-converting enzyme inhibitor (ACEi) if DM and treat HTN
- **First-line treatment:** calcium channel blocker (CCB) or β-blockers
- **Second-line treatment:** combination of CCB + β-blockers
- Long-acting nitrate or nicorandil or ivabridine or ranozaline
- If persistent symptoms are unable to be medically managed, then consider percutaneous coronary intervention (PCI)/coronary artery bypass graft (CABG)

Acute Coronary Syndromes (ACS)

Definition: myocardial ischaemia commonly caused by plaque rupture and thrombosis. Three distinct syndromes:
- **ST-elevation myocardial infarction** (STEMI): infarction with ST elevation on ECG
- **Non ST-elevation myocardial infarction** (NSTEMI): infarction (cell death) without ST elevation on ECG
- **Unstable angina:** ischaemia causing chest pain at rest or minimal exertion OR in a crescendo-like fashion

Buzzwords:
- **Risk factors:** smoking, DM, obesity, HTN, hyperlipidaemia
- **Presentation:** central, crushing chest pain; dyspnoea; nausea; sweating; syncope
  - Silent MIs present without pain and are more common in diabetic patients/older women

Investigations:
- **12-lead ECG**
  - **STEMI** (see Figs 3.6A & 3.7): ST elevation (elevation by one small square (1 mV) in limb leads or two small squares (2 mV) in precordial leads) in specific territories or a new left bundle branch

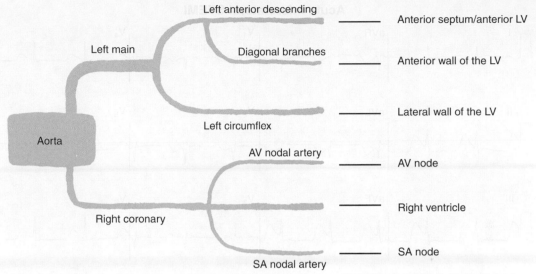

Fig 3.5 Schematic of the Coronary Arteries. (Adapted from Yartsev, 2013; Illustrated by Dr Hollie Blaber.)

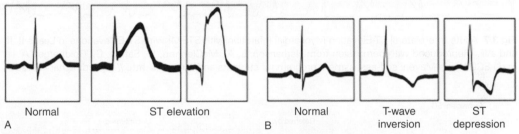

Fig 3.6 (A) ST elevation, (B) T-wave inversion (TWI) and ST depression. (Hanson, M. A., Fareed, M. T., Argenio, S. L., Agunwamba, A. O., & Hanson, T. R. (2013) Coronary artery disease, *Primary Care: Clinics in Office Practice, 40*(1), 1-16, Used with permission of Mayo Foundation for Medical Education and Research, all rights reserved.)

block (LBBB). Reciprocal changes are seen (e.g., ST elevation in anterior leads associated with ST depression in posterior leads)

- **NSTEMI** (see Figs 3.6B & 3.8): ST depression, T-wave inversion, poor R-wave progression
- **Unstable angina:** often a normal ECG tracing
- **Serial troponins**: cardiac blood biomarker released with myocardial necrosis (also raised in renal failure)
  - **STEMI/NSTEMI:** raised
  - **Unstable angina:** not raised
- **Coronary angiography** (if high risk for CV event mortality)

Differentials: musculoskeletal chest pain, costochondritis, AS, acute pericarditis, **acute myocarditis, aortic dissection,** anxiety disorders, gastritis, duodenitis, GORD, oesophagitis/spasm

Management: Unstable angina/NSTEMI (acute management)
- ABCDE
- Analgesia (opiates)
- Nitrates (GTN)
- Aspirin 300 mg, fondaparinux 2.5 mg, ticagrelor 180 mg/clopidogrel 300 mg
- PCI/CABG
  - Dependent on the GRACE score (mortality prediction post-MI)

Management: STEMI (acute management)
- ABCDE
- Analgesia (opiates)
- Nitrates (GTN)
- Aspirin 300 mg, ticagrelor 180 mg/clopidogrel 300 mg

Acute Inferolateral STEMI

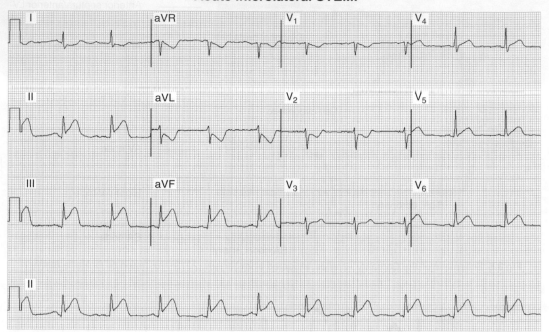

Fig 3.7 Acute Inferolateral ST-Elevation Myocardial Infarction with STEMI with ST Eelevations in Leads II, III and aVF. (Reproduced with permission from Nathanson, L. A., McClennen, S., Safran, C., Goldberger, A. L., (n.d.) ECG Wave-Maven: self-assessment program for students and clinicians. http://ecg.bidmc.harvard.edu.)

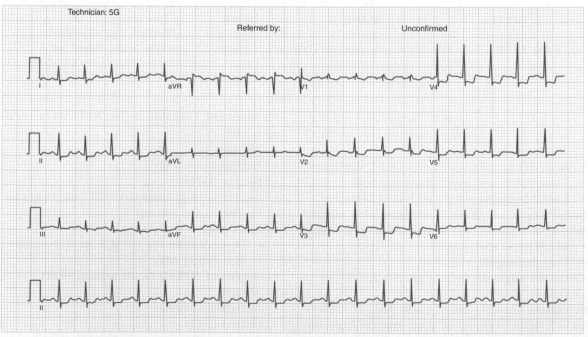

Fig 3.8 Non-ST-Elevation Myocardial Infarction with ST Depression in Leads V2 to V6. (With permission from Fryearson, J., & Adamson, D. L. (2014). *Best practice & research clinical obstetrics & gynaecology* (Fig. 2). Elsevier. Copyright © 2014 Published by Elsevier Ltd.)

- Primary PCI/thrombolysis (depending on facilities and access to primary PCI service)

Long-term management

- Drug treatment: ACEi, b-Blocker, statin, dual-antiplatelet therapy
- Primary care monitoring of CV risk factors, cardiac rehabilitation

Heart Failure

Definition: insufficient cardiac output to meet the body's needs. This condition is a clinical state triggered by many potential causes and not a diagnosis in its own right. Common causes include MI, IHD, arrythmias, valvular dysfunction, cardiomyopathies and infection.

Classifications:

- Left ventricular failure (LVF): causes include IHD, MI
- Right ventricular failure (RVF): causes include chronic lung disease, pulmonary stenosis, LVF

Buzzwords:

- **Risk factors:** smoking, obesity, DM, hypercholesterolaemia
- **Presentation:**
  - LVF: dyspnoea (see Table 3.3), orthopnoea, paroxysmal nocturnal dyspnoea (PND), low exercise tolerance (excess fluid in lungs)
  - RVF: peripheral oedema (excess fluid around body)
  - Diagnosis of CCF is made using the Framingham criteria: two major criteria or one major + two minor (see Table 3.4)

Investigations:

- **Chest x-ray (CXR): (ABCDEF)** **A**lveolar oedema, **B** lines, **C**ardiomegaly, **D**ilated upper vessels, **E**ffusions, **F**luid in fissure (see Fig 3.9)
- **ECG:** ischaemia, arrhythmias, hypertrophy
- **Echocardiogram:** ventricular dysfunction, valvular disease
- **Blood:** brain natriuretic peptide (BNP) (normal value can reliably rule out heart failure), U&Es, FBC, LFTs, thyroid function tests (TFTs)

Differentials: community-acquired pneumonia (CAP) (developing oxygen requirement, particularly if in 'cold sepsis' with indeterminate CXR signs), acute respiratory distress syndrome (ARDS) (sudden onset provoked respiratory distress with infiltrates on CXR)

Management: Acute heart failure

- ABCDE, treat reversible causes (e.g., arrhythmias, sepsis)

TABLE 3.3   New York Heart Association Categories

New York Heart Association Category	Description
I	No limitation of physical activity
II	Slight limitation. Relieved by rest
III	Less than ordinary activity brings on symptoms, comfortable at rest
IV	Unable to carry out activities. Rest symptoms

TABLE 3.4   Framingham Criteria

Major	Minor
Paroxysmal nocturnal dyspnoea	Bilateral ankle oedema
Positive abdominojugular reflux	Shortness of breath on exertion
Neck vein distension	HR >120 bpm
S3	Nocturnal cough
Basal crepitations	Hepatomegaly
Cardiomegaly	Pleural effusion
Active pulmonary oedema	30% reduction vital capacity
Elevated central venous pressure (>16 cmH$_2$O)	
Weight loss >4.5 kg in 5 days 2° to Rx	

- IV diuretics (monitor renal function, weight loss, oxygen requirement)
- Non-invasive ventilation may be indicated

Management: Chronic heart failure:

- Lifestyle advice: reduce CV risk factors (e.g., smoking, weight loss, salt intake)
- Vaccines: annual influenza, one-off pneumococcal
- Treat reversible causes (arrhythmias, valvular disease)
- Medical:
  - First line: diuretics, ACEi, β-blocker
  - Second line: consider spironolactone if symptoms uncontrolled

Heart Failure with Preserved Ejection Fraction (HFpEF)

Definition: Heart pumps normally but is too stiff to fill properly (aka 'diastolic heart failure'), resulting

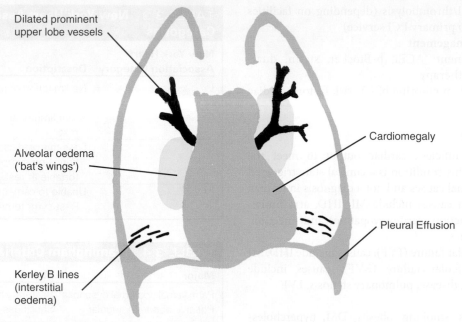

Dilated prominent upper lobe vessels

Cardiomegaly

Alveolar oedema ('bat's wings')

Pleural Effusion

Kerley B lines (interstitial oedema)

Fig 3.9 Cardinal Signs of Heart Failure Seen on Chest X-ray. (Adapted from Wilkinson et al., 2017a, 2017b, 2017c, 2017d, 2017e; Illustrated by Dr Hollie Blaber.)

in clinical signs of heart failure with normal/near-normal left ventricular function (LVEF >50% (normally 60% in good health)). This condition has a complex pathophysiology featuring impaired ventricular relaxation, decreased LV compliance and increased LV stiffness.

Buzzwords:
- **Risk factors**: >70 years, female, HTN, obesity, CKD, DM, CAD, AF
- **Presentation**: exertional dyspnoea, also orthopnoea/PND, fatigue, fluid retention, diastolic impairment (narrowed pulse pressure)

Investigations:
- **Bloods:** BNP – in ambulatory setting (sensitivity>specificity), U&Es, LFTs, TFTs, FBC
- **Echocardiogram**: Normal ejection fraction with impaired diastolic function (increased left atrial size)

Differentials: anaemia, CKD, AF, CAD, valvular heart disease, pulmonary hypertension, restrictive cardiomyopathies, amyloidosis, constrictive pericarditis

Management:
- Nonacute: risk factor management – guideline-directed treatment of HTN and hyperlipidaemia

- Acute, with overload: treat overload with diuretics
- Acute, with hypertension: consider use of β-blockers (carvedilol), ACEi
- CAD: offer revascularisation
- Multidisciplinary team (MDT) approach: improve exercise capacity and physical functioning
- Avoid: spironolactone, ARBs, nitrates, digoxin (in >65 s)

Heart Failure with Reduced Ejection Fraction (HFrEF)

Definition: left ventricular ejection fraction (LVEF) is ≤40%, accompanied by clinical heart failure with progressive left ventricular dilatation, adverse cardiac remodelling (upregulation of the RAAS system) and fluid retention.

Buzzwords:
- **Risk factors:** Same as HFpEF, less common in females and with atrial fibrillation (AF)
- **Presentation:**
  - Symptoms (very similar to HFpEF): dyspnoea, orthopnoea/PND, reduced exercise tolerance, fatigue, peripheral oedema (ankles)
  - Signs: S3 (gallop rhythm), elevated jugular venous pressure (JVP), positive abdominojugular reflex, displaced apex beat

Investigations:

- **CXR: ABCDEF of heart failure** (**A**lveolar oedema, **B** lines, **C**ardiomegaly, **D**ilated upper vessels, **E**ffusions, **F**luid in fissures - See Fig 3.9)
- **Echocardiogram**: Ejection fraction (EF) <40%
- **Blood**: BNP, U&Es, LFTs, TFTs, FBC

Differentials: any cardiopulmonary condition: COPD, pneumonia; other causes of volume overload: nephrotic syndrome, anaemia, hypothyroidism, obesity and deconditioning, HFpEF

Management:

- ACEi/ARB and β-blocker (carvedilol, bisoprolol). Titrate doses up according to side effects and with U&Es monitoring
- Spironolactone
- Specialist use: ivabradine, sacubitril valsartan, hydralazine, digoxin

Vasovagal Syncope

Definition: A transient loss of consciousness (TLoC) due to neural reflex vasodilation and/or bradycardia, leading to a fall in the systemic arterial pressure and cerebral hypoperfusion.

Buzzwords:

- **Risk factors:** dehydration, exposure to triggers
- **Presentation:** vasovagal **3 P's**
  - Posture: prolonged standing or similar episodes that have been prevented by lying down
  - Provoking factors: pain, medical procedures
  - Prodromal symptoms: sweating or feeling warm/hot before TLoC
  - Other features: TLOC followed by a rapid, spontaneous recovery; brief seizure-like activity (but NOT suggestive of epilepsy)

Investigations: (A detailed history and witness account required!)

- **Lying-standing BP:** normal (rule out orthostatic hypotension)
- **ECG:** exclude arrythmias
- **Blood** (identify exacerbating factors): ↓ Hb, CBG, βHCG
- **Carotid sinus massage** if >40 years: asystole ventricular pause >3 s and/or a fall in systolic BP of >50 mmHg = carotid sinus hypersensitivity (CSH). Caution if Hx of CVA/carotid stenosis
- **Echocardiogram:** exclude structural heart disease

- ***Tilt-table test:** 65% sensitive, >90% specific – response: induction of reflex hypotension (<60 mmHg systolic blood pressure)/bradycardia
- **Insertable loop recorder**: Exclude paroxysmal arrhythmias

Differentials: seizure, orthostatic hypotension, arrhythmias, valvular disease (e.g., aortic stenosis)

Management:

1. Patient education (avoid triggers/volume depletion)
2. Strategies for reducing long-term syncope recurrence include:
   - Physical techniques to improve orthostatic tolerance
   - Pharmacological interventions to prevent depletion of intravascular volume and/or enhance arterial and venous tone
   - Cardiac pacing to avert bradycardia or refractory CSH

Infective Endocarditis

Definition: A serious infection of the endocardium including the heart valves. Common causative organisms include *Streptococcus viridans*, *Staphylococcus aureus*, Enterococci, *Coxiella burnetti* and HACEK organisms. The Duke criteria (see Table 3.5) are used to guide diagnosis:

- **Definite diagnosis**: ×2 major, or ×1 major and ×3 minor, or ×5 minor.
- **Possible diagnosis**: ×1 major + ×1 minor or ×3 minor

Buzzwords:

- **Risk factors:**
  - **Normal valves:** intravenous drug use (IVDU), skin breeches, immunosuppression, DM, renal failure
  - **Abnormal valves:** rheumatic fever, valvular disease, coarctation, patent ductus arteriosus, ventricular septal defect, prosthetic valve
- **Presentation:** fever with new murmur, chills, night sweats, arthralgia, malaise, weight loss, clubbing, Janeway lesions, splinter haemorrhages, Osler nodes, Roth spots
- **Complications:** systemic septic emboli, stroke, infectious (mycotic) aneurysms, splenic infarct, myo-pericarditis, CCF, arrythmias, AKI

Investigations:

- **Blood cultures:** ×3 separate sets obtained before antibiotics to identify characteristic organisms

TABLE 3.5   Duke Criteria

Major Criteria	Minor Criteria
1. Blood cultures positive for infective endocarditis 2. Evidence of endocardial involvement (echocardiogram detects a vegetation, abscess, or new partial dehiscence of proethetic valve; new valvular regurgitation)	1. Predisposing factor (intravenous drug use or predisposing heart condition: murmur/echo not meeting major criterion) 2. Temperature >38°C 3. Vascular phenomena: major arterial emboli, septic emboli, pulmonary infarcts, mycotic aneurysm, intracranial haemorrhage, conjunctival haemorrhage, and painless skin lesions (Janeway's lesions) 4. Immunologic phenomena: glomerulonephritis, painful nodes (Osler's nodes), retinal haemorrhages with small, clear centres (Roth's spots) and positive RhF 5. Microbiologic evidence: positive blood cultures not meeting a major criterion or serologic evidence of an active infection with an organism known to cause infective endocarditis

- **Blood:** FBC (anaemia, leucocytosis), CRP/ESR elevated, U&Es, rheumatoid factor
- **Urinalysis:** RBC casts, WBC casts, proteinuria
- **Echocardiogram:** may show vegetations. First line: transthoracic echocardiogram (TTE); gold standard: transoesophageal echocardiogram (TOE) is diagnostic

Differentials: sepsis, TB, rheumatic fever, atrial myxoma, Libman-Sacks endocarditis

Management:
- IV antibiotics for 4–6 weeks
  - Native valve: amoxicillin and gentamicin
  - Prosthetic valve: vancomycin, rifampicin and gentamicin
- Surgery to repair valve if: severe valvular incompetence, aortic abscess, treatment resistance, recurrent emboli
- Prophylactic treatment for high-risk patients is no longer recommended.

Myocarditis

Definition: inflammation of the myocardium (acute or chronic) resulting in a variety of presentations, including an incidental ECG finding to fulminant cardiac failure, arrhythmias and sudden cardiac death. Most commonly caused by viral infection but may also be bacterial, protozoal (Chagas), fungal, autoimmune or due to toxic exposure.

Buzzwords:
- **Risk factors:** infection (non-HIV viral/bacterial), HIV, smallpox vaccination, autoimmune/immune-mediated diseases
- **Presentation:** chest pain, palpitations, heart failure

Investigations:
- **Bloods:** ↑CRP, ↑ESR (both often also raised in pericarditis), ↑↑ troponin
- **ECG:** abnormal, but not specific/sensitive. ST elevation, T wave inversion, QT prolongation
- **Echocardiogram:** rule out regional wall abnormalities, dilated cardiomyopathies and valvular dysfunction
- **CMRI:** evidence of myocardial inflammation/oedema and fibrosis (late gadolinium enhancement)
- **Endomyocardial biopsy** (EMB): used very infrequently and only in specialist centres if there is doubt about aetiology

Differentials: pericarditis, MI, Chagas disease, various cardiomyopathies (including Takotsubo cardiomyopathy)

Management:
1. Treat underlying cause, arrhythmias and heart failure
2. Cardiopulmonary assist devices if haemodynamically unstable
3. Avoid exercise and exertion until recovery

4. Immunomodulatory/immunosuppressive therapies only if indicated by EMB

Prognosis: resolves in 2–4 weeks in 50% of cases, 25% progress to acute ventricular dysfunction

Pericarditis

Definition: inflammation of the pericardium
Buzzwords:

- **Risk factors:** viral infection (Coxsackie), TB, trauma, post MI (2–6 weeks: Dressler's syndrome), connective tissue disease, vasculitides, malignancy, uraemia, drugs
- **Presentation:** pleuritic chest pain relieved when leaning forward, pericardial rub, ±pericardial effusion, nonproductive cough

Investigations:

- **ECG** (see Fig 3.10): widespread saddle-shaped ST elevation, PR depression
- **Echocardiogram:** effusion
- **CMRI:** evidence of pericardial inflammation/oedema and fibrosis (late gadolinium enhancement), effusion

Differentials: acute gastritis, angina, MI, oesophageal spasm

Management:

1. Treat underlying cause
2. NSAIDs or aspirin + gastroprotection
3. Colchicine

Pericardial Effusion

Definition: Accumulation of fluid in the pericardial sac (normally >50 mL)
Buzzwords:

- **Risk factors:** pericarditis, myocardial rupture, malignancy, idiopathic
- **Presentation:** dyspnoea, elevated JVP (prominent x descent), bronchial breathing at left base ± tamponade

Investigations:

- **CXR:** enlarged, globular heart (and clear lungs)
- **ECG:** low-voltage QRS complexes, alternating QRS amplitude (electrical alternans)
- **Echocardiogram:** echo-free zone around heart

Management:

1. Assess haemodynamic compromise, treat as cardiac tamponade if present
2. Treat cause (pericarditis: aspirin/NSAIDs, colchicine, etc.)

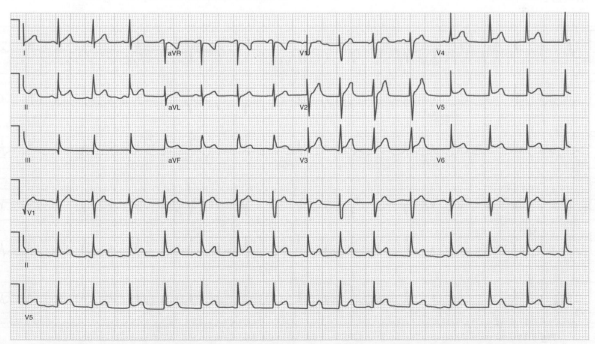

Fig 3.10 Widespread ST Elevation in Pericarditis. (With permission from Dudzinski, D. M., Mak, G. S., & Hung, J. W. (2012). *Current problems in cardiology* (Fig. 2). Elsevier. Copyright © 2012 Published by Elsevier Inc.)

3. Pericardiocentesis may be diagnostic (purulent/tuberculous: culture, ZN stain, cytology) or therapeutic (tamponade)

Cardiac Tamponade

Definition: a life-threatening compression of the heart from pericardial accumulation of fluid, pus, blood, clots or gas. Effusion raises the intrapericardial pressure, reducing ventricular filling and decreasing cardiac output, which can rapidly lead to cardiac arrest. Causes include inflammation, trauma, rupture of the heart or aortic dissection.

Buzzwords:

- **Risk factors:** pericarditis, TB, iatrogenic (PCI, invasive procedure related, postcardiac surgery), trauma, neoplasm
- **Presentation:** Beck's triad (↑ JVP, muffled heart sounds, hypotension), electrical alternans (variable QRS complex size), tachycardia, pulsus paradoxus (inspiratory decrease in systolic arterial pressure of 10 mmHg during normal breathing), Kussmaul's sign (paradoxical rise in JVP on inspiration)

Investigations:

- **ECG (see Fig 3.11):** low voltage, electrical alternans, signs of pericarditis

- **Echocardiogram:** echo-free zone around heart, diastolic collapse of the RA and RV, swinging of heart

Differentials: PE, MI, Type A aortic dissection, tension pneumothorax

Management:

1. ABCDE in acute setting
2. Urgent pericardiocentesis (under fluoroscopic/echocardiographic guidance)

VALVULAR DISEASE

- A group of conditions that generally produce symptoms of right or left-sided heart failure (except aortic stenosis (AS)), depending on which valve is affected
- Can be acute or chronic and stenotic or regurgitant
- On examination, a murmur may be heard, and echocardiography is generally diagnostic

Murmurs

Definition: Sound created by turbulent blood flow, often across a valve. Detectable by auscultation of the precordium.

Valve locations (see Fig 3.12): mnemonic – **All Patients Take Medicine** (**A**ortic, **P**ulmonic, **T**ricuspid, **M**itral)

Character of heart sounds see Fig 3.13:

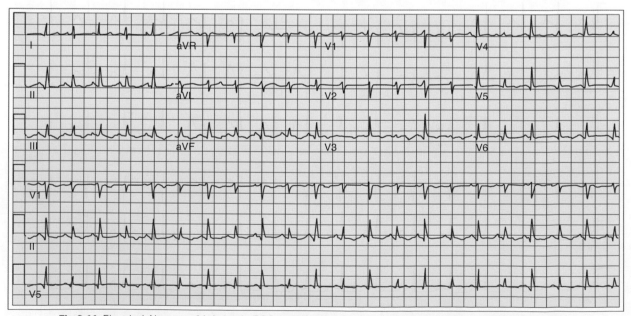

Fig 3.11 Electrical Alternans (Variation in QRS Amplitude) in Cardiac Tamponade. (With permission from Lewinter, M. M., & Imazio, M. (2019). Pericardial diseases (Fig. 83.4, Chapter 83). In *Braunwald's heart disease: A textbook of cardiovascular medicine, 2-volume set.* Elsevier. Copyright © 2019 Elsevier Inc. All rights reserved.)

AUSCULTATING HEART VALVE SOUNDS

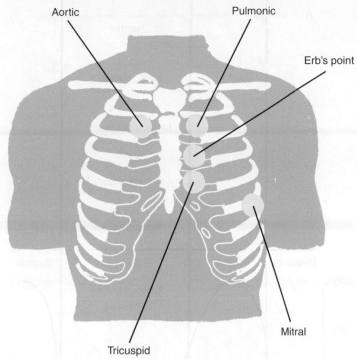

Fig 3.12 Location of Heart Sounds. (Adapted with permission from Zerwekh, Claborn & Miller, 2007; Illustrated by Dr Hollie Blaber.)

Radiation:
- AS: radiates to carotids
- Mitral regurgitation (MR): radiates to axilla

Accentuating manoeuvres:
- Expiration: left-sided murmurs
- Leans forward: aortic regurgitation (AR)
- Left lateral position: mitral stenosis (MS)

Aortic Stenosis

Definition:
- **Aortic sclerosis:** thickening of the valve leaflets without a functional narrowing of the aortic valve opening. Often precedes AS, although can progress to AR instead
- **Aortic stenosis:** a narrowing of the aortic valve opening. This is a very common condition and causes include DM, HTN, smoking and dyslipidaemia (same as atherosclerosis!).

Buzzwords:
- **Risk factors:** degenerative senile calcification (age >55 years), congenital (age <55 years), e.g., bicuspid valve, rheumatic heart disease (RHD)

Presentation:
- Aortic sclerosis: asymptomatic, ESM **does not radiate** to carotids
- AS: mnemonic **SAD** – Syncope, Angina, Dyspnoea
- **Signs:** systolic ejection murmur, radiates to carotids, ejection click, split S2, slow-rising pulse, narrow pulse pressure, aortic thrill, signs of LVF (lung crepitations)

Investigations:
- *Echocardiogram: leaflet thickening, Doppler to assess pressure gradient (>40 mmHg indicates a need for surgery), bicuspid morphology
- **ECG:** left ventricular hypertrophy, left axis deviation, often with secondary repolarization abnormalities, can cause AF
- **CXR:** left ventricular border and apex rounding, normal cardiac size
- **CMRI:** left ventricular hypertrophy, interstitial myocardial fibrosis, reduced aortic valve with increased velocity, aortic valve morphology

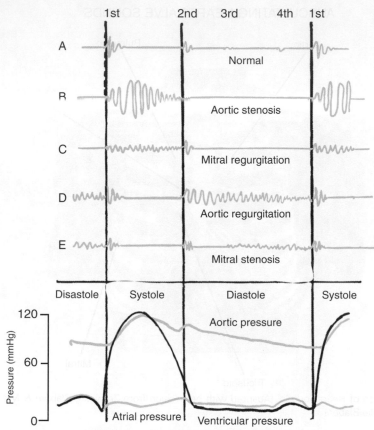

Fig 3.13 Auscultogram. (Copyright Dr Ari Horton.)

Differentials: aortic sclerosis, Williams syndrome, subacute bacterial endocarditis, hypertrophic obstructive cardiomyopathy (HOCM)

Management:

- Serial examinations and monitoring, avoid heavy exertion
- Medical approach controversial: little evidence for statins/ACEi, otherwise treat for atherosclerosis risk factors
- Surgical: surgical aortic valve replacement (AVR) (definitive: perform early), balloon valvuloplasty (not definitive), transcatheter aortic valve implantation (TAVI) (lower risk and useful in patients who are not suitable for surgery)

Aortic Regurgitation (AR)

Definition: leakage of blood during diastole from the aorta back into the LV due to poor leaflet apposition. AR causes progressive LV dilatation with resultant systolic dysfunction. Patients may present acutely or remain asymptomatic for decades before experiencing irreversible myocardial damage.

Buzzwords:

- **Risk factors**: RHD, intrinsic/congenital valve disease, IE, Type A aortic root dissection, autoimmune/connective tissue disease
- **Presentation**:
  - **Acute AR**: rapid-onset, disabling dyspnoea/pulmonary oedema
  - **Chronic AR**: long-latency exertional dyspnoea. Sometimes with symptoms of heart failure, including orthopnoea/PND
  - **Signs:** early decrescendo diastolic murmur (sitting forward), collapsing pulse, wide pulse pressure, Corrigan's sign (carotid pulsation), De Musset's (head nodding), Quincke's (capillary pulsation in nail beds), Traube's (pistol-shot sound over femorals)

Investigations:

- ***Echocardiogram:** valve pathology, jet analysis, LV function, aortic root assessment
- **ECG:** left ventricular hypertrophy
- **CXR:** cardiomegaly
- **CT aortogram:** if high suspicion of a Type A dissection (particularly if associated with intense chest pain)
- **CMRI:** valve pathology, jet analysis, LV function, aortic root assessment, aortic regurgitant fraction

Differentials: MR, hyperdynamic circulation (thyrotoxicosis, severe anaemia)

Management:

- Serial examinations and monitoring
- Medical approach: vasodilators/inotropes (uncertain merits, temporising pre-surgery)
- Surgical: surgical AVR (definitive: perform at symptom onset or with LV function deterioration) ± aortic replacement surgery

Mitral Regurgitation (MR)

Definition: incomplete mitral valve closure causing leakage back into the LA with contraction of the LV. Causes include:

- Primary (organic) MR: abnormalities of the mitral valve apparatus
- Secondary (functional and ischaemic) MR: LV disease and remodelling (e.g., MI)

Buzzwords:

- **Risk factors**: degenerative MR, papillary muscle/chordae rupture in acute MI, infective endocarditis or trauma
- **Presentation**:
  - **Acute:** caused by rupture, characterised by tachycardia, acute dyspnoea/pulmonary oedema, CCF
  - **Chronic** (trivial in the healthy): gradually decompensating heart failure, decreased exercise tolerance/dyspnoea
  - **Signs:** pansystolic murmur, high-pitched and loudest at the apex (radiating to axilla), displaced apex beat

Investigations:

- ***Echocardiogram:** assess presence, grade (severity), mechanism. Defined by a regurgitant jet into the LA, quantified using Doppler (TOE is best)
- **ECG:** signs of left ventricular and left atrial hypertrophy (broad P wave). AF is common, Q waves if ischaemic

- **CXR:**
  - Acute: pulmonary oedema
  - Chronic: cardiomegaly
- **CMRI:** if echocardiography suboptimal
- **Coronary angiography:** to exclude ischaemia

Differentials: calcified AS, TR, ventricular septal defect (paediatric)

Management:

- Serial examinations and monitoring for chronic disease
- Optimise risk factors: statins, treat HTN, DM, AF (rate control and anti-coagulation)
- Medical (acute): nitrates, diuretics, sodium nitroprusside, positive inotropic agents and intra-aortic balloon pump
- Medical (chronic): drugs to treat afterload for symptomatic relief (ACEis, or β-blocker (carvedilol), diuretics)
- Surgical: valve replacement or repair. Urgent if acute presentation. Indications: severe symptomatic MR with HF, severe asymptomatic MR but with diastolic dysfunction: ↓ EF

Mitral Stenosis (MS)

Definition: Narrowing of the mitral valve orifice, almost exclusively caused by rheumatic valvulitis (rare in the West due to the eradication of RHD), producing a fusion and thickening of valve leaflets. MS results in decreased left ventricular filling, which increases the left atrial pressure and leads to heart failure.

Buzzwords:

- **Risk factors**: RHD, age and other CV RFs, HTN, AS, CKD, may be associated with other heart valve lesions (TR)
- **Presentation**:
  - **Chronic**: gradual appearance over years, shortness of breath on exertion, embolic events (cerebral), pAF becoming chronic, hoarseness (recurrent laryngeal nerve palsy), triggers (e.g., emotional stress, sexual intercourse, infection)
  - **Signs:** low-volume pulse; low-pitched, mid-late diastolic murmur at non-displaced apex; loud S1; opening snap; mitral facies with intermittent malar flushes; jugular distension; RV heave ± signs of pulmonary hypertension

Investigations:

- **Echocardiogram (TTE):** measures the size of valves (<1 cm = severe) and mean transvalvular gradient.

Also pulmonary arterial pressure, associated MR and left atrial size

- **ECG**: AF is common. RAD with widened and notched (bifid) P wave if in sinus rhythm (LA dilation: P-mitrale)
- **Stress testing**: exercise echocardiography (or dobutamine if exercise not feasible)

Differentials: left atrial myxoma, infective endocarditis

Management:
- Serial testing
- Medical: diuretics transiently ameliorate dyspnoea. Digoxin, β-blocker or rate-regulating CCBs can improve exercise tolerance. If AF, needs anticoagulation
- Surgical: percutaneous mitral balloon commissurotomy (PMC) is mainstay, valve replacement for degenerative MS

Tricuspid Stenosis (TS)

Definition: Narrowing of the tricuspid orifice due to thickening and sclerosis of valve leaflets. This condition is commonly associated with both TR and left-sided valvular lesions (MS) that dominate the presentation. This is less commonly seen due to falls in cases of RHD.

Buzzwords:
- **Risk factors**: Hx of RHD, TR
- **Presentation**: low-output symptoms of fatigue, anorexia, wasting, peripheral cyanosis and cold skin. Increased venous pressure results in the symptoms of right heart failure
  - **Signs**: low-intensity diastolic murmur at left sternal border that increases with inspiration, preceded by a subtle opening snap (often accompanied by TR producing paradoxical septal motion (PSM) in same location), oedema, presystolic jugular distension, systemic venous congestion (hepatic distension end pulsation, ascites: severe compared to the degree of dyspnoea)

Investigations:
- **Echocardiogram (TTE)**: tricuspid leaflets are thickened
- **ECG**: tall peaked P waves (right atrial/biatrial hypertrophy); atrial fibrillation/flutter common
- **CXR**: enlarged cardiac silhouette with right (and commonly left) atrial enlargement

Differentials: congenital tricuspid atresia, tumours in the RA, carcinoid syndrome (endomyocardial fibrosis)

Management:
- Treat any underlying conditions (e.g., IE) and associated arrythmias
- Medical: diuretics may reduce oedema but have limited efficacy
- Surgical: conservative surgery or valve replacement preferred over PMC, performed with interventions for other valves

Tricuspid Regurgitation (TR)

Definition: retrograde flow through tricuspid valve, usually during systole. This may be caused by:
- Primary: abnormal valve morphology
- Secondary: Tricuspid annular dilation occurs due to left-sided cardiac disease but with normal valve morphology

Buzzwords:
- **Risk factors** (if primary): IE, history of RHD, carcinoid, myxomatous disease
- **Presentation:** well tolerated (often an incidental finding on TTE), fatigue and effort intolerance, dyspnoea, palpitations, abdominal distension, early satiety, dyspepsia or indigestion
  - **Signs:** high-pitched pansystolic murmur along the left sternal border, increasing with inspiration (Carvallo's sign); systolic jugular vein expansion ('v' wave); pulsatile, enlarged liver; hepatojugular reflux exacerbated on exercise

Investigations:
- ***Echocardiogram (TTE)**: assess for structural abnormalities of the valve to distinguish between primary and secondary.
- **ECG**: may show tall, peaked P waves (right atrial/biatrial hypertrophy); incomplete right bundle branch block (RBBB) and AF common
- **CXR**: cardiomegaly
- **Blood**: FBC, LFTs, U&Es – assess for anaemia/thrombocytopaenia, liver congestion and renal abnormalities
- **CMRI** and **coronary angiography**

Differentials: MR, Ebstein's anomaly, cor pulmonale

Management:
- Do not treat mild TR, treat the underlying cause (e.g., IE) and any resulting arrythmias
- Medical: diuretics to reduce congestion, ACEi, digoxin
- Surgical: tricuspid annuloplasty, considered at time of left-sided valve replacement

ECG BASICS

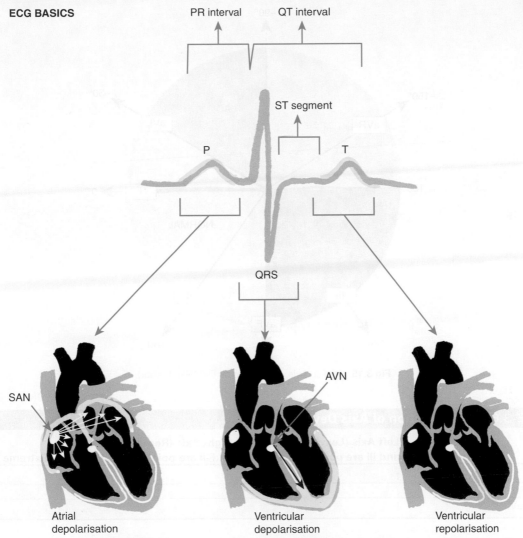

PR interval   QT interval

ST segment

P   T

QRS

SAN

AVN

Atrial depolarisation   Ventricular depolarisation   Ventricular repolarisation

Fig 3.14 Component Parts of an ECG. (Illustrated by Dr Hollie Blaber).

ECGs

ECG BASICS

See Table 3.1 and Fig 3.2 for the lead territories and Fig 3.14 for the components of an ECG.

Rate:

Calculated by:

• 300/number of large squares between R waves (each large square is 0.2 seconds)

• Number of R waves × 6 (ECG sheet is 10 seconds long)

Rhythm:

• Are QRS complexes regular/regularly irregular/irregularly irregular?

Axis:

• The normal axis of the heart is between –30º and +90º (see Fig 3.15)

• Axis deviation is suggestive of an underlying pathology

• There are many methods to assess axis deviation, with the simplest being to look at leads I, II and III/aVF and decide if the QRS complex is mostly positive or negative (see Table 3.6).

P Waves:

Represents atrial depolarisation:

• Are they present? (or flutter/fibrillation/no activity)

• Are they normal? (e.g., atrial ectopic)

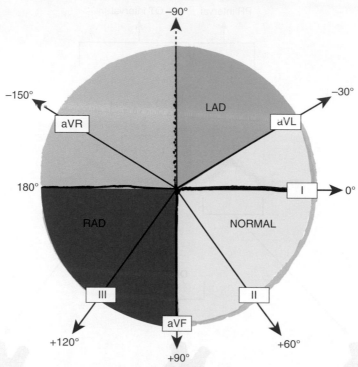

Fig 3.15 Cardiac Axis. (Illustrated by Dr Hollie Blaber).

TABLE 3.6	**Interpretation of Axis Deviation**			
	Normal Axis	**Left Axis (Leaving – Leads I and III are pointing away)**	**Right Axis (Reaching – Leads I and III are pointing towards)**	**Extreme Axis**
Lead I	↑	↑	↓	↓
Lead II	↑	↓	↑	↓
Lead III/aVF	↑	↓	↑	↓

- Are they each associated with a QRS complex? (think of heart blocks)

PR Interval:

Normal interval is 120–200 ms (3–5 small squares)

- Short (<120 ms): consider pre-excitation (e.g., Wolff-Parkinson-White (WPW), look for delta wave (slurred upstroke to R wave))
- Prolonged (>200 ms): atrio-ventricular block (see later for more details)
  - First degree: fixed, lengthened PR interval
  - Second degree type I: progressive lengthening of PR until a ventricular beat (QRS complex) is missed
  - Second degree type II: fixed PR interval with occasional missed ventricular beats

- Third degree: no association between atrial beats (P waves) and ventricular beats (QRS complexes)

QRS Complex:

Represents ventricular depolarisation. A normal QRS complex is <120 ms (<3 small squares)

- Broad (>120 ms): abnormal ventricular depolarisation (e.g,. ventricular ectopic, bundle branch block)
- Tall complexes: may suggest left ventricular hypertrophy
- R-wave progression: R waves should become more positive from V1 to V6

ST Segment:

- Is it elevated/depressed? (STEMI, NSTEMI, pericarditis)

T Waves:

Represent repolarisation of the ventricles

- Are they inverted? (negative T waves are normal in V1)
- Are they tall? (hyperkalaemia, STEMI)

BRADYCARDIAS

First-degree Heart Block

Definition: a conduction delay at the atrioventricular (AV) node causing a consistently lengthened PR interval of >0.2 ms.

Buzzwords:

- **Risk factors:** previous MI, AV-blocking drugs, athletes
- **Presentation:** asymptomatic
- **ECG changes:** prolonged PR interval (See Fig 3.16)

Management: treat reversible causes. No indication for a pacemaker unless causing symptoms.

Second-degree Heart Block (Type I)

Definition: block in AV node causes progressive lengthening of the PR interval before a P wave fails to conduct through the AV node, resulting in a dropped QRS complex. Also known as **Mobitz type I** or **Wenckebach** phenomenon.

Buzzwords:

- **Risk factors:** inferior MI, AV-blocking drugs, athletes, cardiac surgery

- **Presentation:** asymptomatic or (pre-) syncope
- **ECG changes:** irregular rhythm, progressive lengthening of PR interval resulting in dropped QRS complex, narrow QRS complexes (see Fig 3.17A)

Management: monitoring. Pacemaker indicated if symptomatic

Second-degree Heart Block (Type II)

Definition: block at the AV node, His bundle or bundle branches, which causes occasionally dropped QRS complexes in a repeating cycle (e.g., 4:1). The PR interval is regular. This condition has a high risk of progression to a third-degree (complete) heart block. Also known as **Mobitz type II**.

Buzzwords:

- **Risk factors:** MI, cardiac surgery, autoimmune conditions, AV-blocking drugs, amyloidosis, fibrosis
- **Presentation:** palpitations, presyncope, syncope
- **ECG changes:** regularly irregular rhythm (see Fig 3.17B), consistent PR interval with occasionally dropped QRS complexes. QRS complexes may be narrow (if block is proximal to the His bundle) or broad (if block is distal to His bundle)

Management:

1. Admit patient
2. Cardiac monitoring
3. Temporary pacing
4. Treat reversible causes or insert permanent pacemaker.

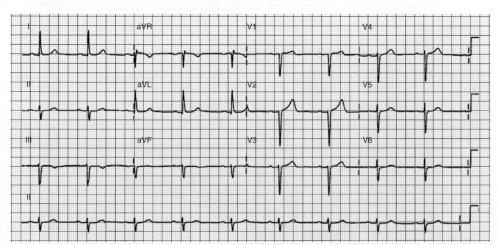

Fig 3.16 First-degree Heart Block with a Regular Rhythm, Lengthened PR Interval and Narrow QRS Complex. (With permission from Meyerson, A. CC BY-SA 3.0, via Wikimedia Commons. https://upload.wikimedia.org/wikipedia/commons/6/65/First_Degree_AV_Block_ECG_Unlabeled.jpg.)

Third-degree (Complete) Heart Block

Definition: complete dissociation of atrial and ventricular beats due to a complete loss of conduction through the AV node.

Buzzwords:

- **Risk factors:** cardiac surgery, structural heart disease, previous MI, endocarditis, autoimmune disease
- **Presentation:** syncope, heart failure, chest pain, palpitations
- **ECG changes** (see Fig 3.17C): regular P waves dissociated from regular QRS complexes. Escape QRS complexes can be narrow (originating from above the His bundle) or broad (originating from below the His bundle). Ventricular rate often <40 bpm

Management:

- Admit patient, cardiac monitoring. Temporary pacing until permanent pacemaker available
- NB: co-prescription of a β-blocker (e.g., propranolol) and a non-dihydropyridine CCB (e.g., verapamil) can result in complete heart block

Right Bundle Branch Block (RBBB)

Definition: blockade of the right bundle branch, below the His bundle.

Buzzwords:

- **Risk factors:** IHD, cor pulmonale, PE, congenital heart disease, myocarditis
- **Presentation:** can present as any of the above conditions.
- **ECG changes** (see Fig 3.18): broad QRS complex (>120 ms), second R wave (R') in leads V1/V2, broad S wave in leads V1, V5, V6. (More easily remembered as the MaRRoW pattern)

Management: treat cause

Left Bundle Branch Block (LBBB)

Definition: blockade of the left bundle branch, below the His bundle.

Buzzwords:

- **Risk factors:** IHD, HTN, dilated cardiomyopathy
- **Presentation:** new-onset LBBB is associated with MI. The left bundle branch is supplied by the left anterior descending (LAD) artery
- **ECG changes** (see Fig 3.18): broad QRS complex (>120 ms), broad R wave in leads V1, V5, V6, with no Q waves in leads V5 and V6. (More easily remembered as the WiLLiaM pattern)

Management: Treat as STEMI if new onset

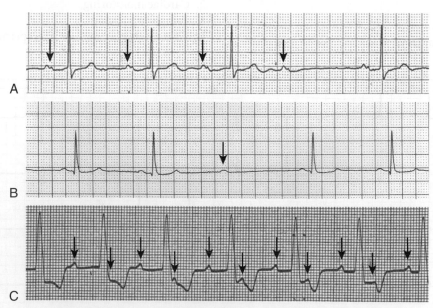

Fig 3.17 (A) Second-degree heart block (type I), (B) Second-degree heart block (type II), (C) Complete heart block. (With permission from Birnbaum, I, Birnbaum, Y, & Levine, G. N. (2018) Electrocardiography (Fig. 3.2, Chapter 3). In *Cardiology secrets*. Elsevier. Copyright © 2018 Elsevier Inc. All rights reserved.)

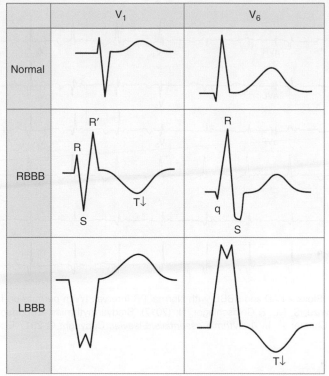

Fig 3.18 ECG Changes Seen in Right Bundle Branch Block (RBBB) and Left Bundle Branch Block (LBBB) in Leads V1 and V6. (From Goldberger, A. L., Goldberger, Z. D., & Shvilkin, A. (2017). *Goldberger's clinical electrocardiography: a simplified approach* (9th ed.). Philadelphia: Elsevier.)

Bifascicular Block

Definition: conduction delay in two of the three fascicles. This may be:

- RBBB and left anterior fascicle block (LAFB) – left axis deviation
- RBBB with left posterior fascicle block (LPFB) – right axis deviation

Buzzwords:

- **Risk factors:** as for bundle branch blocks
- **Presentation:** MI, CV instability
- **ECG changes:** broad QRS complex (>120 ms), broad R wave in leads V1, V5, V6, with no Q waves in leads V5 and V6. Axis deviation (see Fig 3.19)

Management: treat cause

Trifascicular Block

Definition: RBBB with LAFB or LPFB and AV block. An ECG will show a RBBB with a left axis or right axis deviation depending on the fascicle **AND** a first/second/third-degree heart block, depending on the location of the atrioventricular block.

Buzzwords:

- **Risk factors:** as for bundle branch blocks
- **Presentation:** MI, CV instability, bradycardia, syncope
- **ECG changes (see figure 3.20):** broad QRS complex (>120 ms), broad R wave in leads V1, V5, V6, with no Q waves in leads V5 and V6. Left axis deviation. Long PR interval or atrioventricular dissociation. (RBBB, left axis or right axis deviation and prolonged PR interval)

Management:

1. Treat cause
2. May need permanent pacemaker

EXTRA BEATS

Atrial Ectopic/Premature Atrial Complex (PAC)

Definition: when electrical activity originates at a point within the atrium other than the sinus node. This often conducts through the AV node and results in a normal

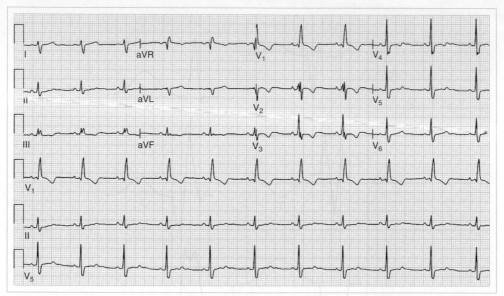

Fig 3.19 Bifasciular Block – LAD and RBBB with Normal PR Interval. (With permission from Olshansky, B., Chung, M. K., Pogwizd, S. M., & Goldschlager, N. (2017). Bradyarrhythmias – Conduction system abnormalities (Fig. 2.18, Chapter 2). In *Arrhythmia essentials*. Elsevier. Copyright © 2017 Elsevier Inc. All rights reserved.)

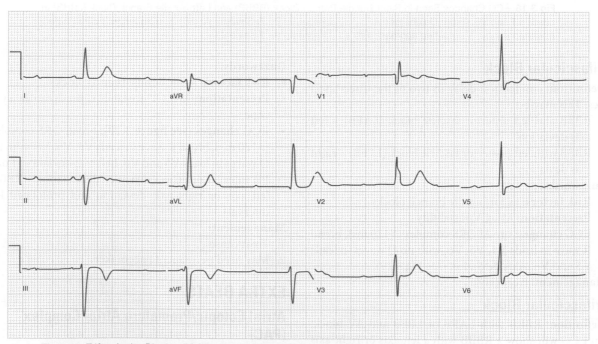

Fig 3.20 Trifascicular Block – RBBB with LAFB and third-degree Heart Block. (With permission from Garcia, D., Mattu, A., Holstege, C. P., & Brady, W. J. (2009). Intraventricular conduction abnormality – an electrocardiographic algorithm for rapid detection and diagnosis (Fig. 13). *The American Journal of Emergency Medicine*. Elsevier. Copyright © 2009 Elsevier Inc. All rights reserved.)

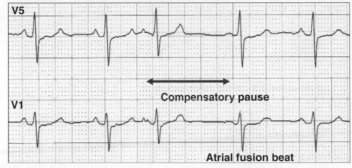

Fig 3.21 Atrial Ectopic Beat (note different P-wave morphologies) Followed by a Compensatory Pause. (With permission from Mond, H. G., & Haqqani, H. M. (2019). The electrocardiographic footprints of atrial ectopy (Fig. 1). *Heart, Lung and Circulation*. Elsevier. Crown Copyright © 2019 Published by Elsevier B.V. on behalf of Australian and New Zealand Society of Cardiac and Thoracic Surgeons (ANZSCTS) and the Cardiac Society of Australia and New Zealand (CSANZ). All rights reserved.)

QRS complex followed by a compensatory pause as the sinoatrial (SA) node resets.

Buzzwords:

- **Risk factors:** increased age, HTN, increased body habitus, anxiety, β-blockers
- **Presentation:** asymptomatic (majority), palpitations, increased risk of AF and other tachyarrhythmias
- **ECG changes:** an abnormal P wave followed by a normal QRS complex. If unifocal (from one source), these abnormal P waves are the same; if multifocal (more than one source), these can vary (see Fig 3.21)

Management:

- Risk factor modification, lifestyle advice
- Treat tachyarrhythmia if present

Junctional Escape

Definition: electrical activity originating from the AV junction causing a premature beat, which propagates through the physiological His-Purkinje system resulting in normal ventricular depolarisation.

Buzzwords:

- **Risk factors:** often physiological
- **Presentation:** often asymptomatic, palpitations
- **ECG changes:** premature, narrow QRS complex not associated with a preceding P wave and followed by a compensatory pause (see Fig 3.22)

Management: if isolated or rare, no treatment is needed

Ventricular Ectopic/Premature Ventricular Complex (PVC)

Definition: when electrical activity spontaneously originates at a point within the ventricle, causing abnormal depolarisation (not through the His-Purkinje system) and a broad QRS complex.

Buzzwords:

- **Risk factors:** anxiety, caffeine, electrolyte disturbance
- **Presentation:** palpitations or asymptomatic. A PVC can also trigger arrhythmias, such as ventricular tachycardia (VT) and SVTs
- **ECG changes:** an isolated, broad QRS complex. The next QRS will be normal and exactly two R-R interval lengths after the previous normal complex. (See Fig 3.23)

Management:

- If isolated or rare: no investigation or treatment is needed
- If symptomatic or frequent: treatment may include risk factor modification (e.g., reducing caffeine intake) or β-blockade

NARROW-COMPLEX TACHYCARDIAS

Sinus Tachycardia

Definition: rate of >100 bpm, originating at the SA node and propagating through the AV node and physiological His-Purkinjie conduction network.

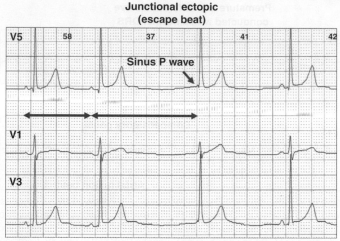

Fig 3.22 Junctional Ectopic Beat Following a Pause. (With permission from Mond, H. G., & Haqqani, H. M. (2019). The electrocardiographic footprints of atrial ectopy (Fig. 2). *Heart, Lung and Circulation*. Elsevier. Crown Copyright © 2019 Published by Elsevier B.V. on behalf of Australian and New Zealand Society of Cardiac and Thoracic Surgeons (ANZSCTS) and the Cardiac Society of Australia and New Zealand (CSANZ). All rights reserved.)

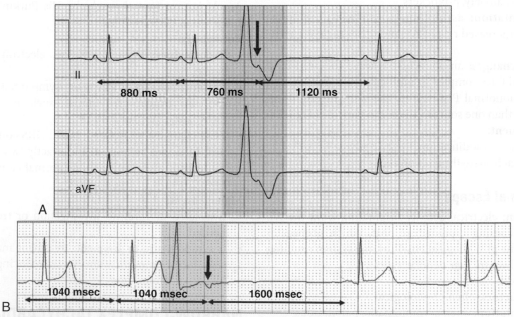

Fig 3.23 (A) Ventricular Ectopic (*red*) with a P Wave Within the Complex (*red arrow*). (B) Ventricular Ectopic Followed by a Nonconducted P Wave (*red arrow*). (With permission from Mond, H. G., & Haqqani, H. M. (2020). The electrocardiographic footprints of atrial ectopy (Fig. 8). *Heart, Lung and Circulation*. Elsevier. Crown Copyright © 2019 Published by Elsevier B.V. on behalf of Australian and New Zealand Society of Cardiac and Thoracic Surgeons (ANZSCTS) and the Cardiac Society of Australia and New Zealand (CSANZ). All rights reserved.)

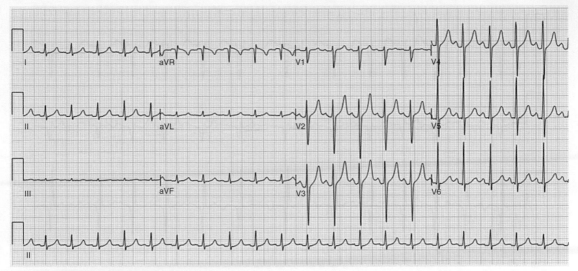

Fig 3.24 Sinus Tachycardia. (With permission from Ewingdo, CC BY-SA 4.0, via Wikimedia Commons. https:// upload.wikimedia.org/wikipedia/commons/1/14/ECG_Sinus_Tachycardia_125_bpm.jpg.)

Buzzwords:

- **Risk factors:** physiological (e.g., pain/exercise/ anxiety/dehydration), pharmacological (e.g., salbutamol), pathological (e.g., PE, hypovolaemia, infection)
- **Presentation:** palpitations. May present alongside other symptoms of pathology
- **ECG changes:** regular rhythm, normal P wave, normal PR interval, associated narrow QRS complex (see Fig 3.24)

Management: treat cause

Atrial Tachycardia

Definition: rate of >100 bpm, originating within the atria (as an ectopic) and propagating through the AV node and physiological His-Purkinjie conduction network.

Buzzwords:

- **Risk factors:** cardiomyopathy, IHD, COPD, digoxin
- **Presentation:** palpitations, can be paroxysmal (benign atrial tachycardia)
- **ECG changes:** regular rhythm if unifocal atrial ectopic. Regular PR interval with associated QRS complex. Multifocal atrial tachycardia results in irregular ventricular rate with a variable P-wave morphology. (See Fig 3.25)

Management: manage CV risks and give lifestyle advice

Atrial Fibrillation (AF)

Definition: rapid, chaotic, irregular electrical activity of the atria. This inconsistent activity does not always lead to conduction through the AV node, resulting in an irregularly irregular ventricular rhythm.

Buzzwords:

- **Risk factors:** IHD, HTN, hyperthyroidism, alcohol excess, idiopathic, sepsis
- **Presentation:** palpitations, paroxysmal (episodes that terminate in <7 days) or sustained, irregularly irregular pulse
- **ECG changes:** irregularly irregular, no P waves (see Fig 3.26)

Management:

- If haemodynamically unstable: electrical cardioversion
- If onset <48 hours without haemodynamic instability: chemical or electrical cardioversion can be attempted (flecainide if no evidence of structural heart disease **or** amiodarone with or without evidence of structural heart disease), offer heparin at first presentation or oral anticoagulation
- If onset >48 hours: anticoagulation for at least 3 weeks and TTE before cardioversion, with rate control as necessary
- If non-acute AF: rate control with a β-blocker, rate-limiting CCB (diltiazem or verapamil) or digoxin

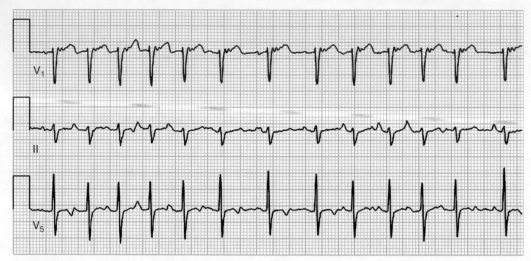

Fig 3.25 Multifocal Atrial Tachycardia. Irregularly irregular, but, unlike atrial fibrillation, there are P waves with at least three different P-wave morphologies. (From Olshansky, B., et al. (2017). *Arrhythmia essentials* (2nd ed.), Philadelphia: Elsevier.)

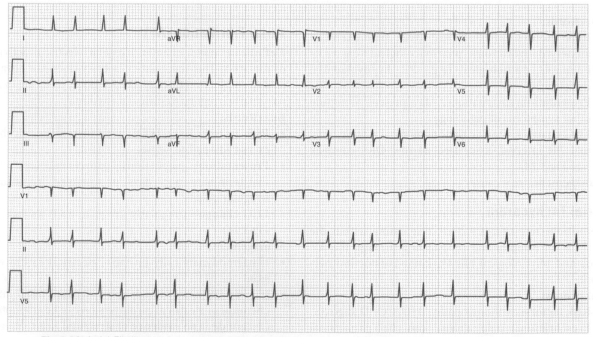

Fig 3.26 Atrial Fibrillation – Irregularly Irregular with No P Waves. (With permission from Atzema, C. L., & Singh, S. S. (2018). Acute management of atrial fibrillation from emergency department to cardiac care unit (Fig. 1). In *Cardiology clinics*. Elsevier. © 2017 Elsevier Inc. All rights reserved.)

(in sedentary patients). Use CHA_2DS_2-VASc to assess stroke risk (if ≥2 or ≥1 in males offer DOAC 1st line for nonvalvular AF), ORBIT bleeding risk score

- If paroxysmal AF: β-blockers; if infrequent episodes, consider 'pill-in-the-pocket' strategy with flecainide or propafenone
- If drug treatment unsuccessful: consider left atrial ablation

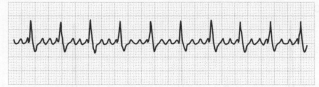

Fig 3.27 Atrial Flutter with 2:1 Conduction. (With permission from McElrath Schwartz, J., Lee, J. K., Hamrick, J. T., Hamrick, J. L., Hunt, E. A., & Shaffner, D. H. (2017). Cardiopulmonary resuscitation (Fig. 54-13, Chapter 54). In *Smith's anesthesia for infants and children*. Elsevier. Copyright © 2017 Elsevier Inc. All rights reserved.)

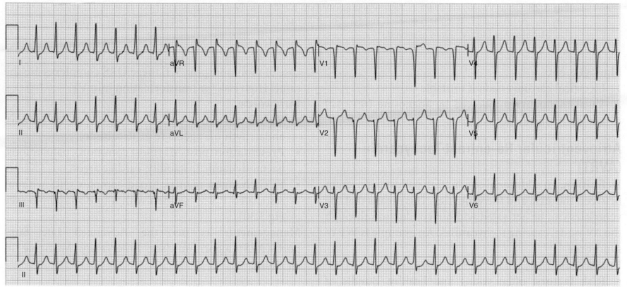

Fig 3.28 AVNRT. (With permission from Ewingdo, CC BY-SA 4.0, via Wikimedia Commons. https://upload. wikimedia.org/wikipedia/commons/d/dd/ECG_AVNRT_181_bpm.jpg).

Atrial Flutter

Definition: presence of a re-entry circuit in the RA. Saw-tooth atrial wave pattern, atrial rate often 300 bpm, with a regular ventricular rate of 150 bpm (2:1 block).

Buzzwords:

- **Risk factors:** IHD, HTN, hyperthyroidism, alcohol excess, idiopathic
- **Presentation:** palpitations, paroxysmal or sustained
- **ECG changes (see Fig 3.27):** broad, saw-tooth P waves (rate of 300 bpm)

Management:

1. If haemodynamically unstable, electrical cardioversion
2. Rate control: see Atrial Fibrillation (AF) section
3. Anticoagulation: see Atrial Fibrillation (AF) section
4. Manage CV risks and give lifestyle advice

5. Refer to cardiology for consideration of cardioversion or flutter ablation

Atrioventricular Nodal Re-entrant Tachycardia (AVNRT)

Definition: a re-entrant circuit is present within the AV node that is made up of two pathways, one slow and one fast. This circuit can be activated by a premature atrial beat before the fast pathway has recovered, resulting in re-entry and tachycardia.

Buzzwords:

- **Risk factors:** often young, healthy females with no structural heart disease
- **Presentation:** palpitations (frequency and duration vary), often paroxysmal, may be haemodynamically unstable
- **ECG changes:** tachycardia, regular P waves may not be visible (buried in complex) or inverted (see Fig 3.28)

C

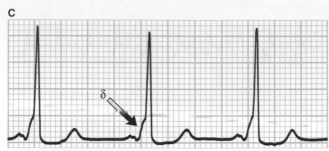

Fig 3.29 Delta Wave, As Seen in Wolff-Parkinson-White Syndrome. (With permission from Bunce, N. H., & Ray, R. (2017). Cardiovascular disease (Chapter 23). In *Kumar and Clark's clinical medicine*. Elsevier. Copyright © 2017 Elsevier Ltd. All rights reserved.)

Management:
1. Electrical cardioversion if unstable
2. Vagal manoeuvres followed by adenosine (6:12:12) are the mainstay of treatment

Atrioventricular Re-entrant Tachycardia (AVRT)

Definition: an additional conduction pathway is present between the atria and the ventricles. This means that the ventricles can be activated without conduction through the AV node, causing tachycardias. An example is WPW syndrome.

Buzzwords:
- **Risk factors:** often young and healthy. Bundle of Kent (WPW) results from a foetal developmental abnormality
- **Presentation:** palpitations, often paroxysmal. May be an incidental ECG finding
- **ECG changes:** shortened PR interval, delta waves (pre-excitation of the ventricles, see Fig 3.29) are seen during sinus rhythm. During tachycardic episodes, there are regular, narrow QRS complexes. P waves may be seen after the QRS complex. *Usually* indistinguishable from an AVNRT ECG at faster rates

Management:
1. Electrical cardioversion if unstable
2. Vagal manoeuvres and adenosine are the mainstay of treatment
3. May require ablation

BROAD-COMPLEX TACHYCARDIAS

Ventricular Tachycardia (VT)

Definition: Consecutive ventricular beats (or extrasystoles) with abnormal, broad QRS complexes. In the case of monomorphic VT, these QRS complexes are the same. High risk for transformation into VF.

Buzzwords:
- **Risk factors:** myocardial damage (e.g., ischaemia), antiarrhythmic agents (e.g., flecainide)
- **Presentation:** post-MI (most common), palpitations, haemodynamic instability, cardiac arrest
- **ECG changes:** regular, broad complex QRS without associated P waves, often with a rate >120 bpm (see Fig 3.30)

Management: as per the Advanced Life Support (ALS) algorithm (see Emergency Medicine in an Hour)

Ventricular Fibrillation

Definition: uncoordinated, irregular and rapid ventricular activity.

Buzzwords:
- **Risk factors:** cardiomyopathy, MI, electrolyte disturbance
- **Presentation:** cardiac arrest
- **ECG changes:** irregular, no detectable P waves or QRS complexes (see Fig 3.31)

Management: as per the ALS algorithm for cardiac arrest (see Emergency Medicine in an Hour)

Torsades de Pointes

Definition: a polymorphic ventricular tachycardia with a variable cardiac axis and amplitude.

Buzzwords:
- **Risk factors:** hypokalaemia, hypomagnesaemia, myocardial ischaemia, antiarrhythmic drugs, long QT
- **Presentation:** electrolyte disturbance, haemodynamic instability, cardiac arrest

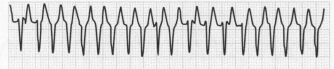

Fig 3.30 Ventricular Tachycardia – Regular, Broad QRS Complexes. (With permission from McElrath Schwartz, J., Lee, J. K., Hamrick, J. T., Hamrick, J. L., Hunt, E. A., & Shaffner, D. H. (2017). Cardiopulmonary resuscitation (Fig. 54-13, Chapter 54). In *Smith's anesthesia for infants and children.* Elsevier. Copyright © 2017 Elsevier Inc. All rights reserved.)

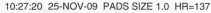

10:27:20 25-NOV-09 PADS SIZE 1.0 HR=137

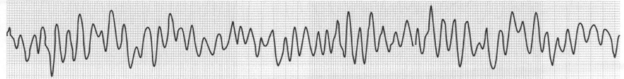

Fig 3.31 Ventricular Fibrillation – Irregular Pattern with No P Waves or QRS Complexes. (With permission from McElrath Schwartz, J., Lee, J. K., Hamrick, J. T., Hamrick, J. L., Hunt, E. A., & Shaffner, D. H. (2017). Cardiopulmonary resuscitation (Fig. 54-18, Chapter 54). In *Smith's anesthesia for infants and children.* Elsevier. Copyright © 2017 Elsevier Inc. All rights reserved.)

- **ECG changes:** cyclical changes in the cardiac axis and amplitude during ventricular tachycardia (see Fig 3.32)

Management:
- Reverse causes (e.g., electrolyte disturbance)
- Intravenous magnesium sulphate (needs expert input and cardiac monitor)
- DC cardioversion if unstable

OTHER IMPORTANT ECGS

Digoxin Toxicity

Definition: a clinical syndrome of symptoms and ECG changes secondary to digoxin. Likelihood increases with a serum digoxin concentration >1.5 micrograms/litre.

Buzzwords:
- **Risk factors:** increased age, decreased renal function, electrolyte imbalance
- **Presentation:** nausea, vomiting, confusion
- **ECG changes:** increased excitability – sinus node dysfunction, premature ventricular complexes, atrial tachycardia, 'reverse tick' sign (see Fig 3.33)

Management:

- Supportive care, correct electrolyte imbalances
- Digoxin-binding (DigiBind, DigiFab) agents if severe

Brugada Syndrome

Definition: autosomal-dominant syndrome associated with sudden cardiac death.

Buzzwords:
- **Risk factors:** genetic mutation, male
- **Presentation:** syncope, VT, sudden cardiac death
- **ECG changes:** can be dynamic. Includes RBBB, ST elevation in V1–V3 (see Fig 3.34)

Management: cardiology advice. Often an implantable cardioverter defibrillator (ICD) is placed

Pulmonary Embolism

Definition, Buzzwords and Management: see Emergency Medicine in an Hour

ECG changes:
- Sinus tachycardia
- Right heart strain (RV hypertrophy, ST depression and T wave inversion)
- SIQIIITIII – rare (except in exams!). S wave in lead I, Q waves and T wave inversion in lead III (see Fig 3.35)

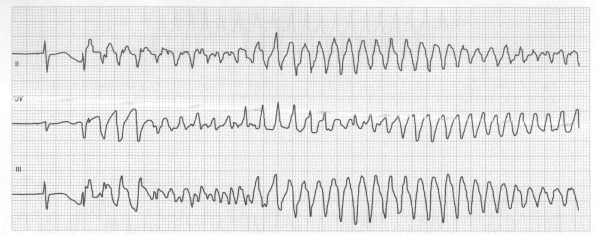

Fig 3.32 Torsades de Pointes – VT with Cyclical Cardiac Axis. (With permission from Agosti, S., Casalino, L., Bertero, G., Barsotti, A., Brunelli, C., & Morelloni, S. (2012). A dangerous fruit juice (Fig. 2). *The American Journal of Emergency Medicine*. Elsevier. Copyright © 2012 Elsevier Inc. All rights reserved.)

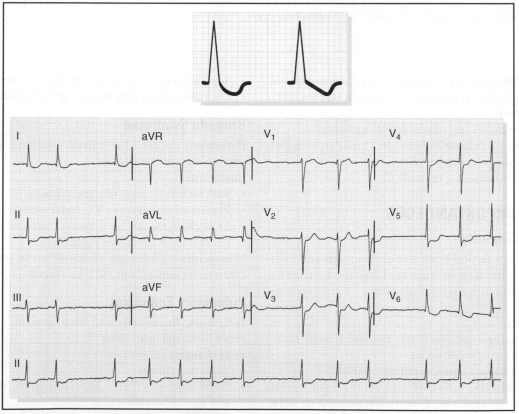

Fig 3.33 Digoxin Toxicity with Reverse Tick Sign in V5 and V6. (From Bonow, R. O., et al. (2012). *Braunwald's heart disease* 9th ed.). Philadelphia: WB Saunders.).

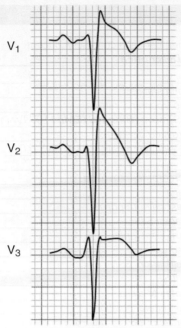

Fig 3.34 Typical ECG in Type 1 Brugada Syndrome. (With permission from PeaBrainC, CC BY-SA 4.0, via Wikimedia Commons. https://upload.wikimedia. org/wikipedia/commons/b/b9/Brugada_syndrome_ECGs.jpg).

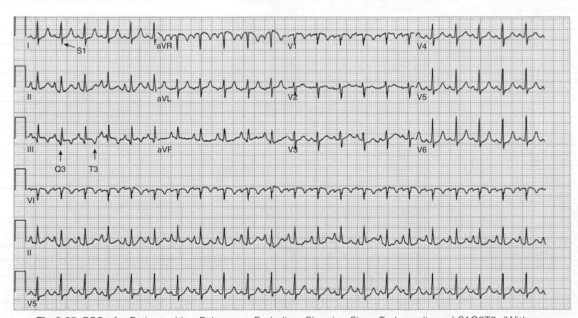

Fig 3.35 ECG of a Patient with a Pulmonary Embolism Showing Sinus Tachycardia and S1Q3T3. (With permission from Santiago, M., Abrams, S., & Truong, J. (2020). Use of US to expedite diagnosis of PE in COVID-19 patient (Fig. 1). *Visual Journal of Emergency Medicine*. Elsevier. © 2020 Elsevier Inc. All rights reserved.

THE ONE-LINE ROUND-UP!

Here are some key words to help you remember each condition/concept.

Condition/Concept	One-line Description
Hypertension	ABPM
Hyperlipidaemia	Lifestyle and statins
IHD	Stable – no troponins, nitrates
ACS	**STEMI:** ↑ ST/new LBBB. **NSTEMI:** ↓ ST, Tw-inv
Heart failure	RHF due to lung disease
HFpEF	EF >50%, elderly, female, ↑ BMI, DM, HTN
HFrEF	EF <40%
Vasovagal syncope	Posture, prodrome, provoked
Infective endocarditis	Duke criteria
Myocarditis	Young chest pain, troponin
Pericarditis	Saddle-shaped ST
Pericardial effusion	Globe heart, clear lungs
Cardiac tamponade	Beck's triad
Aortic stenosis	Senile calcification, ESM, SAD
Aortic regurgitation	Diastolic ULSE
Mitral regurgitation	PSM, radiates to axilla
Mitral stenosis	Chronic, left lateral position
Tricuspid stenosis	Rare, diastolic LLSE
Tricuspid regurgitation	Secondary>primary, due to left heart valvular disease
First-degree heart block	Prolonged PR interval
Second-degree heart block (type 1)	Progressively lengthening PR then dropped
Second-degree heart block (type 2)	Prolonged PR interval, 2:1 block
Third-degree heart block	Dissociated P and QRS complexes
LBBB	WiLLiaM
RBBB	MaRRoW
Bifascicular block	RBBB + LAD or RBBB + RAD
Trifascicular block	Bifascicular block + prolonged PR
Atrial ectopic	Abnormal P wave, narrow QRS
Junctional escape	No P wave, narrow QRS
Ventricular ectopic	Isolated wide QRS
Sinus tachycardia	>100 bpm
Atrial tachycardia	Variable P wave morphology (if multifocal)
Atrial fibrillation	Irregularly irregular, no P waves
Atrial flutter	Saw-tooth P waves
AVNRT	Tachycardia; regular, narrow QRS
AVRT	Delta wave
Ventricular tachycardia	Regular, broad QRS
Ventricular fibrillation	Irregular, no P waves or QRS
Torsades de pointes	Cyclical changes in the cardiac axis and amplitude
Digoxin toxicity	Reverse tick sign
Brugada syndrome	ST elevation in leads V1–V3
Pulmonary embolism	Sinus tachycardia, right heart strain, S1Q3T3

READING LIST: CARDIOLOGY AND ECGS IN AN HOUR

Basic Anatomy and key Concepts
Fig 3.1 Conduction System of the Heart. (Andreoli, Kinney & Packa, 1996; Illustrated by Dr Hollie Blaber). From: Andreoli, K., Kinney, M. & Packa, D. (1996). *Andreoli's comprehensive cardiac care.* Mosby.

Fig 3.2 Coronary Vessels and Their Respective Territories. (ECG Medical Training on Twitter, 2021; Illustrated by Dr Hollie Blaber). From Pinterest. (2021). *ECG medical training on twitter | Medical training, Paramedic school, P wave.* https://www.pinterest.co.uk/pin/216032113351941745/. [Accessed 6 April 2021].

Hypertension
Fig 3.3 Complications of Hypertension. (Idorsia, 2021; Illustrated by Dr Hollie Blaber). From Idorsia. (2021). *Hypertension.* https://www.idorsia.com/about-idorsia/target-diseases/hypertension-ebook. [Accessed 6 April 2021].

Fig 3.4 Treatment Steps for Hypertension. (NICE, 2019). From National Institute of Health and Care Excellence (NICE). (2019). *NG136: Hypertension in adults: diagnosis and management.* https://www.nice.org.uk/guidance/ng136. [Accessed 6 April 2021].

NICE. (2019). *NG136: Hypertension in adults: Diagnosis and management.* https://www.nice.org.uk/guidance/ng136. [Accessed 6 April 2021].

Wilkinson, I. B., Raine, T., Wiles, K., Goodhart, A., Hall, C., & O'Neill, H. (2017). *Oxford handbook of clinical medicine* (10th ed.). Oxford University Press.

Hyperlipidaemia
Grundy, S. M., Stone, N. J., Bailey, A. L., Beam, C., Birtcher, K. K., Blumenthal, R. S., ... Yeboah, J. (2019). AHA/ACC/AACVPR/AAPA/ABC/ACPM/ADA/AGS/APhA/ASPC/NLA/PCNA guideline on the management of blood cholesterol: A Report of the American College of Cardiology/American Heart Association Task Force On Clinical Practice Guidelines. *Circulation, 139,* e1082–e1143. Erratum in: *Circulation.* 2019, 139:e1182-e1186. PMID: 30586774; PMCID: PMC7403606.

Santos, R., Martin, S., & Cardoso, R. (2019). *Hypercholesterolaemia – symptoms, diagnosis and treatment | BMJ best Practice.* https://bestpractice.bmj.com/topics/en-gb/170. [Accessed 6 April 2021].

NICE. (2016). *CG181: Cardiovascular disease: Risk assessment and reduction, including lipid modification.* https://www.nice.org.uk/guidance/cg181. [Accessed 6 April 2021].

Ischaemic Heart Disease
Fig 3.5: Schematic of Coronary Arteries. (Yartsev, 2013; Illustrated by Dr Hollie Blaber). From Yartsev, A. (2013). *Deranged physiology.* https://derangedphysiology.com/main/home. [Accessed 6 April 2021].

NICE. (2016). *CG126: Stable angina: Management.* https://www.nice.org.uk/guidance/cg126. [Accessed 6 April 2021].

Wilkinson, I. B., Raine, T., Wiles, K., Goodhart, A., Hall, C., & O'Neill, H. (2017). *Oxford handbook of clinical medicine* (10th ed.). Oxford University Press.

Acute Coronary Syndromes (ACS)
NICE. (2020). *NG185: Acute coronary syndromes.* https://www.nice.org.uk/guidance/ng185. [Accessed 6 April 2021].

Wilkinson, I. B., Raine, T., Wiles, K., Goodhart, A., Hall, C., & O'Neill, H. (2017). *Oxford handbook of clinical medicine* (10th ed.). Oxford University Press.

Heart Failure
Fig 3.9 Cardinal Signs of Heart Failure Seen on Chest X-ray. XR (Wilkinson et al., 2017; Illustrated by Dr Hollie Blaber). From Wilkinson, I. B, raine, T., Wiles, K., Goodhart, A., Hall, C. & O'Neill, H. (2017). *Oxford handbook of clinical medicine* (10th ed.). Oxford University Press.

NICE. (2018). *NG106: Chronic heart failure in adults: Diagnosis and management.* https://www.nice.org.uk/guidance/ng106. [Accessed 6 April 2021].

Wilkinson, I. B., Raine, T., Wiles, K., Goodhart, A., Hall, C., & O'Neill, H. (2017). *Oxford handbook of clinical medicine* (10th ed.). Oxford University Press.

Heart Failure with Preserved Ejection Fraction (HFPEF)
Yancy, C., Jessup, M., Bozkurt, B., Butler, J., Casey, D., Colvin, M., ... Wilkoff, B. (2017). 2017 ACC/AHA/HFSA Focused Update of the 2013 ACCF/AHA guideline for the management of heart failure. *Journal of Cardiac Failure, 23,* 628–651.

Carr-White, G., & Webb, J. (2019). *BMJ best practice.* https://www.bmj.com/company/bmj-resources/bmj-best-practice/. [Accessed 6 April 2021].

NICE. (2018). *NG106: Chronic heart failure in adults: Diagnosis and management.* https://www.nice.org.uk/guidance/ng106. [Accessed 6 April 2021].

Heart Failure with Reduced Ejection Fraction (HFrEF)
NICE. (2018). *NG106: Chronic heart failure in adults: Diagnosis and management.* https://www.nice.org.uk/guidance/ng106. [Accessed 6 April 2021].

Yusuf, S. (2019). *Chronic congestive heart failure – symptoms, diagnosis and treatment | BMJ Best Practice.* https://bestpractice.bmj.com/topics/en-gb/61. [Accessed 6 April 2021].

Vasovagal Syncope
Brignole, M., Moya, A., de, F., Deharo, J., Elliott, P., Fanciulli, A., Fedorowski, A., ... Gert van Dijk, J. (2018). 2018 ESC Guidelines for the diagnosis and management of syncope. *European Heart Journal, 39,* 1883–1948.

Infective Endocarditis

Habib, G., Lancellotti, P., Antunes, M., Bongiorni, M., Casalta, J., Del Zotti, F., ... Zamorano, J. (2015). 2015 ESC guidelines for the management of infective endocarditis. *European Heart Journal*, *36*, 3075–3128.

Myocarditis

Caforio, A., Pankuweit, S., Arbustini, E., Basso, C., Gimeno-Blanes, J., Felix, S., ... Elliott, P. (2013). Current state of knowledge on aetiology, diagnosis, management, and therapy of myocarditis: A position statement of the European Society of cardiology working group on myocardial and pericardial diseases. *European Heart Journal*, *34*, 2636–2648.

Wilkinson, I. B., Raine, T., Wiles, K., Goodhart, A., Hall, C., & O'Neill, H. (2017). *Oxford handbook of clinical medicine* (10th ed.). Oxford University Press.

Pericarditis

Adler, Y., Charron, P., Imazio, M., Badano, L., Barón-Esquivias, G., Bogaert, J., ... Tomkowski, W. (2015). 2015 ESC Guidelines for the diagnosis and management of pericardial diseases. *European Heart Journal*, *36*, 2921–2964.

Pericardial Effusion

Adler, Y., Charron, P., Imazio, M., Badano, L., Barón-Esquivias, G., Bogaert, J., ... Tomkowski, W. (2015). 2015 ESC Guidelines for the diagnosis and management of pericardial diseases. *European Heart Journal*, *36*, 2921–2964.

Cardiac Tamponade

Adler, Y., Charron, P., Imazio, M., Badano, L., Barón-Esquivias, G., Bogaert, J., ... Tomkowski, W. (2015). 2015 ESC Guidelines for the diagnosis and management of pericardial diseases. *European Heart Journal*, *36*, 2921–2964.

Mahadevan, V., & Agrawal, H. (2019). *Cardiac tamponade - symptoms, diagnosis and treatment | BMJ best Practice.* https://bestpractice.bmj.com/topics/en-gb/459?q=Cardiac%20tamponade&c=suggested. [Accessed 6 April 2021].

VALVULAR DISEASE
Murmurs

Fig 3.13 Locations of Heart Sounds. (Zerwekh, Claborn & Miller, 2007; Illustrated by Dr Hollie Blaber). From Zerwekh, J., Claborn, J. & Miller, J. (2007). *Memory notebook of nursing* (Vol. 1) (3rd ed.). (Nursing Education Consultants).

Fig 3.14 Auscultogram. (Horton, A., Gentles, T. & Remenyi, B., 2020; Illustrated by Dr Hollie Blaber). From Horton, A., Gentles, T. & Remenyi, B. (2020). Chapter 5-Clinical Evaluation and Diagnosis of Rheumatic Heart Disease. In: S. Dougherty, J. Carapetis, L. Zühlke & N. Wilson, (Eds.), *Acute rheumatic fever and rheumatic heart disease*, pp.

69–106. [online] Elsevier. https://doi.org/10.1016/B978-0-323-63982-8.00005-2. [Accessed 6 April 2021].

Aortic Stenosis

Baumgartner, H., Falk, V., Bax, J., De Bonis, M., Hamm, C., Holm, P., ... Zamorano, J. (2017). 2017 ESC/EACTS guidelines for the management of valvular heart disease. *European Heart Journal*, *38*, 2739–2791.

Kalra, G., Dabaliaros, V., & Parker, R. (2020). *Aortic stenosis – symptoms, diagnosis and treatment | BMJ best practice.* https://bestpractice.bmj.com/topics/en-gb/325. [Accessed 6 April 2021].

Aortic Regurgitation

Baumgartner, H., Falk, V., Bax, J., De Bonis, M., Hamm, C., Holm, P., ... Zamorano, J. (2017). 2017 ESC/EACTS guidelines for the management of valvular heart disease. *European Heart Journal*, *38*, 2739–2791.

Wasson, S., & Kalra, N. (2019). *Aortic regurgitation – symptoms, diagnosis and treatment | BMJ best practice.* https://bestpractice.bmj.com/topics/en-gb/324?q=Aortic%20regurgitation. [Accessed 6 April 2021].

Mitral Regurgitation

Baumgartner, H., Falk, V., Bax, J., De Bonis, M., Hamm, C., Holm, P., ... Zamorano, J. (2017). 2017 ESC/EACTS guidelines for the management of valvular heart disease. *European Heart Journal*, *38*, 2739–2791.

Punjabi, P. (2018). *Mitral regurgitation – symptoms, diagnosis and treatment | BMJ best practice.* https://bestpractice.bmj.com/topics/en-gb/322. [Accessed 6 April 2021].

Mitral Stenosis

Baumgartner, H., Falk, V., Bax, J., De Bonis, M., Hamm, C., Holm, P., ... Zamorano, J. (2017). 2017 ESC/EACTS guidelines for the management of valvular heart disease. *European Heart Journal*, *38*, 2739–2791.

Carabello, B. (2020). *Mitral stenosis – symptoms, diagnosis and treatment | BMJ best practice.* https://bestpractice.bmj.com/topics/en-gb/323. [Accessed 6 April 2021].

Tricuspid Stenosis

Baumgartner, H., Falk, V., Bax, J., De Bonis, M., Hamm, C., Holm, P., ... Zamorano, J. (2017). 2017 ESC/EACTS guidelines for the management of valvular heart disease. *European Heart Journal*, *38*, 2739–2791.

Charpie, J., & Zampi, J. (2018). *Tricuspid stenosis – symptoms, diagnosis and treatment | BMJ best practice.* https://bestpractice.bmj.com/topics/en-gb/473. [Accessed 6 April 2021].

Tricuspid Regurgitation

Baumgartner, H., Falk, V., Bax, J., De Bonis, M., Hamm, C., Holm, P., ... Zamorano, J. (2017). 2017 ESC/EACTS guidelines for the management of valvular heart disease. *European Heart Journal*, *38*, 2739–2791.

Akhter, S., & Tang, P. (2019). *Tricuspid regurgitation – symptoms, diagnosis and treatment | BMJ best practice.* https://bestpractice.bmj.com/topics/en-gb/472. [Accessed 6 April 2021].

ECG Basics

Meek, S. (2002). ABC of clinical electrocardiography: Introduction. I – Leads, rate, rhythm, and cardiac axis. *BMJ, 324,* 415–418. https://www.ncbi.nlm.nih.gov/pmc/articles/PMC1122339/. [Accessed 29 April 2021].

BRADYCARDIAS
First-degree Heart Block

Da Costa, D., Brady, W., & Edhouse, J. (2002). ABC of clinical electrocardiography: Bradycardias and atrioventricular conduction block. *BMJ, 324,* 535–538. https://www.ncbi.nlm.nih.gov/pmc/articles/PMC1122450/. [Accessed 29 April 2021].

BMJ Best Practice (2021). *Atrioventricular block.* https://bestpractice.bmj.com/topics/en-gb/728. [Accessed 9 January 2021].

Second-degree Heart Block (Type I)

Da Costa, D., Brady, W., & Edhouse, J. (2002). ABC of clinical electrocardiography: Bradycardias and atrioventricular conduction block. *BMJ, 324,* 535–538. https://www.ncbi.nlm.nih.gov/pmc/articles/PMC1122450/. [Accessed 29 April 2021].

BMJ Best Practice (2021). *Atrioventricular block.* https://bestpractice.bmj.com/topics/en-gb/728. [Accessed 9 January 2021].

Second-degree Heart Block (Type II)

Da Costa, D., Brady, W., & Edhouse, J. (2002). ABC of clinical electrocardiography: Bradycardias and atrioventricular conduction block. *BMJ, 324,* 535–538. https://www.ncbi.nlm.nih.gov/pmc/articles/PMC1122450/. [Accessed 29 April 2021].

BMJ Best Practice (2021). *Atrioventricular block.* https://bestpractice.bmj.com/topics/en-gb/728. [Accessed 9 January 2021].

Third-degree (Complete) Heart Block

Da Costa, D., Brady, W., & Edhouse, J. (2002). ABC of clinical electrocardiography: Bradycardias and atrioventricular conduction block. *BMJ, 324,* 535–538. https://www.ncbi.nlm.nih.gov/pmc/articles/PMC1122450/. [Accessed 29 April 2021].

BMJ Best Practice (2021). *Atrioventricular block.* https://bestpractice.bmj.com/topics/en-gb/728. [Accessed 9 January 2021].

Left Bundle Branch Block

Da Costa, D., Brady, W., & Edhouse, J. (2002). ABC of clinical electrocardiography: Bradycardias and atrioventricular conduction block. *BMJ, 324,* 535–538. https://www.ncbi.nlm.nih.gov/pmc/articles/PMC1122450/. [Accessed 29 April 2021].

Right Bundle Branch Block

Da Costa, D., Brady, W., & Edhouse, J. (2002). ABC of clinical electrocardiography: Bradycardias and atrioventricular conduction block. *BMJ, 324,* 535–538. https://www.ncbi.nlm.nih.gov/pmc/articles/PMC1122450/. [Accessed 29 April 2021].

Bifascicular Block

Da Costa, D., Brady, W., & Edhouse, J. (2002). ABC of clinical electrocardiography: Bradycardias and atrioventricular conduction block. *BMJ, 324,* 535–538. https://www.ncbi.nlm.nih.gov/pmc/articles/PMC1122450/. [Accessed 29 April 2021].

Trifascicular Block

Da Costa, D., Brady, W., & Edhouse, J. (2002). ABC of clinical electrocardiography: Bradycardias and atrioventricular conduction block. *BMJ, 324,* 535–538. https://www.ncbi.nlm.nih.gov/pmc/articles/PMC1122450/. [Accessed 29 April 2021].

EXTRA BEATS
Atrial Ectopic / Premature Atrial Complex (PAC)

BMJ Best Practice (2020). *Assessment of palpitations.* https://bestpractice.bmj.com/topics/en-gb/572/differentials#diff-Common. [Accessed 9 January 2021].

Conen, D., Adam, M., Roche, F., Barthelemy, J., Felber Dietrich, D., Imboden, M., ... Carballo, D. (2012). Premature atrial contractions in the general population. *Circulation, 126,* 2302–2308. https://www.ahajournals.org/doi/pdf/10.1161/CIRCULATIONAHA.112.112300. [Accessed 29 April 2021].

Junctional Escape

Da Costa, D., Brady, W., & Edhouse, J. (2002). ABC of clinical electrocardiography: Bradycardias and atrioventricular conduction block. *BMJ, 324,* 535–538. https://www.ncbi.nlm.nih.gov/pmc/articles/PMC1122450/. [Accessed 29 April 2021].

Ventricular Ectopic / Premature Ventricular Complex (PVC)

BMJ Best Practice (2020). *Assessment of palpitations.* https://bestpractice.bmj.com/topics/en-gb/572/differentials#diff-Common. [Accessed 9 January 2021].

NARROW COMPLEX TACHYCARDIAS
Sinus Tachycardia

Goodacre, S. (2002). ABC of clinical electrocardiography: Atrial arrhythmias. *BMJ, 324,* 594–597. https://www.bmj.com/content/324/7337/594. [Accessed 29 April 2021].

Atrial Tachycardia

BMJ Best Practice (2020). *Focal atrial tachycardia.* https://bestpractice.bmj.com/topics/en-gb/182. [Accessed 9 January 2021].

Goodacre, S. (2002). ABC of clinical electrocardiography: Atrial arrhythmias. *BMJ, 324*, 594–597. https://www.bmj.com/content/324/7337/594. [Accessed 29 April 2021].

Atrial Fibrillation

NICE. (2021). *NG196: Atrial fibrillation: Diagnosis and management*. https://www.nice.org.uk/guidance/ng196/chapter/Recommendations#rate-and-rhythm-control. [Accessed 29 April 2021].

Esberger, D., Jones, S., & Morris, F. (2002). ABC of clinical electrocardiography: Junctional tachycardias. *BMJ, 324*, 662–665. https://www.ncbi.nlm.nih.gov/pmc/articles/PMC1122581/. [Accessed 29 April 2021].

Atrial Flutter

NICE. (2020). *CKS: Palpitations*. https://cks.nice.org.uk/palpitations#!scenario:1. [Accessed 9 January 2021].

Esberger, D., Jones, S., & Morris, F. (2002). ABC of clinical electrocardiography: Junctional tachycardias. *BMJ, 324*, 662–665. https://www.ncbi.nlm.nih.gov/pmc/articles/PMC1122581/. [Accessed 29 April 2021].

Atrioventricular Nodal Re-Entrant Tachycardia (AVNRT)

NICE. (2020). *CKS: Palpitations*. https://cks.nice.org.uk/palpitations#!scenario:1. [Accessed 9 January 2021].

Esberger, D., Jones, S., & Morris, F. (2002). ABC of clinical electrocardiography: Junctional tachycardias. *BMJ, 324*, 662–665. https://www.ncbi.nlm.nih.gov/pmc/articles/PMC1122581/. [Accessed 29 April 2021].

Atrioventricular Re-Entrant Tachycardia (AVRT)

NICE. (2020). *CKS: Palpitations*. https://cks.nice.org.uk/palpitations#!scenario:1. [Accessed 9 January 2021].

Esberger, D., Jones, S., & Morris, F. (2002). ABC of clinical electrocardiography: Junctional tachycardias. *BMJ, 324*, 662–665. https://www.ncbi.nlm.nih.gov/pmc/articles/PMC1122581/. [Accessed 29 April 2021].

BROAD COMPLEX TACHYCARDIAS
Ventricular Tachycardia (VT)

Edhouse, J., & Morris, F. (2002). ABC of clinical electrocardiography: Broad complex tachycardia – Part I. *BMJ, 324*, 719–722. https://www.ncbi.nlm.nih.gov/pmc/articles/PMC1122646/. [April 29 April 2021].

Resuscitation Council UK. (2015). *Guidelines: Peri-Arrest arrhythmias*. https://www.resus.org.uk/library/2015-resuscitation-guidelines/peri-arrest-arrhythmias. [Accessed 29 April 2021].

Ventricular Fibrillation

Morris, F., Brady, W., Camm, J., & Edhouse, J. (2003). *ABC of clinical electrocardiography* (1st ed.). BMJ Books, 61–62.

Resuscitation Council UK. (2015). *Guidelines: Adult Advanced life Support*. https://www.resus.org.uk/library/2015-resuscitation-guidelines/guidelines-adult-advanced-life-support. [Accessed 29 April 2021].

Torsades de Pointes

Edhouse, J., & Morris, F. (2002). ABC of clinical electrocardiography: Broad complex tachycardia – Part I. *BMJ, 324*, 719–722.

BMJ Best Practice (2020). *Sustained ventricular tachycardias*. https://bestpractice.bmj.com/topics/en-gb/537/treatment-algorithm. [Accessed 9 January 2021].

OTHER IMPORTANT ECGS
Digoxin Toxicity

BMJ Best Practice (2020). *Digoxin overdose*. https://bestpractice.bmj.com/topics/en-gb/338. [Accessed 9 January 2021].

BNF. (2021). *Cardiac glycosides*. https://bnf.nice.org.uk/treatment-summary/cardiac-glycosides.html. [Accessed 9 January 2021].

Brugada Syndrome

Francis, J., & Antzelevitch, C. (2005). Brugada syndrome. *International Journal of Cardiology, 101*, 173–178. https://www.ncbi.nlm.nih.gov/pmc/articles/PMC1474051/. [Accessed 29 April 2021].

Edhouse, J., Brady, W., & Morris, F. (2002). ABC of clinical electrocardiography: Acute myocardial infarction – Part II. *BMJ, 324*, 963–966. https://www.ncbi.nlm.nih.gov/pmc/articles/PMC1122906/. [Accessed 29 April 2021].

4

Clinical Epidemiology in an Hour

Hannah Punter and Richard Morris

OUTLINE

KEY DEFINITIONS AND CONCEPTS

Definitions

- **Evidence-based Medicine**: A practice of using the best available evidence to guide clinical management.
- **Observational Study:** Data is collected and observed as it naturally occurs.
- **Interventional Study:** A specific intervention is made to one or more groups of participants.
- **Prospective Study:** A study that observes the development of an outcome after measuring an exposure (study occurs in 'real time').
- **Retrospective Study:** Looks back at data previously collected to assess an exposure once an outcome has already occurred.
- **Bias:** Anything that makes results deviate from the truth, e.g., when comparing two treatments.
- **Causality:** When an exposure directly causes an outcome.
- **Confounding Factor:** A factor that is independently associated with both the exposure and the outcome. This results in an observed association, indicating false causality.
- **PICO:** The format for writing a clinically answerable question. Questions should be specific and include:
  - Population: the population you are studying
  - Intervention: the intervention of interest
- Comparator: a different intervention (e.g., standard practice or placebo)
- Outcome: what you are measuring
- **Primary Outcome:** The main outcome of interest, which should be published prior to the commencement of the trial.
- **Secondary Outcome:** Other outcomes that may be of interest and are recorded during the trial.
- **External Validity:** Are the results generalisable? Can they be applied at a population level?
- **Internal Validity:** Are the research methods reliable?
- **Accuracy:** Represents the true value.
- **Precision:** Repeatable, i.e., the same value is reached each time.
- **Type 1 Error:** False positive. This is closely linked to the p-value. The smaller the p-value, the less likely you are to inappropriately reject a true null hypothesis (i.e., you are less likely to get a significant result by chance).
- **Type 2 Error:** False negative. This is closely linked to the power of a test. The larger the sample size, the less likely you are to make a type 2 error.
- **Audit:** *Are we doing what we should be doing?* In an audit, current clinical practice is compared to a gold standard. We determine if we are following guidelines (e.g., NICE guidelines). A change is then implemented to improve current practice, followed by a reauditing to determine if current clinical practice

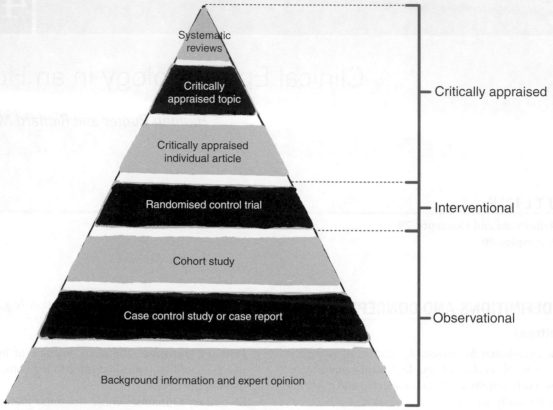

Fig 4.1 Hierarchy of Evidence with the Lowest Quality at the Bottom and the Highest Quality at the Top. (Illustrated by Dr Hollie Blaber.)

is now following the guidelines more closely. Audits need to be officially registered in your hospital.

- **Quality Improvement:** *What could we be doing better?* In a quality improvement project, clinical practice is not compared to a gold standard. Rather, we ask if there is something that can be done to do things better. We then implement a change and collect data again to see if things have improved. Quality improvement projects need to be officially registered in your hospital.
- **Research:** *What is the best way of doing this?* Research investigates novel theories, ideas and interventions to establish an evidence base for the best way of doing things. This evidence can then be used to guide clinical practice.

Hierarchy of Evidence

Definition: the strength of the evidence provided by a study based on the study design and validity (see Fig 4.1). Features to consider in the hierarchy of evidence are:

- **Size of the sample:** the greater the sample size, the more precise
- **Randomisation:** to avoid bias
- **Critical appraisal of data included**

Overview of Trials

Different types of trials are good at answering different types of questions (see Table 4.1).

CASE EXAMPLES

To illustrate each study type, we will use a simple example focusing on **'Coffee addiction'**. Many of us have reached for this warm caffeinated beverage to aid our revisions or to get us through a long stint of lectures during medical school, so hopefully this example will contextualise some of these difficult concepts. All example studies are fictional, and no real data have been included.

TABLE 4.1 Different Type of Trials for Answering Different Types of Questions

Trial Type	Description	Question Type
Systematic review and meta-analysis	Study that combines the numerical data of all published papers (either within a specific database or multiple databases) about a specific topic. Using multiple databases increases the hierarchy.	Treatment or diagnostic tests
Systematic review	Study which finds and appraises all published papers (either within a specific database or multiple databases) about a specific topic.	Any
Literature review	Study that discusses multiple (but not all) published papers about a topic.	Any
Randomised controlled trial (RCT)	Interventional study in which participants are randomised into two (or more) arms: an intervention-of-interest group vs a control group. The outcome is then measured.	Treatment or diagnostic tests
Cohort	Two groups of patients are compared: patients exposed to a specific **risk factor** vs patients not exposed to the **risk factor**. Patients are observed over time to measure the development of an outcome (e.g., a specific disease).	Prognosis
Case-control	Two groups of patients are compared: patients with a specific **outcome (cases)** vs patients **not having the outcome (control)**. Patients are then asked if they were exposed to certain risk factors in the past.	Aetiology
Cross-sectional	Measures the prevalence of exposures and outcomes at a single point in time.	Prevalence
Ecological	Data from whole populations are collated into a single observation for each population. Features of each individual person are not considered.	General trends
Cost effectiveness	Study looking at both the effectiveness and cost of an intervention.	Economics
Qualitative – case studies, focus groups	Research focusing on understanding and interpreting participants' beliefs and actions	Meaning

Basic Structure of a Research Paper and Quantitative Statistical Tools

Introduction:

1. Formulate your question
   Do medical students drink more coffee than other students?
2. Write your **null hypothesis** – a statistical statement saying that no real difference exists:
   'There is no real difference between the amount of coffee medical students drink in comparison to other students'.
3. Write your alternate hypothesis – a statistical statement of the expected difference:
   'Medical students drink different amounts of coffee than other students'.
4. Decide the study type (see Table 4.1)
   In this case, an observational study, such as a cross-sectional study, would be an appropriate way to answer this question, as it can evaluate the prevalence of students who drink coffee.

Methods:

1. Determine how you will carry out your study
2. Determine the type of data you will collect
- **Quantitative:** numerical data
   i. Discrete: integers (*e.g., cups of coffee*)
   ii. Continuous: decimals (*e.g., grams of caffeine consumed*)
- **Qualitative**: non-numerical data (*e.g., symptoms you experience if you don't have your morning coffee*)
- **Type of outcome**
   i. **Clinical:** a measurable clinical outcome, e.g., blood markers, survival or disease recurrence
   ii. **Patient reported:** reported by the patient in the form of a survey
   iii. **Economic/social:** how cost effective is the intervention?

Results:

100 medical students were asked how many cups of coffee they drink each day.

- **Measures of central tendency:**
  - **Mean:** sum of the **variables** divided by the total number of participants *(e.g., the mean was calculated to be 2.6 cups of coffee per day. This value was calculated by adding up the responses of the 100 students (total = 260 cups of coffee) and dividing the total by 100 to get 2.6 cups of coffee drunk by each medical student per day on average.)*
  - **Median:** middle value *(e.g., the median was calculated to be 2.5 cups of coffee. All responses were ordered and the middle (the 50.5th in this case) value gives the median. This figure can be interpreted as meaning that 50% of the students drink less than 2.5 cups and 50% of the students drink more than 2.5 cups of coffee per day.)*
  - **Mode:** the most frequently occurring result *(e.g., the mode for this data set was three cups of coffee. Of all 100 responses, the answer given most often was three cups of coffee.)*
- **Measures of dispersion:**
  - **Range:** the smallest value to the largest value *(e.g., the range was 0–7, since the smallest value given was zero cups of coffee, whilst the largest was seven cups of coffee per day.)*

- **Standard deviation (SD):** measure of variation, no need to memorise this equation! *(e.g., the standard deviation represents how much variation there is in the data by calculating the sum of how far individual values lie from the mean value.)*
- **Standard error (SE):** measure of precision, no need to memorise this equation! *(e.g., a measure of precision that determines the variation of sample means from the true mean. The greater the population size, the greater the n value. This gives a smaller standard error, and the calculated mean is therefore more likely to be closer to the true mean.)*
- **Data distribution** (see Fig 4.2):
  - **Normal distribution:** all values are symmetrically distributed around the mean value, with those closest to the mean occurring more frequently, resulting in a bell-shaped curve. The mean, median and mode all have the same value.
  - **Negative skew:** outliers are predominately in the negative direction and, therefore, the mean< median<mode.
  - **Positive skew:** outliers are predominately in the positive direction and, therefore, the mean> median>mode.

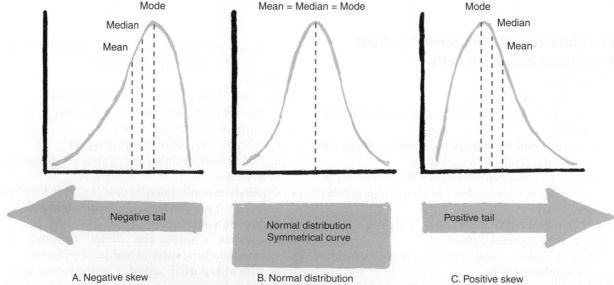

Fig 4.2 Normal Distribution and Skewing. (Illustrated by Dr Hollie Blaber.)

- **Inferred measures:**
  - **Reference range:** 95% of the normal population lies 1.96 × SD away from the mean
    Lower reference = mean - (1.96 × SD)
    2.6 - (1.96 × 1.0) = 0.64
    Upper reference = mean + (1.96 × SD)
    2.6 + (1.96 × 1.0) = 4.56
    The reference range for this population is 0.64 to 4.56 cups of coffee per day. Therefore, 95% of the normal population consume between 0.64 and 4.56 cups of coffee each day.
  - **Confidence intervals:** 95% of the time the population mean will be within 1.96 × SE of the observed sample mean
    "With 95% certainty, I am confident that the true mean lies between the sample mean +/- 1.96 × SE." HINT: This is the same calculation as the reference range; however, the standard error is used instead of the standard deviation.
  - **P-value:** the probability of getting a result just by chance rather than by identifying a true difference
    A p-value of 0.05 indicates that there is only a 5% chance (p-value × 100%) that the result obtained could have occurred by chance, and it is therefore considered to be statistically significant with a true difference between the population (as suggested by the null hypothesis) and the sample mean. This finding allows you to reject the null hypothesis.

Ecological Study

Definition: an observational study in which data from a whole population is analysed as a single group (see Fig 4.3 and Table 4.2). Features of each individual person are not considered. Monitors population health to guide public health interventions.

Example: *Data were collected from all medical schools about student coffee consumption, stress levels and hours of placement per week. Data showed that the highest levels of coffee consumption were in those schools with the greatest number of placement hours. There was no association between coffee drinking and the average level of stress.*

Key concepts:
- **Ecological fallacy:** a relationship between groups is also assumed to be true for an individual.
For example, assuming that an individual medical student with a high level of coffee consumption also attends many hours of placement. You cannot infer causality.

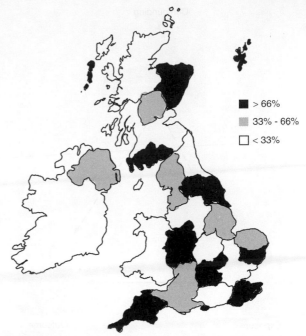

Fig 4.3 Image Illustrating an Ecological Study. UK data showing the percentages of students who drink >2 cups of coffee per day. (Illustrated by Dr Hollie Blaber.)

TABLE 4.2 Strengths and Weaknesses of an Ecological Study

Strength	Weakness
Quick	No causality
Easy	High risk of bias
Good for rare diseases	Confounding
	Ecological fallacy

- **Confounding factor (see Fig 4.4):** a factor that is independently associated with both the exposure and the outcome, which results in an observed association, indicating false causality.
In this situation, we haven't asked about sleep. Sleep could impact both the amount of coffee you drink and how stressed you feel.

Data analysis:
- **Regression analysis:** statistical method to estimate the association between two variables

Cross-sectional Study

Definition: an observational study that measures the prevalence of exposures and outcomes at a single point in time, i.e., a 'snapshot' (see Fig 4.5 and Table 4.4).

Confounding

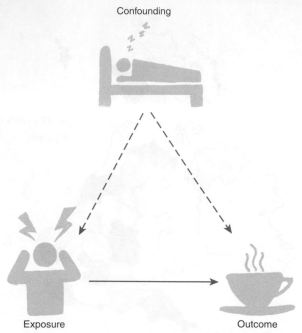

Fig 4.4 Confounding Effect. The amount of sleep you get may impact both how stressed you feel and how much coffee you drink. Therefore, sleep is a confounding factor when considering the link between stress and coffee consumption. (Illustrated by Dr Hollie Blaber.)

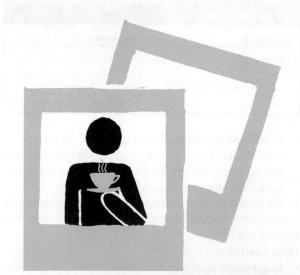

Fig 4.5 Cross-sectional Study. (Illustrated by Dr Hollie Blaber.)

Example: *Bristol Medical School asked all of its medical students to complete a survey about their coffee addiction (**outcome**). Students were also asked about how many hours of sleep they got each night (**exposure**). See Table 4.3*

TABLE 4.3	**Outcomes vs Exposures**		
	Coffee Addiction (Disease)	**No Coffee Addiction (No Disease)**	**TOTAL**
<8 h of sleep (exposed)	60	90	150
>8 h of sleep (unexposed)	10	70	80
TOTAL	70	160	Total population = 230

TABLE 4.4	**Strengths and Weaknesses of a Cross-sectional Study**
Strength	**Weakness**
True burden of disease	**Cannot determine causality:** high risk of reverse causality
Fast and inexpensive	**Cannot determine incidence:** just a snapshot in time
	Measurement bias: current vs historical exposure
	Selection bias: exposure or outcome may impact who replies to studies

for the results. The prevalence of coffee addiction was found to be 30 per 100 students, with an odds ratio of 4.67 seen in those who slept less than 8 hours per night.

Key concepts:

- **Measurement bias:** bias that occurs as a result of data collection

  The student's current levels of sleep may not represent their average amount of sleep. If asked the week after exams, the amount of sleep may be dramatically increased in students, although coffee addiction may still be present.

- **Selection bias:** bias that occurs as a result of selecting the sample of subjects to be enrolled in a study

  If the survey was given out at a 9 a.m. lecture, the students who need more sleep may not be there to complete the survey, resulting in skewed results.

- **Reverse causality:** the disease increases your risk of exposure

  In this case, we are unable to determine if too little sleep leads to the development of a coffee addiction or if a coffee addiction affects your sleep, meaning you sleep less.

Data analysis:

- **Prevalence:** the number of people with a disease divided by the total population at risk, which gives you an indication of how many people in the population currently have the disease. This number will be affected by mortality rates and disease duration.

  Seventy students have a coffee addiction out of a sample of 230, so 70/230 = 0.304 or 30 per 100 students are addicted to coffee.

- $$Odds = \frac{no.\ with\ the\ disease}{no.\ without\ disease}$$

  Look in the totals row (see Table 4.3): 70/160 = 0.44

- $$Odds\ ratio = \frac{odds\ of\ disease\ in\ exposure\ group}{odds\ of\ disease\ in\ unexposed\ group}$$

  This value describes how likely it is to have a disease in the exposed group compared to the unexposed group. *60/90 divided by 10/70 = 4.67. You are therefore 4.67 times more likely to become addicted to coffee if you sleep less than 8 h*

Case-control Study

Definition: an observational study that compares two groups of patients, those with a **specific outcome (cases)** vs those **without the outcome (control)**. Patients are then asked if they were exposed to certain risk factors in the past. (see Fig 4.6 and Table 4.5)

Example: *A group of fifth-year medical students with a coffee addiction (cases) are identified at a self-help group. Another group of similar medical students without a coffee addiction (controls) are identified. Both groups are then interviewed and asked to recall their exercise levels, alcohol consumption, smoking and eating habits over the past 5 years. The results show that smoking is a significant risk factor, with an odds ratio of 2.3, suggesting you are 2.3 times more likely to be a coffee addict if you have a history of smoking. High exercise levels had an odds ratio of 0.8, indicating those with high exercise levels are 0.8 times as likely to be a coffee addict.*

Key concepts:

- **Recall bias:** bias as a result of differing recall between cases and control.

  Those with a coffee addiction may be more aware of and may recall more exposures because their aware-

HISTORY ◄──────── PRESENT

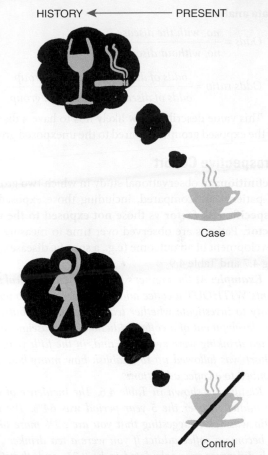

Case

Control

Fig 4.6 Case-control Study. (Illustrated by Dr Hollie Blaber.)

TABLE 4.5	**Strengths and Weaknesses of a Case-control Study**
Strength	**Weakness**
Good for rare conditions	**Selection bias:** bias introduced when selecting cases
Quick	**Recall bias:** bias introduced when recalling exposures
Can test for multiple exposures	**Detection bias:** bias introduced by the interviewer
Good for investigating aetiology	**Reverse causality:** retrospective design

ness may have increased due to their participation in the self-help group.

- **Detection bias:** bias as a result of the detection methods, e.g., the interviewer.

  The interviewer may probe the coffee addicts more than the control group.

Data analysis:

- $Odds = \dfrac{no.\ with\ the\ disease}{no.\ without\ disease}$

- $Odds\ ratio = \dfrac{odds\ of\ disease\ in\ exposure\ group}{odds\ of\ disease\ in\ unexposed\ group}$

This value describes how likely it is to have a disease in the exposed group compared to the unexposed group.

Prospective Cohort

Definition: an observational study in which two groups of patients are compared, including those exposed to a **specific risk factor** vs those **not exposed to the risk factor**. Patients are observed over time to measure the development of an outcome (e.g., a specific disease). See Fig 4.7 and Table 4.9

Example: At the Fresher's Fair, first-year. medical students WITHOUT a coffee addiction were asked to join a study to investigate whether tea drinking contributed to the development of a coffee addiction. The baseline levels of tea drinking were evaluated and, in the fifth year, the cohort was followed up to establish how many had succumbed to a coffee addiction.

Results are shown in Table 4.6. The incidence of coffee addiction over the 5-year period was 64%. The risk ratio was 1.39, suggesting that you are 39% more likely to become a coffee addict if you were a tea drinker. The risk difference was calculated to be 0.21, and, therefore, 21 more cases of coffee addiction per 100 people occurred in tea drinkers.

Key concepts:

- Loss-to-follow-up bias
  Some students may decide that medicine just isn't for them and may switch to a different course therefore not being followed up in the study. This phenomenon may be more common in non-coffee drinkers, since these students may realise that drinking coffee is an important part of becoming a doctor.

PRESENT ⟶ FUTURE

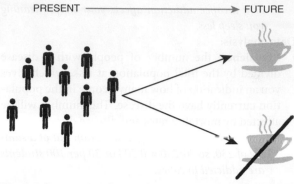

Fig 4.7 Prospective Cohort Study. (Illustrated by Dr Hollie Blaber.)

Data analysis:

- $Incidence = \dfrac{no.\ of\ new\ cases\ in\ a\ set\ time\ period}{total\ population}$

The incidence describes the number of people who develop a disease over a specific time period (see Fig 4.8). It gives you a good indication of the rate at which people are developing a disease and is unaffected by the survival time and average disease duration. This figure is *often* reported as the rate per 100,000 in the population.

To calculate the incidence of coffee addiction, you look at the total number of coffee addiction cases that developed over a 5-year period (160) divided by the total population (250). The calculation is 160 ÷ 250 = 0.64 (see Table 4.6). This finding could be reported as an incidence of 64,000 per 100,000 (or 64%) of the population over 5 years. (NB. This represents a very high incidence.)

- $Risk = \dfrac{no.\ with\ outcome}{total\ population\ at\ risk}$

  To calculate the risk of the exposed group, we take 90 ÷ 120 = 0.75

- $Risk\ ratio = \dfrac{risk\ of\ outcome\ in\ exposed\ group}{risk\ of\ outcome\ in\ unexposed\ group}$

TABLE 4.6	**Exposures vs Outcomes**		
	OUTCOME (AFTER 5-YEAR STUDY)		
	Coffee Addiction	**No Coffee Addiction**	**TOTAL**
Exposure (at start of study) Tea drinker	90	30	120
Non-tea drinker	70	60	130
TOTAL	160	90	250

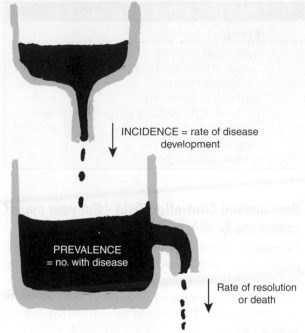

INCIDENCE = rate of disease
development

PREVALENCE
= no. with disease

Rate of resolution
or death

Fig 4.8 Incidence vs Prevalence. (Illustrated by Dr Hollie Blaber.)

To calculate the risk ratio, we calculate the risk of the outcome in the exposed group (90 ÷ 120) and the risk of the outcome in the unexposed group (70 ÷130). We then divide the risk of the exposed group by the risk of the unexposed group to get 1.39. This calculation is (90 ÷ 120) ÷ (70 ÷130). See Table 4.7 for interpretation of the risk ratio.

• Risk difference = risk of outcome in exposed group - risk of outcome in unexposed group

Example: to calculate the risk difference, we subtract the risk of the unexposed group from the risk of the exposed group = (90 ÷ 120) - (70 ÷130) = 0.21. We

can interpret this value by saying that, for every 100 cases of coffee addiction, there are 21 more cases if they were previously tea drinkers than if they weren't. See Table 4.8 for interpretation of risk difference

Retrospective Cohort

Definition: an observational study in which two groups of patients are compared, those exposed to a **specific risk factor** vs those **not exposed to the risk factor**. At the time of the study, the outcome has already occurred, and pre-recorded data (often from electronic health records) or interviews are used to establish the cohort's baseline exposures. A key difference from prospective cohort studies is that, at the time of data collection, **the outcomes have already occurred.** (See Fig 4.9 and Table 4.10)

Example: *A study was designed to see which risk factors may have contributed to the development of a coffee addiction in a cohort of students. All students who started medical school in 2015 were asked to complete a joining questionnaire. One of the questions asked about tea-drinking habits. The final cohort was then interviewed to determine if they had developed a coffee addiction.*

Key concepts:

• **Recall bias:** bias introduced when recalling exposures. These studies rely on records designed for other purposes. Often measures are only recorded if they are directly relevant, e.g., weight is only recorded IF the patient is obese or smoking status is only recorded IF the patient smokes.

• **Selection bias:** the outcome has already occurred, and there is therefore a higher risk of a selection bias.

Data analysis:

• $Incidence = \dfrac{new\ cases\ of\ disease\ in\ a\ given\ time\ period}{population\ at\ risk}$

• $Risk = \dfrac{no\ .\ with\ outcome}{total\ population\ at\ risk}$

TABLE 4.7	**Interpreting the Risk Ratio**	
Risk Ratio (RR)	**Meaning**	**Example**
>1	Exposure increases risk	RR = 1.45: 45% more likely to have outcome if exposed
1	Exposure has no effect on risk	RR = 1: exposure has no effect on outcome
<1	Exposure decreases risk (protective)	RR = 0.67: 33% less likely to have outcome if exposed
NB. If confidence intervals cross 1 (e.g., 0.98–1.05), the results show no significant effect of the exposure on the outcome		

TABLE 4.8 **Interpreting the Risk Difference**

Risk Difference (Rdiff)	Meaning	Example
>0 (positive)	Exposure increases risk	Rdiff = 0.3: for every 100 cases exposed, 30 more of them had the outcome than in the unexposed group
0	Exposure has no effect on risk	Rdiff = 0: no difference
<0 (negative)	Exposure decreases risk	Rdiff = -0.2: for every 100 cases exposed, 20 less of them had the outcome compared to the unexposed group

NB. If confidence intervals cross 0 (e.g., -0.2–0.24), the results show no significant risk difference.

TABLE 4.9 **Strength and Weaknesses of a Prospective Cohort Study**

Strength	Weakness
Reduces risk of reverse causality	Loss-to-follow-up bias: patients may drop out of the study
Less selection bias since the outcome is not yet known	Takes a long time: need to wait for the outcome to develop

HISTORY ← → PRESENT

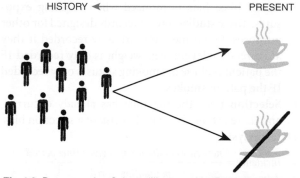

Fig 4.9 Retrospective Cohort. (Illustrated by Dr Hollie Blaber.)

TABLE 4.10 **Strengths and Weaknesses of a Retrospective Cohort Study**

Strength	Weakness
Cheaper and quicker than a prospective study	Selection bias
	Recall bias
Good for rare diseases	Reverse causality

- Risk ratio = $\dfrac{\text{risk of outcome in exposed group}}{\text{risk of outcome in unexposed group}}$

- Risk difference = risk of outcome in exposed group − risk of outcome in unexposed group

Randomised Controlled Trial - *Get your cup of coffee ready, this is a big one!*

Definition: an interventional study in which a sample population is randomly assigned to two arms. Typically, half the participants receive the intervention and the other half do not; however, sometimes there are more than two arms (see Fig 4.10 and Table 4.12). Key steps in an RCT include:

1. **Design** – identify a clinically answerable question and design your study to answer it
2. **Enroll** – select an appropriate population representative of the population you are studying
3. **Allocate** – randomise participants into different arms of the study
4. **Follow up** – collect the results for your study
5. **Analysis** – statistically analyse your results. This may also include an economic analysis to identify how much the intervention will cost
6. **Report** – write up results so they are available to guide clinical practice

Example: *A study was designed to establish the best treatment for coffee addiction. The standard treatment is 'advising more sleep'. However, a new treatment has become available in the form of a tablet called 'co-ffRee' that decreases those coffee cravings. Students with a coffee addiction were recruited and randomised into a control group (advised to have more sleep + placebo) or an intervention group (advised to have more sleep + co-ffRee). Results showed that coffee consumption was 1.5 (95% CI 0.1–2.9, p = 0.04) coffee units lower in those in the intervention group than in those receiving the placebo. Therefore, with 95% certainty, we can say that the true difference lies between 0.1–2.9 coffee units. The risk of coffee addiction in the intervention group was 0.3, whilst, in the control group, it was 0.5. The number needed to*

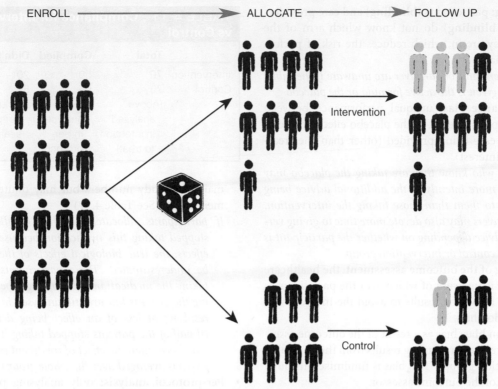

Fig 4.10 Randomised Controlled Trial. (Illustrated by Hollie Blaber.)

treat was calculated to be 5, suggesting that, in every five people treated with Co-ffRee, one reduced their coffee consumption.

Key concepts:

- **Clinical equipoise:** genuine uncertainty in the expert medical community about which treatment is superior. This is required to get ethical approval.

  If there was clear evidence that a treatment worked, it would be unethical to withhold this treatment from the control group.

- **PICO:** to ensure it is a clinically answerable question

- **Cluster trial:** randomisation occurs at an institutional level

  If the intervention involved starting lectures at midday, it would be difficult to implement the study within one university, since participants in the different arms of the study would realise the difference, and the trial would no longer be blinded. In addition, the university would have to hold two sets of lectures, which would be costly! By introducing the intervention at an institutional level, there is less contamination (discussion between control

and intervention arms), and it is logistically more straight forward.

- **Informed consent:** participants voluntarily confirm their willingness to participate in a study after being made aware of all relevant information that could influence their decision to participate

  The student is fully aware prior to the trial starting that he or she may be given the placebo pill or the active pill and of all possible side effects and outcomes.

- **Randomisation:** in an RCT, participants should be **randomly** allocated into the arms

  A random sequence generator determines which participants receive co-ffRee and which receive the placebo.

- **Allocation concealment:** allocation of participants into different treatment arms is concealed from the researchers, which reduces the selection bias

- **Selection bias:** occurs if confounding factors are not equally distributed between the intervention and control groups. This bias is reduced by **randomisation** and **allocation concealment**.

- **Blinding:** participants (**blinding**) and care providers (**double blinding**) do not know which arm of the study they are in, which reduces the risk of performance bias

  The student and/or caregiver are unaware if the tablet being given is the active formula or the placebo.

- **Performance bias:** unequal performance between the groups as a result of the placebo effect or due to unequal care being provided (other than the treatment of interest).

  Students who know they are taking the placebo may listen more intently to the additional advice being given to them than those taking the intervention. Caregivers may also devote more time to giving verbal advice depending on whether the participant is in the control or intervention group.

- **Blinding of the outcome assessment:** the healthcare provider is unaware of which arm the participant is in when recording results to avoid the introduction of detection bias.

- **Detection bias:** bias as a result of the outcome assessor differentially recording results from the control vs intervention groups. This bias is minimised through blinding of the outcome assessor.

- **Attrition bias:** bias occurrence due to a differential loss to follow up between the groups as a result of the impact of the interventions.

  "Co-ffRee" is found to cause diarrhoea, particularly when found to be ineffective at reducing your coffee intake. If those with severe diarrhoea all dropped out and were not included in the analysis, the actual effect of "Co-ffRee" would be overestimated.

- **Outcome-reporting bias:** the preferential reporting of statistically significant results and the lack of reporting of outcomes that are not statistically significant or those perceived as negative.

Data analysis:

- Risk difference and risk ratio can be calculated

- *Number needed to treat to benefit =*

$$\frac{1}{(control\ risk - exposure\ risk)}$$

  In this case, you can calculate it by 1 ÷ (0.5–0.3) = 5. This can be interpreted as, for every five people you treat, one person benefits.

- **Intention-to-treat analysis**: analysing participants in the group to which they have been randomised. This type of analysis respects randomization and

TABLE 4.11	**Compliance for Intervention vs Control**		
	Total	**Complied**	**Didn't Comply**
Intervention	70	50	20
Control	70	65	5
	(Above analysed in intention to treat)	(Above analysed in per-protocol)	(Excluded in per-protocol analysis)

maintains study numbers but may dilute the treatment effect. (See Table 4.11)

If participants allocated to the "Co-ffRee" group stopped taking this medication because of its side effects, the true biological effects of the drug may be underestimated. Those participants no longer taking the medication will no longer be experiencing the benefits but are still analysed in this group, resulting in less of an effect being demonstrated (if half of the patients stopped taking it because of diarrhoea, then the effect of treatment in half of the group is averaged over the whole group).

- **Per-protocol analysis:** only analysing participants who received the treatment they were allocated to (complied). (See Table 4.11)

  This type of analysis only includes data from those who received the treatment they were supposed to, which is effective for looking at the biological effect but is less representative of a 'real-world' intervention and is potentially biased.

- **As-treated analysis:** analysing those who did or didn't receive the treatment regardless of randomisation. (See Table 4.11)

  This type of analysis disregards randomisation, and results are analysed based on what treatment the participant actually received. This results in a high risk of bias.

Economic analysis: analysis of an intervention to determine how effective it is and how much it costs in comparison to standard care (see Fig 4.11). This should include both long-term and short-term costs.

- **Cost effectiveness:** cost per change in a clinically measurable scale (*£100 per 1 less coffee per day*)

- **Cost utility:** number of years lived in full health, measured in quality-adjusted life years (QALYs)

- **Cost benefit:** amount of money saved by the intervention

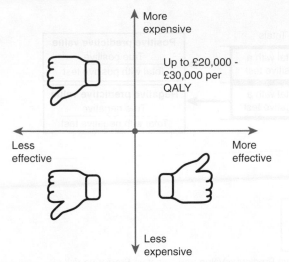

More
expensive

Up to £20,000 -
£30,000 per
QALY

Less
effective

More
effective

Less
expensive

Fig. 4.11 Economic Analysis. (Illustrated by Dr Hollie Blaber.)

TABLE 4.12 Strengths and Weaknesses of a Randomised Controlled Trial	
Strength	**Weakness**
Low risk of bias	Expensive
Selection bias reduced by randomisation and allocation concealment	May be logistically difficult
Measurement bias reduced by blinding	Ethical implications
Evidence of causality	Attrition bias
Reduce effect of confounding factors	
Good for measuring effectivity of an intervention	

- **QALY:** one QALY represents 1 year of perfect health. We calculate how many additional years an intervention may give a patient and weight these years based on a quality-of-life score. The NHS will fund interventions that cost up to £20,000 to £30,000 per QALY.
- *Incremental cost effectiveness (ICER) = $\dfrac{\text{difference in cost}}{\text{difference in effect}}$*
  This can then be plotted on a table (see Fig 4.11) to assist with determining if it is a worthwhile intervention.

Diagnostic Testing - *this is a common exam question calculation**

Definition: research is carried out to determine the sensitivity and specificity of a test, which involves

collecting data about the test result and gold-standard assessment in a typical group of participants. See Fig 4.12 and Table 4.14

- **Sensitivity:** the proportion of people with the disease who have a positive test
- **Specificity:** the proportion of people without the disease who have a negative test
- **Positive predictive value (PPV):** the probability of the patient having the disease if they have a positive test
- **Negative predictive value (NPV):** the probability of the patient NOT having the disease if they have a negative test

Example: *A study was conducted to investigate the reliability of a new test for diagnosing a coffee addiction. The current 'gold-standard' method of diagnosis is self-declaration of drinking more than four cups of coffee per day. The new test measures caffeine levels in the blood from a capillary blood sample.* **Two hundred** *students were randomly selected and tested with both methods.* **One hundred fifty** *students drank more than four cups of coffee per day and were therefore classified as having a coffee addiction. Of those with a coffee addiction,* **140** *also had raised capillary blood caffeine levels. A total of* **40** *patients had a low capillary blood caffeine level. Calculated values are in bold in Table 4.13, with the calculation performed in brackets.*

Step-by-step calculation:
1. *Fill in the missing gaps – read the information carefully*
2. *Calculate sensitivity = e.g., (140/150)*100 = 93.3%. This test has a high* **sensitivity.** *Therefore, if the test result is* **negative,** *you can* **RULE OUT** *the disease from your differentials, which seems a bit paradoxical doesn't it? If the sensitivity is 93.3%, you can say that only 6.7% of people with the disease have a negative test. Therefore a negative test is very likely to be correct and so the disease can be ruled out. You cannot rule in the condition, however, as the sensitivity doesn't tell you how specific it is and therefore the test could be positive for many different conditions.*
3. *Calculate specificity = e.g., (30/50)*100 = 60%. In this case the test has a* **low specificity** *and may give a false-positive result. In this case, if the test is* **positive,** *you cannot* **RULE IN** *coffee addiction, as 40% of positive results may result from other conditions. If a test is highly specific, you could RULE IN the diagnosis, as it is unlikely to be anything other than the specific disease causing the test to be positive.*

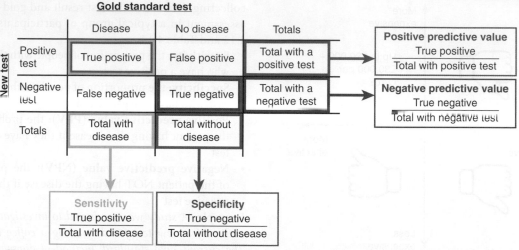

Fig 4.12 Calculation of the Sensitivity, Specificity, Positive Predictive Value and Negative Predictive Value.

TABLE 4.13   Demonstrating the Completion of a Matrix

		GOLD-STANDARD TEST		TOTALS
		Positive = coffee addiction	Negative = NO coffee addiction	
New test – capillary blood caffeine level	Positive test (raised caffeine level)	140	20 (50–30)	160 (140+20)
	Negative test (low caffeine level)	10 (150–140)	30 (40–10)	40
Totals		150	50 (200–150)	200

TABLE 4.14   Strengths and Weaknesses of Diagnostic Testing

Strength	Weakness
Important for guiding clinical practice	Predictive values strongly depend on the prevalence of the condition in the target population, which may differ depending on whether the test is applied in the community, in primary care, or in secondary care

4. *Calculate the PPV = e.g., (140/160)*100 = 87.5%. If the test is positive, there is an 87.5% chance of actually having the disease.*
5. *Calculate the NPV = e.g., (30/40)*100 = 75%. If the test is negative, there is a 75% chance you do not have the disease.*

Systematic Review and Metanalysis

Definition: a **systematic review** systematically searches the literature and appraises all published papers (either within a specific database or in multiple databases) about a specific topic (see Fig 4.13 and Table 4.16). Steps to complete for this type of study include:
1. Design the study (what question are you trying to answer?)
2. Systematic review of the literature
3. Select studies and extract evidence
4. Critically analyse the included studies
5. Analyse the results, which may involve a meta-analysis (see additional steps below)
6. Report your findings
Systematic reviews may also contain a meta-analysis.
A **meta-analysis** aims to combine the numerical results of different studies to determine the effect of an intervention. If the combined studies have similar effects

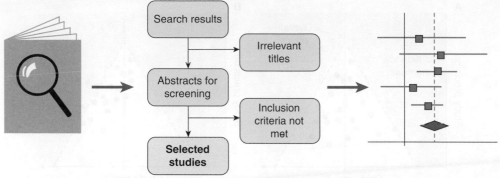

Fig 4.13 Systematic Review. (Illustrated by Dr Hollie Blaber.)

and any variation between the studies is due to random variation (or chance), then we define it as homogeneity. If, on the other hand, the studies show variation in their effects, we define it as heterogeneity. The additional steps include:

1. Determine if the studies show similar effects (homogeneity) or different effects (heterogeneity)
2. Determine the effect size within the population
3. If there is heterogeneity, you can try to adjust for it using a meta-regression analysis
4. Carry out analyses of different groups within your study

Example: *Researchers wanted to investigate the efficacy of 'Co-ffRee' for reducing coffee intake in undergraduate medical students. A literature search was performed which identified 15 studies, of which seven were RCTs. Of these, five studies were deemed to be of high quality, and a meta-analysis was carried out. Heterogeneity between studies was low, with an I² value of 0%. Data showed that CoffRee was associated with a relative risk of 0.76 (p = 0.006, CI: 0.71–0.81), and, therefore, a risk reduction of 24%.*

Key concepts:

- **Design:**
  - Formulate a question
  e.g., does 'Co-ffRee' reduce coffee consumption in medical students? See Table 4.15
- **Literature search:**
  - Compile search terms and combine with operators "AND" and "OR"
  e.g., 'medical student,' 'undergraduate,' 'student,' 'coffee', 'coffee addiction,' 'coffee' 'consumption'
  - Select studies and extract evidence:
    - After your initial searches, you will likely have quite a lot of studies. You will need to read through

TABLE 4.15   Example of PICO Question Formulation

P	Population	*Undergraduate medical students*
I	Intervention	*'Co-ffRee'*
C	Comparison	*Standard management*
O	Outcome	*Reduced coffee consumption*

the titles and determine if they are relevant. Some systematic reviews may only include RCTs in the meta-analysis.

- **Meta-analysis:**
  - **Homogeneity determined** using *I²* **statistic:** The proportion of the total variation in treatment effect that is due to heterogeneity rather than sampling variation. If *I²* is >50%, heterogeneity is present.
  - The treatment effect is estimated using either **Fixed-effect model** (used for when there is homogeneity) or **Random-effect model** (used for when there is heterogeneity)
  - **Meta-regression:** an attempt to quantify how a treatment effect varies with different study or patient-population characteristics
  - **Sub-group analysis:** a meta-analysis performed for each subgroup of studies. This type of analysis can be used if the studies were found to be heterogenous, but different groups of studies were homogenous.
- **Evaluate the quality of evidence:**
  - **Cochrane risk-of-bias tool:** this tool can be used to assess the quality of an RCT with regards to a study's risk of bias
  - **Outcome-reporting bias:** statistically significant trials are more likely to be published, and

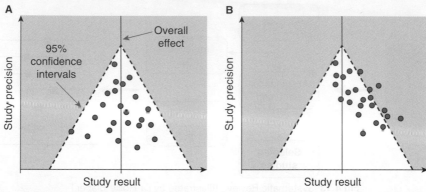

Fig 4.14 Funnel Plots. (A) No reporting bias – symmetrical. (B) Reporting bias - asymmetrical. (Illustrated by Dr Hollie Blaber.)

TABLE 4.16	**Strengths and Weaknesses of a Systematic Review**
Strength	**Weakness**
Very high number of participants, therefore statistically significant	It relies on the quality of trials that have been completed
Cheap and quick	Reporting bias
	Publication bias

positive outcomes are therefore more likely to be reported

If the RCTs looking at Co-ffRee found a really good treatment effect but no effect on overall performance at medical school, they may decide not to report about that outcome. This is why it is important that trial protocols are published prior to trials to avoid an outcome-reporting bias.

- **Publication bias:** large, externally funded studies are more likely to be published quickly in the most accessible forms and are therefore more likely to be included in literature searches than smaller trials. To avoid this, it is important to conduct a thorough search of the literature with inclusive search criteria. Studies with statistically significant results may also be more likely to be published. Funnel plots can be used to determine if publication bias has occurred.
- **Funnel plot** (see Fig 4.14): plots the standard error and the odds ratio of all trials. The plot should be symmetrical.

The trials should produce a symmetrical funnel plot. If they don't, it suggests that trials with less treatment effects

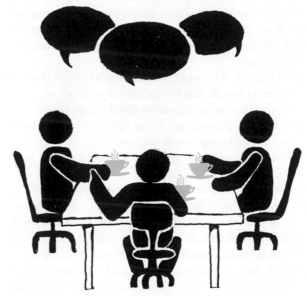

Fig 4.15 Qualitative Research. (Illustrated by Dr Hollie Blaber.)

haven't been published, which could bias our interpretation of the data.

Qualitative Research

Definition: research focusing on understanding and interpreting participants' beliefs and actions (see Fig 4.15 and Table 4.17).

Example: *Researchers wanted to understand how students perceived a coffee addiction in order to identify further areas of research for treatments that could help. A group of 15 students from the coffee addiction self-help group were recruited to be interviewed in order to understand more about their addictions. Interviews were recorded and*

TABLE 4.17 Strengths and Weaknesses of a Qualitative Study

Strength	Weakness
Breadth and depth	Vulnerable to bias
Good for complex situations	
Guide future research	

transcribed verbatim. The data were coded and analysed until saturation was reached. Key themes identified included normalisation of the addiction and improved efficiency.

Key concepts:

- Sampling:
  - **Targeted:** the researcher chooses specific groups of interest

In this case, we have targeted the self-help group, as this is the group we are interested in.

  - **Maximum variation:** sampling extremely contrasting views

In this example, we may decide to also sample the 'anti-coffee' group, since their views would likely be very different and therefore may inform a better understanding of the whole picture.

- Data collection:
  - **Observations:** observe how people behave. This can be biased by the researcher.
  - **Interview:** individually interviewed
  - **Focus group:** thoughts collected in a group setting. This can result in **bias** but is efficient

Data analysis:

- **Coding:** repeated word/idea:

'it's normal', 'everyone else does', 'not much coffee'

- **Theme:** summary of coding

All of the above terms may fit into the theme of 'normalisation'

- Repeat:
  - **Saturation:** continue data collection until no new research themes are identified
  - **Pragmatic:** collect data until a prespecified end point (e.g., after 1 month), even if saturation has not yet been reached

THE ONE-LINE ROUND-UP!

Here are some key words to help you remember each study/concept.

Study/Concept	One-line Description
Ecological	Ecological fallacy
Cross section	Snapshot in time
Case control	Outcome > exposure
Prospective cohort	Exposure > outcome
Retrospective cohort	Looking back in time
RCT	Intervention vs control
Cluster-based RCT	Institutional intervention
Diagnostic testing	Sensitivity and specificity
Economic analysis	Cost vs efficacy
Systematic review	Search all available literature
Meta-analysis	Combine numerical data
Qualitative study	Interviews

THE ONE-LINE ROUND-UP

The Calculations

Calculation	Equation
Mean	$\text{Mean} = \dfrac{\text{sum of variables}}{\text{total number of participants}} \quad \bar{x} = \dfrac{\sum x}{n}$
Standard deviation	$\text{Standard deviation (SD)} = \sqrt{\dfrac{\sum (x - \bar{x})^2}{n-1}}$
Standard error	$\text{Standard error} = \dfrac{SD}{\sqrt{n}}$
Prevalence	$\text{Prevalence} = \dfrac{\text{Number of people with disease}}{\text{Total population at risk}}$

Continued

THE ONE-LINE ROUND-UP—cont'd

Incidence	$$\text{Incidence} = \frac{\text{Number of new cases in a set time period}}{\text{Total population}}$$
Odds	$$\text{Odds} = \frac{\text{Number of people with the outcome}}{\text{Number of people without the outcome}}$$
Odds ratio	$$\text{Odds ratio} = \frac{\text{Odds of disease in exposed group}}{\text{Odds of disease in unexposed group}}$$
Risk	$$\text{Risk} = \frac{\text{Number of people with outcome}}{\text{Total number of people at risk}}$$
Risk ratio	$$\text{Risk ratio} = \frac{\text{Risk of outcome in exposed group}}{\text{Risk of outcome in unexposed group}}$$
Risk difference	$$\text{Risk difference} = \text{Risk of outcome in exposed group} - \text{Risk of outcome in unexposed group}$$
Number needed to treat	$$\text{Number needed to treat} = \frac{1}{\text{Control risk} - \text{Exposed risk}}$$
Sensitivity	$$\text{Sensitivity} = \frac{\text{True positive}}{\text{Total with disease}}$$
Specificity	$$\text{Specificity} = \frac{\text{True negative}}{\text{Total without disease}}$$
PPV	$$\text{Positive predictive value} = \frac{\text{True positive}}{\text{Total with positive test}}$$
NPV	$$\text{Negative predictive value} = \frac{\text{True negative}}{\text{Total with negative test}}$$
Positive likelihood	$$\text{Positive likelihood} = \frac{\text{Sensitivity}}{(1 - \text{Specificity})}$$
Negative likelihood	$$\text{Negative likelihood} = \frac{(1 - \text{Sensitivity})}{\text{Specificity}}$$
ICER	$$\text{ICER} = \frac{\text{Cost of the gold standard} - \text{Cost of the new intervention}}{\text{Efficacy of the gold standard} - \text{Efficacy of the new intervention}}$$

READING LIST: CLINICAL EPIDEMIOLOGY IN AN HOUR

Ranganathan, P., & Aggarwal, R. (2018). Study designs: Part 1 – an overview and classification. *Perspectives in Clinical Research*, 9, 184–186. https://doi.org/10.4103/picr.PICR_124_18.

Aggarwal, R., & Ranganathan, P. (2019). Study designs: Part 2 – descriptive studies. *Perspectives in Clinical Research*, 10, 34–36. https://doi.org/10.4103/picr.PICR_154_18.

Ranganathan, P., & Aggarwal, R. (2019). Study designs: Part 3 – analytical observational studies. *Perspectives in Clinical Research*, 10, 91–94. https://doi.org/10.4103/picr.PICR_35_19.

Aggarwal, R., & Ranganathan, P. (2019). Study designs: Part 4 - interventional studies. *Perspectives in Clinical Research*, 10, 137–139. https://doi.org/10.4103/picr.PICR_91_19.

Basic Structure of a Research Paper and Quantitative Tools

Ali, Z., & Bhaskar, S. B. (2016). Basic statistical tools in research and data analysis. *Indian Journal of Anaesthesia*, 60, 662–669. https://doi.org/10.4103/0019-5049.190623. Published correction appears in *Indian J Anaesth.* 2016, 60, 790.

Ecological Study

Levin, K. (2006). Study design VI – ecological studies. *Evidence Based Dental*, 7, 108. https://doi.org/10.1038/sj.ebd.6400454.

Cross-Sectional Study

Setia, M. S. (2016). Methodology series module 3: Cross-sectional studies. *Indian Journal of Dermatology*, 61, 261–264. https://doi.org/10.4103/0019-5154.182410.

Case-Control Study

Lewallen, S., & Courtright, P. (1998). Epidemiology in practice: Case-control studies. *Community Eye Health*, 11, 57–58.

Prospective Cohort

Kim, H. Y. (2017). Statistical notes for clinical researchers: Risk difference, risk ratio, and odds ratio. *Restorative Dentistry and Endodontics*, 42, 72–76. https://doi.org/10.5395/rde.2017.42.1.72.

Setia, M. S. (2016). Methodology series module 1: Cohort studies. *Indian Journal of Dermatology*, 61, 21–25. https://doi.org/10.4103/0019-5154.174011.

Centers for Disease Control and Prevention. (2012). *Lesson 3: Measures of risk.* https://www.cdc.gov/csels/dsepd/ss1978/lesson3/section2.html. [Accessed July 2020].

Retrospective Cohort Study

Setia, M. S. (2016). Methodology series module 1: Cohort studies. *Indian Journal of Dermatology*, 61, 21–25. https://doi.org/10.4103/0019-5154.174011.

Randomised Controlled Trial (RTC)

Houle, S. (2015). An introduction to the fundamentals of randomized controlled trials in pharmacy research. *Canadian Journal of Hospital Pharmacy*, 68, 28–32. https://doi.org/10.4212/cjhp.v68i1.1422.

NICE

NICE. (2020). *Developing NICE guidelines: the manual.* https://www.nice.org.uk/process/pmg20/chapter/incorporating-economic-evaluation#the-role-of-economics-in-guideline-development. [Accessed July 2020].

NICE. (2015). *How NICE measures value for money in relation to public health interventions.* https://www.nice.org.uk/Media/Default/guidance/LGB10-Briefing-20150126.pdf. https://www.nice.org.uk/glossary?letter=q.

Diagnostic Testing

Parikh, R., Mathai, A., Parikh, S., Chandra Sekhar, G., & Thomas, R. (2008). Understanding and using sensitivity, specificity and predictive values. *Indian Journal of Ophthalmology*, 56, 45–50. https://doi.org/10.4103/0301-4738.37595.

Systematic Reviews

Cochrane. (2019). *Risk of bias tool.* https://sites.google.com/site/riskofbiastool/welcome/rob-2-0-tool/current-version-of-rob-2?authuser=0. [Accessed August 2020].

Higgins, J. P. T., Altman, D. G., Gøtzsche, P. C., Jüni, P., Moher, D., Oxman, A. D., et al. (2011). The Cochrane Collaboration's tool for assessing risk of bias in randomised trials. *BMJ*, 343, d5928.

Qualitative Research

Austin, Z., & Sutton, J. (2014). Qualitative research: getting started. *Canadian Journal of Hospital Pharmacy*, 67, 436–440. https://doi.org/10.4212/cjhp.v67i6.1406.

5

Dermatology in an Hour

Berenice Aguirrezabala Armbruster, James Wiggins,
Nagarjun Konda and Jane Sansom

OUTLINE

INTRODUCTION TO DERMATOLOGY

Skin Layers (see Fig 5.1)

- **Epidermis:** squamous epithelial cell layer
  - Acts as a physical barrier and contains three types of cells: keratinocytes (skin cells), melanocytes (pigment-producing cells), Langerhans cells (immune cells)
- **Dermis:** connective tissue layer. It provides support and consists of:
  - Fibres: collagen (strength) and elastin (elasticity)
  - Cells: fibroblasts (produce collagen), immune cells, muscle cells
- **Subcutis** (a.k.a., subcutaneous tissue, panniculus and hypodermis): contains adipocytes (fat cells), nerves and blood vessels

Types of Lesions (see Fig 5.2)

Flat lesions:
- **Macule:** flat, ≤1 cm
- **Patch:** flat, >1 cm

Lesions involving vessels:
- **Telangiectasia:** superficial capillaries

- **Purpura:** red/purple discolouration, haemorrhage of blood into skin (non-blanching), ≥2 mm
- **Petechiae:** small purpura, <2 mm

Raised lesions:
- **Papule:** raised, solid, ≤5 mm (1 cm in some non-UK definitions)
- **Nodule:** raised, solid, >5 mm (1 cm in some non-UK definitions)
- **Plaque:** flat, elevated, >1 cm

Fluid/pus-containing lesions:
- **Vesicle:** blister, ≤5 mm
- **Bulla:** blister, >1 cm
- **Pustule:** pus-filled papule

Fitzpatrick Skin Types (see Table 5.1)

Topical Corticosteroids (Steroids)

- **Potency:** classified into four types based on their ability to vasoconstrict, reduce inflammation and induce certain side effects (see Table 5.2)
- **Generic name:** official given name
- **Trade name:** name given by manufacturer
- **Fingertip units:** a dose of steroids is prescribed in fingertip units (FTUs). Different amounts are prescribed for different sites (see Fig 5.3).

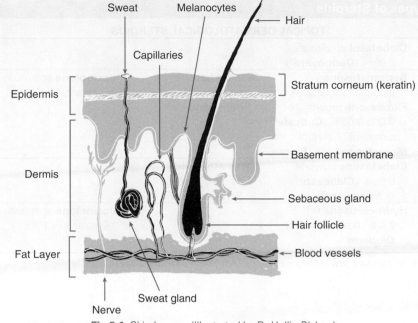

Fig 5.1 Skin Layers. (Illustrated by Dr Hollie Blaber.)

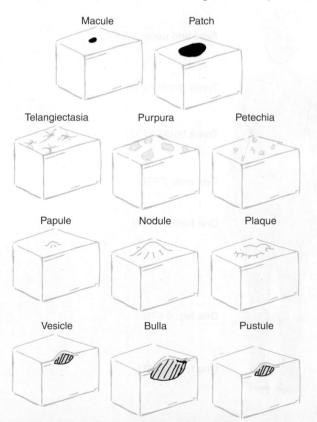

Fig 5.2 Types of skin lesions. (Illustrated by Dr Hollie Blaber.)

TABLE 5.1	**Skin Types**					
	Type 1	**Type 2**	**Type 3**	**Type 4**	**Type 5**	**Type 6**
	Very Fair	**Fair**	**Medium**	**Olive**	**Brown**	**Black**
	Always burns	Usually burns	Sometimes burns	Rarely burns	Never burns	Never burns
	Never tans	Some-times tans	Usually tans	Always tans	Always tans	Always tans

Moisturizers (Emollients) Table

	Composition	**Properties**
Lotion	More water than oil	Evaporates quickly May irritate the skin when applied
Cream	Equal amounts of water and oil	Seals moisture better than lotion May irritate skin when applied
Ointment	More oil than water, paraffin based (NB flammable risk)	Seals moisture better than cream and lotion May lead to acne if long term use Does not irritate skin when applied

TABLE 5.2 **Types of Steroids**

TOPICAL DERMATOLOGICAL STEROIDS		
Very strong	**Clobetasol** propionate 0.05% (**Dermovate**®)	
Strong	**Beclometasone** dipropionate 0.025% **Fluticasone** propionate 0.005–0.05% (**Cutivate**® ointment or cream) **Mometasone** 1% (**Elocon**)	**Betamethasone** valerate 0.1% (**Betnovate**®)	**Fluocinolone** acetonide 0.025% (Synalar®)
Moderate	**Clobetasone** butyrate 0.05% (**Clobavate**® or **Eumovate**®)	**Betamethasone** valerate 0.025% (**Betnovate**-RD®)	
Weak	**Hydrocortisone** 0.1–2.5% (**Dermacort**® or **Dioderm**®)		**Fluocinolone** acetonide 0.0025% (Synalar 1 in 10®)

Adapted from BNF. *Topical steroids.* www.bnf.nice.org.uk [Accessed January 2022]

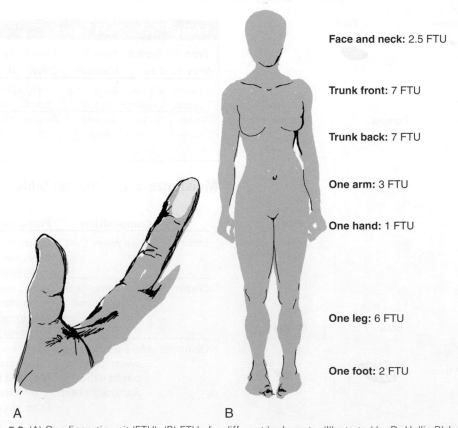

Face and neck: 2.5 FTU

Trunk front: 7 FTU

Trunk back: 7 FTU

One arm: 3 FTU

One hand: 1 FTU

One leg: 6 FTU

One foot: 2 FTU

A   B

Fig 5.3 (A) One fingertip unit (FTU). (B) FTUs for different body parts. (Illustrated by Dr Hollie Blaber.)

DERMATOLOGICAL INFECTIONS

Cellulitis (see Fig 5.4 and 5.5)

Definition: bacterial infection of the dermis and subcutaneous tissue. Most common organisms: *Staphylococcus aureus, Streptococcus pyogenes*

Buzzwords:

- **Risk factors:** break in the skin, venous insufficiency, obesity, pregnancy, oedema, type 2 diabetes mellitus (T2DM)
- **Presentation:** pain, swelling, erythema, warmth +/- systemic symptoms (e.g., fever, malaise, rigors)

Investigations:

- Clinical diagnosis: investigations not required unless uncertain diagnosis. If systemically unwell, consider investigations for sepsis (blood cultures, FBC, U&E, LFTs, CRP, lactate and wound swab if appropriate. Monitor urine output)

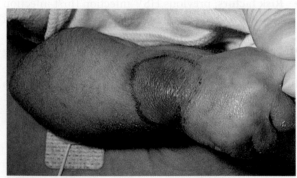

Fig 5.4 Cellulitis in Darker Skin. (With permission from Treat, J., & Fisher B. T. (2015). Bacterial infections (Fig. 12.8). In *Neonatal and infant dermatology*. Elsevier. Copyright © 2015 Elsevier Inc. All rights reserved.)

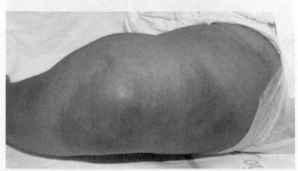

Fig 5.5 Cellulitis in Lighter Skin. (Courtesy of Antonio Torrelo, MD)

- Categorize severity using the Eron classification system:
  - Class I: systemically well and no uncontrolled comorbidities
  - Class II: systemically unwell OR systemically well with uncontrolled comorbidities
  - Class III: severely systematically unwell OR limb-threatening infection
  - Class IV: sepsis OR severe limb-threatening infection (e.g., necrotising fasciitis)

Differentials: erysipelas, impetigo, eczema (contact, venous stasis, atopic), deep vein thrombosis (DVT)/superficial thrombophlebitis, drug reaction, erythema nodosum, insect bite

Management:

1. Decide if patient can be managed in primary care or needs urgent hospital admission:
   - General practitioner (GP): class I
   - Urgent hospital admission: class III or IV (consider class II), immunocompromised, young (<1 year), rapid deterioration, facial/periorbital cellulitis
2. Antibiotics:

- **First-line oral (GP) or IV (hospital) antibiotics:** flucloxacillin (if penicillin allergy: clarithromycin, doxycycline, erythromycin (pregnancy))
- **First-line oral (GP) or IV (hospital) antibiotics if periorbital infection:** co-amoxiclav (if penicillin allergy: clarithromycin with metronidazole)

Impetigo (see Fig 5.6 and 5.7)

Definition: superficial bacterial infection

- **Nonbullous (most common):** caused by *S. aureus, S. pyogenes* or both
- **Bullous (less common):** caused by *S. aureus*

Buzzwords:

- **Risk factors:** close contact with infected individual, sharing of objects with infected individual, preexisting disease, poor hygiene, hot/humid weather
- **Presentation:**
  - **Nonbullous (most common):** presents with small vesicles that rupture, leaving a golden-brown crust
  - **Bullous:** presents with bullae that rupture, leaving a flat, yellow-brown crust

Investigations: clinical diagnosis – investigations not required unless unclear diagnosis

Differentials: cellulitis, erysipelas, eczema (contact, atopic, herpeticum), viral skin infection, staphylococcal scalded skin syndrome, Steven-Johnson syndrome (SJS), toxic epidermal necrolysis (TEN)

Management: primary care management unless complications present (e.g., sepsis) or patient is immunocompromised

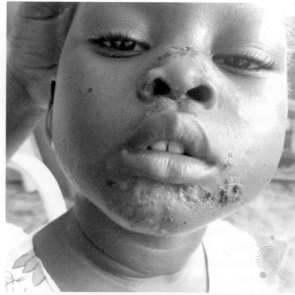

Fig 5.6 Impetigo in Darker Skin. (Skin Deep. (2022). Impetigo.)

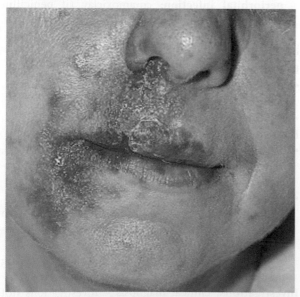

Fig 5.7 Impetigo in Lighter Skin. (With permission from Buttaravoli, P., & Leffler, S. M. (2012) Impetigo (Fig. 172-1). In *Minor emergencies*. Elsevier. Copyright © 2012 Elsevier Inc. All rights reserved.)

- **Localised nonbullous impetigo:** hydrogen peroxide 1% cream (if unsuitable, offer fusidic acid 2% or mupirocin 2%)
- **Widespread bullous impetigo:** short course of a topical antibiotic (fusidic acid 2%) or oral antibiotic (flucloxacillin. If penicillin allergy, clarithromycin or erythromycin)
- **Bullous impetigo:** short course of oral antibiotics (flucloxacillin. If penicillin allergy, clarithromycin or erythromycin)

Herpes Simplex (see Fig 5.8 and Fig 5.9)

Definition:

- Herpes simplex virus serotype 1 (HSV-1): associated with infections of the eyes, lips ('cold sore'), mouth and genitals
- Herpes simplex virus serotype 2 (HSV-2): predominantly associated with genital infections

Buzzwords:

- **Risk factors:** previous HSV infection (first infection is usually the worst), immunosuppression, eczema herpeticum
- **Presentation:** multiple vesicles that rupture, leaving an ulcer that crusts and heals over time

Investigations: clinical diagnosis – no investigations needed unless unclear diagnosis. Viral swabs if diagnosis is unclear

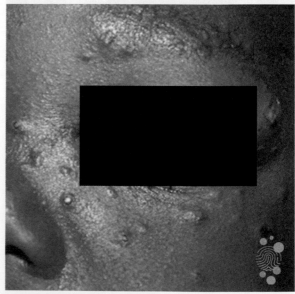

Fig 5.8 Herpes Simplex in Darker Skin. (Skin Deep. (2022). Herpes simplex virus.)

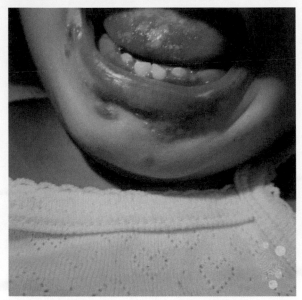

Fig 5.9 Herpes Simplex in Lighter Skin. (Skin Deep. (2022). Herpes simplex virus.)

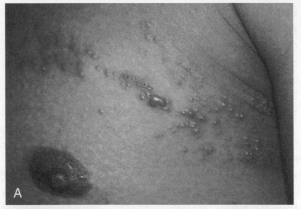

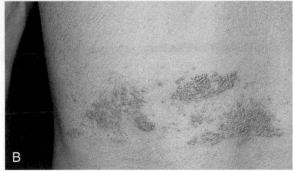

Fig 5.10 (A) Herpes zoster in darker skin, (B) herpes zoster in lighter skin. (With permission from Swartz, M. H. (2014). *Textbook of physical diagnosis* (7th ed.). Philadelphia: Saunders.)

Differentials: Herpes zoster, hand foot and mouth disease, chickenpox, impetigo, sexually transmitted infections (STIs) (genital lesions)

Management:
- **Mild infection:** topical antivirals
- **Severe infection or immunocompromised:** systemic antivirals (e.g., aciclovir, famciclovir or valaciclovir)

Herpes Zoster (Shingles) (see Fig 5.10 A and Fig 5.10 B)

Definition: viral infection of a single nerve and dermatome (skin supplied by that nerve) caused by a reactivation of the varicella-zoster virus (the same virus that causes chickenpox – see Paediatrics in an Hour).

Buzzwords:
- **Risk factors:** elderly, immunocompromised, comorbidities, female, stress
- **Presentation:**
  - Prodrome of pain confined to a single dermatome (burning, stabbing or throbbing)
  - Development of a vesicular rash (dermatomal distribution, does not cross midline, itchy and painful). Vesicles erupt and crust over

- Postherpetic neuralgia can persist >1 month after rash clears

Investigations: clinical diagnosis – investigations not required unless unclear diagnosis. Viral swabs if diagnosis unclear

Differentials: eczema (atopic, herpeticum, contact), herpes simplex, impetigo

Management:
1. Decide if patient can be managed in primary care or needs urgent hospital admission:
   - **GP:** most cases
   - **Hospital care:** complications, ophthalmic distribution of trigeminal nerve affected, immunocompromised
2. Oral antivirals within 72 h of rash appearance. **Always prescribe if** immunocompromised, non-truncal involvement (e.g., rash on face), moderate-to-severe pain/rash. **Consider prescribing if** >50 years of age
3. Analgesia

Candida

Definition: infection with the yeast *Candida albicans*. *C. albicans* is a normal gastrointestinal and vaginal commensal, but transient infections of the oral or vaginal mucosa or between skin folds can occur.

Buzzwords:

- **Risk factors:** skin folds, obesity, diabetes, moisture, inflammation, immunocompromised, drugs (e.g., antibiotics, steroids), other skin conditions, poor hygiene, pregnancy
- **Presentation:** itchy; sore; thin-walled pustules; scaly, white-yellow, curd-like substance; erythematous area

Investigations: clinical diagnosis – investigations not required unless unclear diagnosis

Differentials:

- **Cutaneous:** tinea infection, eczema (contact, atopic, seborrheic), flexural psoriasis, cellulitis, impetigo
- **Oral:** leucoplakia, lichen planus, angular cheilitis, squamous cell carcinoma (SCC)
- **Vaginal:** bacterial vaginosis, trichomoniasis, STIs

Management:

1. Topical antifungals if systemically well and not immunocompromised:
   - Adults: topical imidazoles, such as clotrimazole, econazole, miconazole, ketoconazole or terbinafine
   - Children: same as adults except not ketoconazole or terbinafine
2. Oral antifungals if systemically unwell or severely immunocompromised:
   - Adults and children: oral fluconazole
3. Consider topical hydrocortisone 1% if very itchy
4. Admit to hospital if systemic candidiasis

Pityriasis Versicolor (Tinea Versicolor) (see Fig 5.11 and Fig 5.12)

Definition: yeast infection localised to the *stratum corneum* caused by commensal *Malassezia* species, including *M. globosa* (most common), *M. sympodialis* and *M. furfur*. Most infections occur in healthy individuals.

Buzzwords:

- **Risk factors:** warm/humid environment, excessive sweating, covering of skin by clothes/cream, immunocompromised (although most infections occur in healthy individuals)
- **Presentation:** multiple round/oval macules and confluent patches of hypo- or hyperpigmentation with fine scaling. Asymptomatic usually,

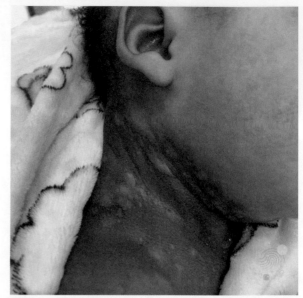

Fig 5.11 Pityriasis Versicolor in Darker Skin. (Skin Deep. (2022). Pityriasis vericolor.)

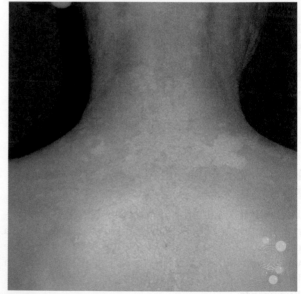

Fig 5.12 Pityriasis Versicolor in Lighter Skin. (Skin Deep. (2022). Pityriasis versicolor.)

sometimes mildly itchy. Usually, young adults in their 20s.

Investigations: clinical diagnosis – investigations not required unless unclear diagnosis. Wood's lamp (ultraviolet (UV) light) examination may show yellow-green fluorescence.

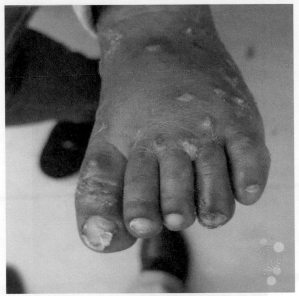

Fig 5.13 Scabies in Darker Skin. (Skin Deep. (2022). Scabies.)

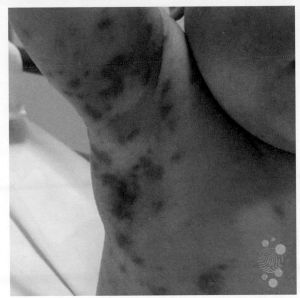

Fig 5.14 Scabies in Lighter Skin. (Skin Deep. (2022). Scabies.)

Differentials: vitiligo, postinflammatory hypopigmentation (e.g., postnummular eczema/guttate psoriasis), pityriasis rosea, tinea corporis

Management:
- **Small area affected:** antifungal creams, such as imidazole creams (e.g., clotrimazole (safe in pregnancy), econazole or ketoconazole)
- **Large area affected:** antifungal shampoo (e.g., ketoconazole 2% or selenium sulphide 2.5% shampoo) or oral itraconazole or fluconazole

Scabies (see Fig 5.13 and Fig 5.14)

Definition: an intensely pruritic rash caused by a skin infestation with the *Sarcoptes scabiei* parasite.

Buzzwords:
- **Risk factors:** close contact with infested individual, crowded environment, female
- **Presentation of scabies:** pruritus (especially at night) with evidence of excoriation, linear burrows, symmetrical erythematous papules (especially in web spaces, fingers, wrist and genitalia), nodules (more likely in long-standing infestation and especially on shaft of penis)
- **Presentation of crusted scabies:** malodorous, thick, erythematous, scaly, crusted lesions containing mites+++, very high risk of transmission

Investigations:
- **Dermoscopy:** triangle or 'delta wing jet' sign of dense head parts of mites

- **Skin scraping and microscopy:** extracted mites/eggs/faecal matter is visible on microscopy

Differentials: insect bites/lice/bedbugs, atopic eczema, folliculitis, dermatitis herpetiformis, eczema (atopic/contact), prurigo nodularis

Management:
1. Permethrin 5% cream (if contraindicated/not tolerated, prescribe malathion aqueous 0.5%)
2. Whole household must be treated. Two treatments, 1 week apart, are necessary to kill mites that have hatched from eggs after the first application. Also, all bed linens need to be washed at high temperatures (60°C wash). Items that cannot be washed or dry cleaned should be sealed in a plastic bag for at least 1 week or put in a freezer.
3. In treatment-resistant scabies, oral systemic treatments such as ivermectin can be used (if >5 years of age, >15 kg, contraindicated in breast feeding/pregnancy).

INFLAMMATORY SKIN CONDITIONS

Atopic Dermatitis (see Fig 5.15 and Fig 5.16)

Definition: atopic dermatitis (eczema) is a chronic inflammatory skin condition characterised by recurrent flares and triggered by multiple factors, including soaps, detergents, animal dander, heat, stress and food.

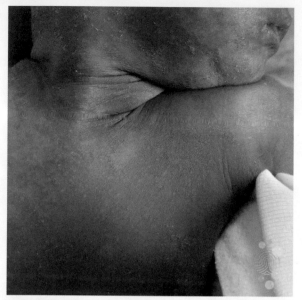

Fig 5.15 Eczema in Darker Skin. (Skin Deep. (2022.) Eczema.)

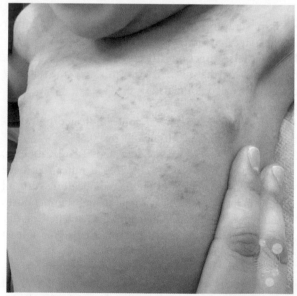

Fig 5.16 Eczema in Lighter Skin. (Skin Deep. (2022). Eczema.)

Buzzwords:
- **Risk factors:** family or personal history of atopy (eczema/asthma/hay fever)
- **Presentation:** dry, itchy rash. It can affect any body site, although commonly affects the extensor surfaces and face in infants. Chronic scratching/rubbing causes lichenification

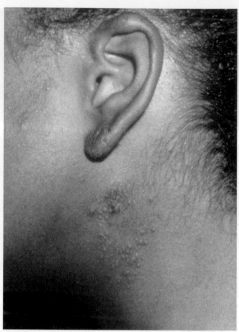

Fig 5.17 Allergic Contact Dermatitis in Darker Skin. (With permission from James, W. D., Elston, D. M., & McMahon, P. J. (2018). Contact dermatitis and drug eruptions (Fig. 5.18A). In *Andrews' diseases of the skin clinical atlas*. Elsevier. Copyright © 2018 Elsevier Inc. All rights reserved.)

Investigations: clinical diagnosis – investigations not required unless unclear diagnosis

Differentials: other types of eczema (contact, seborrheic psoriasis, xerosis, scabies, fungal infection)

Management:
- Conservative: avoidance of triggers/soap, use of soap substitute
- Regular emollients
- Topical steroids (potency depends on location of eczema and severity)

Allergic and Irritant Contact Dermatitis

Definition:
- **Allergic:** type IV (T cell–mediated) delayed hypersensitivity reaction that occurs **after** reexposure to an **allergen,** such as a cosmetic product, metal, topical medication, rubber or plants. A *very small amount* of allergen can provoke a response (see Fig 5.17 and Fig 5.18)
- **Irritant:** immediate inflammatory reaction that occurs **upon direct exposure** to an **irritant,** such as water, detergent, soap, acid or alkali. Response linked to the *intensity/duration of exposure (see Fig 5.19 and 5.20)*

Buzzwords:
- **Risk factors:**
  - **Allergic:** occupational exposure to an allergen (classically hairdressers, beauticians), nickel in jewellery
  - **Irritant:** preexisting dermatitis, recurrent exposure to irritants
- **Presentation:** itchy, erythematous rash and vesiculation (acute phase); dryness, lichenification and fissuring (chronic phase)

Investigations:
- Often a clinical diagnosis for irritant dermatitis
- **Skin patch testing (for allergic dermatitis):** red/pink, itchy and raised area where the substance was applied

Differentials: atopic/seborrheic eczema, psoriasis, infections (e.g., fungal, cellulitis), urticaria, lichen planus

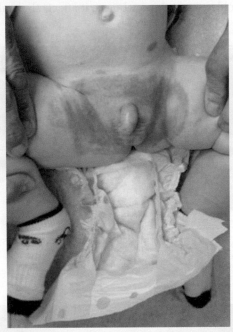

Fig 5.20 Irritant Contact Dermatitis in Lighter Skin. (With permission from James, W. D., Elston, D. M., & McMahon, P. J. (2018). Contact dermatitis and drug eruptions (Fig. 5.15A). In *Andrews' diseases of the skin clinical atlas*. Elsevier. Copyright © 2018 Elsevier Inc. All rights reserved.)

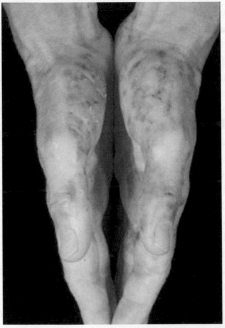

Fig 5.18 Allergic Contact Dermatitis in Lighter Skin. (Courtesy Glen Crawford, MD)

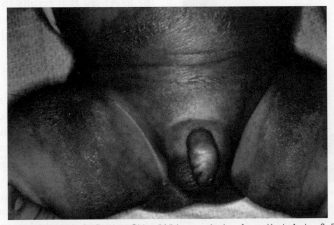

Fig 5.19 Irritant Contact Dermatitis in Darker Skin. (With permission from Krol, A. L., & Bernice R. Krafchik, B. R. (2015). Diaper area eruptions (Fig. 17.1). In *Neonatal and infant dermatology*. Elsevier. *Copyright © 2015 Elsevier Inc. All rights reserved.*)

Management:
1. Identify and avoid irritant/allergen
2. Emollients and topical steroids for acute phase

Seborrhoeic Dermatitis (see Fig 5.21 and Fig 5.22)

Definition: inflammatory skin condition occurring in areas rich in sebaceous glands (e.g., scalp, face, ears, skin folds, chest). In newborns, it affects the scalp and

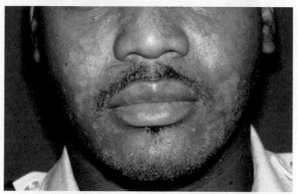

Fig 5.21 Seborrheic Dermatitis in Darker Skin. (Courtesy Scott Norton, MD.)

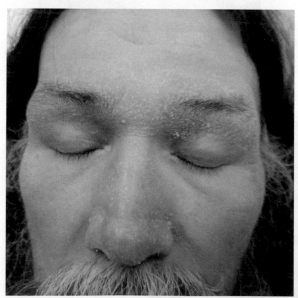

Fig 5.22 Seborrheic Dermatitis in Lighter Skin. (With permission from Cohen, L., Seminario-Vidal, L., & Richard F. Lockey, R. F. (2020). Dermatologic problems commonly seen by the allergist/immunologist. Fig. 2. *The Journal of Allergy and Clinical Immunology: In Practice.* © 2019 American Academy of Allergy, Asthma & Immunology.)

is called cradle cap. Typically occurs in healthy individuals

Buzzwords:
- **Risk factors:** *Malassezia* yeasts, immunocompromised, underlying condition (e.g., Parkinson's disease, stroke, Down syndrome, human immunodeficiency virus (HIV))
- **Presentation:** patches of erythema, flaking of skin, mildly itchy

Investigations: clinical diagnosis – investigations not required unless unclear diagnosis

Differentials: psoriasis, lupus, rosacea, eczema (atopic, contact), tinea capitis, pityriasis (rosea, versicolor)

Management:
- **Adults with scalp and beard involvement:** ketoconazole 2% shampoo. If ineffective, try other shampoos, including those containing zinc pyrithione, coal tar or salicylic acid
- **Adults with face and body involvement:** ketoconazole 2% cream; miconazole 2% + hydrocortisone 1% ('Daktacort')
- **Children with scalp involvement:** topical emollients (e.g., olive oil) and gentle brushing of scales, followed by shampooing. If ineffective, prescribe topical imidazole cream (e.g., clotrimazole 1% or miconazole 2%)
- **Children with body involvement:** imidazole cream or miconazole cream

Venous Eczema (see Fig 5.23 and Fig 5.24)

Definition: venous eczema (a.k.a., varicose eczema or stasis dermatitis) is an inflammatory skin condition of the lower leg that results from valvular incompetence. This condition leads to venous congestion, fluid extravasation and inflammation within the surrounding tissues.

Buzzwords:
- **Risk factors:** overweight, immobility, varicose veins, previous DVT, cellulitis
- **Presentation:** itchy, dry, red, scaly skin in the lower legs that may be painful. Sometimes lipodermatosclerosis (skin thickening) and atrophie blanche (thinning and scarring) may occur

Investigations: clinical diagnosis – investigations not required unless diagnosis is unclear

Differentials: infection (e.g., bacterial, fungal, necrotising fasciitis), DVT, contact dermatitis, vasculitis

Management: weight loss, elevating legs while sitting, compression stockings, topical emollients. Topical steroid for short-term use

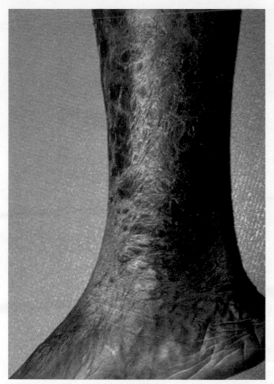

Fig 5.23 Venous Eczema in Darker Skin. (With permission from James, W. D., Elston, D. M., & McMahon, P. J. (2018). Cutaneous vascular diseases (Fig. 35.112). In *Andrews' diseases of the skin clinical atlas*. Elsevier. Copyright © 2018 Elsevier Inc. All rights reserved.)

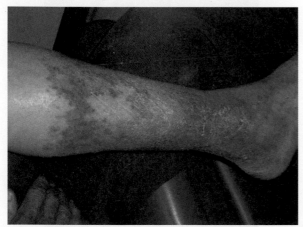

Fig 5.24 Venous Eczema in Lighter Skin. (© Richard P. Usatine)

Discoid Eczema (see Fig 5.25 and Fig 5.26)

Definition: discoid (or 'nummular') eczema is an inflammatory skin condition leading to round areas of inflammation.

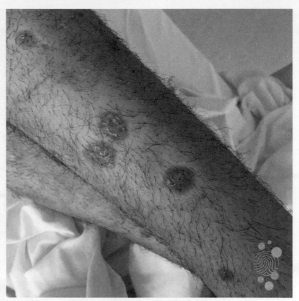

Fig 5.25 Nummular Eczema in Darker Skin. (Skin Deep. (2022). Nummular eczema. https://dftbskindeep.com/all-diagnoses/eczema/#!jig[1]/ML/3614.)

Buzzwords:
- **Risk factors:** adults, male. It can occur in the context of atopic dermatitis
- **Presentation:** coin-shaped and coin-sized pruritic, erythematous plaques. The borders fade gradually (unlike psoriasis)

Investigations: clinical diagnosis – investigations not required unless unclear diagnosis

Differentials: psoriasis (chronic plaque, guttate), pityriasis rosea, tinea corporis, lichen simplex, discoid lupus

Management:
1. Regular emollients
2. Potent or super-potent steroid
3. UV-light therapy
4. Immunosuppressants (e.g., azathioprine, methotrexate, ciclosporin) if extensive or poor response to steroids

Psoriasis (see Fig 5.27 and Fig 5.28)

Definition: immune-mediated, inflammatory skin condition. There are various forms:
- **Chronic plaque psoriasis (most common):** multiple widespread plaques or localised plaques within one region only. If localised, it adopts the name of the region affected (e.g., scalp psoriasis, nail psoriasis, flexural psoriasis).

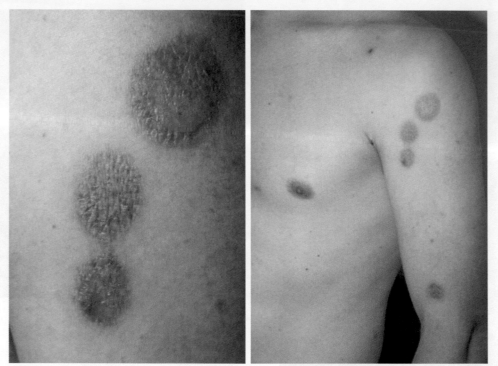

Fig 5.26 Nummular Eczema in Lighter Skin. (With permission from Halberg, M. (2012). Nummular eczema (Fig. 1). *Journal of Emergency Medicine*. Elsevier. Copyright © 2012 Elsevier Inc. All rights reserved.)

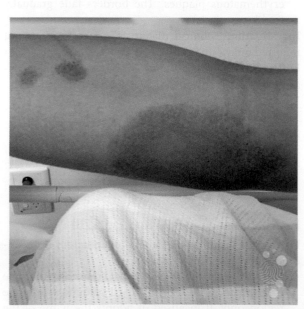

Fig 5.27 Psoriasis in Darker Skin. (Skin Deep. (2022). Psoriasis. https://dftbskindeep.com/all-diagnoses/psoriasis/#!jig[1]/ML/2624.)

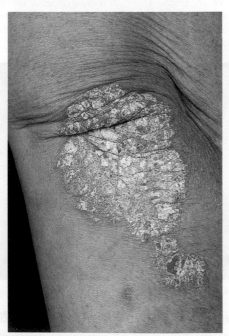

Fig 5.28 Psoriasis in Lighter Skin. (With permission from Cerio, R. (2018). Skin, nails and hair (Fig. 19.5). In: *Hutchison's clinical methods*. Elsevier. Copyright © 2018 Elsevier Ltd. All rights reserved.)

- **Pustular:** chronic plaque psoriasis presenting with pustules. It may present as generalised (medical emergency) or localised to the palms and feet
- **Guttate psoriasis:** psoriasis occurring after an upper respiratory tract infection (URTI) or urinary tract infection (UTI) (classically streptococcal pharyngitis), characterised by multiple small, scaly plaques on the trunk and limbs

Buzzwords:
- **Risk factors:** inherited and environmental factors, such as infection, trauma (Koebner phenomenon), certain medications (e.g., beta blockers, angiotensin-converting enzyme inhibitors (ACEis), antimalarial drugs, lithium), obesity, alcohol, smoking, stress
- **Presentation:** erythematous plaques with silvery-white scale on nail (onycholysis, pitting, salmon patch), scalp, natal cleft, extensor surfaces. Severe cases can be a cause of erythroderma (e.g., after withdrawal of systemic steroids)

Investigations: clinical diagnosis – investigations not required unless unclear diagnosis. Psoriasis Area and Severity Index (PASI) score quantifies severity

Differentials: eczema, tinea corporis, lichen planus, pityriasis rosea, drug eruption, cutaneous T-cell lymphoma, Bowen's disease

Management:
1. **Lifestyle:** smoking cessation, alcohol reduction, weight loss
2. **Topical treatments:** emollients, vitamin D analogues (e.g., calcipotriol), coal tar preparations, topical steroids (especially combined with a vitamin D analogue)
3. **Phototherapy:** used as an additional therapy
4. **Systemic treatments:** immunosuppressants (e.g., ciclosporin, acitretin, methotrexate). **Avoid** systemic steroids due to the risk of severe withdrawal flare

Urticaria, Angioedema and Anaphylaxis

Definition: mast cell immune-mediated reactions leading to raised red rashes, swelling and/or airway problems as a result of exposure to different triggers or allergens. In chronic cases (duration >6 weeks), the trigger often cannot be identified.

Buzzwords:
- **Risk factors:** viral infection, food (e.g., eggs, nuts), insect bites, allergens (e.g., latex), environmental (e.g., sunlight, heat, cold)
- **Presentation:** three types of presentations that may or may not occur simultaneously:

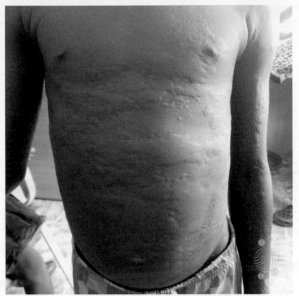

Fig 5.29 Urticaria in Darker Skin. (Skin Deep. (2022). Urticaria. https://dftbskindeep.com/all-diagnoses/urticaria/#!jig[1]/ML/3287.)

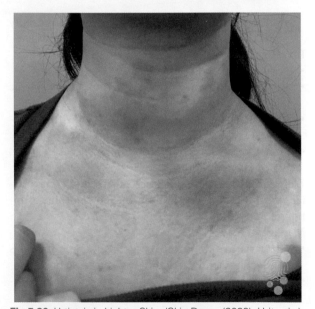

Fig 5.30 Urticaria in Lighter Skin. (Skin Deep. (2022). Uritcaria.)

- Urticaria (a.k.a., hives, wheals, nettle rash): a superficial skin swelling and redness, usually itchy, sometimes with a burning sensation. Duration usually ranges from minutes to 24 h. Can be spontaneous (idiopathic) or inducible (see Fig 5.29 and 5.30)
- Angioedema: a deep skin swelling affecting the face (lips, tongue, eyes), genitalia, feet and hands

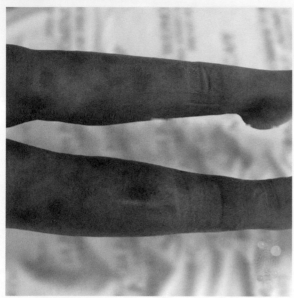

Fig 5.31 Erythema Nodosum in Darker Skin. (Skin Deep. (2022). Erythema nodosum.)

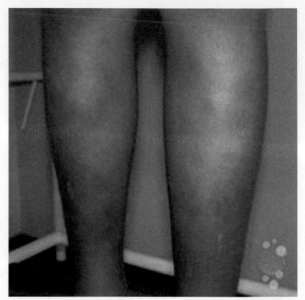

Fig 5.32 Erythema Nodosum in Lighter Skin. (Skin Deep. (2022). Erythema nodosum.)

• Anaphylaxis: a life-threatening hypersensitivity reaction characterised by airway compromise

Investigations:
• None if mild and clear trigger
• Allergy testing: skin prick +/- serum IgE to specific allergens
• Physical challenge (e.g., pressure, cold, dermographism)
• Skin biopsy: if certain conditions suspected (e.g., urticarial vasculitis)

Differentials: eczema (allergic/contact/atopic), urticarial vasculitis, erythema multiforme, polymorphic eruption of pregnancy

Management:
• **Urticaria:** avoid suspected triggers, PO antihistamines (e.g., cetirizine), PO steroids (e.g., prednisolone)
• **Angioedema:** IV/IM chlorphenamine, IV/IM hydrocortisone
• **Anaphylaxis:** see Emergency Medicine in an Hour

Erythema Nodosum (see Fig 5.31 and Fig 5.32)

Definition: a type of panniculitis (inflammation of subcutaneous fat) that results in tender, red nodules, classically on the lower legs.

Buzzwords:
• **Risk factors:** female, infection (e.g., viral/bacterial/fungal), drugs (e.g., oral contraceptive pills (OCPs),

nonsteroidal antiinflammatory drugs (NSAIDs), inflammatory diseases (e.g., irritable bowel disease (IBD), sarcoidosis), malignancy, pregnancy
• **Presentation:** erythematous, tender nodules typically affecting both lower legs but can also affect the thighs and forearms. Spontaneously resolves within 8 weeks in the majority of cases

Investigations: clinical diagnosis – investigations not usually required. Investigate for underlying disorders based on history. Skin biopsy if diagnosis uncertain

Differentials: erysipelas, vasculitis, insect bites, superficial thrombophlebitis, urticaria

Management:
• Treat underlying disease/infection (if present)
• Omit suspected causative medications
• Analgesia (NSAIDs) +/- Colchicine
• Oral steroids (e.g., prednisolone): can be beneficial once infection/malignancy is ruled out

INFLAMMATION OF THE PILOSEBACEOUS UNIT

Acne Vulgaris (see Fig 5.33 and Fig 5.34)

Definition: chronic inflammatory skin condition characterised by open comedones (a.k.a, black heads), closed comedones (a.k.a, white heads), papules, pustules, cysts and/or nodules with background

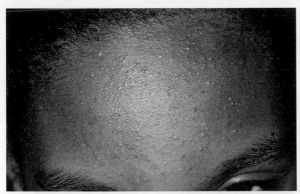

Fig 5.33 Acne in Darker Skin. (With permission from Paller, A. S., & Mancini, A. J. (2016). *Hurwitz clinical pediatric dermatology, a textbook of skin disorders of childhood and adolescence* (5th ed.). Philadelphia: Elsevier.)

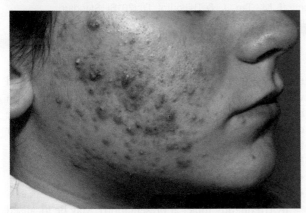

Fig 5.34 Acne in Lighter Skin. (Courtesy Kalman Watsky, MD)

erythema. This condition is caused by excess oil production by sebaceous glands, which is affected by hormones. The bacteria *Cutibacterium acnes* (formerly called *Proprionibacerium acnes)* thrive in this oily environment, causing inflammation and the formation of pustules.

Buzzwords:

- **Risk factors:** puberty, high glycaemic index diet, family history, polycystic ovarian syndrome
- **Presentation:**
  - Mild acne: mainly open and closed comedones with few inflammatory papules and pustules
  - Moderate acne: more inflammatory papules and pustules than in mild acne
  - Severe acne: widespread inflammatory papules, pustules, cysts and nodules

Investigations: clinical diagnosis – investigations not required unless unclear diagnosis

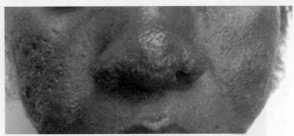

Fig 5.35 Rosacea in Darker Skin. (With permission from Gallo, R. L., Granstein, R. D., Kang, S., Mannis, M., Steinhoff, M., Tan, J., & Thiboutot, D. (2018). Standard classification and pathophysiology of rosacea: The 2017 update by the National Rosacea Society Expert Committee (Fig. 4). *Journal of the American Academy of Dermatology*. Publisher: Elsevier. © 2017 by the American Academy of Dermatology, Inc.)

Differentials: folliculitis, acne rosacea, perioral/seborrheic dermatitis

Management: depends on severity

Mild: topical preparations

- Topical retinoids (e.g., adapalene (Differin 0.1% cream/gel)): avoid in pregnancy
- Benzoyl peroxide wash/gel (Acnecide 5%): safe in pregnancy
- Topical antibiotics: erythromycin, clindamycin

Moderate: systemic preparations

- Oral antibiotics: oxytetracycline or other tetracyclines, such as lymecycline or doxycycline. Erythromycin if contraindicated
- Hormonal agents: combined OCP (COCP), co-cyprindiol

Severe: refer to consultant dermatologist for specialist care

- Oral isotretinoin (teratogenic)

Rosacea (see Fig 5.35 and Fig 5.36)

Definition: chronic inflammatory skin condition causing redness of the face (especially cheeks and nose).

Buzzwords:

- **Triggers:** food/drinks (alcohol, hot drinks, caffeine, cheese), drugs (calcium-channel blockers), environmental (hot shower/bath, sun exposure, warm rooms), topical steroids, oil-based facial creams
- **Presentation:** recurrent episodes of facial flushing, erythema, telangiectasia, papules and pustules, ocular symptoms (dry, gritty, red eyes), scaling, swelling, enlarged nose (rhinophyma, more common in males)

Investigations: clinical diagnosis – investigations not required unless unclear diagnosis

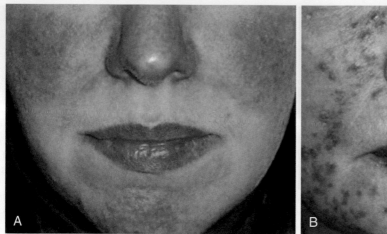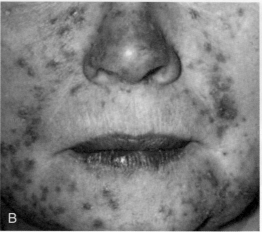

Fig 5.36 Rosacea in lighter skin showing erythema (A) and papules and pustules (B). (With permission from Gallo, R. L., Granstein, R. D., Kang, S., Mannis, M., Steinhoff, M., Tan, J., & Thiboutot, D. (2018). Standard classification and pathophysiology of rosacea: The 2017 update by the National Rosacea Society Expert Committee (Fig. 8). *Journal of the American Academy of Dermatology*. Publisher: Elsevier. © 2017 by the American Academy of Dermatology, Inc.)

Differentials: acne vulgaris, perioral/seborrheic dermatitis, lupus

Management:

1. Conservative: identify and avoid triggers, use of high-factor sunscreen (with both UV-A and UV-B protection), cosmetic camouflage (yellow or green tinting).
2. Manage according to predominant presentation:
- **Erythema:** topical brimonidine 0.5% gel (alpha-adrenergic agonist)
- **Mild-to-moderate papules and/or pustules:** topical preparations only
  - Topical: ivermectin (contraindicated in pregnancy/breastfeeding), metronidazole 0.75%, azelaic acid 15%
- **Moderate-to-severe papules and/or pustules:** topical and oral preparations
  - Topical: same as mild to moderate
  - Oral: doxycycline, oxytetracycline, tetracycline, erythromycin
3. Specialist treatments for severe/resistant cases: oral isotretinoin (teratogenic), laser therapy

IMMUNOBULLOUS DISORDERS

Bullous Pemphigoid (see Fig 5.37)

Definition: autoimmune blistering disorder characterised by autoantibodies (IgG +/- IgE) to collagen type 17 (COL17, a.k.a., BP180), which is associated with the hemidesmosomes located at the junction between the epidermal basement membrane and the dermis, resulting in a loss of adherence and blister formation.

Buzzwords:
- **Risk factors:** elderly
- **Presentation:** thick, tense bullae that do not break easily (frequently intact at presentation). May be localised or widespread on the trunk/proximal limbs/skin folds. Blisters inside the mouth/on genital sites are uncommon. *(Remember – bullous pemphigoiD = Deep (subepidermal) blisters, therefore tense and do not rupture easily)*

Investigations:
- Direct immunofluorescence of biopsy: shows autoantibodies in tissue
- Indirect immunofluorescence of blood sample: shows autoantibodies in blood
- FBC may show eosinophilia

Differentials: pemphigus vulgaris, bullous impetigo, bullous drug eruption, epidermolysis bullosa, linear IgA

Management:
1. Strong topical corticosteroid
2. Tetracycline antibiotics: doxycycline
3. Oral prednisolone in severe/widespread cases: slowly wean until lowest dose achieved
4. Consider immunosuppressive drugs: azathioprine, methotrexate

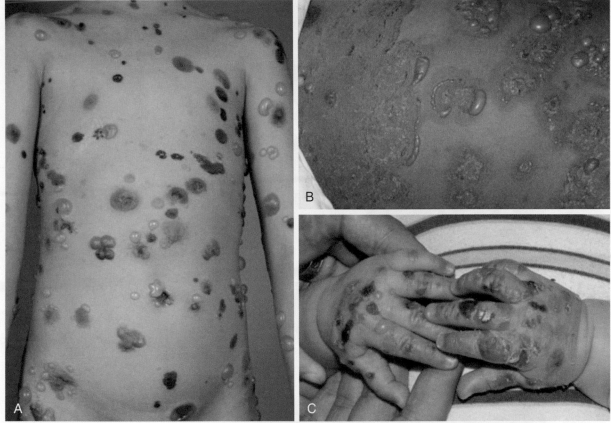

Fig 5.37 Bullous Pemphigoid in Different Skin Tones. (A, With permission from Bernard, P., & Borradori, L. (2018). Pemphigoid group (Fig. 30.7). In *Dermatology: 2-volume set.* Elsevier. Copyright © 2018 Elsevier Ltd. All rights reserved. B,C, Courtesy Julie V Schaffer, MD.)

Pemphigus Vulgaris (see Fig 5.38 and Fig 5.39)

Definition: autoimmune blistering disorder characterised by autoantibodies (IgG) to desmoglein (DSG3, DSG1) proteins present on keratinocytes within the epidermis.

Buzzwords:

- **Risk factors:** adults (40–60 years of age), Jewish and Indian ethnic origins
- **Presentation:** painful blisters of the mucous membranes (e.g., mouth, throat, nose, eyes, genital area) that break easily, leaving an area of erosion. May present with few/no intact blisters. (Remember – pemphigu**S** = **S**uperficial (intraepidermal) blisters, therefore thin-walled and rupture easily)

Investigations:

- For diagnosis: **direct immunofluorescence of biopsy** shows autoantibodies in tissue

- To monitor disease: **indirect immunofluorescence of blood samples** show autoantibodies in serum

Differentials: bullous pemphigoid, other causes of oral ulcers (e.g., Behçet's disease, aphthous), bullous impetigo, Hailey-Hailey disease, bullous drug eruption, linear IgA

Management:

1. Oral corticosteroids
2. Consider immunosuppressive drugs: azathioprine, cyclophosphamide, methotrexate

SKIN CANCER

Basal Cell Carcinoma (BCC)

Definition: most common skin cancer, slow-growing, locally invasive, malignant, keratinocyte-derived (non-melanomatous) skin cancer that rarely spreads and has a

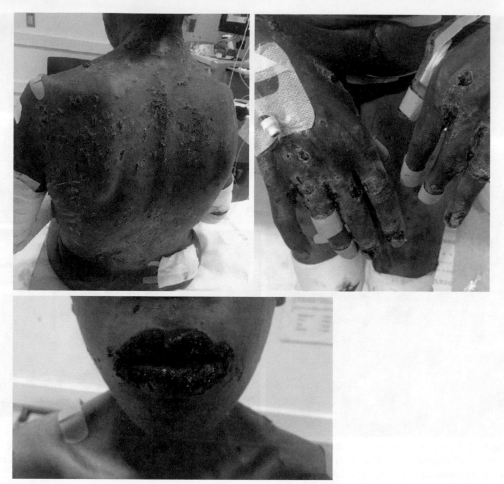

Fig 5.38 Pemphigus Vulgaris in Darker Skin. (With permission from Klufas, D., M., Amerson, E., Twu, O., Clark, L., & Shinkai, K. (2020). Refractory pemphigus vulgaris successfully treated with ofatumumab (Fig. 1). *JAAD Case Reports.* Elsevier. © 2020 by the American Academy of Dermatology, Inc. Published by Elsevier, Inc.)

good prognosis if removed. There are multiple clinical and histological variants. The clinical variants to be aware of include nodular, superficial, morphoeic and basosquamous.

Buzzwords:

- **Risk factors:** sun exposure, sunbeds, Fitzpatrick skin types I and II, previous BCC, genetic conditions (rare, e.g., Gorlin's syndrome, xeroderma pigmentosa)
- **Presentation:**
  - **Nodular BCC** (most commonly facial): pearly nodule, smooth surface, central ulceration, rolled edges (see Fig 5.40), arborising (branching) telangiectasias, incomplete healing
  - **Superficial BCC** (most common in young adults, trunk and shoulders): scaly, irregular plaque; translucent rolled border; multiple microerosions
  - **Morphoeic BCC**: waxy, scar-like, usually midfacial, can infiltrate local nerves
  - **Basosquamous:** mixed basal and squamous

Investigations:

- **Dermoscopy:** arborising vessels, central ulceration
- **Pathology following biopsy or removal:** histological changes consistent with BCC (e.g., positive cytokeratin stain)

Differentials: skin cancers (SCC, amelanotic melanoma), keratoacanthoma, molluscum contagiosum, sebaceous hyperplasia

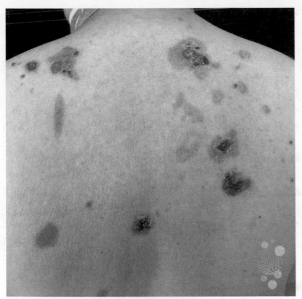

Fig 5.39 Pemphigus Vulgaris in Lighter Skin. (Skin Deep. (2022). Pemphigus vulgaris.)

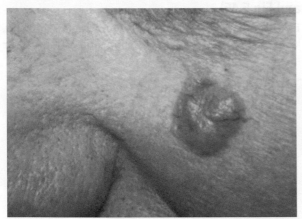

Fig 5.40 Nodular Basal Cell Carcinoma. (Courtesy Stanley J. Miller, MD)

Management:
- **Localised superficial:** options include 5-fluorouracil cream, imiquimod, curettage and cautery, cryotherapy, cream, photodynamic therapy
- **Localised deep:** surgical removal +/- radiotherapy (avoid in young)

Actinic Keratosis (AK) (see Fig 5.41)

Definition: actinic keratosis (a.k.a., solar keratosis) is a precancerous, scaly lesion found on sun-damaged skin. Left untreated, the lesions can progress to SCC, and

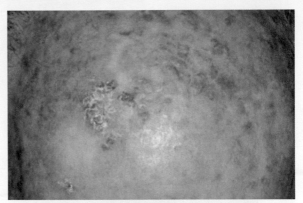

Fig 5.41 Actinic Keratosis in Lighter Skin. (Courtesy H. Peter Soyer, MD)

multiple actinic keratoses predispose to other forms of skin cancer.

Buzzwords:
- **Risk factors:** Fitzpatrick skin types I/II, chronic occupational/recreational sun exposure, increasing age, immunosuppression, bald scalp
- **Presentation:** flat/thickened papule or plaque with white/yellow scaly surface on sun-exposed areas (commonly scalp, ears, face, dorsum of forearm/hand). Can be itchy/tender.

Investigations:
- **Dermoscopy:** surface scales, erythema, irregular shape
- **Skin biopsy:** if diagnosis unclear, to exclude SCC or if treatment is ineffective

Differentials: skin cancers (e.g., SCC, BCC), precancerous conditions (e.g., Bowen's disease)

Management:
- **Conservative:** sun protection, regular moisturiser use
- **Nonsurgical:** cryotherapy (liquid nitrogen); topical treatments: diclofenac, 5-fluorouracil, imiquimod; photodynamic therapy
- **Surgical:** curettage and cautery or excision. Useful if diagnosis unclear (histological confirmation)

Bowen's Disease (SCC In Situ) (see Fig 5.42 and Fig 5.43)

Definition: Bowen's disease (a.k.a., SCC in situ) is a nonhereditary, keratinocyte-derived, premalignant skin lesion, of which around 5% progress to invasive SCC.

Buzzwords:
- **Risk factors:** UV light from sun or sunbeds, Fitzpatrick skin types I and II, immunosuppressed

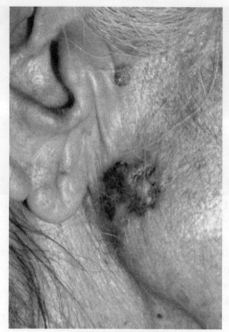

Fig 5.42 Pigmented Bowen's Disease in Darker Skin. (With permission from Verma, S. B. (2011). Dermatology for the elderly: An Indian perspective (Fig. 4). *Clinics in Dermatology.* Elsevier. Copyright © 2011 Elsevier Inc. All rights reserved.)

- **Presentation:** slow growing; red, scaly area; surface catches on clothing. May occasionally look like psoriasis, but, unlike psoriasis, the borders are irregular. Occurs in sun-exposed areas and does not have the symmetry expected with psoriasis

Investigations:

- **Dermoscopy:** red, scaly area with irregular borders
- **Skin biopsy:** histological changes consistent with Bowen's disease

Differentials: skin cancers (e.g., SCC, BCC), inflammatory conditions (e.g., discoid eczema, psoriasis)

Management: consider 2-week wait (2WW) referral if possibility of SCC

- **Localised superficial:** options include curettage and cautery, freezing with liquid nitrogen cryotherapy, 5-fluorouracil (Efudix) cream, imiquimod (Aldara) cream, photodynamic therapy
- **Localised deep:** surgical removal +/- radiotherapy

Squamous Cell Carcinoma (SCC) (see Fig 5.44 and Fig 5.45)

Definition: nonhereditary, slow-growing, malignant, keratinocyte-derived (non-melanomatous) skin cancer

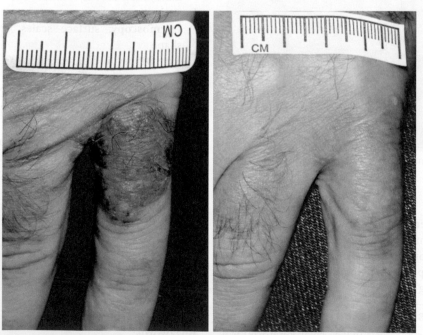

Fig 5.43 Bowen's Disease in Lighter Skin Before and After Photodynamic Therapy. (With permission from Attili, S. K., & Ibbotson, S. H. (2009). How we treat Bowen's disease with topical photodynamic therapy in Dundee (Fig. 3). *Photodiagnosis and Photodynamic Therapy.* Elsevier. Copyright © 2009 Elsevier B.V. All rights reserved.)

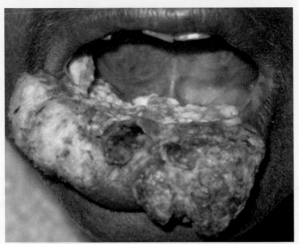

Fig 5.44 Squamous Cell Carcinoma in Darker Skin. (With permission from Verma, S. B. (2011). Dermatology for the elderly: An Indian perspective (Fig. 7). *Clinics in Dermatology*. Elsevier. Copyright © 2011 Elsevier Inc. All rights reserved.)

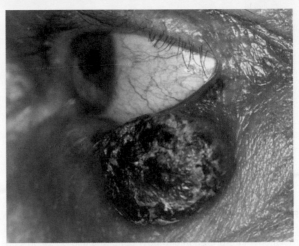

Fig 5.46 Melanoma in Darker Skin. (With permission from Tse, D. T., & Hui, J. I. (2017). Malignant eyelid tumors (Fig. 29.2). In *Cornea, 2-Volume Set*. Elsevier. Copyright © 2017 Elsevier Inc. All rights reserved.)

Investigations:
- **Dermoscopy:** central ulceration/keratin, surrounding erythema
- **Skin biopsy:** histological changes consistent with SCC
- **Imaging** (USS/CT/MRI): if high risk/lymphadenopathy present, assess for metastatic spread

Differentials: skin cancers (BCC, nodular melanoma), Bowen's disease, keratoacanthoma

Management: 2WW referral to dermatologist
- Localised superficial: curettage and cautery
- Localised deep: surgical removal +/- radiotherapy
- Lymph node spread: surgical removal + radiotherapy + chemotherapy

Malignant Melanoma (see Fig 5.46 and Fig 5.47)

Definition: malignant skin cancer caused by an abnormal proliferation of melanocytes that can metastasise to other sites. Subtypes include:
- Superficial spreading melanoma (most common type)
- Nodular melanoma
- Lentigo maligna (a.k.a., melanoma *in situ,* confined to epidermis)
- Lentigo maligna melanoma (invading into the dermis)
- Acral lentiginous melanoma

Buzzwords:
- **Risk factors:** UV light (sun or sunbeds), Fitzpatrick skin types I and II, family/personal history of

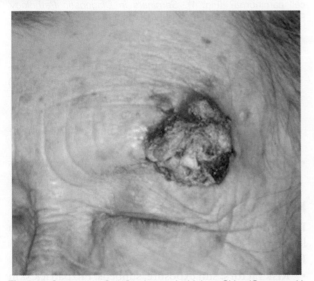

Fig 5.45 Squamous Cell Carcinoma in Lighter Skin. (Courtesy H. Peter Soyer, MD.)

that rarely spreads (more often than BCC). Most common sites for lymphatic spread are the ear and lip.

Buzzwords:
- **Risk factors:** age, sun exposure, sunbeds, Fitzpatrick skin types I and II, previous skin cancer, immunosuppressed, chronic inflammation (e.g., chronic ulceration), preexisting AK/Bowen's
- **Presentation:** scaly, crusted nodule with underlying erythema, located on sun-exposed sites, commonly ulcerates, often tender/painful

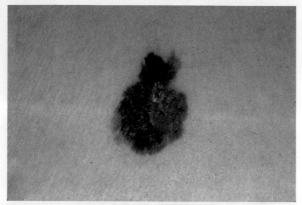

Fig 5.47 Melanoma in Lighter Skin. (With permission from Ricotti, C., Cather, J., & Cockerell, C. J. (2011). Pathology of melanoma interpretation and new concepts (Fig. 27.3). In *Cancer of the skin*. Elsevier. Copyright © 2011 Elsevier Inc. All rights reserved.)

melanoma/non-melanoma skin cancer, increasing age, large number of moles, >5 atypical naevi
- **Presentation:** ABCDE (**A**symmetry, **B**orders irregular, **C**olour uneven, **D**iameter >6 mm, **E**volving lesion)

Investigations:
- **Dermoscopy:** asymmetry, irregular borders, uneven colour, diameter >6 mm
- **Skin biopsy:** staging using the Breslow thickness (BT) to predict the likelihood of spreading:
  - <1mm depth: small chance of spreading
  - >1mm depth: large chance of spreading
- Sentinel lymph node biopsy: staging
- CT/MRI/PET: staging

Differentials: skin cancers (e.g., BCC, especially pigmented BCCs), benign lesions (e.g., atypical naevus, pigmented seborrheic keratosis)

Management: refer any suspected melanoma on 2WW pathway
- **Stage 1 (confined to skin, BT ≤2 mm):** wide local excision (WLE) (1–2 cm around affected area)
- **Stage 2 (confined to skin, BT >2 mm / >1 mm + ulceration):** WLE (>2 cm around affected area)
- **Stage 3 (spread to local lymph node):**
  - Surgery: removal of melanoma and lymphadenectomy
  - If surgery not an option, consider talimogene laherparepvec (or T-VEC, a genetically modified virus) injections directly into tumour to destroy malignant cells

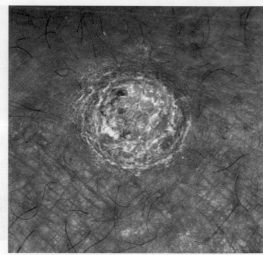

Fig 5.48 Keratoacanthoma in Darker Skin. (With permission from Mandrell, J. C., & Santa Cruz, D. J. (2009). Keratoacanthoma: hyperplasia, benign neoplasm, or a type of squamous cell carcinoma? (Fig. 1). *Seminars in Diagnostic Pathology*. Elsevier. Copyright © 2009 Published by Elsevier Inc.)

- Targeted therapy: if genetics confirm BRAF mutations, consider BRAF inhibitors (e.g., dabrafenib) + MEK inhibitor (e.g., trametinib).
- Immunotherapy: nivolumab, pembrolizumab. Encourages the immune system to target melanoma cells
- **Stage 4 (distant metastasis):** same interventions as stage III + radiotherapy + chemotherapy

Keratoacanthoma (see Fig 5.48 and Fig 5.49)

Definition: nonhereditary, fast-growing benign skin lesion with a good prognosis

Buzzwords:
- **Risk factors:** sun exposure, sunbeds, Fitzpatrick skin types I and II, immunosuppressed, smoking, BRAF inhibitors
- **Presentation:** starts as a pimple-like lesion and rapidly turns into a lump with a crater in the middle (volcano appearance). Most will spontaneously regress (disappear) leaving a scar, but very difficult to distinguish from SCC

Investigations:
- **Dermoscopy:** volcano-like lesions, central keratin
- **Excision biopsy:** histological changes consistent with keratoacanthoma

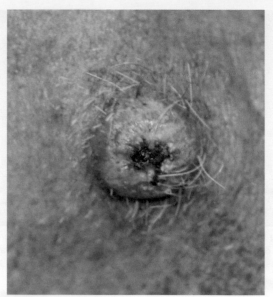

Differentials: skin cancers (e.g., SCC, BCC), benign lesions (e.g., AK, seborrheic keratosis)

Management: 2WW referral to dermatologist to rule out other more serious differentials

- Surgical excision: most common
- Small keratoacanthomas: other options include curettage and cautery or freezing with liquid nitrogen (cryotherapy)

Seborrhoeic Keratosis (see Fig 5.50 and Fig 5.51)

Definition: benign, warty growth that is very common in older age

Buzzwords:
- **Risk factors:** increasing age
- **Presentation:** variable, most commonly a warty, brown plaque (can be skin coloured) with a cerebriform (brainlike) surface and a 'stuck on' appearance, can present anywhere

Investigations:
- **Dermoscopy:** characteristic orange or brown clods (keratin plugs), cerebriform (brainlike) surface
- **Skin biopsy:** features characteristic of seborrheic keratosis

Differentials: warty naevus, skin cancers (e.g., pigmented BCC/melanoma, especially for pigmented seborrheic keratoses)

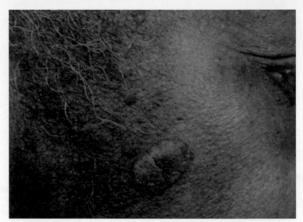

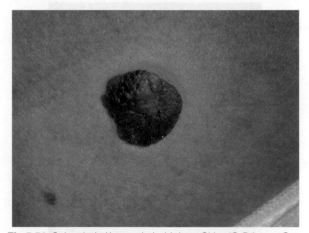

Management:
- **Conservative:** reassurance, education regarding likelihood of growth and more lesions developing
- **Cryotherapy:** used for smaller lesions
- **Excision:** if recurrent irritation or if diagnosis uncertain

PIGMENTARY SKIN DISORDERS

Melasma (see Fig 5.52 and Fig 5.53)

Definition: melasma (a.k.a., chloasma, pregnancy mask) is a non-hereditary, pigmented skin condition characterised by the development of brown/grey areas on the skin.

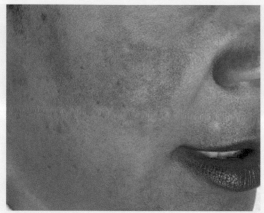

Fig 5.52 Melasma in Darker Skin. (With permission from Bolognia, J. L, Schaffer, J. V., Duncan, K. O., & Ko, K. J. (2014). Disorders of hyperpigmentation (Fig. 55.2). In *Dermatology essentials*. Elsevier. Copyright © 2014 Elsevier Inc. All rights reserved.)

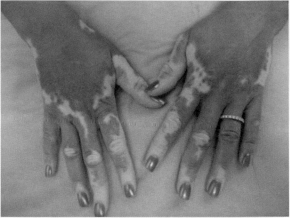

Fig 5.54 Vitiligo in Darker Skin. (With permission from Harris, J., & Rashighi, M. (2018). Vitiligo. In *Treatment of skin disease*. Elsevier. Copyright © 2018 Elsevier Ltd. All rights reserved.)

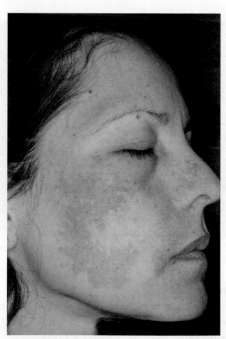

Fig 5.53 Melasma in Lighter Skin. (With permission from Sheth, V. M, & Pandya, A. G. (2011). Melasma: A comprehensive update. Part I (Fig. 3). *Journal of the American Academy of Dermatology*. Elsevier. Copyright © 2010 American Academy of Dermatology, Inc. Published by Mosby, Inc. All rights reserved.)

Buzzwords:
- **Risk factors:** pregnancy, COCP, thyroid disorders, UV light exposure
- **Presentation:** flat brown/grey areas of pigmentation

Investigations: clinical diagnosis – investigations not required unless unclear diagnosis

Differentials: acanthosis nigricans, inflammatory (e.g., lupus, post-inflammatory hyperpigmentation), drug-induced photosensitivity

Management: there is no cure for melasma; rather, treatments aim to improve the appearance and prevent further areas of pigmentation. If it occurs during pregnancy, it may resolve after childbirth. Cessation of COCP may also help

1 Avoid triggers, sun protection and skin camouflage
2 Skin-lightening creams and procedures (e.g., chemical peels, microneedling, laser therapy)

Vitiligo (see Fig 5.54 and Fig 5.55)

Definition: hereditary autoimmune skin condition targeting melanocytes, resulting in a loss of normal skin pigmentation

Buzzwords:
- **Risk factors:** other autoimmune conditions, repeated trauma
- **Presentation:** white/pink areas of depigmentation, can occur in any skin type but is more visible in Fitzpatrick skin types IV–VI

Investigations: clinical diagnosis – investigations not required unless unclear diagnosis

Differentials: fungal infection (e.g., pityriasis versicolour), post-inflammatory hypopigmentation, leprosy

Management: there is no cure; rather, treatments aim to improve pigmentation

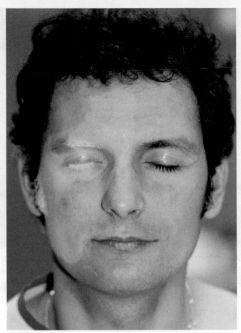

Fig 5.55 Vitiligo in Lighter Skin. (With permission from Ezzedine, K., Eleftheriadou, V., Whitton, M., & van Geel, N. (2015). Vitiligo (Fig. 1). *The Lancet*. Elsevier. Copyright © 2015 Elsevier Ltd. All rights reserved.)

- Topical treatments: sun cream, topical corticosteroids, topical vitamin D analogue, skin camouflage
- Other options: laser treatment, phototherapy

HAIR LOSS

Alopecia Areata (see Fig 5.56)

Definition: hair loss due to inflammation. The cause of the inflammation is unknown, but the condition is associated with other autoimmune conditions such as thyroid disease.

Buzzwords:
- **Risk factors:** family history
- **Presentation:** nonscarring, noninflamed areas of hair loss

Investigations: none if characteristic clinical changes
- **Hair-pull test:** positive test (≥3 hairs pulled away)

Differentials: tinea capitis, telogen effluvium, trichotillomania (hair pulling), androgenic alopecia

Management:
1. Topical treatments: steroid creams/injections, topical immunosuppressants
2. Psoralen plus UVA light therapy (PUVA)

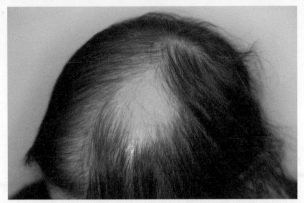

Fig 5.56 Alopecia. (With permission from Paller, A. S., & Mancini, A. J. (2016). *Hurwitz clinical pediatric dermatology, a textbook of skin disorders of childhood and adolescence* (5th ed.). Philadelphia: Elsevier.)

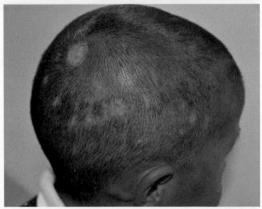

Fig 5.57 Tinea Capitis. (With permission from Tang, J., Ran, X., & Ran, Y. (2017). Ultraviolet dermoscopy for the diagnosis of tinea capitis (Fig. 1). *Journal of the American Academy of Dermatology*. Elsevier. © 2016 by the American Academy of Dermatology, Inc.)

3. Systemic treatment: steroid tablets, oral immunosuppressants
4. Conservative options: wigs and hair pieces

Tinea Capitis (see Fig 5.57)

Definition: tinea capitis (a.k.a., scalp ringworm) is a fungal infection of the scalp that can lead to hair loss.

Buzzwords:
- **Risk factors:** children, close contact with infected individual (e.g., sharing towels)
- **Presentation:** itchy, red, **scaly** scalp; hair loss

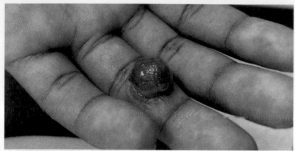

Fig 5.58 Pyogenic Granuloma in Darker Skin. (With permission from Allen, R., Shah, K., & Jayanth, A. (2021). Slam dunk diagnosis: Pyogenic granuloma after basketball injury. *Journal of Emergency Medicine*. Elsevier. Date: April 2021. Figure 1 © 2020 Elsevier Inc. All rights reserved.)

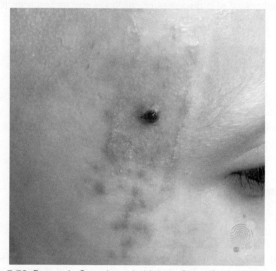

Fig 5.59 Pyogenic Granuloma in Lighter Skin. (SKINDEEP.)

Investigations: scale/hair sample for culture shows fungal infection
Differentials: alopecia areata, eczema (atopic, seborrheic), psoriasis, trichotillomania
Management: oral antifungals AND antifungal shampoo. Good hygiene (avoid sharing of towels)

VASCULAR DERMATOLOGY

Pyogenic Granuloma (see Fig 5.58 and Fig 5.59)

Definition: harmless overgrowth of blood vessels due to an unknown cause but sometimes triggered by minor trauma
Buzzwords:
- **Risk factors:** children, young adults, trauma, retinoids

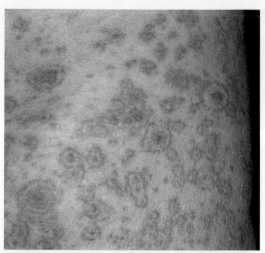

Fig 5.60 Erythema Multiforme in Lighter Skin. (With permission from Avarbock, A., & Jorizzo, J. L. Erythema multiforme, Stevens-Johnson syndrome, and toxic epidermal necrolysis (Fig. 11-1). In *Dermatological signs of systemic disease*. Elsevier. Copyright © 2017 Elsevier Inc. All rights reserved.)

- **Presentation:** red skin lump (like a raspberry) most commonly on the fingers, scalp and face that may bleed easily after minor trauma
Investigations: clinical diagnosis – investigations not required unless unclear diagnosis
Differentials: skin cancers (e.g., BCC, SCC, melanoma), congenital haemangioma
Management: curettage and cautery or excision

DERMATOLOGY EMERGENCIES

Erythema Multiforme (EM) (see Fig 5.60, Fig 5.61 and Fig 5.62)

Definition: hypersensitivity skin reaction commonly triggered by infections. Causes include HSV 1 and 2, *Mycoplasma* pneumonia, fungal infections, drugs (e.g., NSAIDs, penicillins, barbiturates, anticonvulsants – less common cause)
Buzzwords:
- **Risk factors:** 20–40 years of age, male, HLA-DQw3
- **Presentation:** target lesions +/- mucosal, genital and conjunctival involvement, Köebner's phenomenon
Investigation: clinical diagnosis – investigations not required unless unclear diagnosis
Differentials: erythroderma, burns, staphylococcal scalded skin syndrome, SJS, TEN

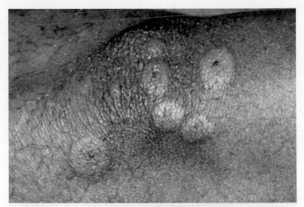

Fig 5.61 Erythema Multiforme in Darker Skin. (With permission from James, W. D., Elston, D. M., & McMahon, P. J. (2018). Contact dermatitis and drug eruptions (Fig. 7.9). In *Andrews' diseases of the skin clinical atlas.* Elsevier. Copyright © 2018 Elsevier Inc. All rights reserved.)

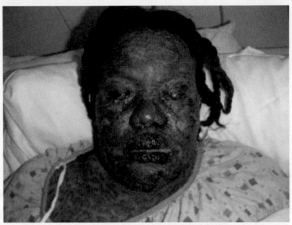

Fig 5.63 Toxic Epidermal Necrolysis in Darker Skin. (Courtesy of Barry Hahn, MD, Department of Emergency Medicine, Staten Island University, Norwell Health.)

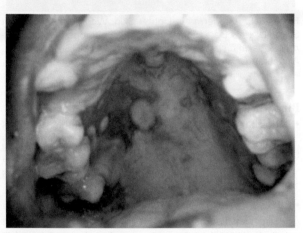

Fig 5.62 Erythema Multiforme of the Palate. (With permission from Silverman, S. (2007). Mucosal lesions in older adults (Fig. 5). *The Journal of the American Dental Association.* Elsevier. Copyright © 2007 American Dental Association. Published by Elsevier Inc. All rights reserved.)

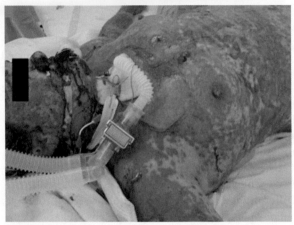

Fig 5.64 Toxic Epidermal Necrolysis in Lighter Skin. (With permission from Downey, A., Jackson, C., Harun, N., et al. (2012). Toxic epidermal necrolysis: Review of pathogenesis and management. *Journal of the American Academy of Dermatology* 66, 995–1003.)

Management: treat underlying cause (e.g., cyclovir for HSV, stop offending drugs). Erythema multiforme usually resolves in 3–5 weeks without complications

Stevens-Johnson Syndrome and Toxic Epidermal Necrolysis (see Fig 5.63 and Fig 5.64)

Definition: SJS and TEN are drug-related, severe, immune complex–mediated hypersensitivity skin reactions characterised by skin and mucosal loss. SJS and TEN are classified according to the percentage of the body surface area that is detached. SJS is characterised

by <10% epidermal detachment, while TEN is a lot more severe, with >30%. Causes include antibiotics (e.g., penicillin and cephalosporins), sulphonamides (e.g., cotrimoxazole, trimethoprim and sulfasalazine), anticonvulsants (e.g., phenytoin, valproic acid, lamotrigine), NSAIDs and salicylates.

Buzzwords:
- **Risk factors:** females > males, 100× more common in individuals with HIV
- **Presentation:** lesions commonly affect the extensor surfaces, dorsum of hand, palms or trunk. Widescale erythema, target lesions (as in erythema

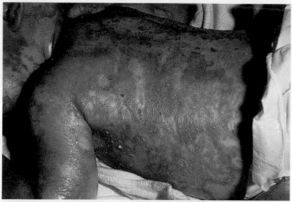

Fig 5.65 Erythroderma in Darker Skin. (With permission from Levy, M. L. (2015). Erythrodermas, immunodeficiency, and metabolic disorders (Fig. 18.14). In *Neonatal and infant dermatology*. Elsevier. Copyright © 2015 Elsevier Inc. All rights reserved.)

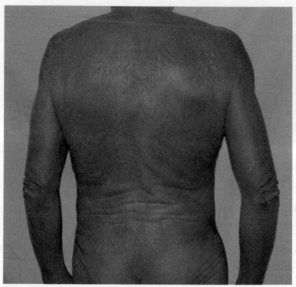

Fig 5.66 Erythroderma in Lighter Skin. With permission from Shim, T. N., & Berth-Jones, J. (2018). Erythroderma. In *Treatment of skin disease*. Elsevier. Copyright © 2018 Elsevier Ltd. All rights reserved.

multiforme), flaccid blisters and erosions. Mucosal involvement (e.g., mouth ulcers; red, crusted lips), eye involvement (e.g., conjunctivitis, corneal ulcers), genital involvement (e.g., balanitis, erosive vulvovaginitis)

Investigations: clinical diagnosis – investigations usually not required unless unclear diagnosis
- Blood: anaemia, ↓ WCC, ↓ neutrophils, ↓ lymphocytes, ↑ eosinophils
- Skin biopsy

Differentials: erythema multiforme, erythroderma, bullous pemphigoid, burns, pemphigus vulgaris, staphylococcal scalded skin syndrome

Management:
1. Remove causative drug immediately and perform A–E assessment
2. Assess criteria using SCORTEN. Patients with SCORTEN >3 should be managed in the ICU
3. Consider transfer to a burn centre to supplement supportive treatment with surgical measures
4. Supportive treatment involves fluid replacement, analgesia, ophthalmology assessments, frequent skin assessment for infection, tissue debridement and dressing

Erythroderma (see Fig 5.65 and Fig 5.66)

Definition: widespread and intense inflammatory reddening of the skin with associated severe itching and pain affecting >90% of the skin surface

Buzzwords:
- **Risk factors:** worsening psoriasis, unstable psoriasis + infection/new drug/stopping corticosteroids, drug eruption (e.g., antibiotics, ACEi, anticonvulsants, NSAIDs, tricyclics), atopic dermatitis and pityriasis rubra pilaris
- **Presentation:** may be preceded by a morbilliform eruption (measles-like) followed by generalised erythema. Skin may be tender, hot and itchy. Lichenification and scaling may be seen after the acute stage.

Investigations: clinical diagnosis–investigations not required unless unclear diagnosis

Differentials: cutaneous T-cell lymphoma (Sézary's syndrome), eczema (atopic, contact, seborrheic)

Management:
1. **Initial:** A–E assessment
2. **Supportive treatment:** IV fluid replacement, nutritional replacement, warm environment to prevent excessive fluid loss, prophylactic venous thromboembolism, strict fluid input/output monitoring
3. **Skin-specific treatments:** wet dressings, emollients, mild topical steroids
4. Antibiotics for super-added bacterial infection and antihistamines for itching

THE ONE-LINE ROUND-UP!

Here are some key words to help you remember each condition/concept.

Condition	One-line Description
Cellulitis	Staphylococcus aureus *or* Streptococcus pyogenes
Impetigo	*Golden crust*
Herpes simplex	*Multiple vesicles that rupture and crust*
Herpes zoster	*Dermatomal distribution*
Candida	*Curd-like white coating*
Pityriasis versicolor	*Hypopigmentation with scales*
Scabies	*Linear burrows in the web space*
Atopic dermatitis	*Emollients and steroids*
Contact dermatitis	*Identify the trigger*
Seborrheic dermatitis	*Cradle cap*
Venous eczema	*Dry, scaly, lipodermatosclerosis*
Discoid eczema	*Coin-shaped erythematous plaques*
Psoriasis	*Silvery-white scale, onycholysis, pitting, salmon patch*
Urticaria	*Hives and wheals*
Angioedema	*Swelling of eyes, lips and tongue*
Erythema nodosum	*Large, tender nodules*
Acne vulgaris	*Comedones, pustules, cysts and nodules*
Rosacea	*Red cheeks and nose*
Bullous pemphigoid	*Tense, intact bullae*
Pemphigus vulgaris	*Pemphig**S** = **S**uperficial*
BCC	*Pearly nodule with arborising vessels*
Actinic keratosis	*Scaly plaque, sun-exposed areas*
Bowen's disease	*Red and scaly with irregular border*
SCC	*Crusty nodule with ulceration*
Malignant melanoma	*ABCDE*
Keratoacanthoma	*Volcano appearance*
Seborrheic keratosis	*Stuck on appearance*
Melasma	*Brown/grey pigmentation*
Vitiligo	*Depigmentation, symmetrical*
Alopecia areata	*Nonscarring*
Tinea capitis	*Scalp ring worm*
Pyogenic granuloma	*Like a raspberry*
Erythema multiforme	*HSV, target lesions*
Stevens Johnson Syndrome	*<10% of epidermal detachment*
Toxic epidermal necrolysis	*>30% of epidermal detachment*
Erythroderma	*Psoriasis*

READING LIST: DERMATOLOGY IN AN HOUR

Introduction to Dermatology
DermNet, N. Z. (2007). *Structure of normal skin.* http://www.dermnetnz.org. [Accessed 2020].

British Association of Dermatologists. *Student Handbook.* https://www.bad.org.uk/shared/get-file.ashx?item-type=document&id=6595.

Table 5.2 Steroids. (Adapted from National Eczema Society).

National Eczema Society. (2019). *Topical steroids fact sheet.* https://eczema.org/wp-content/uploads/Topical-steroids-Sep-19-1.pdf.

Infections
Cellulitis
NICE. (2019). *CKS: Cellulitis.* http://www.cks.nice.org.uk. [Accessed June 2020].

Impetigo
NICE. (2020). *CKS: Impetigo.* http://www.cks.nice.org.uk. [Accessed June 2020].

Herpes Simplex
BAD. (2019). *Herpes Simplex.* http://www.cks.nice.org.uk. [Accessed June 2020].

BNF. *Herpesvirus infection.* http://www.bnf.nice.org.uk. [Accessed June 2020].

Herpes Zoster
NICE. (2019). *CKS: Shingles.* http://www.cks.nice.org.uk. [Accessed June 2020].

Candida
NICE. (2017). *CKS: Candida.* http://www.cks.nice.org.uk. [Accessed June 2020].

Pityriasis Versicolor
NICE. (2020). *CKS: Pityriasis versicolor.* http://www.cks.nice.org.uk. [Accessed June 2020].

DermNet, N. Z. (2020). *Pityriasis versicolor.* http://www.dermnetnz.org/topics/pityriasis-versicolor. [Accessed January 2021].

Scabies
NICE. (2017). *CKS: Scabies.* http://www.cks.nice.org.uk. [Accessed June 2020].

Inflammatory Skin Conditions
Atopic Dermatitis
NICE. (2018). *Atopic dermatitis.* http://www.cks.nice.org.uk. [Accessed June 2020].

Allergic And Irritant Contact Dermatitis
NICE. (2018). *CKS: Allergic contact dermatitis.* http://www.cks.nice.org.uk. [Accessed June 2020].

BAD. (2020). *Patch testing.* http://www.bad.org.uk. [Accessed Sep 2020].

NICE. (2018). *CKS: Irritant contact dermatitis.* http://www. cks.nice.org.uk. [Accessed June 2020].

Seborrheic Dermatitis
NICE. (2019). *CKS: Seborrheic dermatitis.* http://www.cks. nice.org.uk. [Accessed June 2020].

Venous Eczema
BAD. (2019). *Venous eczema* http://www.bad.org.uk. [Accessed July 2020].

Discoid Eczema
BAD. (2019). *Discoid eczema.* http://www.bad.org.uk. [Accessed July 2020].

Psoriasis
NICE. (2018). *CKS: Psoriasis.* http://www.cks.nice.org.uk. [Accessed June 2020].

DermNet, N. Z. (2020). *Psoriasis.* http://www.dermnetnz.org. [Accessed February 2021].

Urticaria, Angioedema and Anaphylaxis
NICE. (2018). *CKS: Urticaria.* http://www.cks.nice.org.uk. [Accessed June 2020].

NICE. (2018). *CKS: Angioedema and anaphylaxis.* http:// www.cks.nice.org.uk. [Accessed June 2020].

Resus. (2016). *Emergency treatment of anaphylactic reactions.* http://www.resus.org.uk. [Accessed June 2020].

Erythema Nodosum
DermNet, N. Z. (2019). *Erythema nodosum.* http://www. dermnetnz.org. [Accessed February 2021].

Inflammation of the Pilosebaceous Unit

Acne
NICE. (2019). *CKS: Acne vulgaris.* http://www.cks.nice.org. uk. [Accessed June 2020].

BAD. (2020). *Acne.* http://www.bad.org.uk. [Accessed Sep 2020].

Rosacea
NICE. (2018). *CKS: Rosacea.* [https://cks.nice.org.uk/topics/ rosacea/ - Accessed June 2020]

Immunobullous Disorders

Bullous Pemphigoid
Patient info. (2015). *Bullous pemphigoid.* http://www.patient. info. [Accessed June 2020].

DermNet, N. Z. (2016). *Bullous pemphigoid.* http://www. dermnetnz.org/topics/bullous-pemphigoid. [Accessed February 2021].

Pemphigus Vulgaris
BAD. (2018). *Pemphigoid vulgaris.* http://www.bad.org.uk. [Accessed June 2020].

Skin Cancer and Important Differentials

Basal Cell Carcinoma (BCC)

BAD. (2018). *Basal cell carcinoma.* http://www.bad.org.uk. [Accessed February 2021].

DermNet, N. Z. (2015). *Basal cell carcinoma.* http://www. dermnetnz.org. [Accessed Sep 2020].

Actinic Keratosis
DermNet, N. Z. (2015). *Actinic keratosis.* http://www.dermnetnz.org. [Accessed February 2021].

Bowen's Disease (SCC IN SITU)
BAD. (2020). *Bowen's disease.* http://www.bad.org.uk. [Accessed June 2020].

Squamous Cell Carcinoma (SCC)
BAD. (2018). *Squamous cell carcinoma.* http://www.bad.org. uk. [Accessed June 2020].

DermNet, N. Z. (2015). *Squamous cell carcinoma.* http://www. dermnetnz.org. [Accessed February 2021].

Malignant Melanoma
BAD. (2019). *Melanoma.* http://www.bad.org.uk. [Accessed June 2020].

Keratoacanhoma
BAD. (2019). *Keratoacanthoma.* http://www.bad.org.uk. [Accessed June 2020].

Seborrheic Keratosis
DermNet NZ. 2016. [https://dermnetnz.org/topics/seborrhoeic-keratosis#:~:text=Seborrhoeic%20keratosis%20 is%20a%20harmless,%2C%20wisdom%20wart%2C%20 or%20barnacle. - Accessed February 2021].

Pigmentary Disorders
Melasma
BAD. (2018). *Melasma.* http://www.bad.org.uk. [Accessed June 2020].

Vitiligo
BAD. (2019). *Vitiligo.* http://www.bad.org.uk. [Accessed June 2020].

Hair Loss
Alopecia Areata
BAD. (2019). *Alopecia areata.* http://www.bad.org.uk. [Accessed June 2020].

NICE. (2018). *CKS: Alopecia.* http://www.cks.nice.org.uk. [Accessed Sep 2020].

Tinea Capitis
BAD. (2017). *Tinea capitis.* http://www.bad.org.uk. [Accesed June 2020].

Vascular Dermatology
Pyogenic Granuloma
BAD. (2018). *Pyogenic granulomas.* http://www.bad.org.uk. [Accessed June 2020].

Dermatological Emergencies

Erythema Multiforme

Patient info. (2014). *Erythema multiforme*. http://www.patient.info. [Accessed December 2020].

DermNet, N. Z. (2015). *Erythema multiforme*. http://www.dermnetnz.org. [Accessed December 2020].

Steven Johnson Syndrome and Toxic Epidermal Necrolysis

Patient info. (2016). *Stevens-Johnson syndrome*. http://www.patient.info. [Accessed December 2020].

DermNet, N. Z. (2016). *Stevens–Johnson syndrome*. http://www.dermnetnz.org. [Accessed December 2020].

DermNet, N. Z. (2016). *Toxic epidermal necrolysis*. http://www.dermnetnz.org. [Accessed December 2020].

British Association of Dermatologists. (2016). *UK guidelines for the management of Stevens-Johnson syndrome*. http://www.bad.org.uk. [Accessed December 2020].

Erythroderma

Patient info. (2015). *Erythrodermic psoriasis*. http://www.patient.info. [Accessed December 2020].

DermNet, N. Z. (2016). *Erythroderma*. http://www.dermnetnz.org. [Accessed December 2020].

6

Ear, Nose and Throat (ENT) and Ophthalmology in an Hour

Mark Lam, Claire Langton-Hewer, Berenice Aguirrezabala Armbruster, Dominic Mahoney and Denize Atan

OUTLINE

ENT

ANATOMY

See Fig 6.1 for ear anatomy

ENT SPECIAL TESTS AND INVESTIGATIONS

Rinne and Weber Tests

Use: to differentiate between **conductive and sensorineural** hearing loss (see Fig 6.2 and Table 6.1)

Conductive loss:
- **Definition:** sound does not transmit effectively between the outer ear, external auditory canal, tympanic membrane and middle ear
- **Causes:**
  - **Outer ear:** earwax, otitis externa
  - **Middle ear:** acute otitis media (OM), perforated tympanic membrane, cholesteatoma, tympanosclerosis

Sensorineural loss:
- **Definition:** dysfunction of the cochlea or the vestibulocochlear nerve (**CN VIII**)
- **Causes:**
  - **Genetic:** nonsyndromic hearing loss and deafness (DFNB1), neurofibromatosis type 2 (NF2), Alport syndrome, Waardenburg syndrome, Usher syndrome
  - **Acquired:** infection (e.g., rubella, CMV, toxoplasmosis, bacterial meningitis), presbycusis, noise induced, Ménière's disease, ototoxic medications (e.g., aminoglycosides, cisplatin, nonsteroidal anti-inflammatory drugs (NSAIDs), loop diuretics), trauma, stroke

TOP TIP: Start with the Weber test first, as the results of this test can influence a **false-negative Rinne test** (when bone conduction transmits through the skull to the opposite ear and is detected).

Example 1

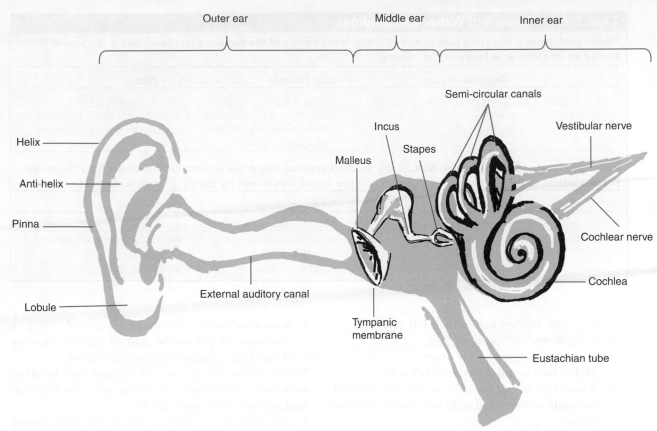

Fig 6.1 Ear Anatomy. (Illustrated by Dr Hollie Blaber.)

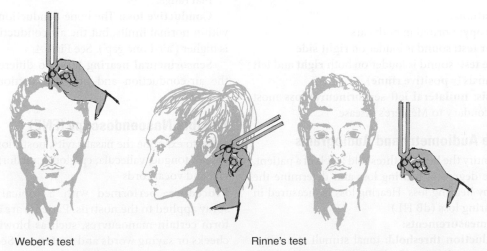

Weber's test

Rinne's test

Fig 6.2 Weber and Rinne Tests. (Illustrated by Dr Hollie Blaber.)

TABLE 6.1   Rinne and Weber Test Findings

Weber test: place a vibrating tuning fork (512 Hz) in the centre of the patient's forehead. Ask if the sound is louder on one side or is heard in the midline.

	Negative Weber	Right Weber	Left Weber
Patient response	Sound in midline	Sound is louder on right	Sound is louder on left
Interpretation	Normal	Unilateral right conductive loss or unilateral left sensorineural loss	Unilateral left conductive loss or unilateral right sensorineural loss

Rinne test: place vibrating tuning fork on the mastoid process. When the patient can no longer hear the sound, place it lateral to the ear canal. Ask the patient if the sound was louder by the ear or on the mastoid process.

	Positive Rinne	Negative Rinne	Equal Rinne
Patient response	Sound louder by ear canal	Sound louder on mastoid	Sound equal
Interpretation	Air conduction>bone conduction = Normal or sensorineural loss	Bone conduction>air conduction = Conductive loss	Air conduction=bone conduction= Mild conductive loss

Patient reports hearing loss in their **left ear.**

- **Investigations:**
  - **Otoscopy:** bulging left ear drum
  - **Weber test:** sound is louder on **left side**
  - **Rinne test:** sound is louder on the **left mastoid** (=negative rinne) and **right ear canal** (=positive rinne)
- **Diagnosis: unilateral left conductive loss** most likely secondary to otitis media

Example 2

Patient reports hearing loss, ringing and fullness in their **left ear.**

- **Investigations:**
  - **Otoscopy:** normal in both ears
  - **Weber test:** sound is louder on **right side**
  - **Rinne test:** sound is louder on both **right** and **left** ear canals (=**positive rinne**)
- **Diagnosis: unilateral left sensorineural loss** most likely secondary to Ménière's disease

Pure-Tone Audiometry and Audiograms

Uses: to identify the hearing threshold levels of a patient, quantify the degree of hearing loss and determine the nature of any hearing loss. Hearing loss is measured in decibels hearing loss (dB HL)

Important measurements:

- **Air-conduction threshold:** tonal stimuli at a range of frequencies delivered by headphones

- **Bone-conduction threshold:** measured using a transducer placed on the mastoid process. Masking of the other ear prevents cross-stimulation.

Patients respond to the sound by raising their hands or via a button, and results are plotted on an **audiogram.** **Audiograms show (see Fig 6.3):**

- Air conduction is plotted with an "O" representing the right ear and an "X" representing the left ear
- Bone conduction is plotted with "<" representing the right ear and ">" representing the left ear
- Any sounds heard at 20 dB or less are within the normal range.

Conductive loss: The bone-conduction threshold is within normal limits, but the air-conduction threshold is higher ('air-bone gap'). See Fig 6.4

Sensorineural hearing loss: no difference between the air-conduction and bone-conduction thresholds. See Fig 6.5

Flexible Nasoendoscopy (FNE)

Uses: to examine the nasal cavity, posterior nasal space, base of tongue, vallecula, epiglottis, piriform fossae, larynx and vocal cords

Procedure: performed with a topical anaesthetic spray applied to the nostrils. Patients are asked to perform certain manoeuvres, such as blowing out their cheeks or saying words and sentences. See Fig 6.6 and Fig 6.7.

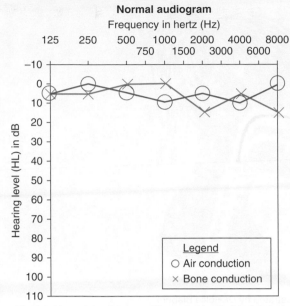

Fig 6.3 Normal Audiogram. (Illustrated by Dr Mark Lam.)

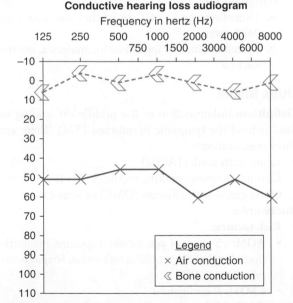

Fig 6.4 Audiogram with Conductive Loss. (Illustrated by Dr Mark Lam.)

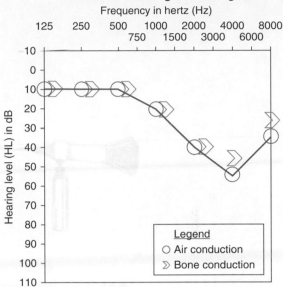

Fig 6.5 Audiogram with Sensorineural Loss. (Illustrated by Dr Mark Lam.)

EAR CONDITIONS

Otitis Externa (OE)

Definition: inflammation of the external auditory canal (EAC). This condition can be localised (e.g., infected hair follicle), diffuse (involving the external ear and tympanic membrane) or malignant (also known as necrotising, involving the mastoid and temporal bones).

Buzzwords:
- **Risk factors:** swimming, eczema, diabetes mellitus (DM), immunosuppression (malignant)
- **Infective organisms:** *Pseudomonas aeruginosa, Staphylococcus aureus, Aspergillus, Candida albicans*
- **Presentation:** itchy, severe disproportionate pain (worse when moving the tragus/pinna), discharge, scaly, inflamed EAC and tympanic membrane, whitish strands or black/white balls (fungal), granulation tissue/exposed bone and facial nerve palsy (malignant), **conductive loss**

Investigations:
- Clinical diagnosis
- **Swab with microbiology, culture and sensitivities** (M, C & S) if unresponsive to treatment/recurrent episodes
- **CT middle ear** (if evidence of malignant OE): thickened EAC soft tissue and bony erosion

Differentials: otitis media (OM), impacted ear wax, cholesteatoma, mastoiditis

Management:
1. **General management:** manage underlying skin conditions, analgesia, aural toilet (syringing, dry swabbing, microsuction)

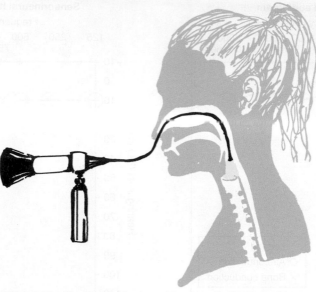

Fig 6.6 Flexible Nasoendoscopy. (Illustrated by Dr Hollie Blaber.)

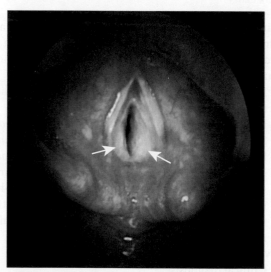

Fig 6.7 Nasoendoscopic View of a Patient with Croup (*arrows highlight subglottic mucosal oedema*). (With permission from Gurgel H., & Harnsberger H. R. (1979). Croup. In *Imaging in otolaryngology*. Elsevier. Copyright © 2018 Elsevier Inc. All rights reserved.)

2. **Localised OE**: topical acetic acid 2% spray
3. **Acute diffuse OE**: topical antibiotic (e.g., ciprofloxacin, chloramphenicol, neomycin or gentamicin) + topical corticosteroid
4. **Chronic diffuse OE**: topical steroid + antifungal (e.g., clotrimazole 1%)

5. **Malignant OE**:
   a. Urgent referral to ENT for further investigations: MRI, swab
   b. IV ceftazidime + ciprofloxacin, analgesia, microsuction

Otitis Media

Definition: inflammation of the middle ear leading to fluid behind the tympanic membrane (TM). There are three presentations:
- Acute otitis media (AOM)
- Chronic suppurative otitis media (CSOM)
- Otitis media with effusion (OME) or 'glue ear'

Buzzwords:
- **Risk factors:**
  - **AOM:** <5 years of age, smoke exposure, malnutrition, allergies, *Haemophilus influenzae*, *Streptococcus pneumoniae*, RSV
  - **CSOM:** *P. aeruginosa*
  - **OME:** cleft palate, Down syndrome, previous acute OM
- **Presentation:**
  - **AOM: rapid-onset** earache, ear tugging, bulging TM (see Fig 6.8), air-fluid level, perforation, **conductive loss**
  - **CSOM:** 6–12 weeks of recurrent otorrhoea, hearing loss, tinnitus, perforation (see Fig 6.9), **conductive loss**

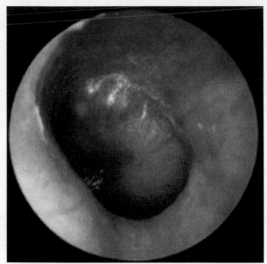

Fig 6.8 Acute Otitis Media. (With permission from Pichichero, M. E. (2013). Otitis media (Fig. 4). In *Pediatric clinics*. Elsevier. Copyright © 2013 Elsevier Ltd. All rights reserved.)

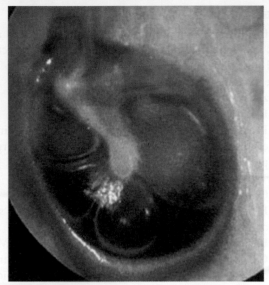

Fig 6.10 Otitis Media with Effusion. (With permission from Pichichero, M. E. (2013). Otitis media (Fig. 5). In *Pediatric clinics*. Elsevier. Copyright © 2013 Elsevier Ltd. All rights reserved.)

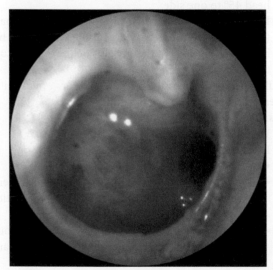

Fig 6.9 Chronic Suppurative Otitis Media with Perforation. (With permission from Chole, R. A., & Sharon, J. D. (2021) Chronic otitis media, mastoiditis, and petrositis (Fig. 140.4, Chapter 140). In *Cummings otolaryngology*. Elsevier. Copyright © 2013 Elsevier Ltd. All rights reserved.)

- **OME:** fluid without signs of acute inflammation, hearing loss, inattention, speech and language delay, loss of light reflex, air fluid level, retracted TM (see Fig 6.10), **conductive loss**

Investigations:
- Clinical diagnosis

- **Pure-tone audiometry:** conductive loss

Differentials: OE, impacted ear wax, mastoiditis, cholesteatoma

Management:
1. **AOM:**
- Reassurance and analgesia
- Admit to hospital if: severe systemic illness, neurological complications, <3 months of age **AND** temp ≥38.0°C.
- If not requiring hospital admission but systemically unwell/high risk of complications: amoxicillin 5–7-day course
- If otorrhoea or <2 years of age with bilateral infection: conservative, delayed antibiotic script or amoxicillin
2. **CSOM:**
   Refer to ENT for aural microsuction and antibiotic-steroid ear drops (e.g., ciprofloxacin and dexamethasone)
3. **OME:**
- Active observation for 6–12 weeks and, if present, treatment of underlying rhinitis and eustachian tube dysfunction with topical nasal steroids (e.g., beclomethasone, mometasone, fluticasone). If no improvement, refer to ENT
- Medical: hearing aid, auto inflation
- Surgical: myringotomy and grommet insertion

Mastoiditis

Definition: inflammation of the mastoid lining and air cell system. Usually secondary to the spread of a bacterial infection from a pre-existing OM but can also be due to cholesteatoma.

Buzzwords:
- **Risk factors:** see AOM section
- **Presentation:** earache, post-auricular swelling, erythema, pinna protrusion, purulent discharge, pyrexia, headache, facial nerve palsy

Investigations:
- Clinical diagnosis
- **Ear swab + M, C & S** (if discharge present): see organisms for AOM
- **Blood cultures** (if febrile): see organisms for AOM
- **CT petrous bones and brain** (if signs of extra/intra-cranial involvement or unresponsive to antibiotics): opacified mastoid cells, bony erosion, cerebral abscess

Differentials: OM, malignant OE, cholesteatoma

Management:
1. Primary care: immediate hospital admission for specialist assessment
2. IV ceftriaxone + IV metronidazole
3. If evidence of subperiosteal abscess: myringotomy/grommet + cortical mastoidectomy
4. If signs of neurological involvement: refer to neurosurgery

Cholesteatoma

Definition: abnormal accumulation of keratinising squamous epithelium within the middle ear or mastoid air cell spaces that can become infected and erode the surrounding structures.

Buzzwords:
- **Risk factors:** male, previous acute OM, middle ear surgery, cleft palate, Down syndrome
- **Presentation:** foul discharge, hearing loss, facial nerve palsy, TM retraction, keratin debris, white/brown mass in posterosuperior (attic) region on otoscopy, **conductive loss**

Investigations:
- Clinical diagnosis
- **Audiometry:** conductive loss
- **High-resolution CT temporal bones:** middle ear bony erosion

Differentials: OM, malignant OE, mastoiditis

Management:
1. Semi-urgent referral to ENT
2. Excision +/- tympanoplasty +/- mastoidectomy

Benign Paroxysmal Positional Vertigo

Definition: inner ear disorder characterised by repeated episodes of positional vertigo due to dislodged otoliths migrating into the semicircular canals, producing vertigo-like symptoms.

Buzzwords:
- **Risk factors:** older age, head injury, prolonged recumbent position (recent visit to hairdresser or dentist), ear surgery
- **Presentation:** room spinning, head movement (trigger), nausea, vomiting, seconds to minutes, **no hearing loss**

Investigations:
- ***Dix-Hallpike manoeuvre (Fig 6.11)*:** positive result = vertigo and rotatory nystagmus towards **affected ear**
1. Position patient sitting upright and turn his or her head 45° to one side
2. In one swift motion, whilst supporting the neck, have the patient go from sitting to supine with his or her head over the edge of the bed 30° below the horizontal

Differentials: labyrinthitis, vestibular neuronitis, Ménière's disease, cerebellar stroke

Management:
1. Watchful waiting
2. Epley manoeuvre (Fig 6.11):
   - **Steps 1 and 2:** see Dix-Hallpike manoeuvre
   - **Step 3:** Turn patient's head 90° to the contralateral side, >45° past the midline and maintain position for 30 sec
   - **Step 4:** Ask patient to roll on to his or her shoulder (on the side to which the head is turned) and rotate the head to face the floor for 30 sec
   - **Step 5:** Return patient to sitting, keeping the head rotated sideways
   - **Step 6:** Once sitting up, return the head to the midline with the neck flexed (not shown)
3. Brandt-Daroff exercises (patient can perform at home)

Labyrinthitis and Vestibular Neuronitis

Definition: Labyrinthitis and vestibular neuronitis were previously used interchangeably but are now considered to be two separate entities. Labyrinthitis is an

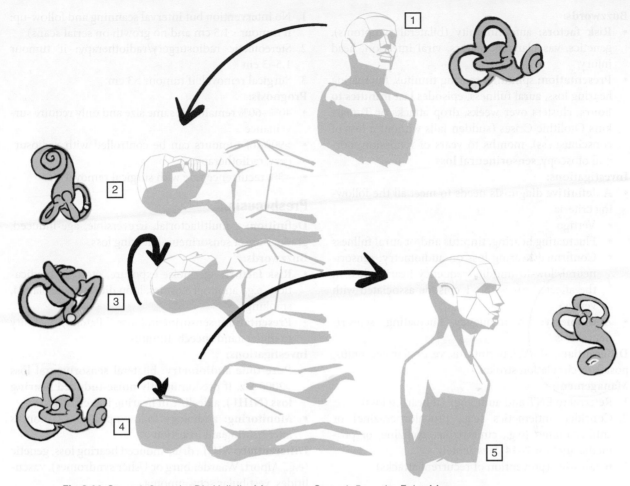

Fig 6.11 Steps 1–2 are the Dix-Hallpike Manoeuvre, Steps 1–5 are the Epley Manoeuvre.

inflammation of the labyrinth, while vestibular neuronitis is an inflammation of the vestibular nerve.

Buzzwords:

- **Risk factors:** preceding viral illness, allergies, head injury, vertebrobasilar ischaemia, meningitis, ototoxic medication.
- **Presentation:** nausea, vomiting, falls, hearing loss, tinnitus (labyrinthitis>vestibular neuronitis, rotational vertigo, horizontal nystagmus, **symptoms for 72 h** (may take 6 weeks for full recovery), normal otoscopy, **sensorineural loss**, hyperacute onset, unremitting symptoms (think posterior circulation stroke)

Investigations: primarily a **clinical diagnosis** based on history and examination. A **HiNTS exam** (**H**ead impulse, **N**ystagmus, **T**est of **S**kew) can differentiate a **peripheral** (e.g., labyrinthitis and vestibular neuronitis) from a **central** (e.g., posterior circulation stroke) cause,

with an **abnormal** head impulse, **unidirectional** or **no nystagmus** and **no vertical skew** supporting a **peripheral cause**. (See Fig 6.12 & Fig 6.13)

Differentials: benign paroxysmal position vertigo (BPPV), Ménière's disease, posterior circulation stroke

Management:

1. Antiemetics or antihistamines: prochlorperazine (buccal if severe) or an antihistamine (e.g., cinnarizine, cyclizine, or promethazine) for up to 3 days
2. Referral to balance specialist if atypical symptoms or persistent symptoms for >1 week with treatment (or if >6 weeks in total)

Ménière's Disease

Definition: a condition of the inner ear involving overproduction or impaired reabsorption of endolymph, affects balance and hearing.

Buzzwords:

- **Risk factors:** autoimmunity (bilateral symptoms), genetics, vascular risk factors, viral infection, head injury
- **Presentation:** spinning, roaring tinnitus, fluctuating hearing loss, aural fullness, episodes **last minutes to hours**, clusters over weeks, drop attacks or Tumarkin's Otolithic Crises (sudden falls without a loss of consciousness), months to years of remission, normal otoscopy, **sensorineural loss**

Investigations:

- A **definitive diagnosis** needs to meet all the following criteria:
  - Vertigo
  - Fluctuating hearing, tinnitus and/or aural fullness
  - Confirmed hearing loss on audiometry: sensorineural, low-to-middle frequency hearing loss in the affected ear with >1 episode associated with vertigo
- **Audiometry:** low-frequency, fluctuating, sensorineural loss

Differentials: BPPV, labyrinthitis, vestibular neuronitis, posterior circulation stroke

Management:

1. Referral to ENT and audiology (if hearing loss)
2. Consider antiemetics (e.g., prochlorperazine) or antihistamines (e.g., cinnarizine, cyclizine, or promethazine) for 7–14 days acutely
3. Betahistine (prevention of recurrent attacks)

Vestibular Schwannoma (Acoustic Neuroma)

Definition: benign, slow-growing tumour arising from the Schwann cells surrounding the vestibular branch of the vestibulocochlear nerve (CN VIII).

Buzzwords:

- **Risk factors:** NF2
- **Presentation:** unilateral sensorineural loss/tinnitus, headache, cerebellar signs, facial nerve palsy, normal otoscopy, cranial nerve palsies

Investigations:

- **Pure-tone audiometry:** high-frequency sensorineural loss
- *MRI*: lesion suggestive of vestibular schwannoma, bilateral tumours (seen in NF2)
- **Monitoring:** MRI a few months after surgery then yearly for 5 years

Differentials: meningioma, BPPV, Ménière's disease, stroke

Management:

1. No intervention but interval scanning and follow-up: if tumour <1.5 cm and no growth on serial scans)
2. Stereotactic radiosurgery/radiotherapy: if tumour 1.5–3 cm
3. Surgical removal: if tumour >3 cm

Prognosis:

- 40%–60% remain the same size and only require surveillance
- >90% of tumours can be controlled with radiosurgery/radiotherapy
- <5% recurrence rate with surgical removal

Presbycusis

Definition: a multifactorial, irreversible, age-induced, gradual-onset sensorineural hearing loss.

Buzzwords:

- **Risk factors:** age, noise exposure, ototoxic medication (e.g., aminoglycosides, loop diuretics, cisplatin), smoking
- **Presentation:** sensorineural loss (bilateral), inability to understand speech, tinnitus

Investigations:

- **Pure-tone audiometry:** bilateral sensorineural loss >2000 Hz. If predominantly **noise-induced hearing loss (NIHL)**, a decline in hearing is seen at 4 kHz
- **Monitoring:** audiology follow-up at 6–12 months after hearing aid insertion

Differentials: NIHL, drug-induced hearing loss, genetic (e.g., Alport, Waardenburg or Usher syndromes), vasculitides, vestibular schwannoma

Management: hearing aid

Childhood Hearing Loss

Definition: a hearing threshold of >25 dB in both ears. This condition can be graded as mild, moderate, severe or profound.

Buzzwords:

- **Risk factors:** congenital (e.g., Down, Waardenburg, Usher, Alport's, Turner's, Klinefelter's and TORCH syndromes), neonatal problems (e.g., prematurity, low birth weight), infection (e.g., meningitis, mumps, HIV)
- **Presentation:** speech problems, language delay, behavioural problems, inattention

Investigations:

- **Otoacoustic emission** (OAE): performed at 4–5 weeks
- **Auditory brainstem response** (ABR): if OAE results are unclear

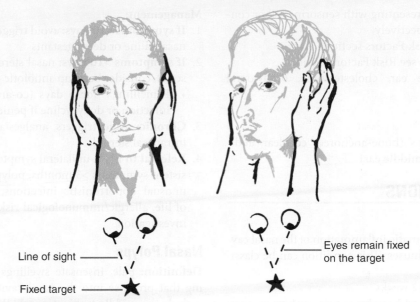

Fig 6.12 Head-impulse Test. In a normal response, the eyes stay fixed on target. (Illustrated by Dr Hollie Blaber.)

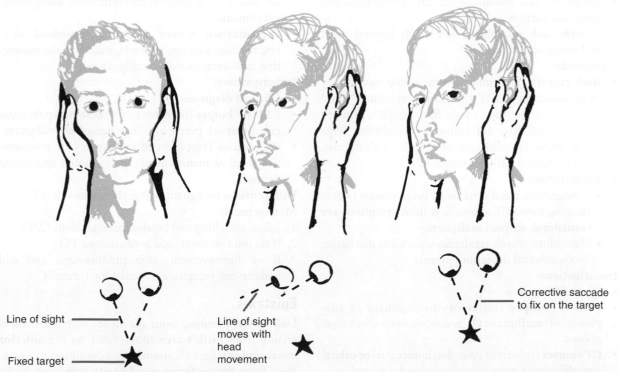

Fig 6.13 Head-impulse Test. In an abnormal response, the eyes are dragged off target before corrective saccades. (Illustrated by Dr Hollie Blaber.)

- **MRI or CT:** if presenting with sensorineural or conductive loss, respectively
- **Serology:** see Risk Factors section
- **Genetic testing:** see Risk Factors section

Differentials: glue ear, cholesteatoma, behavioural issues

Management:
1. Hearing aids
2. Hearing implants (bone-anchored, cochlear, auditory brainstem, middle ear)

NOSE CONDITIONS

Rhinosinusitis

Definition: symptomatic inflammation of the nasal cavity and paranasal sinuses. This condition can be classified as:
- Acute: lasting <12 weeks
- Chronic: lasting >12 weeks, recurrent (four or more episodes/year)
  - Can be subcategorised as being with or without nasal polyps (see Nasal Polyps section)
- Uncomplicated: inflammation stays within nasal and paranasal cavities
- Complicated: inflammation extends beyond nasal and paranasal cavities

Buzzwords:
- **Risk factors:** anatomical, viral upper respiratory tract infection (URTI), asthma, smoking, nasal obstruction, allergies, cystic fibrosis (CF), primary ciliary dyskinesia, autoimmune vasculitides (e.g., eosinophilic granulomatosis with polyangiitis, granulomatosis with polyangiitis)
- **Presentation:**
  - Congestion, nasal drip, facial pain/pressure (worse leaning forward), anosmia. **If these symptoms are unilateral, suspect malignancy**
  - Periorbital/cheek tenderness, purulent discharge, polyps, septal deviation, pyrexia

Investigations:
- Clinical diagnosis
- **FNE +/- biopsy** (refractory to treatment or suspicion of malignancy): mucopurulent discharge, polyps
- **CT sinuses** (recurrent episodes, intracranial or orbital complications): bony erosion, abscess formation

Differentials: URTI, nasal foreign body, sinonasal tumour, migraine, dental pain

Management:
1. **If symptoms <10 days:** avoid triggers, analgesia, trial nasal saline or decongestants
2. **If symptoms >10 days:** nasal steroid (e.g., mometasone), consider back-up antibiotic prescription.
   - Penicillin V for 5 days (co-amoxiclav if severe infection or doxycycline if penicillin allergic)
3. **Chronic:** avoid triggers, analgesia, nasal irrigation, intranasal steroids
4. **Referral to ENT:** unilateral symptoms (urgent), persistent symptoms >3 months, polyps, recurrent OM, unusual opportunistic infections, affecting quality of life, allergic/immunological risk factors requiring investigation

Nasal Polyps

Definition: pale, insensate swellings of the nasal lining that prolapse into the nasal cavity. Common sites include the middle turbinates, middle meatus and ethmoids (see Fig 6.14).

Buzzwords:
- **Risk factors:** chronic rhinosinusitis, asthma, aspirin sensitivity, CF, Churg-Strauss syndrome, allergic fungal sinusitis
- **Presentation:** watery discharge, postnasal drip, obstruction, snoring, anosmia, mobile, pale, insensitive, unilateral (possible malignancy)

Investigations:
- **Clinical diagnosis.**
- **FNE +/- biopsy** (if unable to visualise polyp on nasal examination): polyp, histology benign or malignant
- **CT sinuses** (suspicion of malignancy or preoperative surgical management): polyp noted and extent defined

Differentials: malignant polyp, rhinosinusitis, CF

Management:
1. Saline douching and betamethasone drops (2/52)
2. If no improvement, add prednisolone PO
3. If no improvement, stop prednisolone and add leukotriene-receptor antagonist for 1 month

Epistaxis

Definition: bleeding from the nose, with most cases arising from **Little's area** (80%–95%) on the **anterior nasal septum**. Less commonly, this condition can originate from the **posterior nasal cavity** (branches of the sphenopalatine artery).

Buzzwords:

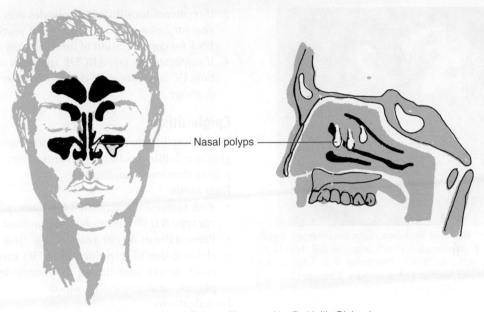

Fig 6.14 Nasal Polyps. (Illustrated by Dr Hollie Blaber.)

Nasal polyps

- **Risk factors:** trauma, post-nasal surgery, nasal steroids, anticoagulants, nasal oxygen, hereditary haemorrhagic telangiectasia (HTT), coagulopathy, malignancy
- **Presentation:** acutely or as recurrent episodes. Bleeding gums (secondary to myeloma, leukaemia or HHT), syncope and lightheaded (hypovolaemia).

Investigations:
- Clinical diagnosis
- **Blood:** coagulopathy, ↓ Hb requiring transfusion
- **CT angiography** (CTA): localise the source of bleeding prior to vessel embolisation

Differentials: haemoptysis, haematemesis

Management:
- ABCDE, resuscitation, treat reversible causes (anticoagulation)
- **First aid:** sit head forward, pinch soft part of nose for 20 min, suck ice/place on forehead or nape of neck, spit out blood
- **If anterior:** chemical (e.g., silver nitrate) or electrocautery
- **If anterior or posterior:** nasal packing (e.g., Merocel or Rapid Rhino)
- If no improvement: ligation of sphenopalatine artery under general anaesthesia
- If no improvement: arterial embolisation

THROAT CONDITIONS

Pharyngitis and Tonsillitis

Definition: inflammation of the pharynx and/or tonsils.

Buzzwords:
- **Risk factors:** viral URTI, bacterial URTI (*S. pyogenes* or Group A *Streptococcus* (GAS)), Epstein-Barr virus (EBV)
- **Presentation:** fever, sore throat, dysphagia, odynophagia, headache, nausea and vomiting, drooling (epiglottitis), exudate, cervical lymphadenopathy, swollen tonsils (see Fig 6.15), 'hot potato voice' (peritonsillar abscess or quinsy)

Investigations:
- **Clinical diagnosis** utilising the FeverPAIN score (see Table 6.2) or Centor (as recommended by NICE) (see Table 6.3). **If FeverPAIN score of 4 or 5 OR Centor score 3 or 4:**
  - **Rapid antigen test for GAS:** positive
  - **Throat culture:** growth of GAS
  - **Blood:** ↑ WCC and CRP, positive Monospot test for EBV
- **CT neck with contrast** (if suspected parapharyngeal abscess): evidence of collection in parapharyngeal space

Differentials: viral or bacterial epiglottitis, peritonsillar abscess, infectious mononucleosis, Lemierre's syndrome

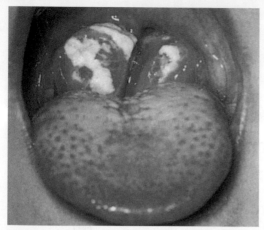

Fig 6.15 Acute Bacterial Tonsillitis. Grossly enlarged tonsils with exudate. (With permission from Jeannon, J-P., Narula, A., Saleh, H., & Sandhu, G. (2013). The throat (Fig. 3.48). In *Ear, nose and throat and head and neck surgery*. Elsevier. Copyright © 2013 Elsevier Ltd. All rights reserved.)

TABLE 6.2 FeverPAIN Score

FeverPAIN	Interpretation
Fever in past 24 h	Each FeverPAIN criteria scores 1 point (max score of 5):
Purulent tonsils	
Attend rapidly (≤3 days of symptom onset)	0 or 1 = no antibiotic
Severely Inflamed tonsils	2 or 3 = no antibiotic or back up antibiotic
No cough or coryza	4 or 5 = immediate antibiotic or back up prescription

TABLE 6.3 Centor Score

Centor Criteria	Interpretation
Tonsillar exudate	Each of the Centor criteria scores 1 point (max score of 4):
Tender cervical lymphadenopathy	0, 1 or 2 = no antibiotic
History of fever (>38°C)	3 or 4 = immediate antibiotic or back-up prescription
Absence of cough	

(internal jugular vein thrombophlebitis commonly secondary to *Fusobacterium necrophorum* infection)

Management:
1. Self-care (e.g., fluid intake, analgesia, saltwater gargles)
2. If GAS suspected (FeverPAIN score 4 or 5; Centor score 3 or 4): phenoxymethylpenicillin (clarithromycin if penicillin allergic)

3. If recurrent tonsillitis (>7 episodes over 1 year, 5 per year for 2 years, or 3 per year for 3 years): referral to ENT for consideration of tonsillectomy
4. If suspected quinsy: ABCDE approach and resuscitation, IV ceftriaxone, IV dexamethasone, incision and drainage

Epiglottitis

Definition: life-threatening condition caused by supraglottic cellulitis, leading to inflammation, swelling and potential airway compromise.

Buzzwords:
- **Risk factors:** unvaccinated for *Haemophilus influenzae* type B (Hib), immunocompromised
- **Presentation:** 40–50 years of age (less common in children due to introduction of Hib vaccine); acute-onset, severe sore throat; dysphagia; drooling; dysphonia; stridor; tripod position

Investigations:
- **Clinical diagnosis:** do not delay early airway control for investigations
- **Laryngoscopy (during intubation):** swelling of supraglottic structures
- **Lateral neck x-ray (if patient not in extremis):** thumbprint sign

Differentials: croup, bacterial tracheitis, pharyngitis, tonsillitis, peritonsillar abscess

Management:
1. Keep patient calm, do not examine the oral cavity
2. Stable patient without impending airway compromise: consider Heliox, nebulised adrenaline, IV antibiotics, IV steroids
3. Unstable patient with impending airway compromise: contact senior anaesthetist and ENT surgeon, urgent tracheal intubation in theatre, may require surgical airway

Obstructive Sleep Apnoea (OSA)

Definition: repetitive irregular breathing at night and symptoms of sleep disturbance with excessive daytime sleepiness.

Buzzwords:
- **Risk factors:** male, obesity, neck circumference (>43 cm), family history, smoking, hypothyroidism, acromegaly, large tonsils, craniofacial abnormalities, Down syndrome
- **Presentation:** snoring and daytime sleepiness, mood changes, nocturia

Investigations:

- **Epworth sleepiness questionnaire:** abnormal daytime sleepiness
- ***Polysomnography*:** five episodes of apnoea and/or hypopnoea per hour of sleep

Differentials: insufficient sleep, narcolepsy, depression, hypothyroidism, drug-induced apnoea

Management:

1. **Conservative:** weight loss, exercise, smoking cessation, change sleeping position
2. **Medical:** continuous positive airway pressure (CPAP), intraoral devices (e.g., mandibular advancement)
3. **Surgical:** adenotonsillectomy (if secondary to adenotonsillar hypertrophy)

ANTERIOR TRIANGLE NECK LUMPS

Branchial Cyst

Definition: congenital mass resulting from incomplete branchial cleft obliteration

Buzzwords:

- **Risk factors:** 10–40 years of age, post-trauma or infection
- **Presentation:** painless (but may become infected), slow growing, smooth, fluctuant (see Fig 6.16)

Investigations:

- **US neck:** well-defined cystic mass with enhancing rim
- **Fine-needle aspiration cytology (FNAC):** thick, yellow, pus-like fluid, **contains cholesterol**

Differentials: epidermoid cyst, lymphadenopathy, carotid body tumour

Management:

- Medical: antibiotics (if infected), sclerotherapy
- Surgical excision

Pharyngeal Pouch

Definition: oesophageal wall herniation at Killian's dehiscence (between the thyropharyngeal and cricopharyngeal muscles)

Buzzwords:

- **Risk factors:** >50 years of age, chronic acid reflux, smoking, excess alcohol, stroke, oesophageal surgery
- **Presentation:** soft and painless swelling, dysphagia, gurgling, halitosis, regurgitation, coughing, chest infection

Investigations:

- ***Barium swallow or video fluoroscopy*:** diverticulum from midline or posterior pharyngeal wall

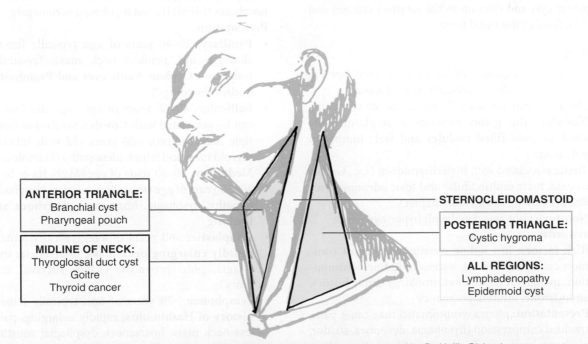

ANTERIOR TRIANGLE:
Branchial cyst
Pharyngeal pouch

MIDLINE OF NECK:
Thyroglossal duct cyst
Goitre
Thyroid cancer

STERNOCLEIDOMASTOID

POSTERIOR TRIANGLE:
Cystic hygroma

ALL REGIONS:
Lymphadenopathy
Epidermoid cyst

Fig 6.16 Neck Lump Regions and Common Conditions. (Illustrated by Dr Hollie Blaber.)

Differentials: oesophageal cancer, lymphadenopathy, epidermoid cyst

Management:

- **Conservative** (if medically unfit or asymptomatic)
- **Surgery:** endoscopic or open cricopharyngeal myotomy or endoscopic stapling/laser diverticulectomy

MIDLINE NECK LUMPS

Thyroglossal Duct Cyst

Definition: benign cyst formed from an incomplete closure of the thyroglossal duct, which extends from the foramen caecum (base of the tongue) to the pyramidal lobe of the thyroid gland.

Buzzwords:

- **Risk factors:** first decade of life
- **Presentation:** painless (unless infected), fluctuant, mobile, **moves up with tongue protrusion**

Investigations:

- **US neck:** well-defined, thin-walled anechoic lesion
- **CT neck:** cystic, thin-walled, homogeneously fluid-dense with capsular enhancement

Differentials: goitre, thyroid nodules, thyroid cancer, dermoid cyst

Management: Sistrunk's operation: removal of the thyroglossal cyst and duct up to the foramen caecum and middle third of the hyoid bone

Goitre

Definition: enlargement of the thyroid gland (see Fig 6.17). Goitres can be described in several ways:

- **Diffuse:** entire gland swells and is smooth to touch
- **Nodular:** the gland contains a single/multiple solid or fluid-filled nodules and feels lumpy on palpation
- **Toxic:** associated with hyperthyroidism (e.g., Grave's disease, toxic multinodular and toxic adenoma) (see Endocrinology in an Hour chapter).
- **Non-toxic:** not associated with hyperthyroidism

Buzzwords:

- **Risk factors:** low iodine consumption (most common cause worldwide), excessive iodine consumption, malignancy, radiation, smoking, family history, amiodarone, lithium, pregnancy
- **Presentation:** often asymptomatic, may cause pain, tracheal compression (dysphagia, dyspnoea, stridor, plethora, hoarseness), stigmata of hyperthyroidism

or hypothyroidism (see Endocrinology in an Hour chapter), thyroid gland moves with swallowing, may be firm, single or multinodular, bruit, lymphadenopathy

Investigations: see Hyperthyroidism, Hypothyroidism (Endocrinology in an Hour chapter) and Thyroid Cancer sections

Differentials: thyroid cancer, thyroid nodules, thyroglossal duct cyst

Management: dependent upon underlying cause:

- No treatment: small goitre and benign nodule
- Antithyroid drugs: hyperthyroidism
- Thyroid replacement: hypothyroidism
- Thyroidectomy: malignancy

Thyroid Cancer

Definition: a rare cancer that develops from tissues of the thyroid gland. The main types are:

- Papillary (most common and better prognosis)
- Follicular (including Hürthle cell)
- Medullary
- Anaplastic (worst prognosis)
- Lymphoma (least common)

Buzzwords:

- **Risk factors:** <20 or >60 years of age, benign thyroid disease (e.g., adenoma, goitre, thyroiditis), radiation, family history (e.g., thyroid cancer, multiple endocrine neoplasias (MEN) IIa and b), obesity, acromegaly
- **Presentation:**
  - **Papillary:** 20–40 years of age; typically female; slow-growing, painless neck mass; favourable prognosis; **Orphan Annie eyes and Psammoma bodies (histology)**
  - **Follicular:** 40–60 years of age, typically female, can be associated with **Cowden syndrome** (multiple hamartomas), >60 years old with bilateral thyroid mass and lymphadenopathy (Hürthle cell)
  - **Medullary:** 20–30 years of age (MEN IIa or b) or 40–50 years of age (sporadic), cervical lymphadenopathy, dysphagia, hoarseness, **diarrhoea and flushing**
  - **Anaplastic:** >60 years of age, typically female, **rapidly enlarging neck mass**, hoarseness, dysphagia, poor prognosis (<10% survival at 5 years)
  - **Lymphoma:** >70 years of age; typically female; **history of Hashimoto's**; rapidly enlarging, painless neck mass; hoarseness; dysphagia; constitutional symptoms

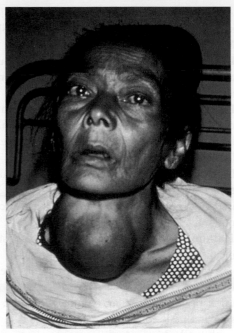

Fig 6.17 Endemic Goitre Caused by Iodine Deficiency. (With permission from Raftery, A. T., Lim, E., & Östör, A. J. K. (2014). Goitre (Fig. 25). In *Churchill's pocketbook of differential diagnosis*. Elsevier. Copyright © 2014 Elsevier Ltd. All rights reserved.)

Investigations:
- **Blood:** ↔ Thyroid-stimulating hormone (TSH), ↑ calcitonin and carcinoembryonic antigen (only if medullary suspected)
- **US neck:** see Table 6.4
- **FNAC:** histological features of malignancy (see Table 6.5)
- **Monitoring:** raised thyroglobulin (recurrence of papillary, follicular or Hürthle cell), raised calcitonin (recurrence of medullary), hypocalcaemia (parathyroid injury)

Differentials: benign thyroid nodule, goitre, thyroglossal duct cyst

Management:
1. Depending upon type and stage of cancer, options include:
   - Surgery: hemithyroidectomy or total thyroidectomy +/- neck dissection
   - Radiotherapy (unresectable tumours and residual disease post-thyroidectomy)
   - Chemotherapy (lymphomas)

TABLE 6.4 U Grading of Thyroid Nodules

U Grading of Thyroid Nodules	Findings	Management
U1 normal	Normal	No follow-up required
U2 benign	Halo, iso-echoic, cystic change, peripheral calcification and vascularity	No follow-up required – FNAC not recommended unless high level of clinical suspicion of thyroid cancer
U3 equivocal	Homogenous, hyper-echoic, solid, halo, cystic change, mixed vascularity	FNAC
U4 suspicious	Solid, hypo-echoic, disrupted peripheral calcification, lobulated	FNAC
U5 malignant	Solid, hypo-echoic, irregular, micro-calcification, intranodular vascularity	FNAC

FNAC, Fine-needle aspiration cytology.

TABLE 6.5 Thyroid Fine-needle Aspiration Cytology Grading

Thyroid FNAC Grading	Findings	Management
Thy 1	Non-diagnostic	Repeat FNAC
Thy 2	Non-neoplastic	No follow-up if no suspicious US or clinical features
Thy 3F	Follicular lesion	Hemithyroidectomy or total if mass >4 cm
Thy 3A	Atypia present	Repeat US and FNAC
Thy 4	Suspicious of thyroid cancer	MDT discussion and hemithyroidectomy
Thy 5	Diagnostic of thyroid cancer	MDT, staging scans, total thyroidectomy +/- central node clearance (if high risk)

FNAC, Fine-needle aspiration cytology; MDT, multidisciplinary team; US, ultrasound.

- Radioiodine therapy (tumour >1 cm and post-total or near-total thyroidectomy)
2. If total or near-total thyroidectomy: prescribe levothyroxine

Prognosis:
- Overall survival rate of 90% after 1 year for all types and stages of thyroid cancer
- Prognoses associated with type of cancer: papillary>follicular>medullary>lymphoma>anaplastic

POSTERIOR TRIANGLE NECK LUMPS

Cystic Hygroma

Definition: benign, fluid-filled sac caused by a lymphatic system malformation

Buzzwords:
- **Risk factors:** Turner's syndrome, Down syndrome, trisomy 13 and 18, aortic coarctation, foetal alcohol syndrome
- **Presentation:** infants, increase in size with coughing/crying, **transilluminates brightly**

Investigations:
- **US neck:** multilocular, cystic, variable-thickness septations
- **CT neck:** poorly circumscribed, multi-loculated, hypodense masses with fluid attenuation

Differentials: lymphadenopathy, epidermoid cyst, lipoma

Management:
1. Medical: sclerotherapy
2. Surgical: excision

NECK LUMPS: ALL REGIONS

Lymphadenopathy

Definition: enlarged lymphoid tissue containing the B and T cells responsible for filtering foreign antigens (see Fig 6.18)

Buzzwords:
- **Risk factors:** mnemonic MIAMI:
  - Malignancy: head and neck cancer, lymphoma, leukaemia, metastatic disease
  - Infection: bacterial (e.g., *Streptococcus*, *Staphylococcus*, TB), viral (e.g., URTI, Herpes simplex, Herpes zoster, EBV, HIV), other (e.g., Lyme disease, toxoplasmosis)

- Autoimmune: rheumatoid arthritis (RA), Sjogren syndrome, systemic lupus erythematosus (SLE)
- Miscellaneous: amyloidosis, sarcoidosis
- Iatrogenic: medications (e.g., phenytoin, allopurinol, atenolol, hydralazine, penicillin, cephalosporins)
- **Presentation:**
  - **Likely benign or inflammatory:** acute enlargement, painful, soft, mobile, no progression, generalised (see Infection and Autoimmune, and Lymphoma sections)
  - **Likely malignant:** slow growing, painless, unilateral, hard, fixed, progressive enlargement, localised (left supraclavicular node, a.k.a., Virchow's node=likely gastric cancer)

Investigations: clinical diagnosis. If not diagnostic for a specific disorder, further testing is required:
- **Blood:** anaemia, leucocytosis, neutropenia in leukaemia, positive viral serology
- **Chest x-ray (CXR):** hilar lymphadenopathy, nodules, cavitating lesions, lung mass
- *Lymph node biopsy*: differentiates benign from malignant histology
- **CT or MRI:** abnormal lymphadenopathy, identifies tumour site

Differentials: epidermoid cyst, lipoma, carotid body tumour

Management: treat underlying cause.

Epidermoid Cyst

Definition: a benign cyst derived from the upper portion of the hair follicle, encapsulated in a thin layer of squamous epithelium, typically filled with keratin and fatty deposits. Most common cutaneous cyst.

Buzzwords:
- **Risk factors:** 3rd to 4th decade of life, Gardner syndrome, *S. aureus*
- **Presentation:** firm, fixed, central punctum, compressible, cheesy discharge, asymptomatic (unless infected)

Investigations: clinical diagnosis

Differentials: lipoma, dental abscess, salivary gland pathology

Management:
1. Conservative (asymptomatic; small, uncomplicated cysts)
2. Incision and drainage (if acutely infected)
3. Surgical excision (definitive)

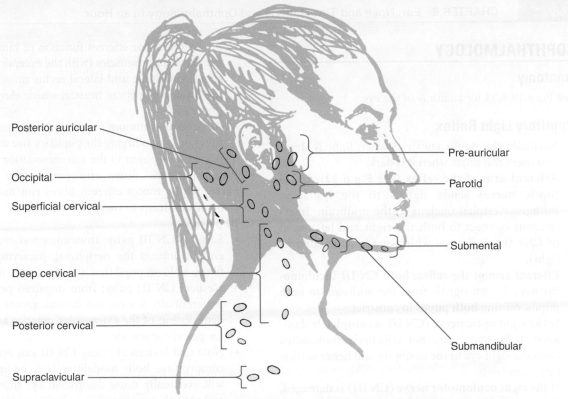

Posterior auricular

Occipital

Superficial cervical

Deep cervical

Posterior cervical

Supraclavicular

Pre-auricular

Parotid

Submental

Submandibular

Fig 6.18 Lymph Nodes of the Head and Neck. (Illustrated by Hollie Blaber.)

THE ONE-LINE ROUND-UP!

Here are some key words to help you remember each condition/concept.

Condition/Concept	One-line Description
Otitis externa	Swimmer's ear
Malignant otitis externa	Immunosuppression
Acute otitis media	Bulging tympanic membrane
Chronic suppurative otitis media	Perforated tympanic membrane
Otitis media with effusion	Fluid level behind tympanic membrane
Mastoiditis	Mastoid swelling with protruding pinna
Cholesteatoma	Keratin debris in attic region
BPPV	Worse on head movement
Labyrinthitis/vestibular neuronitis	Vertigo and sensorineural loss lasting days to weeks
Meniere's disease	Aural fullness
Vestibular schwannoma	Bilateral tumours=NF2
Presbycusis	Bilateral sensorineural loss
Childhood hearing loss	OAE 1st line, ABR 2nd line
Rhinosinusitis	Postnasal drip
Nasal polyps	Unilateral=think malignancy

Condition/Concept	One-line Description
Epistaxis	Little's area
Pharyngitis and tonsillitis	Fever PAIN
Epiglottitis	Haemophilus influenza B
Obstructive sleep apnoea	Polysomnography
Pharyngeal pouch	Barium swallow
Branchial cyst	Cholesterol contents
Thyroglossal duct cyst	Upward movement with tongue protrusion
Goitre	Upward movement on swallowing
Papillary	Psammoma bodies
Follicular	Cannot differentiate benign and malignant = thyroidectomy
Medullary	MEN II
Anaplastic	Rapidly enlarging poor prognosis
Lymphoma	Hashimoto's
Cystic hygroma	Transilluminates
Lymphadenopathy	Firm, fixed, painless = think malignancy
Epidermoid cyst	Central punctum

OPHTHALMOLOGY

Anatomy

See Fig 6.19-6.21 for anatomy of the eye.

Pupillary Light Reflex

- Normally, the pupils constrict when light is shone into them and dilate when it is dark.
- **Afferent arm of the reflex (see Fig 6.22): CN II (optic nerve)** sends signals to the ipsilateral Edinger-Westphal nucleus in the midbrain. Interneurons connect to both the right and left nuclei of CN3 (regardless of which eye is stimulated by light).
- **Efferent arm of the reflex: both CN III (oculomotor nerve)** send signals from the midbrain to **both** pupils, causing **both** pupils to constrict.
- **If the right optic nerve (CN II) is completely damaged,** light signals are not effectively transmitted from the right eye to the midbrain and hence neither pupil constricts.
- **If the right oculomotor nerve (CN III) is damaged,** light signals are transmitted correctly, but the right pupil cannot constrict because it is damaged, whilst the left pupil can constrict.

Direct Pupillary Reflex vs Consensual Pupillary Reflex

- **Direct response:** pupillary response of the eye into which light is being directly shone
- **Consensual response:** pupillary response of the eye contralateral to that into which light is being shone

Relative Afferent Pupillary Defect

A relative afferent pupillary defect (RAPD) indicates that there is damage to the optic nerve on one side more than the other. The deficit is best observed during a 'swinging light test', in which the examiner shines a light from one eye to the other. When the light is shone into the better eye, there is an immediate ipsilateral constriction of the pupil. When the light is shone into the affected eye, there is an initial dilation of the ipsilateral pupil before it constricts to direct light.

CRANIAL NERVES

CN III Palsy

Definition:
- The oculomotor nerve has two functions:

- A general motor efferent function of innervating the extraocular muscles (with the exception of the superior oblique and lateral rectus muscles) and the levator palpebrae muscle, which elevates the upper eyelid
- A general autonomic efferent/parasympathetic function of modifying the pupillary size and altering the lens power in the accommodation reflex
- Parasympathetic fibres run peripherally in the nerve, whilst motor efferent fibres run more centrally, which leads to two distinctive patterns of CN III palsies:
  - Surgical CN III palsy: from compression; preferentially injures the peripheral, parasympathetic fibres→ blown pupil that is unreactive to light
  - Medical CN III palsy: from impaired perfusion; preferentially injures the central, motor fibres→ denervation of the extraocular muscles and levator palpebrae muscle
  - Note that lesions affecting CN III can eventually compromise both modalities (i.e., compression will eventually cause disordered eye movements and ptosis)

Buzzwords:
- **Risk factors:** surgical palsy = trauma, posterior communicating artery (PComA) aneurysm; medical palsy = hypertension (HTN), DM, smoking, hyperlipidaemia
- **Presentation:** dilated pupil that is unreactive to light (consensual response intact), ptosis and paretic eye directed 'down-and-out' because the lateral rectus and superior oblique muscles 'win the tug of war' against the denervated muscles (see Fig 6.23)

Investigations:
- **Blood:** HbA1c, lipids
- **Blood pressure (BP)**
- **Urgent CT head/angiogram:** potential aneurysm, trauma

Differentials: PComA aneurysm, trauma, HTN, DM

Management:
- Surgical: urgent referral to neurosurgical team for PComA aneurysm/raised intracranial pressure (ICP)
- Medical: address vascular risk factors to reduce probability of further microvascular event
- Diplopia: prisms +/- squint surgery

CN IV Palsy

Definition: Trochlear nerve palsies can be very subtle. The inferior oblique muscle exerts two actions on the

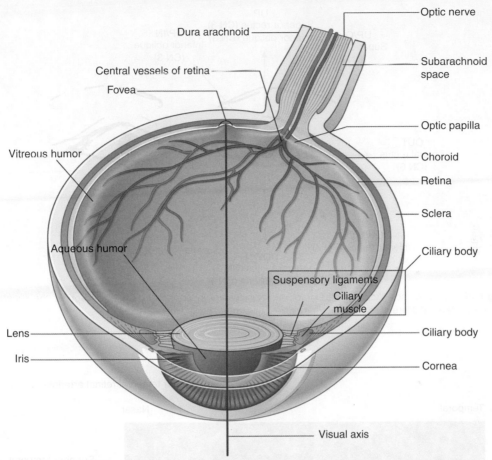

Fig 6.19 The Eyeball. (From Mtui, E. (2016) *Fitzgerald's clinical neuroanatomy* (7th ed.). Fig. 28.2. Philadelphia: Elsevier.)

eye: pulls the eye up when adducted and intorts the eye (rotates it toward the nose – clockwise for the right eye and counter clockwise for the left eye).

Buzzwords:

- **Risk factors:** very fragile and prone to injury intra-operatively and following trauma (due to its long intracranial course)
- **Presentation:** diplopia when walking downstairs or reading a book (looking down), extortive and upward drift of affected eye (see Fig 6.24), head tilt **away** from affected side (to straighten up their vision)

Investigations: clinical diagnosis

Differentials: congenital, trauma, postsurgical CN IV palsy

Management: prisms or squint surgery

CN VI Palsy

Definition: CN VI innervates the lateral rectus, which abducts the eye. If this muscle is denervated, the affected eye will be unable to abduct and may drift medially when looking straight ahead (see Fig 6.25).

Buzzwords:

- **Risk factors:** raised ICP, vascular risk factors, multiple sclerosis (MS), tumours in the cavernous sinus or orbit
- **Presentation:** diplopia (particularly on looking towards the affected side), impaired abduction.

Investigations:

- **BP**
- **Blood:** HbA1c, lipids

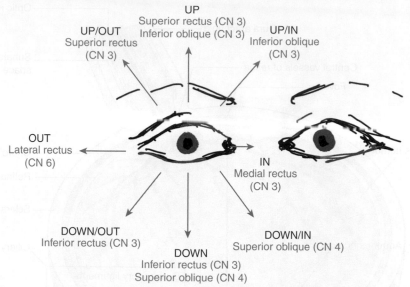

UP
Superior rectus (CN 3)
Inferior oblique (CN 3)

UP/OUT
Superior rectus
(CN 3)

UP/IN
Inferior oblique
(CN 3)

OUT
Lateral rectus
(CN 6)

IN
Medial rectus
(CN 3)

DOWN/OUT
Inferior rectus (CN 3)

DOWN/IN
Superior oblique (CN 4)

DOWN
Inferior rectus (CN 3)
Superior oblique (CN 4)

Fig 6.20 Ocular Muscle Actions. All extraocular muscles are innervated by CN III except for the superior oblique (CN IV) and lateral rectus (CN VI) muscles. (Illustrated by Dr Hollie Blaber.)

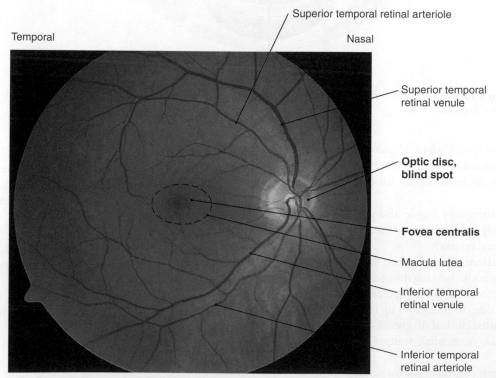

Temporal

Nasal

Superior temporal retinal arteriole

Superior temporal retinal venule

Optic disc, blind spot

Fovea centralis

Macula lutea

Inferior temporal retinal venule

Inferior temporal retinal arteriole

Fig 6.21 Right-eye Ophthalmoscopic View. (From Paulsen, F. & Waschke, J. (2018). *Sobotta atlas of human anatomy* (16th ed.). © Elsevier 2018 GmbH, Urban & Fischer, Munich.)

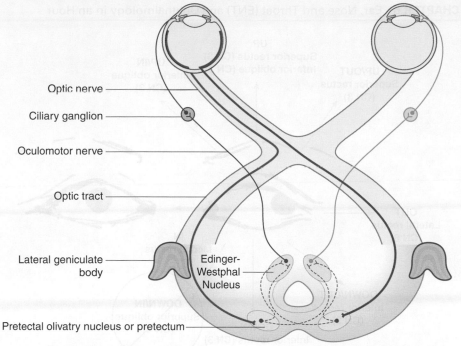

Optic nerve

Ciliary ganglion

Oculomotor nerve

Optic tract

Lateral geniculate body

Edinger-Westphal Nucleus

Pretectal olivatry nucleus or pretectum

Fig 6.22 Pupillary Light Reflex. (With permission from Kargon, R. (2011). Regulation of light through the pupil (Fig. 25.3). In *Adler's physiology of the eye*. Elsevier. Copyright © 2011 Elsevier Inc. All rights reserved.)

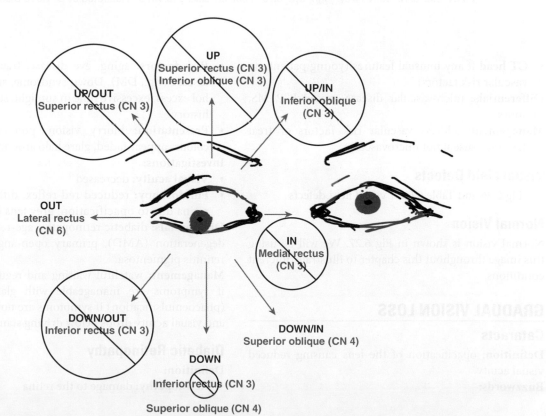

UP/OUT
Superior rectus (CN 3)

UP
Superior rectus (CN 3)
Inferior oblique (CN 3)

UP/IN
Inferior oblique (CN 3)

OUT
Lateral rectus (CN 6)

IN
Medial rectus (CN 3)

DOWN/OUT
Inferior rectus (CN 3)

DOWN/IN
Superior oblique (CN 4)

DOWN
Inferior rectus (CN 3)
Superior oblique (CN 4)

Fig 6.23 Cranial Nerve III Palsy. Right eye 'down and out' on looking forward. (Illustrated by Dr Hollie Blaber.)

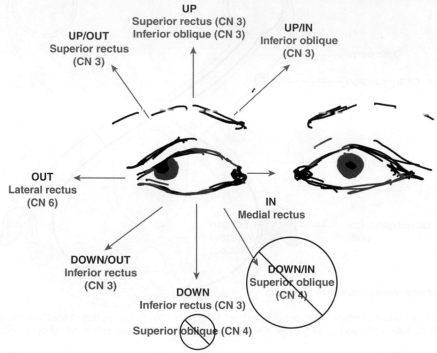

Fig 6.24 Cranial Nerve IV Palsy. Right eye 'up and out' on looking forward. (Illustrated by Dr Hollie Blaber.)

- **CT head** if any unusual features (young patient, no vascular risk factors)

Differentials: microvascular disease, raised ICP, MS, tumours

Management: address vascular risk factors or treat underlying cause if not microvascular

Visual Field Defects

See Fig 6.26 and Table 6.6 for visual field defects

Normal Vision

Normal vision is shown in Fig 6.27. We will be using this image throughout this chapter to illustrate different conditions.

GRADUAL VISION LOSS

Cataracts

Definition: opacification of the lens causing reduced visual acuity

Buzzwords:

- **Risk factors:** aging, eye disease, trauma, systemic disease (e.g., DM), Down syndrome, smoking, alcohol excess, excessive time in sunlight, steroids, family history
- **Presentation:** blurry vision, poor night vision, colours appear faded, glare halo around lights

Investigations:

- **Visual acuity:** decreased
- **Fundoscopy:** reduced red reflex, difficulty seeing retina due to opacification, grey lens (see Fig 6.28)

Differentials: diabetic retinopathy, age-related macular degeneration (AMD), primary open-angle glaucoma, retinitis pigmentosa.

Management: watchful waiting and regular follow-up if symptoms are manageable with glasses. Surgery (phacoemulsification) if symptoms are not manageable, and visual acuity drops below driving standards.

Diabetic Retinopathy

Definition:

- **Retinopathy:** damage to the retina

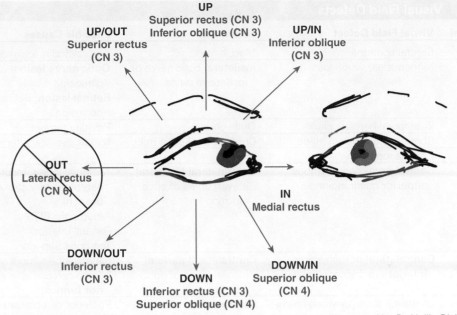

UP
Superior rectus (CN 3)
Inferior oblique (CN 3)

UP/OUT
Superior rectus
(CN 3)

UP/IN
Inferior oblique
(CN 3)

OUT
Lateral rectus
(CN 6)

IN
Medial rectus

DOWN/OUT
Inferior rectus
(CN 3)

DOWN
Inferior rectus (CN 3)
Superior oblique (CN 4)

DOWN/IN
Superior oblique
(CN 4)

Fig 6.25 Cranial Nerve VI Palsy. Right eye 'in' on looking straight ahead. (Illustrated by Dr Hollie Blaber.)

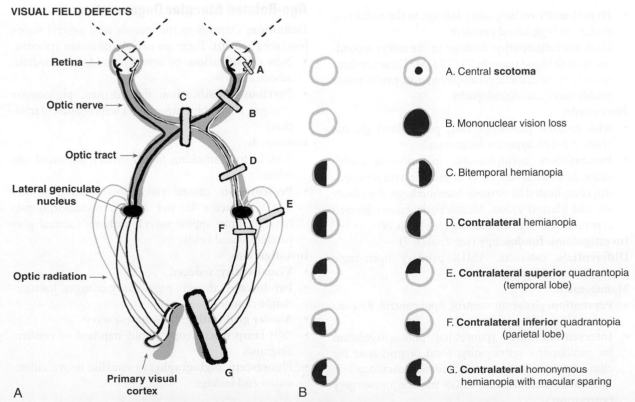

VISUAL FIELD DEFECTS

Retina

Optic nerve

Optic tract

Lateral geniculate
nucleus

Optic radiation

Primary visual
cortex

A

A. Central **scotoma**

B. Mononuclear vision loss

C. Bitemporal hemianopia

D. **Contralateral** hemianopia

E. **Contralateral superior** quadrantopia
(temporal lobe)

F. **Contralateral inferior** quadrantopia
(parietal lobe)

G. **Contralateral** homonymous
hemianopia with macular sparing

B

Fig 6.26 (A) Site of lesion. (B) Visual field defect. (Illustrated by Dr Hollie Blaber.)

TABLE 6.6   Visual Field Defects

Diagram Label	Visual Field Defect	Lesion Site	Possible Causes
A	Central scotoma	Macula	Age-related macular degeneration
B	Mononuclear vision loss	**Ipsilateral** optic nerve or **ipsilateral** retina	**Optic nerve lesion:** optic neuritis, glaucoma **Retinal lesion:** Retinal artery occlusion
C	Bitemporal hemianopia	Optic chiasm	Pituitary tumour
D	Contralateral homonymous hemianopia	**Contralateral** optic tract	Middle cerebral artery stroke (**stem**)
E	**Contralateral** homonymous **superior** quadrantanopia	**Contralateral temporal** (lower) fibres of optic radiation	Temporal lobe tumour or middle cerebral artery stroke (**inferior branch**) *Mnemonic:* PITS Parietal Inferior Temporal Superior
F	**Contralateral** homonymous **inferior** quadrantanopia	**Contralateral parietal** (upper) fibres of optic radiation	Parietal lobe tumour Middle cerebral artery stroke (**superior branch**)
G	Contralateral homonymous hemianopia with macular sparing	**Contralateral** optic radiation in the **occipital lobe**	Posterior cerebral artery stroke

- **Hypertensive retinopathy:** damage to the retina secondary to high blood pressure
- **Diabetic retinopathy:** damage to the retina secondary to high blood sugar in T1/T2 DM. There are three main types of diabetic retinopathy: non-proliferative, proliferative and maculopathy

Buzzwords:

- **Risk factors:** prolonged DM, poor blood glucose control, HTN, hypercholesteremia
- **Presentation:** asymptomatic in non-proliferative cases. In more severe cases of proliferative retinopathy, complicated by vitreous haemorrhage, then floaters and blurred vision. Maculopathy causes blurred central vision, e.g., for reading (see Fig 6.29)

Investigations: fundoscopy (see Table 6.7)

Differentials: cataracts, AMD, primary open-angle glaucoma, retinitis pigmentosa

Management:

- **Prevention:** glycaemic control, lipid control, BP control
- **Intervention:** laser (panretinal photocoagulation for proliferative retinopathy; focal or grid laser for clinically significant non-ischaemic maculopathy), intravitreal steroids, anti-VEGF medication, surgery (vitrectomy)

Age-Related Macular Degeneration

Definition: Damage to the macula with central vision loss (see Fig 6.30). There are two classification systems:

- **New classification:** by severity (mild, intermediate, advanced)
- **Previous classification:** dry (drusen, pigmentary changes, geographic atrophy) vs wet (neovascularisation)

Buzzwords:

- **Risk factors:** smoking, family history, advanced age, white
- **Presentation:** central vision loss (gradual in dry AMD, subacute in wet AMD), metamorphopsia (straight lines appear wavy), scotoma (central grey patch in visual field)

Investigations:

- **Visual acuity:** reduced
- **Fundoscopy:** drusen, pigmentary changes, haemorrhagic changes
- **Amsler grid testing:** lines appear wavy
- ***Slit-lamp microscopy*:** gold standard to confirm diagnosis
- **Fluorescein angiography:** to visualise neovascularisation and leakage

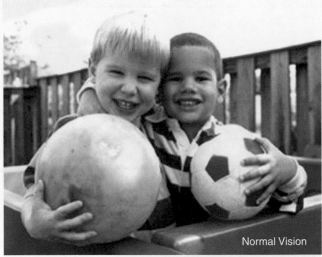

Fig 6.27 Normal Vision. (From Wikimedia Commons.)

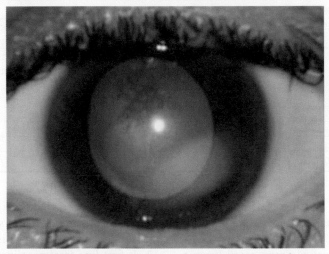

Fig 6.28 Cataract. (With permission from Thompson, J., & Lakhani, N. (2015). Cataracts (Fig. 5). In *Primary care: clinics in office practice*. Elsevier. Copyright © 2015 Elsevier Inc. All rights reserved.)

- **Optical coherence tomography (OCT):** to confirm the diagnosis and monitor the treatment response

Differentials: cataracts, diabetic retinopathy, primary open-angle glaucoma, retinitis pigmentosa

Management:
- Urgent referral to ophthalmologist if suspected (to be seen within 1 week)
- **Dry AMD:** manage risk factors (e.g., quit smoking), nutritional supplements
- **Wet AMD:** intravitreal injection of anti-VEGF drugs (e.g., ranibizumab, bevacizumab, and aflibercept)

Primary Open-Angle Glaucoma

Definition: reduced drainage of aqueous humour from the eye through the trabecular meshwork leading to a gradual increase in intraocular pressure and optic nerve damage.

Buzzwords:

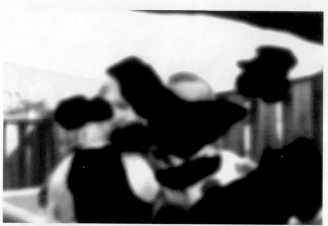

Fig 6.29 Diabetic Retinopathy. (With permission from National Eye Institute, National Institutes of Health. Public domain, via Wikimedia Commons.)

TABLE 6.7   Fundoscopy Findings in Diabetic Retinopathy

Type	Subtype	Fundoscopy Findings
Nonproliferative	Mild	≥1 microaneurysms
	Moderate	Microaneurysms or intraretinal haemorrhage +/- cotton wool spots, venous beading, intraretinal microvascular abnormalities
	Severe	Same as in moderate but need to be present in a specific number of quadrants (4-2-1 rule)
		Microaneurysms or intraretinal haemorrhages in 4 quadrants
		Venous beading in ≥2 quadrants
		Intraretinal microvascular abnormalities in ≥1 quadrant
Proliferative	N/A	Same as non-proliferative but with neovascularisation
Maculopathy	Focal	Leakage + circular ring of exudate (drusen = lipid deposits)
	Diffuse	Retinal oedema but no leakage
	Ischaemic	Confirmed with fluorescein angiography

- **Risk factors:** increased age, myopia (near-sighted), African American/Hispanic/Latino background, family history
- **Presentation:** asymptomatic in most cases. If symptomatic, may present with halos and tunnel vision

Investigations:
- **Visual fields:** tunnel vision (see Fig 6.31)
- **Fundoscopy:** cupping of optic disc
- **Goldmann applanation tonometry:** to check intraocular pressure

Differentials: cataracts, diabetic retinopathy, AMD, retinitis pigmentosa

Management: start treatment if intraocular pressure ≥21 mm Hg
1. First-line topical treatment: prostaglandin analogue (e.g., latanoprost, travoprost, bimatoprost). Other topical drugs include beta blockers (e.g., timolol), carbonic anhydrase inhibitors (e.g., dorzolamide, brinzolamide) and alpha-2-agonists (e.g., brimonidine).
2. If first-line treatment ineffective: switch to a different topical treatment, combine topical treatments or consider selective laser trabeculoplasty or surgery (trabeculectomy)

Retinitis Pigmentosa

Definition: Rare inherited genetic condition causing degeneration of the photoreceptors of the retina (rods mainly, cones are affected later). More than 50 genes are implicated in causing this disorder. Retinitis pigmentosa can be inherited in three ways: autosomal dominant, autosomal recessive and X linked.

Buzzwords:

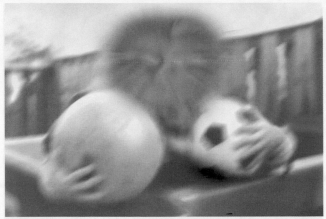

Fig 6.30 Macular Degeneration. (With permission from National Eye Institute, National Institutes of Health. Public domain, via Wikimedia Commons.)

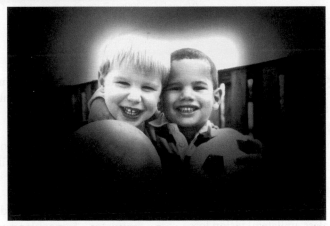

Fig 6.31 Glaucoma. (With permission from National Eye Institute, National Institutes of Health. Public domain, via Wikimedia Commons.)

- **Risk factors:** family history, associated syndromes (e.g., Usher syndrome)
- **Presentation:** gradual onset in childhood or adulthood depending on the gene implicated. Rod degeneration causes a loss of peripheral vision ('tunnel vision') and a loss of night vision.

Investigations:

- **Visual acuity:** decreased late in disease
- **Visual fields:** loss of peripheral vision
- **Fundoscopy:** shows *bone spicule-shaped* pigment in periphery with peripheral retinal atrophy (see Fig 6.32)
- **Electroretinogram (ERG):** decreased electrical responses of photoreceptors to light

- **Genetic testing:** to identify the specific gene defect, which determines the prognosis

Differentials: cataracts, diabetic retinopathy, AMD, glaucoma

Management:

- No specific intervention available to stop progression
- **Improve function:** low-vision aids, guide dog
- Gene therapy is available for *RPE65* mutations (Luxterna)
- Other recent developments are in the clinical trial stage:
  - Gene therapy for other gene mutations
  - Epiretinal electrode microarray ('bionic eye')

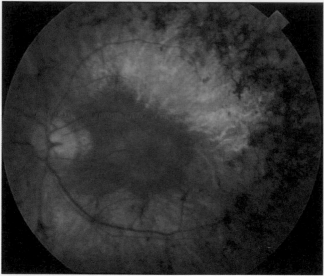

Fig 6.32 Retinitis Pigmentosa on Fundoscopy. (Hamel, C. (2006). Retinitis pigmentosa. *Orphanet J Rare Dis* 1, 40. https://doi.org/10.1186/1750-1172-1-40.)

ACUTE PAINLESS VISION LOSS

Central Retinal Artery Occlusion

Definition: blocked central artery by an embolus (painless) or inflammation secondary to giant cell arteritis (GCA) (painful).

Buzzwords:
- **Risk factors:** atrial fibrillation (AF), atherosclerosis, GCA
- **Presentation:** acute, painless, unilateral vision loss

Investigations:
- **Visual acuity:** decreased
- **Fundoscopy:** pale retina, cherry-red spot (see Fig 6.33), RAPD

Differentials: central retinal vein occlusion, vitreous haemorrhage, retinal detachment

Management:
1. Emergency referral to ophthalmologist
2. Ocular massage or anterior paracentesis to try to dislodge clot
3. Long term: treat underlying vascular risk factors

Retinal Vein Occlusion

Definition: blocked central vein by thrombosis leading to retinal haemorrhages and exudates
- **Central retinal vein occlusion:** widespread retinal haemorrhages affecting the whole retina
- **Branch retinal vein occlusion:** localised retinal haemorrhages in the distribution of one branch vein (see Fig 6.34)

Buzzwords:
- **Risk factors:** atherosclerosis, HTN, DM
- **Presentation:** sudden painless vision loss

Investigations:
- Visual acuity: decreased
- Fundoscopy: flame and blot haemorrhages and exudates +/- macular oedema and neovascularisation

Differentials: central retinal artery occlusion, vitreous haemorrhage, retinal detachment

Management:
- Urgent referral to ophthalmologist
- Laser photocoagulation, anti-VEGF therapies (e.g., ranibizumab, aflibercept or bevacizumab), steroids (e.g., a dexamethasone intravitreal implant) to treat neovascularisation/macula oedema

Vitreous Haemorrhage

Definition: bleeding into the vitreous gel

Buzzwords:
- **Risk factors:** proliferative diabetic retinopathy, retinal detachment, posterior vitreous detachment, anticoagulation medications or trauma
- **Presentation:** acute painless vision loss, floaters

Investigations:
- **Visual acuity:** decreased
- **Fundoscopy:** haemorrhage in vitreous gel

Differentials: central retinal artery occlusion, central retinal vein occlusion, retinal detachment

Management:
1. Emergency referral to ophthalmologist to rule out retinal detachment
2. Observation if no retinal detachment present – vitreous haemorrhage clears on its own in weeks

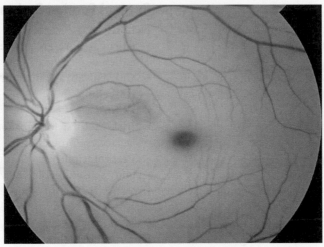

Fig 6.33 Central Retinal Artery Occlusion. (With permission from sidthedoc, CC BY-SA 4.0, via Wikimedia Commons.)

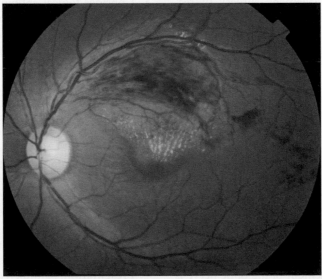

Fig 6.34 Branch Retinal Vein Occlusion. (From Yong, K. C., Kah, T. A., & Ghee, Y. T., et al. (2011). Branch retinal vein occlusion associated with quetiapine fumarate. *BMC Ophthalmol 11*, 24. https://doi.org/10.1186/1471-2415-11-24.)

3. If patient has a retinal detachment, then vitrectomy is required
4. Patients with proliferative diabetic retinopathy may need vitrectomy if the haemorrhage does not clear within 12 weeks

Retinal Detachment

Definition: retina separates and lifts up from the back of the eye allowing serous fluid to accumulate underneath. Usually occurs due to a retinal tear.
Buzzwords:
- **Risk factors:** posterior vitreous detachment, proliferative diabetic retinopathy, trauma, cataract surgery, myopia
- **Presentation:** acute painless vision loss, floaters, flashes, blurred vision, shadow/curtain

Investigations:
- Visual field loss
- **Fundoscopy:** asymmetrical red reflex, retinal detachment

Differentials: central retinal artery occlusion, central retinal vein occlusion, vitreous haemorrhage
Management: immediate referral to an ophthalmologist
- Retinal tear management (without detachment): laser therapy or cryotherapy
- Retinal detachment management: surgery (vitrectomy plus pneumatic retinopexy or scleral buckle)

ACUTE PAINFUL VISION LOSS

Optic Neuritis

Definition: inflammation of the optic nerve
Buzzwords:
- **Risk factors:** young females
- **Presentation:** subacute blurred vision, reduced colour vision, eye pain at rest and on eye movement

Investigations:
- **Cranial nerve examination:** RAPD, reduced colour vision, visual field loss
- **Fundoscopy:** often normal appearance of optic nerve (retrobulbar optic neuritis), but may be swollen
- **MRI:** sometimes enhancement of the optic nerve is visible, may show other evidence of MS (see Fig 6.35)

Differentials: MS, neuromyelitis optica, anterior ischaemic optic neuropathy, acute glaucoma

Management: referral to an ophthalmologist and/or neurologist. High-dose oral or IV methylprednisolone if patient already has poor vision in the other eye or bilateral disease

RED EYE

Corneal Foreign Body and Corneal Abrasion

Definition:
- **Corneal foreign body:** dust or other particles adhered to surface of the cornea
- **Corneal abrasion:** traumatic break in the corneal epithelium

Buzzwords:
- **Risk factors:** foreign body, trauma, contact lenses, lack of eye protection
- **Presentation:** red, painful eye; lacrimation; foreign body sensation; blurred vision

Investigations: slit-lamp examination for diagnosis. Fluorescein stain to check for abrasion or foreign body. (see Fig 6.36)
Differentials: other causes of red eye
Management:
- Emergency (same-day referral) to ophthalmology
- Remove foreign body under topical anaesthesia with sterile cotton bud, needle or burr
- Consider topical antibiotic prophylaxis (e.g., chloramphenicol QDS for 5 days)
- Do not wear contact lenses during treatment
- Systemic analgesia for first 24 h (e.g., ibuprofen) or very limited supply of topical anaesthesia for home
- Consider cycloplegia to prevent pupil spasm (e.g., cyclopentolate 0.1% BD).

Keratitis

Definition: inflammation of the cornea. Causes include infection (e.g., viral, bacterial, fungal, *Acanthamoeba*) and non-infectious causes (e.g., autoimmune conditions, foreign bodies like contact lenses).
Buzzwords:
- **Risk factors:** contact lenses, immunodeficiency, steroid use, autoimmune diseases (e.g., RA)
- **Presentation:** painful, red eye; photophobia; reduced visual acuity

Investigation:
- **Slit-lamp examination** (see Fig 6.38) for diagnosis

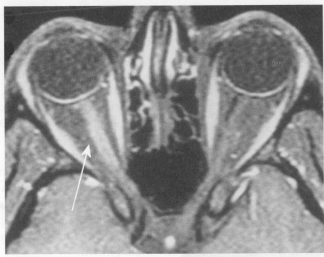

Fig 6.35 Axial T1-weighted, Fat-suppressed, Gadolinium-enhanced Orbital MRI in Optic Neuritis. (With permission from Pineles, S. L., & Balcer, L. J. (2019). Visual loss optic neuropathies (Fig. 5.32). In *Liu, Volpe, and Galetta's neuro-ophthalmology*. Elsevier. Copyright © 2019 Elsevier Inc. All rights reserved.)

- **Fluorescein stain:** may show dendritic ulcers in HSV 1 or 2 keratitis (see Fig 6.37)

Differentials: other causes of red eye

Management:

- Emergency (same-day) referral to ophthalmologist
- **Bacterial keratitis:** topical fluoroquinolone (e.g., ofloxacin, levofloxacin or moxifloxacin)
- **Acanthamoeba keratitis:** topical polyhexamethylene biguanide 0.02% or chlorhexidine 0.02% and propamidine 0.1% (Brolene)
- **Viral keratitis:** topical occ. aciclovir
- **Fungal keratitis:** topical natamycin 5%
- **Non-infectious keratitis:** treat underlying cause

Anterior Uveitis (Iritis)

Definition: inflammation of the uveal tract (iris, ciliary body, choroid)

Buzzwords:

- **Risk factors:** autoimmune disorders, trauma, infection, HLA B27, juvenile RA
- **Presentation:** red, painful eye; photophobia; lacrimation; synechiae; ciliary flush

Investigation: slit-lamp examination (ciliary flush, keratic precipitates, posterior synechiae (see Fig 6.39), hypopyon)

Differentials: other causes of red eye

Management:

- Emergency (same-day) referral to ophthalmology

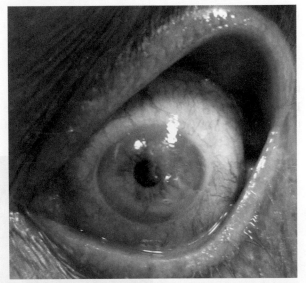

Fig 6.36 Corneal Abrasion Highlighted by Fluorescein Staining. (With permission from Heilman, J. CC BY-SA 3.0, via Wikimedia Commons.)

- Topical corticosteroids to reduce inflammation
- Cycloplegic-mydriatic drug (e.g., cyclopentolate) to paralyse ciliary body
- In severe or chronic cases, intravitreal steroid implants or systemic immunosuppressive drugs (e.g.,

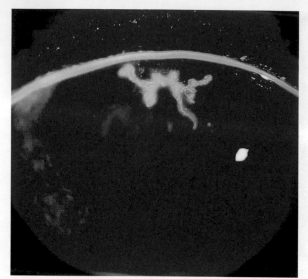

Fig 6.37 Dendritic Pattern after Fluorescein Staining. (With permission from Imrankabirhossain. CC BY-SA 4.0, via Wikimedia Commons.)

prednisolone, methotrexate, mycophenolate mofetil), TNF inhibitors (e.g., adalimumab), laser phototherapy, cryotherapy or vitrectomy

Primary Angle-Closure Glaucoma

Definition: complete closure of the angle between the iris and cornea prevents drainage of the aqueous fluid of

the eye, leading to an increased intraocular pressure and optic nerve damage.

Buzzwords:

- **Risk factors:** increased age, female, Asian ethnicity, hyperopia (long-sighted)
- **Presentation:** acute red, painful eye; hazy cornea; blurred vision; lacrimation; firm eyeball; fixed mid-dilated pupil (see Fig 6.40)

Investigation:

- **Visual acuity:** decreased
- **Fundoscopy:** optic disc cupping
- ***Goldmann applanation tonometry*:** gold standard to check intraocular pressure

Differentials: corneal foreign body, corneal abrasion, keratitis, anterior uveitis, scleritis

Management:

- Emergency (same-day) referral to ophthalmologist
- Miotic agent (e.g., pilocarpine) to open the angle between the iris and cornea
- Oral or intravenous carbonic anhydrase inhibitor (e.g., acetazolamide) to reduce production of aqueous humour
- Analgesia
- YAG laser peripheral iridotomy

Scleritis

Definition: inflammation of the sclera

Buzzwords:

- **Risk factors:** systemic inflammatory disease (e.g., RA, SLE, sarcoidosis, irritable bowel disease (IBD))

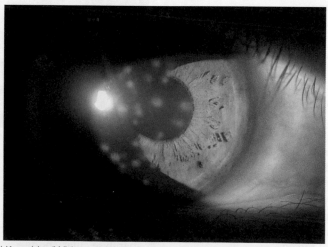

Fig 6.38 Adenoviral Keratitis. (With permission from Imrankabirhossain. CC BY-SA 4.0, via Wikimedia Commons.)

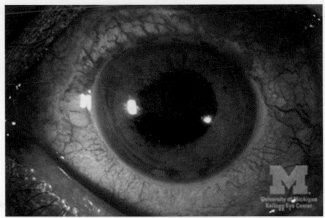

Fig 6.39 Anterior Uveitis with Posterior Synechiae. (With permission from Trobe, J. CC BY 3.0, via Wikimedia Commons.)

- **Presentation:** extremely painful red eye (localised or diffuse - see Fig 6.41), photophobia, lacrimation, visual loss
- Note painless scleritis can occur in RA, which can lead to a perforation of the globe (scleromalacia perforans)

Investigation: visual acuity is decreased. Further investigations for systemic inflammatory disease

Differentials: other causes of red eye

Management:
- Emergency (same-day) referral to ophthalmologist
- NSAIDs (topical/systemic)
- Steroids (topical/systemic)
- Immunosuppression for chronic or frequently relapsing cases (e.g., methotrexate, azathioprine)

Orbital and Preseptal Cellulitis

Definition:
- **Orbital cellulitis (see Fig 6.43):** inflammation of tissues lying posterior to the orbital septum, most commonly due to local/systemic bacterial infection (e.g., *Streptococcus*, *S. aureus*, *H. influenzae*)
- **Preseptal cellulitis (see Fig 6.42):** inflammation limited to structures anterior to the orbital septum, usually confined to the eyelid. Five times more common than orbital cellulitis

Buzzwords:
- **Risk factors:** URTI, sinusitis, trauma, eye surgery, dental abscess
- **Presentation:**
  - **Both:** red, swollen eyelid and conjunctiva +/- fever and malaise

- **Orbital:** proptosis (protrusion of eyeball), red eye, pain, limited eye movements, reduced visual acuity, +/- RAPD, reduced colour vision, progression to involve the central nervous system (CNS)

Investigations:
- **Visual acuity:** normal (preseptal cellulitis), decreased (orbital cellulitis)
- **Eye movements:** normal (preseptal cellulitis), limited (orbital cellulitis)
- **CT sinuses and orbit:** only indicated for orbital cellulitis
- **Blood:** only indicated for orbital cellulitis. Includes FBC, blood cultures

Differentials: other causes of red eye

Management:
- Emergency (same-day) referral to ophthalmologist and ENT
- **Orbital cellulitis:** admission and IV antibiotics (co-amoxiclav in non-penicillin allergy). Consider surgery if abscess detected on CT scan
- **Preseptal cellulitis:** consider admission if systematically unwell. Antibiotics (co-amoxiclav in non-penicillin allergy)
- **In children:** admit and treat as orbital cellulitis until proven otherwise

Thyroid Eye Disease

Definition: inflammation of the muscles and soft tissues of the orbit, caused by Grave's disease. Patients can be hyperthyroid, euthyroid or hypothyroid.

Buzzwords:
- **Risk factors:** female, myasthenia gravis, smoking

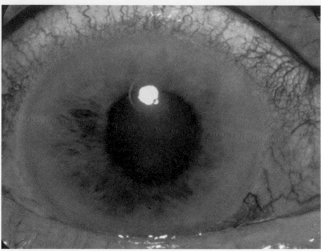

Fig 6.40 Acute Angle-closure Glaucoma. (With permission from Trobe, J. CC BY 3.0, via Wikimedia Commons.)

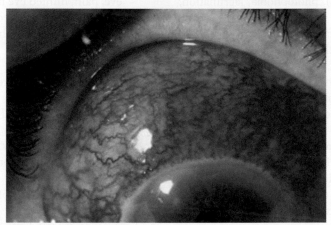

Fig 6.41 Diffuse Anterior Scleritis. (With permission from Galor, A., & Thorne, J. E. (2007). Scleritis and peripheral ulcerative keratitis (Fig. 2). In *Rheumatic disease clinics of North America*. Elsevier. Copyright © 2007 Elsevier Inc. All rights reserved.)

- **Presentation:** unilateral or bilateral symptoms, eyelid retraction (see Fig 6.44), proptosis (bulging eyes), lagophthalmos (inability to close eyes completely), reduced eye movements, photophobia, gritty eyes, painful eye (especially on movement), excessive tearing or dry eyes in some cases.

Investigations:
- **Blood:** thyroid function tests (hyper/hypo/euthyroid) and anti-thyroid antibodies (see Endocrinology in an Hour chapter)
- **CT/MRI scan of orbits:** increase in the size of extraocular muscles/increase in the orbital fat volume

Differentials: physiological exophthalmos
Management:
- **Mild cases:** artificial tears
- **Moderate to severe cases:** systemic (oral or IV) steroids +/- surgery (decompression surgery, eye muscle surgery, eyelid surgery)

Conjunctivitis

Definition: inflammation of conjunctiva. Three main causes: bacterial, viral and allergic
Buzzwords:
- **Risk factors:** depends on cause (see below)

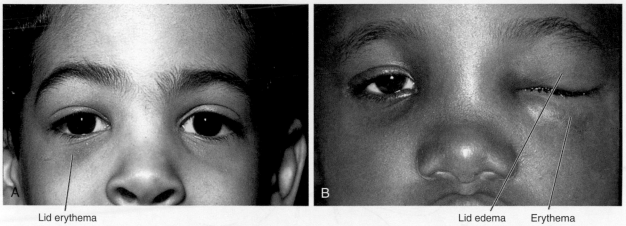

Lid erythema

Lid edema   Erythema

Fig 6.42 Preseptal cellulitis (A) in lighter skin, (B) in darker skin. (With permission from Neil J. Friedman, N. J., Kaiser, P. K., & Pineda, R, II. (2021). Orbit (Figs. 1.10 and 1.11). In *The Massachusetts Eye and Ear Infirmary illustrated manual of ophthalmology*. Elsevier. Copyright © 2021 Elsevier Inc. All rights reserved.)

Lid edema/erythema

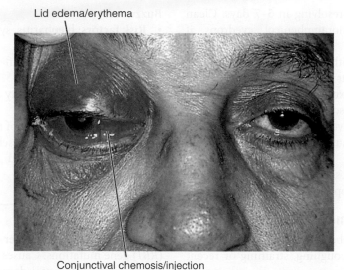

Conjunctival chemosis/injection

Fig 6.43 Orbital Cellulitis. (With permission from Neil J. Friedman, N. J., Kaiser, P. K., & Pineda, R, II. (2021). Orbit (Fig. 1.12). In *The Massachusetts Eye and Ear Infirmary illustrated manual of ophthalmology*. Elsevier. Copyright © 2021 Elsevier Inc. All rights reserved.)

- **Bacterial:** contact lenses, poor hygiene, close contact (sexually transmitted chlamydia/gonorrhoea)
- **Viral:** poor hygiene, close contact (school), URTI
- **Allergic:** contact with allergen (e.g., grass pollen, animal dander)
- **Presentation (see Fig 6.45):**
  - **Bacterial:** starts in one eye and then spreads to the other. Red, burning, grittiness, **purulent discharge**, crusting (eyelids get stuck during sleep)

- **Gonococcal:** rare – as above, but with risk of progression to disseminated infection/vision loss
- **Viral:** same as bacterial but discharge is clear
- **Allergic:** one or both eyes affected. Eyelid oedema, chemosis (swelling of conjunctiva), itching, lacrimation

Investigations: clinical diagnosis. Eye swab to identify organism

Differentials: other causes of red eye

Management:

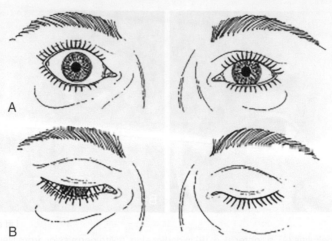

Fig 6.44 Thyroid Eye Disease. (A) Eyelid retraction. (B) lagophthalmos. (With permission from Cockerham, K. P., & Chan, S. S. (2010). Thyroid eye disease. In *Neurologic clinics*. Elsevier. Copyright © 2010 Elsevier Inc. All rights reserved.)

- **Bacterial:** usually self-resolving in 5–7 days. Clean eyelids regularly. Chloramphenicol eyedrops if needed.
  - **Chlamydia:** oral azithromycin/doxycycline, tracing of sexual contacts
  - **Gonococcal:** ceftriaxone IM/azithromycin PO
- **Viral:** usually self-resolving within 1–2 weeks. Antivirals are ineffective against *Adenovirus* infection (most common cause). Artificial tears can help relieve symptoms
- **Allergic:** usually self-resolving in a few hours. Consider antihistamines (topical/systemic)

Subconjunctival Haemorrhage

Definition: bleed into subconjunctival space (see Fig 6.46) caused by trauma, coughing, straining or recent eye surgery
Buzzwords:
- **Risk Factors:** contact sports, HTN, anticoagulation, bleeding disorder, trauma, DM
- **Presentation:** may be asymptomatic or mild ache
Investigations:
- **Visual acuity:** normal
- **BP:** may be raised
Differentials: other causes of red eye
Management: reassurance. Self-resolving in 5–10 days. Haemorrhage will usually turn yellow then disappear

Episcleritis

Definition: episcleral inflammation (see Fig 6.47)

Buzzwords:
- **Risk factors:** blepharitis, systemic inflammatory disease (e.g., RA, SLE, IBD)
- **Presentation:** one eye affected, mild ache, red eye (localised or diffuse)
Investigations: Visual acuity and fundoscopy are normal
Differentials: other causes of red eye
Management: reassurance (self-resolving in 7–10 days). Artificial tears can be offered

MALIGNANCY

Retinoblastoma

Definition: childhood cancer caused by retinoblastoma (*RB1*) gene mutations. Causes include:
- Inherited (autosomal-dominant) mutations: usually affects both eyes
- Non-inherited mutations: usually affects one eye
Buzzwords:
- **Risk factors:** family history, low birth weight, prematurity
- **Presentation:** leukocoria (white pupillary reflex instead of red - see Fig 6.48), strabismus
Investigations:
- **Fundoscopy:** leukocoria, white retinal mass
- **Ocular ultrasound and MRI:** characterise tumour/spread
Differentials: congenital cataract, retinal detachment, uveitis, corneal opacity

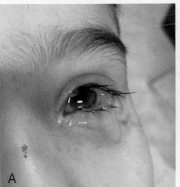
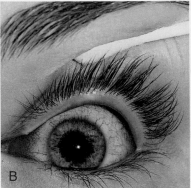
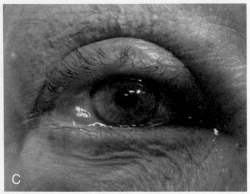

Fig 6.45 (A) Bacterial conjunctivitis (*left*). (B) Viral conjunctivitis (*middle*). (C) Allergic conjunctivitis (*right*). (With permission from (A) Gzzz. CC BY-SA 4.0, via Wikimedia Commons; (B) Joyhill09. CC BY-SA 3.0, via Wikimedia Commons; (C) Heilman, J. CC BY-SA 4.0, via Wikimedia Commons.)

Management:
- Urgent referral (2-week wait) to ophthalmologist
- Specialist management: laser, cryotherapy or plaque radiotherapy for small tumours; surgery, radiotherapy and chemotherapy for large tumours

EYELID PROBLEMS
Blepharitis
Definition: inflammation of eyelid margins (often bilateral). Two types:
- **Anterior blepharitis:** inflammation of the base of the eyelashes (see Fig 6.49)
- **Posterior blepharitis:** inflammation of meibomian glands

Buzzwords:
- **Risk factors:** dry eye disease, seborrheic dermatitis, acne rosacea
- **Presentation:** bilateral burning, itching, crusting of eyelids (worst in the morning)

Investigations: clinical diagnosis
Differentials: chalazion, conjunctivitis, dry eye disease, preseptal cellulitis
Management:
1. Eyelid hygiene and warm compresses
2. If first step ineffective, consider antibiotics:
    - Anterior blepharitis: topical chloramphenicol

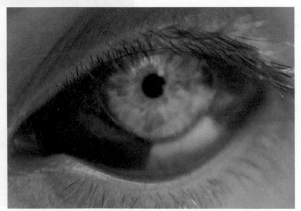

Fig 6.46 Subconjunctival Haemorrhage. (With permission from Therealbs (2002). CC BY-SA 3.0, via Wikimedia Commons.)

- Posterior blepharitis: oral doxycycline or tetracycline
3. Advise patient that blepharitis is a chronic, intermittent condition
4. Artificial tears

Stye (Hordeolum)
Definition: infection and inflammation of the tear glands of the eyelids (usually unilateral, see Fig 6.50). Two types:
- External stye: present on eyelid margin
- Internal stye: present on conjunctival side of the eyelid
Buzzwords:

- **Risk factors:** chronic blepharitis, acne rosacea
- **Presentation:** unilateral swelling and pus affecting the eyelid, presents over days

Investigations: clinical diagnosis

Differentials: blepharitis, xanthelasma, papilloma

Management:

- Reassurance; self-resolving
- Warm compresses
- If it doesn't resolve, refer to ophthalmologist for incision and drainage

Chalazion (Meibomian Cyst)

Definition: obstruction of sebaceous gland that causes the gland to enlarge (see Fig 6.51). Sometimes the chalazion ruptures, releasing lipids into the surrounding tissue and stimulating an inflammatory response.

Buzzwords:

- **Risk factors:** other eyelid problems (e.g., blepharitis, stye), skin problems (e.g., acne rosacea, seborrheic dermatitis)
- **Presentation:** unilateral swelling of upper eyelid (more common), painless, develops over weeks

Investigations: clinical diagnosis

Differentials: blepharitis, stye, sebaceous gland carcinoma

Management:

1. Warm compresses and gentle massage
2. If no improvement in 6 months, refer to ophthalmologist

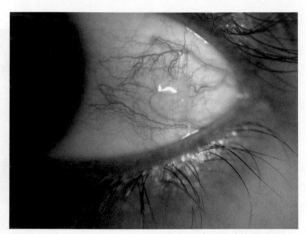

Fig 6.47 Episcleritis. (With permission from Imrankabirhossain. CC BY-SA 4.0, via Wikimedia Commons.)

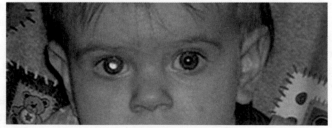

Fig 6.48 Leukocoria, Right Eye. (With permission from Parulekar, M. V. (2010). Retinoblastoma – Current treatment and future direction (Fig. 3). In *Early human development*. Elsevier. Copyright © 2010 Elsevier Ireland Ltd. All rights reserved.)

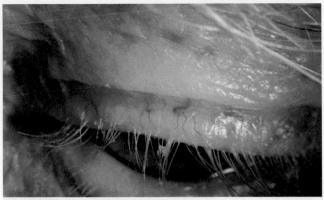

Fig 6.49 Anterior Blepharitis. (With permission from Isteitiya, J., Gadaria-Rathod, N., Fernandez, K. B., & Asbell, P. A. (2019). Blepharitis. In *Ophthalmology*. Elsevier. Copyright © 2019 Elsevier Inc. All rights reserved.)

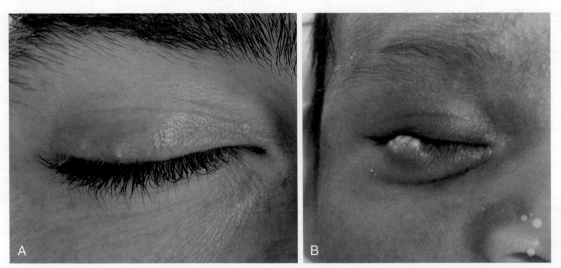

Fig 6.50 (A) External stye in lighter skin. (B) Internal stye in darker skin. (With permission from (A) Heilman, J. CC BY-SA 4.0, via Wikimedia Commons; (B) SKIN DEEP. Red swollen lesion with yellowish spots on the lower lid. https://dftbskindeep.com/all-diagnoses/stye/#!jig[1]/ ML/3449.)

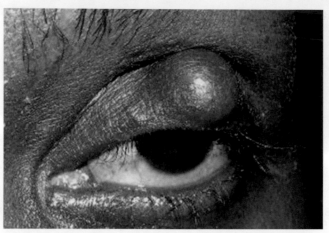

Fig 6.51 Chalazion, Upper Lid. (Courtesy of Dr Mark Mannis.)

THE ONE-LINE ROUND-UP!

Here are some key words to help you remember each condition/concept.

Condition/Concept	One-line Description
RAPD	Affected eye – initially dilates with swinging light test
CN III palsy	Dilated, ptosis, down and out
CN IV palsy	Diplopia walking down the stairs
CN VI palsy	Medial deviation, cavernous sinus tumours
Visual field defect	Bitemporal – optic chiasm, homonymous hemianopia – stroke, PITS
Cataracts	Old age/DM – lens opacification
Diabetic retinopathy	Non-proliferative vs proliferative = neovascularisation
Age-related macular degeneration	Central vision loss, VEG-F
Primary open-angle glaucoma	Tunnel vision, raised intraocular pressure, prostaglandin analogues
Retinitis pigmentosa	Loss of night vision, family history, bone spicule pigment

Condition/Concept	One-line Description
Central retinal artery occlusion	Cherry red spot, pale retina, AF
Retinal vein occlusion	Flame-shaped haemorrhages
Vitreous haemorrhage	Floaters, DM, anticoagulation
Retinal detachment	Flashers, shadow/curtain
Optic neuritis	RAPD, loss of colour vision, MS
Corneal FB/abrasion	Fluorescein staining
Keratitis	Contact lenses, dendritic pattern in HSV
Anterior uveitis	Autoimmune conditions, synechiae, photophobia
Primary angle-closure glaucoma	Fixed dilated pupil, hazy cornea, haloes around light
Scleritis	Very painful, systemic inflammatory disease, photophobia
Orbital/preseptal cellulitis	Inflammation – behind or in front of orbital septum
Thyroid eye disease	Proptosis, lagophthalmos, Grave's disease
Conjunctivitis	Bacterial = purulent, viral/allergic = clear discharge

THE ONE-LINE ROUND-UP!—cont'd

Subconjunctival haemorrhage	Painless red eye following coughing/trauma	Blepharitis	Inflammation of eyelid margin, crusting
Episcleritis	Mildly irritated, normal acuity, self-resolving	Stye (hordeolum)	Infection of tear gland in eyelid, warm compresses
Retinoblastoma	Leukocoria (loss of red reflex)	Chalazion (meibomian cyst)	Sebaceous gland obstruction, lump in eyelid

READING LIST: ENT

Otitis Externa (OE)
NICE. (2018). *CKS: Otitis externa.* https://cks.nice.org.uk/topics/otitis-externa/. [Accessed April 2021].
ENT UK. (2020). *Guideline on necrotising otitis externa.* https://www.entuk.org/sites/default/files/files/Necrotising%20otitis%20externa.pdf. [Accessed April 2021].

Otitis media (OM)
NICE. (2018). *CKS: Otitis media acute.* https://cks.nice.org.uk/topics/otitis-media-acute/. [Accessed April 2021].
NICE. (2017). *CKS: Otitis media chronic suppurative.* https://cks.nice.org.uk/topics/otitis-media-chronic-suppurative/. [Accessed April 2021].
NICE. (2016). *CKS: Otitis media with effusion.* https://cks.nice.org.uk/topics/otitis-media-with-effusion/. [Accessed April 2021].
BNF. (2020). *Ear infections, antibacterial therapy.* https://bnf.nice.org.uk/treatment-summary/ear-infections-antibacterial-therapy.html. [Accessed April 2021].

Mastoiditis
British Society of Otology. (2020). *Mastoiditis.* https://www.entuk.org/sites/default/files/files/Mastoiditis%20flowchart%20v7.pdf. [Accessed April 2021].
Patient info. (2015a). *Mastoiditis.* https://patient.info/doctor/mastoiditis. [Accessed April 2021].

Cholesteatoma
NICE. (2019). *CKS: Cholesteatoma.* https://cks.nice.org.uk/topics/cholesteatoma/. [Accessed April 2021].
BMJ Best Practice. (2019). *Cholesteatoma.* https://bestpractice.bmj.com/topics/en-gb/1033. [Accessed April 2021].

Benign Paroxysmal Positional Vertigo (BPPV)
NICE. (2017). *CKS: Benign paroxysmal positional vertigo.* https://cks.nice.org.uk/topics/benign-paroxysmal-positional-vertigo/. [Accessed April 2021].

Labyrinthitis and Vestibular Neuronitis
NICE. (2017). *CKS: Vestibular neuronitis.* https://cks.nice.org.uk/topics/vestibular-neuronitis/. [Accessed April 2021].
Australian Family Physician. (2016). *An approach to vertigo in general practice.* https://www.racgp.org.au/afp/2016/april/an-approach-to-vertigo-in-general-practice/. [Accessed April 2021].

Ménière's Disease
NICE. (2017). *CKS: Ménière's disease.* https://cks.nice.org.uk/topics/menieres-disease. [Accessed April 2021].
BMJ Best Practice. (2019). *Ménière's disease.* https://bestpractice.bmj.com/topics/en-gb/155. [Accessed April 2021].

Vestibular Schwannoma (Acoustic Neuroma)
NHS Commissioning Board. (2013). *Clinical commissioning policy: Vestibular schwannoma and other cranial nerve neuromas.* https://www.england.nhs.uk/wp-content/uploads/2018/07/Stereotactic-radiosurgery-radiotherapy-for-vestibular-schwannoma-and-other-cranial-nerve-neuromas.pdf. [Accessed April 2021].
BMJ Best Practice. (2020). *Vestibular schwannoma.* https://bestpractice.bmj.com/topics/en-gb/731. [Accessed April 2021].

Presbycusis
NICE. (2019). *CKS: Hearing loss in adults.* https://cks.nice.org.uk/topics/hearing-loss-in-adults/. [Accessed April 2021].

Childhood Hearing Loss
Collier, J., Etheridge, L., Longmore, M., Bonner, A., & Amarakone, K. (2013). Ear, nose, and throat. In *Oxford handbook of clinical specialties* (9th ed.). Oxford University Press.
British Association of Audiovestibular Physicians. (2018). *Guidelines for aetiological investigation into progressive permanent childhood hearing impairment.* https://www.baap.org.uk/uploads/1/1/9/7/119752718/guideline_progressive_hl_final.pdf. [Accessed April 2021].

Rhinosinusitis

NICE. (2018). *CKS: Rhinosinusitis*. https://cks.nice.org.uk/
topics/sinusitis/. [Accessed April 2021].

Nasal Polyps

British Society for Allergy & Clinical Immunology. (2008).
Rhinosinusitis & nasal polyposis. https://www.bsaci.org/
wp-content/uploads/2020/01/RhinosinusitisPolypo-
sis2008.pdf. [Accessed April 2021].

BMJ Best Practice. (2020). *Nasal polyps*. https://bestpractice.
bmj.com/topics/en-gb/1130. [Accessed April 2021].

Epistaxis

NICE. (2019). *CKS: Epistaxis*. https://cks.nice.org.uk/topics/
epistaxis-nosebleeds/. [Accessed April 2021].

Pharyngitis and Tonsillitis

NICE. (2018). *NG84: Sore throat (acute): Antimicrobial
prescribing*. https://www.nice.org.uk/guidance/ng84.
[Accessed April 2021].

ENT UK. (2020). *COVID-19 adult tonsillitis & quinsy guide-
lines*. https://www.entuk.org/sites/default/files/ENT%20
UK%20COVID-19%20Tonsillitis%20%26%20Quinsy%20
Guidelines%20FINAL.pdf. [Accessed April 2021].

Epiglottitis

BMJ Best Practice. (2020). *Epiglottitis*. https://bestpractice.
bmj.com/topics/en-gb/452. [Accessed April 2021].

Entsho.com. (2019). *Epiglottitis and supraglottitis*. https://
entsho.com/epiglottitis-supraglottitis. [Accessed April
2021].

Infectious Mononucleosis

NICE. (2020). *CKS: Glandular fever (infectious mononucleosis)*. https://cks.nice.org.uk/topics/glandular-fever-
infectious-mononucleosis/. [Accessed April 2021].

Rezk, E., Nofal, Y. H., Hamzeh, A., Aboujaib, M. F., Al
Kheder, M. A., & Al Hammad, M. F. (2015). Steroids for
symptom control in infectious mononucleosis. *Cochrane
Database of Systematic Reviews*, *11*, CD004402. https://
www.cochranelibrary.com/cdsr/doi/10.1002/14651858.
CD004402.pub3/full. [Accessed April 2021].

Obstructive Sleep Apnoea (OSA)

NICE. (2015). *CKS: Obstructive sleep apnoea*. https://cks.
nice.org.uk/topics/obstructive-sleep-apnoea-syndrome/.
[Accessed April 2021].

Branchial Cyst

Collier, J., Etheridge, L., Longmore, M., Bonner, A., & Amarakone, K. (2013). Ear, nose, and throat. In *Oxford handbook
of clinical specialties* (9th ed.). Oxford University Press.

Branchial Cyst

Collier, J., Etheridge, L., Longmore, M., Bonner, A., & Amarakone, K. (2013). Ear, nose, and throat. In *Oxford handbook
of clinical specialties* (9th ed.). Oxford University Press.

Thyroglossal Duct Cyst

BMJ Best Practice. (2020). *Assessment of thyroid mass*. https://
bestpractice.bmj.com/topics/en-gb/1200. [Accessed April
2021].

Goitre

Patient info. (2020a). *Thyroid lumps including goitre*. https://
patient.info/doctor/thyroid-lumps-including-goitre.
[Accessed April 2021].

Thyroid Cancer

Mitchell, A., Gandhi, A., Scott-Coombes, D., & Perros, P.
(2016). Management of thyroid cancer: United Kingdom national multidisciplinary guidelines. *The Journal
of Laryngology & Otology*, *130*, S150–S160. https://doi.
org/10.1017/S0022215116000578

Cancer Research UK. (2018). *Thyroid cancer – survival*.
https://www.cancerresearchuk.org/about-cancer/thyroid-
cancer/survival. [Accessed April 2021].

Cystic Hygroma

NICE. (2016). *CKS: Neck lump*. https://cks.nice.org.uk/topics/
neck-lump/. [Accessed April 2021].

Lymphadenopathy

BMJ Best Practice. (2020). *Assessment of lymphadenopathy*.
https://bestpractice.bmj.com/topics/en-gb/838. [Accessed
April 2021].

NICE. (2016). *CKS: Neck lump*. https://cks.nice.org.uk/topics/
neck-lump/. [Accessed April 2021].

Epidermoid Cyst

Patient info. (2018). *Epidermoid and pilar cysts (sebaceous
cysts)*. https://patient.info/skin-conditions/epidermoid-and-
pilar-cysts-sebaceous-cysts-leaflet. [Accessed April 2021].

READING LIST: OPHTHALMOLOGY

Cranial Nerve Palsy
Cranial Nerve III Palsy

Binder, D. K., Sonne, D. C., & Fischbein, N. J. (2010). *Cranial
nerves: Anatomy, pathology and imaging*. Thieme.

Cranial Nerve VI Palsy

Binder, D. K., Sonne, D. C., & Fischbein, N. J. (2010). *Cranial
nerves: Anatomy, pathology and imaging*. Thieme.

Cranial Nerve VI Palsy

Binder, D. K., Sonne, D. C., & Fischbein, N. J. (2010). *Cranial nerves: Anatomy, pathology and imaging.* Thieme.

Visual Field Defect

Patient info. (2021). *Visual field defects.* https://patient.info/doctor/Visual-Field-Defects. [Accessed June 2020]

Mansbridge, C. (2018). *The OSCE revision guide for medical students.* OSCEstop.com.

Vivekananda, U. (2019). *Crash course: Neurology.* Elsevier.

Doulgas, G., Nicol, E. F., Robertson, C., Britton, R., & Danielson, E. (2013). *Mucleod's clinical examination.* Livingstone/Elsevier

Gradual Vision Loss
Cataracts

NICE. (2020). *CKS: Cataracts.* https://cks.nice.org.uk/topics/cataracts/. [Accessed June 2020].

National Eye Institute. (2019). *Cataracts.* https://www.nei.nih.gov/learn-about-eye-health/eye-conditions-and-diseases/cataracts.

National Eye Institute. (2020). *Age related macular degeneration.* https://www.nei.nih.gov/learn-about-eye-health/eye-conditions-and-diseases/age-related-macular-degeneration. [Accessed June 2020].

Primary Open-Angle Glaucoma

NICE. (2019). *CKS: Glaucoma.* https://cks.nice.org.uk/topics/glaucoma/. [Accessed June 2020].

National Eye Institute. (2020). *Glaucoma.* https://www.nei.nih.gov/learn-about-eye-health/eye-conditions-and-diseases/glaucoma. [Accessed June 2020].

Retinitis Pigmentosa

Patient info. (2019). *Retinitis pigmentosa.* https://patient.info/doctor/retinitis-pigmentosa. [Accessed June 2020].

National Eye Institute. (2019). *Retinitis pigmentosa.* https://www.nei.nih.gov/learn-about-eye-health/eye-conditions-and-diseases/retinitis-pigmentosa. [Accessed June 2020].

Acute Painless Vision Loss
Central Retinal Artery Occlusion

Patient info. (2016). *Retinal artery occlusions.* https://patient.info/doctor/retinal-artery-occlusions. [Accessed June 2020].

Broadway, D. C. (2012). How to test for a relative afferent pupillary defect (RAPD). *Community Eye Health, 25,* 58–59. PMID: 23520419; PMCID: PMC3588138.

Vanderah, T. W., & Gould, D. J. (2021). *Nolte's the human brain: An introduction to its functional anatomy.* https://www.clinicalkey.com/dura/browse/bookChapter/3-s2.0-C2018000609X.

Retinal Vein Occlusion

The Royal College of Ophthalmologists. (2015). *Retinal vein occlusion guidelines.* https://www.rcophth.ac.uk/resources-listing/retinal-vein-occlusion-rvo-guidelines/ [Accessed June 2020].

Vitreous Haemorrhage

Patient info. (2015). *Vitreous hemorrhage.* https://patient.info/doctor/vitreous-haemorrhage-pro. [Accessed June 2020].

Retinal Detachment

NICE. (2019). *CKS: Retinal detachment.* https://cks.nice.org.uk/topics/retinal-detachment/. [Accessed June 2020].

Acute Painless Vision Loss
Optic Neuritis

Patient info. (2014). *Acute optic neuritis.* https://patient.info/doctor/acute-optic-neuritis. [Accessed June 2020].

Red Eye
Corneal Foreign Body and Corneal Abrasion

College of Optometrists Guidance. (2020). *Corneal abrasion.* https://www.college-optometrists.org/clinical-guidance/clinical-management-guidelines/cornealabrasion. [Accessed June 2020].

Keratitis

College of Optometrists Guidance. (2019). *Herpes simplex keratitis.* https://www.college-optometrists.org/clinical-guidance/clinical-management-guidelines/herpessimplexkeratitis_hsk. [Accessed June 2020].

Tuft, S., & Burton, M. (2013). *Microbial keratitis. Focus.* Moorfields Eye Hospital NHS Foundation Trust. http://www.rcophth.ac.uk.

Singh, P., Gupta, A., & Tripathy, K. (2020). *Keratitis.* StatPearls. StatPearls Publishing. https://www.ncbi.nlm.nih.gov/books/NBK559014/.

Anterior Uveitis

NICE. (2019). *CKS: Anterior uveitis.* https://cks.nice.org.uk/topics/uveitis/. [Accessed June 2020].

Primary Angle-Closure Glaucoma

NICE. (2019). *CKS: Primary angle-closure glaucoma.* https://cks.nice.org.uk/topics/glaucoma/diagnosis/primary-angle-closure-glaucoma/. [Accessed June 2020].

Scleritis

College of Optometrists Guidance. (2018). *Scleritis.* https://www.college-optometrists.org/clinical-guidance/clinical-management-guidelines/scleritis. [Accessed June 2020].

Orbital and Preseptal Cellulitis

Patient info. (2020). *Orbital and pre-septal cellulitis.* https://patient.info/doctor/orbital-and-preseptal-cellulitis. [Accessed June 2020].

College of Optometrists Guidance. (2021). *Cellulitis, preseptal and orbital*. https://www.college-optometrists.org/clinical-guidance/clinical-management-guidelines/cellulitis_preseptalandorbital. [Accessed June 2020].

BNF. (2021). *Skin infections*. https://bnf.nice.org.uk/treatment-summary/skin-infections.html. [Acessed June 2021].

Thyroid Eye Disease

British Thyroid Foundation. (2019). *Thyroid eye disease*. https://www.btf-thyroid.org/thyroid-eye-disease. [Accessed June 2020].

American Thyroid Association. (2021). *Grave's eye disease*. http://thyroid.org/wp-content/uploads/patients/brochures/Graves_brochure.pdf [Accessed June 2020].

Conjunctivitis

College of Optometrists Guidance. (2018). *Conjunctivitis (bacterial)*. https://www.college-optometrists.org/clinical-guidance/clinical-management-guidelines/conjunctivitis_bacterial [Accessed June 2020].

College of Optometrists Guidance. (2019). *Conjunctivitis (viral, non-herpetic)*. https://www.college-optometrists.org/clinical-guidance/clinical-management-guidelines/conjunctivitis_viral_non-herpetic. [Accessed June 2020].

College of Optometrists Guidance. (2019). *Conjunctivitis (acute allergic)*. https://www.college-optometrists.org/clinical-guidance/clinical-management-guidelines/conjunctivitis_acuteallergic. [Accessed June 2020].

Costumbrado, J., Ng, D. K., & Ghassemzadeh, S. (2021). *Gonococcal conjunctivitis*. StatPearls. StatPearls Publishing. https://www.ncbi.nlm.nih.gov/books/NBK459289.

Subconjunctival Haemorrhage

College of Optometrists Guidance. (2019). *Subconjunctival haemorrhage*. https://www.college-optometrists.org/clin-ical-guidance/clinical-management-guidelines/sub-con-junctivalhaemorrhage. [Accessed June 2020].

Episcleritis

College of Optometrists Guidance. (2018). *Episcleritis*. https://www.college-optometrists.org/clinical-guidance/clinical-management-guidelines/episcleritis. [Accessed June 2020].

Malignancy
Retinoblastoma

Patient info. (2016). *Retinoblastoma*. https://patient.info/doctor/retinoblastoma-pro. [Accessed June 2020].

Medscape. (2019). *Retinoblastoma differential diagnoses*. https://emedicine.medscape.com/article/1222849-differential. [Accessed June 2020].

Eyelid Problems
Blepharitis

NICE. (2019). *CKS: Blepharitis*. https://cks.nice.org.uk/topics/blepharitis/. [Accessed June 2020].

Emedicine Medscape. (2019). *Adult blepharitis differential diagnoses*. https://emedicine.medscape.com/article/1211763-differential. [Accessed June 2020].

Stye

NICE. (2019). *CKS: Stye*. https://cks.nice.org.uk/topics/styes-hordeola/. [Accessed June 2020].

Chalazion

NICE. (2019). *CKS: Meibomian cyst (chalazion)*. https://cks.nice.org.uk/topics/meibomian-cyst-chalazion/. [Accessed September 2020].

7

Emergency Medicine in an Hour

Thomas Brankin-Frisby, Nagarjun Konda, Charlotte Hayden and Jason Louis

OUTLINE

RESPIRATORY EMERGENCIES

Anaphylaxis

Definition: a severe and life-threatening systemic hypersensitivity reaction characterised by rapid-onset airway, breathing and circulatory problems that develop in response to a trigger, e.g., food, medicines and insect stings.

Buzzwords:

- **Risk factors:** previous anaphylaxis
- **Presentation:** acute onset, urticaria, angio-oedema, dyspnoea, wheezing, stridor, hypotension, syncope, abdominal pain, diarrhoea

Investigations: clinical diagnosis – do not delay treatment

- **Mast cell tryptase:** typically raised (except from food-induced reactions)
- **Serum C4 level:** low in hereditary angio-oedema/bradykinin-mediated angio-oedema, normal in other cases

Differentials: other shock states, asthma, hereditary angio-oedema/bradykinin-mediated angio-oedema, foreign body aspiration

Management: (see Table 7.1)

1. Remove trigger

2. Adrenaline IM – repeat at 5-min intervals until an adequate response
3. Hydrocortisone and chlorphenamine IV
4. Salbutamol nebuliser if wheezing develops

Tension Pneumothorax

Definition: condition in which air is drawn into the pleural cavity but cannot escape, causing pressure to build up and compressing the mediastinum (containing the great vessels). May lead to cardiorespiratory compromise/arrest.

Buzzwords:

- **Risk factors:** trauma, non-invasive/invasive ventilation, lung disease (particularly asthma and chronic obstructive pulmonary disease (COPD))
- **Presentation:** dyspnoea, tachycardia, reduced breath sounds over affected side, distended neck veins, hypotension, tracheal deviation away from affected side

Investigations: clinical diagnosis – investigations should NOT delay treatment

Differentials: pulmonary embolism (PE), anaphylaxis, cardiac tamponade, septic or cardiogenic shock, haemothorax

Management:

1. High-flow oxygen

TABLE 7.1 Anaphylaxis Drugs in Order of Priority (from Left to Right)

Age Group	Adrenaline IM 1:1000	Hydrocortisone IM/IV	Chlorphenamine IM/IV	Salbutamol Nebuliser
Child <6 months	150 µg (0.15 mL)	25 mg	250 µg/kg	2.5 mg
Child 6 months to 6 years	150 µg (0.15 mL)	50 mg	2.5 mg	2.5 mg
Child 6–12 years	300 µg (0.3 mL)	100 mg	5 mg	5 mg
Adult or child ►12 years	500 µg (0.5 mL)	200 mg	10 mg	5 mg

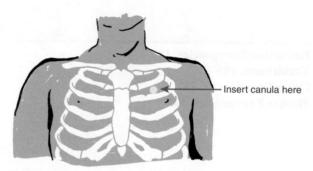

Insert canula here

Fig 7.1 Insertion of Cannula into the 2nd Intercostal Space at the Midclavicular Line. (Illustrated by Dr Hollie Blaber.)

2. Insert a large-bore cannula into the 2nd intercostal space at the midclavicular line (see Fig 7.1)
3. Intercostal drain in the safe triangle, confirm positioning with chest x-ray (CXR)

Pneumothorax

Definition: air within the pleural cavity. This condition can be classified into:
- **Primary spontaneous**: no underlying lung disease
- **Secondary spontaneous:** associated with underlying lung disease (e.g., congenital bullae, COPD, >50 years of age with a significant smoking history)
- **Iatrogenic:** caused by a medical treatment (e.g., lung biopsy via transthoracic needle aspiration, central line placement, thoracocentesis, pleural biopsy, mechanical ventilation)

Buzzwords:
- **Risk factors:**
  - **Primary:** smoking, tall stature, Marfan's syndrome, family history
  - **Secondary:** COPD, malignancy, sarcoidosis, cystic fibrosis (CF), tuberculosis (TB), pulmonary fibrosis, acquired immunodeficiency syndrome

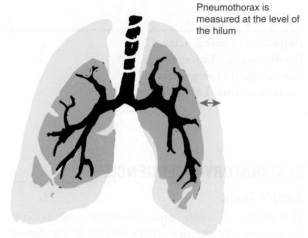

Pneumothorax is measured at the level of the hilum

Fig 7.2 Measurement of a Pneumothorax. (Illustrated by Dr Hollie Blaber.)

(AIDS) patients with *Pneumocystis jiroveci* pneumonia (PJP)
- **Presentation:** sudden onset, dyspnoea, pleuritic chest pain, breathlessness, hyperresonant percussion, reduced breath sounds over affected side, may be asymptomatic

Investigations:
- **CXR:** air in pleural cavity (see Fig 7.2 and Radiology in an Hour)
- **CT chest** (in complex cases): air in pleural cavity
- Important to exclude other differentials

Differentials: acute exacerbation of COPD or asthma, PE, pleural effusion

Management:
- Acute management: see Fig 7.3
- Post-acute event:
  - **Safety netting:** no air travel for 1–2 weeks after full resolution confirmed with CXR. Scuba diving should be avoided for life unless managed with a bilateral surgical pleurectomy

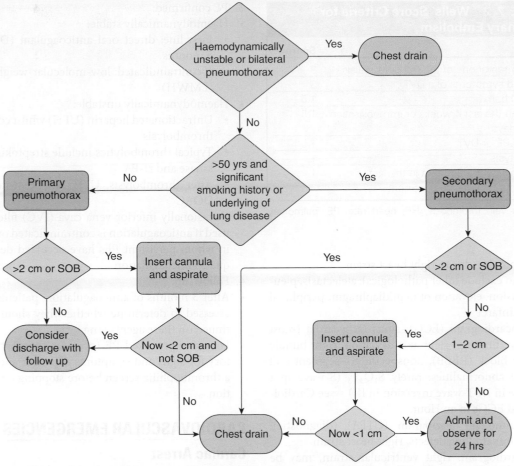

Fig 7.3 Flow Diagram of Management of a Spontaneous Nontension Pneumothorax Based on British Thoracic Society Guidelines. (Illustrated by Dr Tom Brankin-Frisby; Adapted from MacDuff, A., Arnold, A., & Harvey, J. (2010). Management of spontaneous pneumothorax: British Thoracic Society pleural disease guideline 2010. *Thorax*, 65, ii18–ii3.)

- **Pleurodesis:** if recurrent or failure of chest drain to achieve lung reexpansion. Two options:
- **Medical pleurodesis:** If not fit for surgery, a sclerosing agent such as tetracycline or talc is passed into the pleural cavity to cause adhesions between the lungs and chest wall
- **Surgical pleurodesis:** Pleurectomy has the lowest recurrence rate of all methods

Pulmonary Embolism

Definition: obstruction of the pulmonary arterial system by an embolus or emboli, typically a venous blood clot arising from the deep leg veins.

Buzzwords:

- **Risk factors:** see Wells' criteria (see Table 7.2), lower limb trauma, pregnancy and up to 6 weeks postpartum, combined oral contraceptive pill (COCP) or hormone replacement therapy (HRT), long-distance travel, obesity, thrombophilia (e.g., factor V Leiden), increasing age
- **Presentation:** dyspnoea, pleuritic chest pain, haemoptysis, presyncope, syncope, tachypnoea, tachycardia, hypoxia, pyrexia, elevated jugular venous pressure, gallop rhythm, pleural rub, hypotension, and shock

Investigations:

- Arterial blood gas (ABG): ↓PO_2, ↓PCO_2
- D-dimer: ↑

TABLE 7.2 Wells' Score Criteria for Pulmonary Embolism

Criteria	Score
PE is the top or one of the top differentials	3
Signs and symptoms of a DVT	3
HR >100 bpm	1.5
Surgery in the last 4 weeks or immobilisation for ≥3 days	1.5
Previous PE or DVT	1.5
Haemoptysis	1
Malignancy with treatment in the last 6 months or palliative treatment	1

DVT, Deep vein thrombosis; HR, heart rate; PE, pulmonary embolism.

- Troponin: $\uparrow/\leftrightarrow$ due to right heart strain
- CXR (to exclude other pathologies): atelectasis, pleural effusion, elevation of hemidiaphragm, peripheral wedge infarct
- Electrocardiogram (ECG): sinus tachycardia (most sensitive finding), right axis deviation, right bundle branch block (RBBB), nonspecific ST-segment and T-wave abnormalities, rarely $S_1Q_3T_3$ (S-wave in I Q-wave in III T-wave inversion in III) – see Cardiology and ECGs in an Hour.
- CT pulmonary angiogram (CTPA) (diagnostic): intraluminal filling defects, right heart strain
- Echocardiogram: right ventricular strain, may be useful in unstable patients

Differentials: acute coronary syndrome (ACS), pneumonia, pneumothorax, acute exacerbation of COPD, gastro-oesophageal reflux disease (GORD), acute congestive heart failure, musculoskeletal chest wall pain, aortic dissection, pericarditis

Management:
1. Oxygen if needed
2. Two-level Wells' score to guide management: (see Table 7.2)
- **Wells' score >4:** immediate CTPA and therapeutic-dose anticoagulation initiated
- **Wells' score ≤4:** perform a D-dimer blood test
  - Positive result: immediate CTPA, interim therapeutic anticoagulation if there is delay
  - Negative result: stop therapeutic anticoagulation if started and consider alternative diagnosis
Interim therapeutic-dose anticoagulation if results from either test are not available within 4 h

3. PE confirmed:
- Haemodynamically stable:
  - First line: direct oral anticoagulant (DOAC) for 3 months
  - If contraindicated: low-molecular-weight heparin (LMWH)
- Haemodynamically unstable:
  - Unfractionated heparin (UFH) whilst considering thrombolysis
  - Typical thrombolytics include streptokinase, urokinase and rt-PA
  - After thrombolysis, UFH can be switched to a DOAC
- Occasionally inferior vena cava (IVC) filters can be used if anticoagulation is contraindicated or for those in whom persistent PEs have occurred despite adequate anticoagulation
4. Follow-up:
- After 3 months of anticoagulation, patients are then assessed to determine whether they should be continued on these agents long term
- For an unprovoked PE (no clear cause), take a history for signs and symptoms of cancer and consider a thrombophilia screen before stopping anticoagulation

CARDIOVASCULAR EMERGENCIES

Cardiac Arrest

Definition: sudden loss of cardiac output leading to circulatory collapse and eventually death
Buzzwords:
- Reversible causes:
  - **4 H's:** Hypoxia, Hypovolaemia, Hyper/Hypokalaemia, Hypothermia
  - **4 T's:** Tension pneumothorax, (cardiac) Tamponade, Toxins (drugs, poisons), Thrombus (PE, myocardial infarction (MI))
- **Presentation:** cardiorespiratory arrest, absent carotid pulse
Investigations: should not delay management but are performed to identify reversible causes:
- **ABG:** hypoxia, hyper/hypokalaemia
- **Bloods:** electrolyte disturbances
- **Echocardiogram:** cardiac tamponade
Management: (in adults)
1. Call for help: ask the nearest colleague to place a 2222 call and fetch the resus trolley

2. Cardiopulmonary resuscitation (CPR) 30:2
3. Attach defibrillator and assess rhythm:
- **If shockable rhythm** (ventricular fibrillation (VF)/ pulseless ventricular tachycardia (VT)):
  - One shock and resume CPR
  - Rhythm check at 2 min
  - Adrenaline 1 mg IV **1:10,000** every 3–5 min
  - Amiodarone 300 mg IV after three shocks
- **If nonshockable rhythm** (pulseless electrical activity (PEA)/asystole):
  - Resume CPR
  - Adrenaline 1 mg IV **1:10,000** every 3–5 min
  - Rhythm check at 2 min
4. Treat reversible causes
5. Post-cardiac arrest: oxygen, analgesia, ECG, intensive care support

Major Haemorrhage

Definition:
- $\geq$ total blood volume within 24 h **or**
- $\geq$ 50% of total blood volume lost in less than 3 h **or**
- $\geq$ 150 mL/min

Causes include childbirth, ruptured abdominal aortic aneurysm (AAA), bleeding varices, trauma and surgery

Buzzwords:
- **Risk factors:** coagulopathy, hypothermia, acidosis, and anticoagulant and antiplatelet medications
- **Presentation:** tachycardia, hypotension, pallor, raised capillary refill time (CRT), weak pulse, altered consciousness. 'On the floor, plus four more' – blood may not always be visible, but think: thorax, abdomen, pelvis and long bones

Investigations:
- **Bloods:** coagulation screen ($\uparrow$ PT, $\uparrow$ APPT), $\downarrow$ fibrinogen, FBC ($\downarrow$ Hb), G&S, crossmatch
- **Venous blood gas (VBG):** possible acidosis, $\uparrow$ lactate, $\downarrow$ Hb

Differentials: septic/cardiogenic/obstructive shock, dehydration, hypothermia

Management:
1. Activate major haemorrhage protocol (fast bleep 2222 – depends on hospital)
2. Direct haemorrhage control (pressure/tourniquet or immediate transfer to surgery)
3. Warm IV fluid bolus until blood arrives
4. Transfuse red blood cells (RBCs) and fresh frozen plasma (FFP) at a ratio of at least 2:1

5. If trauma <3 h prior, give a tranexamic acid 1g IV bolus over 10 min then 1 g IV over 8 h
6. Give blood products based on lab results:
- Low Hb: give more RBCs
- APPT or PT ratio >1.5: give more FFP
- Low fibrinogen: give cryoprecipitate
- Platelets $<50 \times 10^9$/L: give 1 adult platelet dose
7. Avoid lethal triad: hypothermia, acidosis, coagulopathy
8. Consider permissive hypotension (70–90 mm Hg systolic) to reduce risk of rebleeding

Sepsis

Definition: a clinical syndrome of potentially life-threatening organ dysfunction characterised by a dysregulated host inflammatory response to infection. If you are considering sepsis in the differential diagnosis, remember the 'Sepsis 6' – give 3 (O_2, fluids, antibiotics), take 3 (cultures, lactate, urine output)

Buzzwords:
- **Risk factors:** <1 year or >75 years of age, frailty, impaired immunity, invasive procedures
- **Presentation:** $\uparrow$ HR, $\uparrow$ RR, $\downarrow$ SpO$_2$, $\downarrow$ BP, $\downarrow$ urine output, mottled or ashen appearance, cyanosis, confusion

Investigations:
- **Blood culture:** to isolate specific organism
- **Bloods:** FBC ($\uparrow$ WCC, $\uparrow$ CRP, $\downarrow$ eosinophils), U&E ($\uparrow$ creatinine, $\uparrow$ urea)
- **Blood gas:** $\uparrow$ lactate, $\downarrow$ pH
- **Urine output**
- Further tests depending on clinical suspicion of source: midstream specimen of urine (MSU), wound swab, CXR, abdominal ultrasound scan (USS), lumbar puncture (LP), ascitic or pleural aspiration

Differentials: alcohol withdrawal, pancreatitis, poisoning, anaphylaxis, thyrotoxicosis, serotonin syndrome, acute adrenal (Addisonian) crisis

Management:
1. Oxygen
2. IV antibiotics within 1 h (local guidance for antibiotic choice depending on likely source)
3. IV fluids: aim for 30 mL/kg within the first 3 h
4. Fluid-balance monitoring

NEUROLOGICAL EMERGENCIES
Convulsive Status Epilepticus

Definition: a single seizure exceeding 5 min OR multiple seizures without full recovery exceeding a 5-min period. Causes include CNS pathologies (e.g., malignancy, infection, epilepsy, stroke), drug intoxication/withdrawal, hypoglycaemia, electrolyte derangement, sleep deprivation, hypoxia, preeclampsia

Buzzwords:

- **Risk factors:** age extremes, brain injury, poor medication concordance
- **Presentation:** loss of consciousness with repeated contraction and extension of arms and legs

Investigations: carried out to determine cause

- Capillary blood glucose (CBG)
- VBG: ↑ lactate
- Bloods: FBC, U&E, LFTs, CRP
- CT head
- Pregnancy test and blood pressure (BP)
- LP

Differentials: nonepileptiform attacks

Management:

1. Treat reversible causes
2. Benzodiazepines after 5 min
- 4 mg IV lorazepam *or*
- 10 mg buccal midazolam *or*
- 10 mg PR diazepam
3. Repeat benzodiazepines after 10 min
4. Phenytoin after 25 min
- Loading therapy: 20 mg/kg phenytoin mixed with 0.9% NaCl
- Maintenance therapy: 100 mg IV phenytoin TDS
5. Consider anaesthesia after 45 min

Acute Alcohol Withdrawal

Definition: a syndrome that occurs after the abrupt cessation of alcohol intake, typically 6–8 h after last alcohol consumption. Can progress to **delirium tremens,** which has a significant mortality rate if untreated

Buzzwords:

- **Risk factors:** alcohol use disorder, previous episodes of delirium tremens or alcohol withdrawal seizures, liver disease, poor nutrition
- **Presentation:**
  - **Alcohol withdrawal:** occurs 6–8 h after cessation, anxiety, restlessness, tremor, insomnia, tachycardia, nausea and ataxia
  - **Delirium tremens:** occurs 48–72 h after cessation, more significant autonomic hyperactivity including hypertension (HTN); hyperreflexia; fever; visual, auditory or tactile hallucinations; confusion; disorientation; delusions. Death usually

follows arrythmias, seizures and cardiovascular collapse

The CIWA-Ar assessment tool is routinely used to quantify the severity of alcohol withdrawal and to stratify treatment. Patients are scored based on the severity of their signs and symptoms using a 67-point scale. Proformas are typically available on the ward or can be found online

Investigations:

- **CBG** (to rule out hypoglycaemia): may be low anyway due to disease process
- **VBG:** mixed results – respiratory alkalosis (hyperventilation), hypochloraemic metabolic acidosis (with vomiting), metabolic acidosis with high anion gap (if in alcoholic ketoacidosis)
- **FBC & CRP** (to rule out infection): ↓ platelets, ↔ CRP, ↔ WCC
- **Serum ammonia** (to rule out hepatic encephalopathy): normal
- Consider **CT-head** and **LP** if history is unclear

Differentials: intracranial bleed (e.g., subdural haemorrhage), hypoglycaemia, hepatic encephalopathy, delirium, CNS infection, Wernicke's encephalopathy, sympathomimetic intoxication, benzodiazepine withdrawal

Management:

1. IV thiamine (Pabrinex)
2. Correct hypoglycaemia (only after Pabrinex to minimise risk of precipitating Wernicke's encephalopathy) and electrolyte imbalances
3. Those with a CIWA score ≥10:
- Oral benzodiazepines (chlordiazepoxide)
- Consider IV lorazepam if oral route of administration not feasible
- If psychotic symptoms persist, consider olanzapine or haloperidol
4. Referral to alcohol support services: never advise sudden cessation without pharmacological support because it can precipitate acute alcohol withdrawal and seizures

Wernicke-Korsakoff Syndrome

Definition: Wernicke's encephalopathy and Korsakoff syndrome are both complications of chronic alcohol excess caused by a thiamine deficiency, often presenting with a mixed picture. Untreated Wernicke's encephalopathy can lead to Korsakoff syndrome. In the absence of replenishment, the body's thiamine stores only last about 2 weeks

Buzzwords:

- **Risk factors:** alcohol excess, poor nutrition, chemotherapy, gastrointestinal insufficiency
- **Presentation:**
  - **Wernicke's encephalopathy:** classically presents as a triad of ocular disturbance (e.g., ophthalmoplegia, gaze palsies, nystagmus), ataxia, confusion
  - **Korsakoff syndrome:** profound retrograde and anterograde amnesia with relative preservation of other intellectual abilities, confabulation. This condition is permanent

Investigations:

- Serum thiamine and folate: low
- Serum ammonia (to rule out hepatic encephalopathy)

Differentials: alcohol intoxication, alcohol withdrawal, viral encephalitis, hepatic encephalopathy, Miller-Fisher syndrome

Management:

1. IV thiamine replacement (Pabrinex): improvement of Wernicke's symptoms
2. Alcohol cessation with support
3. Ongoing oral thiamine replacement and nutritional support

GASTROINTESTINAL EMERGENCIES

Upper GI Bleed

Definition: bleeding from the oesophagus, stomach or duodenum (see Fig. 7.4 for vascular anatomy). Causes include:

- Peptic/duodenal ulcer
- Oesophageal varices
- Mallory-Weiss tear
- Erosive duodenitis or gastritis
- Malignancy
- Vascular malformation/Dieulafoy's lesions
- Portal hypertensive gastropathy

Buzzwords:

- **Risk factors:** alcohol abuse, chronic renal failure, increasing age, nonsteroidal antiinflammatory drug (NSAID) and steroid use, cirrhosis with portal hypertension, anticoagulants, antiplatelets, haematological disorders causing thrombocytopaenia
- **Presentation:** depends on site and rate of bleeding. Haematemesis, coffee-ground vomiting, melaena, haematochezia, signs of anaemia and shock. Signs of underlying pathology

TABLE 7.3   Blatchford Score Criteria

Blatchford Score Criteria:	Possible Scores:
Blood urea (higher urea = higher score)	0, 2, 3, 4, 6
Haemoglobin (gender-specific, lower haemoglobin = higher score)	1, 3, 6
Initial systolic blood pressure (lower blood pressure = higher score)	0, 1, 2, 3
Heart rate (higher heart rate = higher score)	0, 1
Melaena present	0, 1
Recent syncope	0, 2
Hepatic disease history	0, 2
Cardiac failure present	0, 2
Total	0–23

Investigations:

- **Endoscopy:** to visualise and treat source of bleeding (see Figs 7.5 and 7.6)
- **FBC:** ↓ Hb, often ↓ platelets in alcoholic liver disease
- **U&Es:** ↑ urea (digested blood)
- **Clotting screen:** ↑ PT and ↑ APPT often seen in liver disease
- **H. pylori testing:** samples taken during endoscopy

Differentials: epistaxis, haemoptysis, other causes of hypovolaemic shock

Management:

1. Resuscitate, activate major haemorrhage protocol if necessary
2. Correct coagulopathy, if present
3. Blatchford score at first assessment (see Table 7.3)
4. Rockall scoring is performed after endoscopy
5. Endoscopy should be performed on all patients within 24 h (if Blatchford score of zero, can be considered for early discharge and outpatient endoscopy)

Nonvariceal:

- Acute:
  - Endoscopic treatment, one of: clips +/- adrenaline, thermal coagulation with adrenaline or fibrin with adrenaline
  - Offer urgent interventional radiology or surgery to unstable patients who rebleed after endoscopic treatment

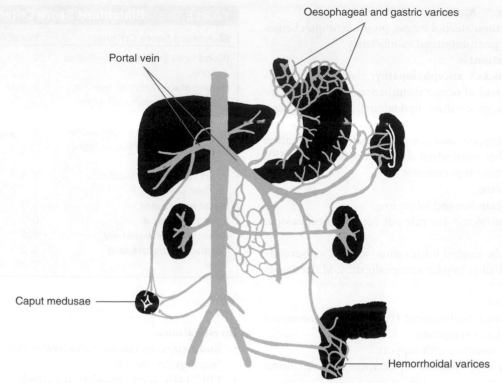

Fig 7.4 Portal Vein Collaterals. (Illustrated by Dr Hollie Blaber.)

- Proton pump inhibitor (PPI) after endoscopy
- *H. pylori* eradication therapy (if relevant)
- Long term:
  - Consider repeat endoscopy for patients at high risk of rebleeding

Variceal:
- Acute:
  - IV terlipressin
  - IV broad-spectrum prophylactic antibiotics
  - Oesophageal varices: endoscopic band ligation
  - Gastric varices: endoscopic sclerotherapy
  - Oesophageal balloon tamponade (Sengstaken-Blakemore tube) should be considered as a temporary measure in an unstable patient with oesophageal bleeding who requires advanced airway support
- Long term:
  - Beta blocker
  - Consider transjugular intrahepatic portosystemic shunt (TIPS) procedure if bleeding is still not controlled

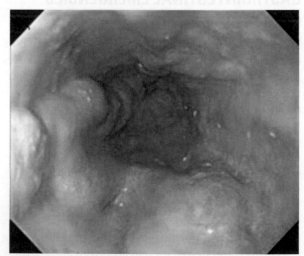

Fig 7.5 Oesophageal Varices. (From Akiyama, T., Abe, Y., Iida, H., et al. Endoscopic therapy using an endoscopic variceal ligation for minute cancer of the esophagogastric junction complicated with esophageal varices: a case report. *Journal of Medical Case Reports 4*, 149 (2010).)

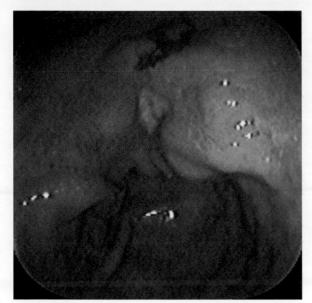

Fig 7.6 Peptic Ulcer. (With permission from Lash R. H., Lauwers, G. Y., Odze, R. D., & Genta, R. M. (2015). Inflammatory disorders of the stomach (Fig. 15.35). In *Odze and Goldblum surgical pathology of the GI tract, liver, biliary tract and pancreas.* Elsevier. *Copyright © 2015 Elsevier Inc. All rights reserved.*)

ENDOCRINE EMERGENCIES

Hypoglycaemia

Definition: Hypoglycaemia is defined as a CBG <4 mmol/L. Normal CBG levels:

- **Pre-meals:** 4–7 mmol/L
- **Post-meals:** 5–9 mmol/L

Buzzwords:

- **Risk factors:**
  - **Diabetes mellitus (DM) related:** insulin overdose (most common), oral hypoglycaemics (typically sulfonylureas and SGLT2 inhibitors), renal failure, alcohol, delayed meals, exercise
  - **Nondiabetic:** insulinoma (multiple endocrine neoplasias (MEN)-1), acute liver failure, pituitary/adrenal insufficiency, renal failure
- **Presentation:**
  - Early: sweating, flushing, fatigue, agitation, tremors and palpitations (adrenaline-mediated; therefore, beta blockers inhibit some of these effects and can reduce awareness)
  - Moderate: confusion, reduced consciousness
  - Severe: seizures, coma

Investigations:

- **CBG:** <4 mmol/L. If clearly caused by diabetic medication, no further investigation is required
- **Bloods:** LFTs (deranged if liver failure), U&Es (acute kidney injury (AKI) may impair excretion of diabetic drugs)
- **Fasting insulin and C-peptide levels:** High insulin indicates an insulinoma or exogenous insulin use, whereas an elevated C-peptide excludes exogenous insulin use.
- **Morning cortisol:** low level indicates adrenal or pituitary insufficiency

Differentials: delirium, epilepsy, alcohol or drug intoxication, alcohol withdrawal

Management:

1. **If safe to swallow:** 15–20 g of short-acting oral carbohydrate (e.g., glucose/dextrose, glucose tablets, gel, shot, high-sugar drink/juice)
2. **If unable to swallow safely, there are two options:**
   - Stat IV glucose infusion: typically 10% or 20% dextrose
   - 1 mg glucagon IM/SC: will not work if malnourished/depleted glycogen stores and may cause rebound hyperglycaemia
3. **Post-acute management:**
   - Meal containing complex carbohydrates
   - Continue obtaining regular CBGs until blood glucose levels stabilise
   - Review insulin dosing/investigate cause of hypoglycaemia

Diabetic Ketoacidosis (DKA)

Definition: DKA is diagnosed when there is:

- Hyperglycaemia
- Significant ketosis
- Acidaemia

An inadequate serum insulin level in a patient with DM means that glucose is unable to pass into cells from the blood. Cells metabolise fatty acids as an alternative energy source, producing acidic metabolites including ketones. This condition may be how an individual with type 1 DM (T1DM) first presents.

Buzzwords:

- **Risk factors:** nearly exclusively in T1DM, inadequate administration of insulin, intercurrent illness, history of eating disorders (diabulimia – some avoid using their insulin as a means to lose weight). SLG2 inhibitors can cause euglycemic DKA.

- **Presentation:** fruity-smelling breath, fatigue, confusion, abdominal pain, thirst, polyuria, polydipsia, Kussmaul's respirations (deep, laboured gasping)

Investigations:
- **CBG:** hyperglycaemia >11 mmol/L
- **Ketones:** blood ketones >3.0 mmol/L or urine ketones ++/+++
- **VBG:** acidosis (pH <7.3) and/or bicarbonate <15 mmol/L
- **Investigate precipitant:** include septic screen (CXR, urine culture and bloods) and screen for MI (ECG and troponins)

Differentials: hyperglycaemic hyperosmolar state (HHS), alcoholic ketoacidosis

Management:
1. **Fluid resuscitation** then maintenance: 1 L of normal saline over 1 h, then over 2 h, 2 h, 4 h, 4 h and then 6 h (1-2-2-4-4-6)
2. **Potassium monitoring:** VBG every 2 h. If serum potassium falls below 5.5 mmol/L, add **KCl** to the maintenance fluids
3. **STOP short-acting insulin and START a fixed-rate insulin infusion** of 0.1 units/kg/h, adjust infusion rate to blood ketone and glucose concentrations
4. **CONTINUE or start long-acting insulin therapy**
5. **When CBG is <14 mmol/L, give 10% glucose** by IV infusion in addition to the normal saline already started
6. **Continue insulin infusion until:**
   1. Blood ketones <0.3 mmol/l
   2. pH is >7.3
   3. Able to eat and drink so that the usual (or amended) SC insulin regimen can be resumed safely

Hyperosmolar Hyperglycaemic State (HHS)

Definition: HHS is diagnosed when there is:
- **Severe** hyperglycaemia
- No significant ketosis
- No significant acidosis
- High serum osmolality

HHS predominantly affects patients with type II DM (T2DM), often when they fall ill, and it typically occurs over a period of several days. Osmotic diuresis is often coupled with poor fluid intake, which leads to profound hypovolaemia

Buzzwords:
- **Risk factors:** dementia, sedative drugs, poor medication concordance, hot environment, immunocompromised, intercurrent illness and infection, corticosteroids, thiazide diuretics
- **Presentation:** malaise, muscle cramps, nausea, visual disturbance, focal neurology, confusion, seizures, polyuria, polydipsia, signs of severe dehydration (e.g., dry mucous membranes, tachycardia, reduced skin turgor, hypotension)

Investigations:
- **CBG:** hyperglycaemia (but not always) ≥30 mmol/L
- **Serum osmolarity:** >320 mOsm/kg
- **Ketones:** no significant ketosis (blood ketones <3mmol/L or urine ketones negative/+)
- **VBG:** no significant acidosis (pH >7.3, bicarbonate >15 mmol/L)
- **U&Es:** hyper/hyponatraemia or hyper/hypokalaemia, dehydration
- **Investigate precipitant:** include septic screen (CXR, urine culture and bloods) and screen for MI (ECG and troponins)

Differentials: DKA, alcoholic ketoacidosis

Management:
1. Fluids: resuscitation if necessary and then slow rehydration (to avoid cerebral oedema) using 0.9% saline at around 0.5 L/h
2. Low-dose fixed-rate IV insulin: 0.05 units/kg/h only once glucose is no longer falling with fluids alone (except if ketosis is present)
3. Venous thromboembolism (VTE) prophylaxis
4. Treat any underlying precipitant

Adrenal Crisis

Definition: life-threatening deficiency of glucocorticoids. Causes include:
- Abrupt withdrawal of long-term exogenous steroid therapy (most common)
- Untreated/undiagnosed primary adrenal insufficiency (Addison's disease)
- Intercurrent illness with primary adrenal insufficiency, increasing the body's demand for glucocorticoids

Buzzwords:
- **Risk factors:** infections, surgery, pregnancy, trauma, hypoglycaemia, pregnancy, MI, missed steroid medication

- **Presentation:** malaise, myalgia, nausea, abdominal pain, low-grade fever, hypoglycaemia, confusion, hypotension, shock

Investigations:

- **CBG:** possible hypoglycaemia
- **U&Es:** hyponatraemia, hyperkalaemia
- **Morning cortisol:** low
- **Adrenocorticotropic hormone (ACTH) stimulation test:**
  - A synthetic ACTH derivative (Synacthen) is given via IV/IM routes, and the cortisol level is subsequently measured at 0 min, 30 min and 60 min
  - Subsequent serum cortisol <500 nanomol/L is indicative of adrenal insufficiency
- **Investigate precipitant:** drug history is important. Include a septic screen (CXR, urine culture and bloods) and screen for MI (ECG and troponins)

Differentials: septic shock, hypothyroidism (myxoedema coma)

Management:

1. 100 mg stat dose of hydrocortisone IV – do not wait for investigation results
2. Correct hypoglycaemia if present
3. IV fluid resuscitation
4. Investigate and treat underlying precipitant

Hyperthyroid Crisis (Thyrotoxic Storm)

Definition: a rare complication of hyperthyroidism resulting from severe overproduction of thyroid hormones

Buzzwords:

- **Risk factors:** infection, recent thyroid surgery, trauma, pregnancy, MI, stroke, excessive thyroid medication intake
- **Presentation:** hyperthermia, hypertension, nausea, diarrhoea, acute abdomen, tachycardia, atrial fibrillation (AF), heart failure, hypotension, agitation, confusion, coma

Investigations:

- Thyroid function tests (TFTs): TSH low, T3 and T4 raised
- CBG: potentially low as glycogen stores may become depleted
- ECG: Thyrotoxicosis may precipitate arrythmias
- Investigate precipitant: drug history is important. Include septic screen (CXR, urine culture and bloods) and screen for MI (troponins)

Differentials: sepsis, poisoning or overdose, phaeochromocytoma, malignant hyperthermia, neuroleptic malignant syndrome

Management: do not wait for investigation results!

1. 5 Bs:
   1. Block synthesis: carbimazole
   2. Block release: aqueous iodine solution 4 h after carbimazole (e.g., Lugol's solution)
   3. Block T4 into T3 conversion: hydrocortisone
   4. Beta blocker: propranolol
   5. Block enterohepatic circulation: cholestyramine
2. Sedation if severe agitation
3. Cooling may be required
4. Treat underlying precipitant
5. If medical therapy fails, consider plasma exchange or thyroidectomy

Prognosis: ~10% mortality

TOXIDROMES

Paracetamol Overdose

Definition: ingestion of >75 mg/kg requires referral to hospital and assessment of paracetamol levels

Buzzwords:

- **Risk factors:** unsupervised children, young adults, history of self-harm
- **Presentation:** asymptomatic initially, nausea, vomiting and right upper quadrant (RUQ) tenderness at 24 h, altered level of consciousness later or with higher overdoses

Investigations:

- **Plasma paracetamol concentration** (4 h from last ingestion): ↑ paracetamol level
- **Bloods:** ↑ ALT, ↑ PT/INR, ↑ creatinine
- **VBG:** if severe, may show lactic acidosis
- **Salicylate level** (to rule out salicylate overdose)

Differentials: acute drug-induced hepatitis, ischaemic hepatitis, viral hepatitis

Management:

1. Activated charcoal: consider if patient presents within 1 h of overdose
2. Acetylcysteine IV infusions are given in the following cases:

- Plasma paracetamol concentration lies on or exceeds the treatment line on the paracetamol treatment graph (see Fig 7.7)

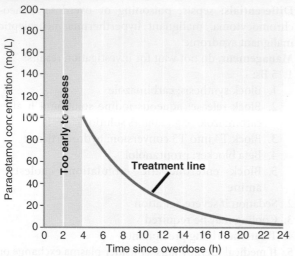

Fig 7.7 Paracetamol Treatment Nomogram. (With permission from Thomas S. H. L. (2018). Poisoning (Fig. 7.2). In *Davidson's principles and practice of medicine*. Elsevier. Copyright © 2018 Elsevier Ltd.)

- Ingestion over 150 mg/kg and measurement of plasma paracetamol concentration cannot be performed or is delayed >8 h
- >24-h post-ingestion with any of the following: jaundice, hepatic tenderness, raised ALT, raised INR or detectable paracetamol level
- Staggered dose (significant quantities taken over a time period of >1 h)
3. Haemodialysis: consider if very high serum paracetamol concentration (>700 mg/L) associated with coma and elevated blood lactate concentrations
4. Consider referral to transplant centre if meeting King's College criteria

Lithium Toxicity

Definition: serum lithium level >1.2 mmol/L
Buzzwords:
- **Risk factors:** long-term lithium use (tissues already saturated), accidental or deliberate overdose of medication, dehydration, renal impairment, diarrhoea and vomiting, co-prescription of drugs that interfere with lithium excretion (e.g., angiotensin-converting enzyme inhibitors (ACEis), diuretics, NSAIDs)
- **Presentation:**
  - **Mild intoxication:** nausea, vomiting, restlessness, gross tremor, diarrhoea, polyuria, lethargy

- **Moderate intoxication:** dysarthria, ataxia, delirium
- **Severe intoxication:** seizures, coma, hypotension, arrythmias
- **Renal failure:** depends on premorbid renal function as well as plasma lithium concentration

Investigations:
- **ECG:** sinoatrial (SA) and atrioventricular (AV) block, QT prolongation, ST changes, T-wave inversion
- **CBG** (to rule out hypoglycaemia) ↔
- **Serum lithium level:** >1.2 mmol/L
- **Bloods:** hypernatremia, deranged TFTs

Differentials: hypoglycaemia, alcohol toxicity, delirium tremens, neuroleptic malignant syndrome, anticholinergic poising, stroke
Management:
1. Hold lithium
2. Gastric lavage should be considered if significant lithium ingestion has occurred within 1 h
3. IV fluids
4. Renal replacement therapy: consider with severe toxicity (serum concentration >2.0 mmol/L) or severe symptoms
5. Consider whole-bowel irrigation if significant lithium ingestion (>4 g)

Serotonin Syndrome

Definition: an uncommon, life-threatening, drug-induced condition caused by excessive central and peripheral serotonergic activity
Buzzwords:
- **Risk factors:** initiation or increase of a serotonergic drug, including antidepressants (e.g., selective serotonin reuptake inhibitors (SSRIs) and monoamine oxidase inhibitors (MAOIs)), analgesics (e.g., tramadol), herbal remedies (e.g., St John's wort) and recreational drugs (e.g., MDMA)
- **Presentation:** typically characterised by a triad of:
  - Autonomic hyperactivity: hypertension, mydriasis, tachycardia, hyperthermia, diarrhoea
  - Neuromuscular abnormality: clonus, hypertonicity, tremor, hyperreflexia
  - Mental status changes: agitation, mania, confusion, altered consciousness

Investigations: clinical diagnosis, investigations to rule out differentials and identify complications

- **Creatine kinase (CK)** (monitor for rhabdomyolysis): may be raised
- **LP** (to rule out encephalitis)
- **Urine drug screen** (if unclear history): serotonergic drugs

Differentials: encephalitis, neuroleptic malignant syndrome, anticholinergic toxicity

Management:
1. Stop causative drug
2. Supportive care, sedation if necessary: may require HDU/ITU care
3. Serotonergic antagonist: consider cyproheptadine

Neuroleptic Malignant Syndrome

Definition: a rare, life-threatening idiosyncratic reaction to treatment with antipsychotic drugs or cessation of dopamine agonists

Buzzwords:
- **Risk factors:** antipsychotics (especially 'typical' antipsychotics, e.g., haloperidol and chlorpromazine), genetic susceptibility, withdrawal from dopaminergic Parkinson's disease medications, other medications with central D_2 antagonist effects (e.g., metoclopramide)
- **Presentation:** hyperthermia, altered consciousness, muscle rigidity, tremor, autonomic dysfunction (pallor, tachycardia, tachypnoea, labile blood pressure, incontinence)

Investigations: clinical diagnosis, investigations to rule out differentials and identify complications.
- **CT head** (to rule out intracranial lesions)
- **CK** (monitor for rhabdomyolysis): typically raised
- **U&Es:** possible AKI secondary to rhabdomyolysis
- **Septic screen (CXR, blood and urine cultures)** (to rule out infection)
- **LP** (to rule out encephalitis and meningitis)

Differentials: serotonin syndrome, heat stroke, catatonia, sepsis, encephalitis, vasculitis, stroke

Management:
1. Stop causative agent (effects may last 5–7 days after drug discontinuation)
2. If agitated: IV lorazepam
3. Supportive care: rehydration, cooling if hyperthermia
4. Dopamine agonist, bromocriptine, and muscle relaxant, dantrolene, are often used; however, there is little evidence to support their use

Poisoning of Unknown Origin and Common Toxidromes

Definition: poisoning without a clear enough history to identify a particular agent

Buzzwords:
- **Risk factors:** occupational exposure, young children, learning difficulties, concomitant intoxication with alcohol or other drugs, malicious intent
- **Presentation:** see Table 7.4 for signs and symptoms of common toxidromes

Investigations: should be directed by signs, symptoms and history
- **Bloods:** salicylate/paracetamol levels
- **CBG** (to rule out hypoglycaemia)
- **CT head** (to rule out intracranial lesions)
- **CRP and FBC** (to rule out infection)
- **Urine toxin screen:** positive for particular toxins. Can take days to come back, not all drugs can be screened for

Differentials: hypoglycaemia, head injury, encephalopathy and infection can mimic an intoxication by causing neurological impairment.

Management: treatment is often commenced based on a high degree of clinical suspicion in the absence of a specific test for a specific poison
1. Check Toxbase (www.toxbase.org) for management advice
2. Supportive care: fluids, airway management
3. Methods to reduce absorption of a poison:
   - Activated charcoal: given within 1 h of ingestion can be useful for binding some toxins, although beware because not all toxins can bind to charcoal, and ingestion is unpleasant
   - Whole-bowel irrigation: limited use for extended-release preparations as well as iron and lithium
4. Specific antidotes if poison known (see Table 7.4)
5. Psychiatric assessment (if relevant)

OTHER EMERGENCIES

Hyperthermia (Heat Stroke)

Definition: a state of hyperthermia (typically >40ºC) in which CNS dysfunction and widespread tissue damage is manifested

Buzzwords:
- **Risk factors:** heat and humidity exposure, alcohol use or withdrawal, cardiac disease, intense exercise,

TABLE 7.4 Common Poisons

Toxin	Buzzwords	Management/Antidote
Adder bites	Grey/brown snake, puncture marks, abdominal pain, vomiting	European viper venom antiserum (VipraTAb), admit for 24-h observation period
Anticholinergics – atropine, TCAs, glyoopyrronium, oxybutynin	Dry mucous membranes, flushing, urinary retention, altered mental status, dilated pupils (mydriasis)	Supportive, benzodiazepine for agitation
Beta blockers – propranolol, bisoprolol, etc.	Bradycardia, hypotension, syncope	Glucagon. Inotropes, vasopressors and IV insulin (with dextrose) can be considered
Benzodiazepines – diazepam (Valium), temazepam, chlordiazepoxide, etc.	Drowsiness, ataxia, dysarthria, nystagmus	Flumazenil – should be used with extreme caution due to epileptogenic effect. Rarely used
Carbon monoxide – incomplete combustion in boilers, cars, stoves	Headache, nausea and vomiting, dizziness, confusion, blisters, tachycardic, tachypnoeic	100% oxygen
Digoxin	Arrythmias (AV block with paroxysmal atrial tachycardia), hyperkalaemia, yellow visual halos	Digoxin-specific antibody fragments (Digibind)
Ethylene glycol or methanol – antifreeze, 'homemade' alcohol	Initially mimics ethanol poisoning, later stages with cardiac failure, blindness and neurological symptoms. Metabolic acidosis with high anion gap and osmolar gap	Fomepizole (not to be confused with flumazenil, fomepizole → glycol, methanol). If unable to obtain, ethanol can also be used
Heparin – unfractionated or low molecular weight	Bleeding	Protamine
Hydrogen cyanide	Bitter almond smell, headache, anxiety, lactic acidosis	Oxygen and dicolbalt edetate or hydroxocobalamin
Iron	Nausea, vomiting, abdominal pain, GI haemorrhage, metabolic acidosis	Desferrioxamine
Local anaesthetic – lidocaine, bupivacaine, etc.	Numbness of mouth and tongue, tinnitus, confusion, convulsions, arrythmias and coma	Lipid emulsion (Intralipid)
Opioids – morphine, diamorphine (heroin), fentanyl	Respiratory depression, reduced GCS score, pinpoint pupils (miosis)	Naloxone
Organophosphates – insecticides (think farmers)	Inhibits cholinesterase Fluids out ++ → salivation lacrimation urination diarrhoea, pinpoint pupils (miosis), bradycardia	Atropine and pralidoxime or obidoxime
Salicylates – aspirin	Nausea, tinnitus, respiratory alkalosis leading to metabolic acidosis	Correct acidosis with sodium bicarbonate Dialysis if critically unwell
Sympathomimetics – cocaine, amphetamine, MDMA (ecstasy)	Mydriasis – big pupils, agitation, delirium, hyperthermia, seizures	Supportive, benzodiazepines for agitation, nitrates, e.g., GTN for chest pain/hypertension
TCAs – amitriptyline, imipramine, nortriptyline	Antidepressant, neuropathic pain, long-QT, hypotension, wide QRS, metabolic acidosis	Sodium bicarbonate – if wide QRS or arrythmia

AV, Atrioventricular; GCS, Glasgow Coma Scale; GI, gastrointestinal; GTN, Glyceryl trinitrate; TCA, tricyclic antidepressant.

use of stimulants, dehydration, elderly and young children

- **Presentation:**
  - **Skin:** sweating, although skin may feel cool due to vasoconstriction
  - **CNS:** confusion, delirium, seizures, coma, muscle rigidity, cerebellar dysfunction and dilated pupils
  - **CVS:** tachycardia, hypotension and arrhythmias
  - **Clotting:** purpura, conjunctival haemorrhages and petechiae

Investigations:
- Core body temperature (rectal or oesophageal): >40°C
- U&Es: possible hyponatraemia
- CXR: may show pulmonary oedema
- TFTs (exclude thyrotoxic crisis)
- Clotting profile (exclude disseminated intravascular coagulation (DIC)):
  - **FBC:** may show low platelets and Hb, especially low if DIC
  - **PT and APPT:** may show long PT and APTT, especially long if DIC
  - **Fibrinogen:** especially low if DIC
  - **D-dimer:** may be raised, especially high in DIC

Differentials: malignant hyperthermia, delirium tremens, neuroleptic malignant or serotonin syndromes, thyrotoxic crisis

Management:
1. Remove from external heat source
2. Fluids PO/IV
3. Correct hypoglycaemia
4. Rapid cooling:
- External: preferred method is evaporative by wetting the skin with tepid water, ice packs can also be placed around the axilla and groin
- Internal: gastric, rectal and bladder lavage
5. Benzodiazepines can be used to control shivering and seizures

Hypothermia

Definition: core body temperature below 35°C
Buzzwords:
- **Risk factors:** environmental exposure, alcohol and other sedatives, general anaesthetic, Parkinson's disease, older age, infants/young children, gram-negative septicaemia
- **Presentation:**

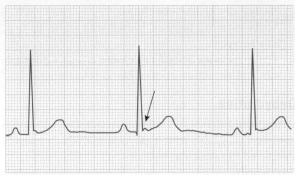

Fig 7.8 J-waves (*arrow*) on Electrocardiogram. (With permission from Nicol, A. J., & Navsaria, P. H. (2013). The J-wave: A new electrocardiographic sign of an occult cardiac injury. *Injury.* Elsevier. *Copyright © 2013 Elsevier Ltd. All rights reserved.*)

- Mild: shivering (not a reliable sign), tachypnoea, tachycardia, hypertension
- Moderate: altered mental status, bradycardia, bradypnoea
- Severe: coma, apnoea
- Miscellaneous: frost bite, cold-induced diuresis, ventricular fibrillation (VF)

Investigations:
- **Core body temperature** (rectal or oesophageal): <35°C (severe: <30°C)
- **ECG:** sinus bradycardia; J-wave (see Fig 7.8); prolonged PR, QTc and QRS intervals; AF; cardiac arrest due to VF, VT or asystole
- **CXR:** normal or may show pulmonary oedema
- **U&Es:** hypokalaemia
- **Clotting screen:** raised PT and APPT
- **FBC:** raised Hb due to haemoconcentration, potentially low platelets due to sequestration in spleen
- **CBG:** Varied, can be low or high

Differentials: intoxication, sepsis and hypothyroidism
Management:
1. Remove person from the cold environment/wet garments and dry skin
2. Warm humidified oxygen
3. Warm IV fluids. Hypotension is common during rewarming as vasodilation occurs
4. Rewarm the patient (passive, active external or active core). Beware of active warming because it can cause hypotension and pulmonary/cerebral oedema. Must be done in higher care areas

- Passive: dry blankets or clothes
- Active external: blankets heated with warm air (e.g., Bair Hugger)
- Active core: peritoneal or colonic lavage with warm saline. Also, extracorporeal blood rewarming

Dehydration

Definition: a deficit of total body water. Dehydration is not interchangeable with hypovolaemia, which refers to a depleted intravascular volume

Buzzwords:
- **Risk factors:**
  - **Reduced fluid intake**: reduced consciousness, advanced age, dementia, self-neglect
  - **Increased losses**:
  - **Sensible losses:** diarrhoea, vomiting, high-output stoma, dialysis, increased diuresis (diuretics, e.g., furosemide, diabetes insipidus, nephrotic syndrome, hyperglycaemia including DKA and HHS)
  - **Insensible losses:** burns, exercise, environmental exposure, tachypnoea, fever
- **Presentation:** thirst, dry mucous membranes, reduced skin turgor, hypotension, reduced capillary refill time, tachycardia, oliguria, fatigue, sunken eyes

Investigations:
- **U&Es:** raised urea, raised creatinine and often hypernatremia
- **Urine output:** reduced
- **Investigate precipitant:** drug history is important.

Differentials: other causes of shock (e.g., sepsis, Sjögren syndrome), urinary retention or obstruction

Management:
1. If significantly hypotensive, correct with IV isotonic fluid bolus/es
2. Review medications and suspend any culprit drugs, such as furosemide or bendroflumethiazide, as necessary
3. Replace fluid
- Oral replacement if possible
- Consider oral rehydration salt solution (e.g., Dioralyte) in cases of electrolyte depletion seen with persistent diarrhoea or vomiting. Selective electrolyte replacement (using Sando K for example), can be done with reference to up-to-date U&Es
- Avoid large shifts in sodium as this can lead to central pontine myelinosis

- Practise caution in those with heart failure or chronic kidney disease, as they may become fluid overloaded
4. Treat precipitant

Bites

Definition: injury inflicted by the teeth of an animal or human, carrying a risk of puncture, crush injuries and infection.

Buzzwords:
- **Risk factors:**
  - **Risk of being bitten:** pets, farms, domestic violence, bare-knuckle boxing, communities with a high incidence of stray animals
  - **Susceptibility to infection:** delayed presentation, poor hygiene, DM, alcoholism, immunocompromised
- **Presentation:**
  - **Early:** superficial trauma, neurovascular damage, haemorrhage
  - **Late:** wound site infection, sepsis, tetanus, viral hepatitis, HIV, rabies

Investigations: clinical diagnosis. Consider:
- **X-ray:** possible foreign bodies (e.g., tooth fragments), fractures, air in tissue, soft tissue injury
- **Wound swab:** possible growth of pathogenic organisms
- **Serum virology** to be considered

Differentials: other trauma

Management:
1. **Clean:** explore under appropriate anaesthesia and debride if necessary, wash with normal saline
2. **Closure:** avoid closing puncture wounds. Facial wounds or those with tendon or joint involvement should be referred to a specialist
3. **Antibiotic prophylaxis:** broad-spectrum antibiotics with anaerobic cover (e.g., co-amoxiclav) recommended for most animal and **all** human/cat bites that have broken the skin. Seek advice for esoteric animal bites (e.g., seals)
4. **Tetanus prophylaxis:** consider, depending on the immunisation status of the patient and the degree of contamination of the wound
5. **Hep B, C and HIV risk assessment:** only required in human bites that have broken the skin
6. Escalate any safeguarding concerns

TABLE 7.5 Description and Presentation of Burns

Classification	Description	Presentation
Superficial epidermal	Only epidermis	Erythematous, painful, no blisters, capillary refill blanches with rapid filling
Superficial dermal	Epidermis and upper layer of dermis	Moist, painfully hypersensitive, potentially blistered, homogenously pink, capillary refill blanches, slower filling
Deep dermal	Epidermis and all layers of dermis	Drier, less painful, potentially blistered, red or mottled in appearance, does not blanch to touch
Full thickness	All skin layers and into the subcutaneous tissue. If severe, extending to muscle and bone	Leathery, translucent, or waxy white, surface is painless to light touch or pin prick and is dry, does not blanch to touch

PLASTICS EMERGENCIES

Burns

Definition: burns are injuries caused by exposure to various forms of energy, including thermal, electrical, chemical and radiation. Causes include thermal (e.g., sunburn, oil, fires), electrical (e.g., lightning, household current), chemical (e.g., strong acids) and radiation (e.g., radiotherapy, UV rays).

Buzzwords:

- **Risk factors:** occupational exposure
- **Presentation:** See Table 7.5 and Figs 7.9 and 7.10
  Investigations: clinical diagnosis
- **ABG:** ↑ carboxyhaemoglobin (HbCO) in inhalational injury

Differentials: Staphylococcal scalded skin syndrome, erythroderma, Steven-Johnson syndrome (SJS), toxic epidermal necrolysis (TEN), necrotising fasciitis

Management:

- Consider admission if >5% of total body surface area affected (see Fig 7.11), deep, dermal, full-thickness, complex burns (electrical/chemical)
- **Minor injury:** irrigate with normal saline for 20–30 min, layer of clingfilm to cover burn, elevate to reduce oedema, analgesia
- **Severe injury:**
  - Airway control and oxygenation
  - Aggressive fluid resuscitation (according to Parkland formula)
  - IV analgesia
  - Consider surgery: escharotomy, skin grafting
  - Regular wound dressings and warming to prevent excess fluid and heat loss

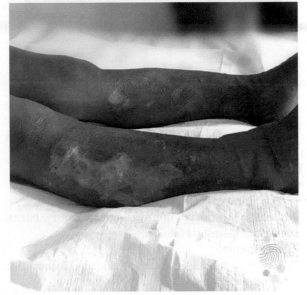

Fig 7.9 Burns in Darker Skin. (With permission from SKINDEEP.)

- Check for and treat any associated injuries

Frostbite

Definition: injury to skin and underlying tissue caused by exposure to cold environments. Most common affected sites are the digits, nose and ears.

Buzzwords:

- **Risk factors:** low temperature, immobilisation, open wounds, moisture, extremes of age, drug intoxication, cognitive impairment
- **Presentation:**
  - **First degree:** oedema and hyperaemia, no necrosis

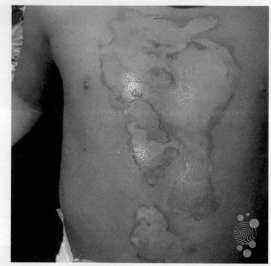

Fig 7.10 Burns in Lighter Skin. (With permission from SKINDEEP.)

- **Second degree:** large, clear vesicle formation, partial skin necrosis (see Fig 7.12)
- **Third degree:** skin and subcutaneous tissue necrosis
- **Fourth degree:** involves muscle and bone with gangrene (see Fig 7.13)

Investigations:
- Low-reading thermometer: temperature <35°C
- ECG: J waves

Differentials: frostnip, nonfreezing cold injury, burns, trench foot, perniosis (chilblains)

Management:
1. Rewarm with warm water and added chlorhexidine or iodine, air dry
2. Analgesia
3. Debridement and drainage for blisters
4. Consider amputation for gangrene
   Treat associated conditions, such as hypoglycaemia, sepsis, drug or alcohol ingestion

Crush Injury

Definition: trauma and ischaemia to soft tissues and skeletal muscle after a long period of severe crushing characterised by hypovolaemic shock and hyperkalaemia. Injury to muscle tissue releases large amounts of intracellular potassium, phosphate, CK, urate and myoglobin. The excess myoglobin is nephrotoxic and can lead to AKI.

Buzzwords:

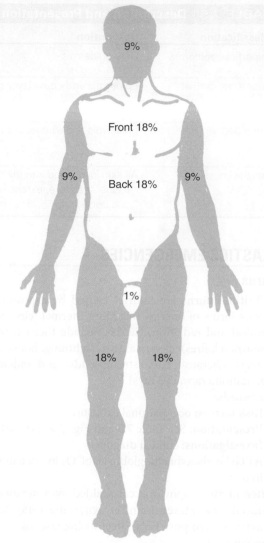

Fig 7.11 Percentage of Total Body Surface Area (TBSA) Mapped Using Wallace's Rule of Nines. (Illustrated by Dr Hollie Blaber.)

- **Risk factors:** occupational hazards, extreme sports, fall and long lie
- **Presentation:** oedema, sensory and motor disturbances, rhabdomyolysis with myoglobinuria causing dark, amber-coloured urine (with CK >10,000 U/L) (see Fig 7.14), hypovolaemic shock

Investigations:
- **ABG:** metabolic acidosis, ↑ lactate
- **Bloods:** ↑ potassium, ↑ urea, ↑ creatinine, ↑ CK, ↑ myoglobin, ↑ phosphate, ↓ calcium, deranged FBC/clotting (DIC)

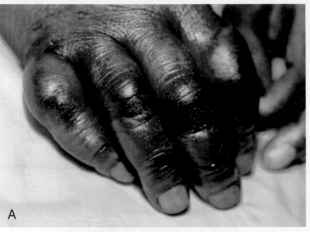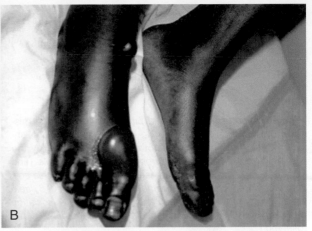

Fig 7.12 Second-degree Frostbite in Darker Skin. (With permission from Manson, P. N. (2020). Management of frostbite, hypothermia, and cold injuries (Fig. 2). In *Current surgical therapy*. Elsevier. *Copyright © 2020 Elsevier Inc. All rights reserved.*)

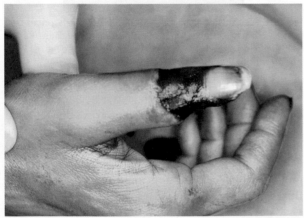

Fig 7.13 Third- and Fourth-degree Frostbite with Tissue Death in Lighter Skin. (From Cameron J. L., Cameron A. M. (2011). *Current surgical therapy* (10th ed.). Philadelphia: WB Saunders.)

- **ECG:** hyperkalaemia changes
- **Trauma CT/X-ray** to exclude fracture and other injuries

Differentials: compartment syndrome, cellulitis, degloving injury, traumatic fracture

Management:
- **Medical:**
  - Aggressive IV fluid management and analgesia
  - Treat hyperkalaemia
  - Urinary alkalinisation with sodium bicarbonate to prevent AKI
  - Treat DIC (see Haematology in an Hour)

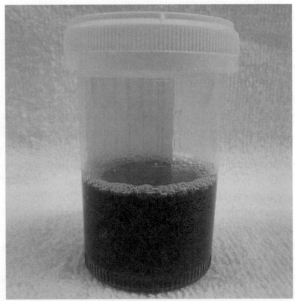

Fig 7.14 Myoglobinuria. (With permission from James Heilman, MD, CC BY-SA 3.0 via Wikimedia Commons.)

- **Surgical:** grafting to restore function, amputation for unsalvageable crush injury

Necrotising Fasciitis (NF)

Definition: severe, life-threatening spread of infection from the subcutaneous tissue along fascial planes. There are four main types:

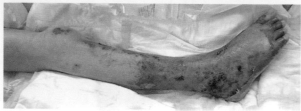

Fig 7.15 Necrotising Fasciitis in Lighter Skin. (With permission from Endo, A., Matsuoka, R., Mizuno Y., Doi, A, & Nishioka, H. (2016). Sequential necrotizing fasciitis caused by the monomicrobial pathogens *Streptococcus equisimilis* and extended-spectrum beta-lactamase-producing *Escherichia coli*. *Journal of Infection and Chemotherapy.* Elsevier. © 2016 Japanese Society of Chemotherapy and The Japanese Association for Infectious Diseases. Published by Elsevier Ltd. All rights reserved.)

- **Type 1 (most common in the UK):** polymicrobial infection with an anaerobe (*Bacteroides* or *Peptostreptococcus*) along with a facultative anaerobe (*Enterobacterales* or non-group A *Streptococcus*), usually in immunocompromised patients
- **Type 2:** monomicrobial, usually with group A *Streptococcus* (*Streptococcus pyogenes*)
- **Type 3:** Gram negative, usually *Vibrio spp.*
- **Type 4:** Fungal, usually *Candida spp.* in immunocompromised

Buzzwords:

- **Risk factors:** trauma, surgery, DM, peripheral vascular disease, immunocompromised, IV drug use, CKD, hepatic disease
- **Presentation: PAIN++ out of proportion,** numbness, systemic illness, severe oedema and necrosis/gangrene (see Figs 7.15 and 7.16). It can affect any part of the body. Fournier's gangrene refers to NF affecting the perineal, perianal and genital areas.

Investigations: if high clinical suspicion (e.g., pain is out of proportion), do not delay treatment

- **Bloods:** ↑ WCC, ↑ CRP, ↑ CK, ↑ lactate, ↑ urea, cultures
- ***Deep tissue biopsy + culture:** to target antibiotics*
- **X-ray, CT and MRI:** to visualise extent of spread

Differentials: cellulitis, osteomyelitis, erysipelas, impetigo, gas gangrene

Management:

1. IV fluids
2. Urgent, extensive surgical debridement
3. Antibiotics: broad spectrum initially, followed by narrow spectrum based on cultures and microbiology advice

Prognosis: mortality, even following surgery, is between 10%–40%

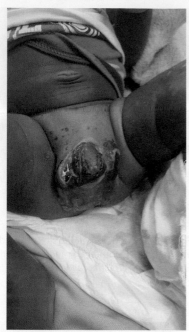

Fig 7.16 Necrotising Fasciitis in Darker Skin. (Reference: Delport, J. E., & Makamba, K. (2020). Necrotising fasciitis in a ten month old infant (Fig. 1). *Urology case reports.* Elsevier. © 2020 The Author(s). Published by Elsevier Inc.)

Compartment Syndrome

Definition: compartment syndrome arises due to raised pressure in the fascial compartments, often affecting the limbs. As a result, there is decreased tissue perfusion and damage to muscles and nerves. Causes include fractures, prolonged limb compression, infection and haematoma.

Buzzwords:

- **Risk factors:** crush injury, burns, trauma, bleeding disorders, anticoagulant use, open fractures
- **Presentation:**
  - 6 Ps: Pain +++ (early), pressure (muscle tightness, early), paraesthesia (early), pulselessness (late), pallor (late), paralysis (late)
  - Significant pain on passive stretching of the muscle is a useful early sign

Investigations:

- **Bloods:** ↑ CK
- **Urine:** ↑ myoglobin
- Compartment pressure measurement using a manometer: ↑
- Important to rule out other differentials

Differentials: NF, DVT, acute limb ischaemia, haematoma, muscle rupture

Management:

1. Immediate removal of any dressings, casts and splints
2. Strong analgesia (e.g., patient-controlled analgesia)
3. Surgical management: fasciotomy release and debridement of tissue necrosis

READING LIST: EMERGENCY MEDICINE IN AN HOUR

Respiratory
Anaphylaxis

Best Practice, B. M. J. (2020). *Anaphylaxis*. http://www.best-practice.bmj.com. [Accessed 17 November 2020].

THE ONE-LINE ROUND-UP!

Here are some key words to help you remember each condition/concept.

Condition/Concept	One-line Description
Anaphylaxis	*500 micrograms of adrenaline for adults at 5-min intervals*
Tension pneumothorax	*Large-bore canula, midclavicular line, 2nd intercostal space*
Pneumothorax	*Primary vs secondary*
Pulmonary embolism	*Wells' score to guide treatment*
Cardiac arrest	*Help, CPR, 4 Hs and 4 Ts*
Major haemorrhage	*On the floor and 4 more: thorax, abdomen, pelvis and long bones*
Sepsis	*Give 3 (O_2, fluids, Abx), take 3 (cultures, lactate, urine output)*
Convulsive status epilepticus	*Loss of consciousness due to seizure activity for over 5 min. 1st line: IV lorazepam, buccal midazolam or rectal diazepam*
Acute alcohol withdrawal	*First IV thiamine and then benzodiazepines for those with a CIWA ≥10*
Wernicke's and Korsakoff syndromes	*Wernicke's encephalitis is reversible, Korsakoff syndrome is not*
Upper-GI bleed	*Blatchford first, Rockall's post-endoscopy*
Hypoglycaemia	*CBG <4 mmol/L*
DKA	*CBG >11 mmol/L, blood ketones >3 mmol/L or ≥++ urine ketones and pH <7.3 or bicarb <15 mmol/L*
HHS	*Hyperglycaemia and high serum osmolality without ketosis or acidosis*
Adrenal crisis	*IV hydrocortisone stat*
Hyperthyroid crisis	*5 Bs for management - Block synthesis, block release, block T4/T3 conversion, beta blocker, block enterohepatic circulation*
Paracetamol overdose	*Acetylcysteine IV if over treatment line*
Lithium toxicity	*>1.2 mmol/L in serum*
Serotonin syndrome	*Autonomic hyperactivity, neuromuscular abnormality, mental status change*
Neuroleptic malignant syndrome	*Antipsychotics or withdrawal of dopaminergic drugs*
Poisoning of unknown origin	*Use Toxbase!*
Hyperthermia (heat stroke)	*Core temp >40°C (with CNS dysfunction for heat stroke)*
Hypothermia	*Core temp <35°C*
Dehydration	*Reduced intake or increased losses*
Bites	*Prophylactic antibiotics*
Burns	*Wallace's rule of nines, Parkland formula*
Frostbite	*Warming and debridement if necessary*
Crush injuries	*Myoglobinuria, acute tubular necrosis*
Necrotising fasciitis	*Pain out of proportion*
Compartment syndrome	*6 Ps*

NICE. (2018). *CKS; Angio-oedema and anaphylaxis.* http://www.cks.nice.org.uk. [Accessed 5 October 2020].

Resuscitation Council UK. (2008). *Emergency treatment of anaphylactic reactions.* http://www.resus.org.uk. [Accessed 9 November 2020].

Tension Pneumothorax

MacDuff, A., Arnold, A., & Harvey, J. (2010). Management of spontaneous pneumothorax: British Thoracic Society pleural disease guideline 2010. *Thorax, 65,* ii18–ii31.

Payne, D. (2017). *Pneumothorax | Doctor.* Patient info. http://www.patient.info. [Accessed 6 October 2020].

Pneumothorax

MacDuff, A., Arnold, A., & Harvey, J. (2010). Management of spontaneous pneumothorax: British Thoracic Society pleural disease guideline 2010. *Thorax, 65,* ii18–ii31.

Payne, D. (2017). *Pneumothorax | Doctor.* Patient. info. http://www.patient.info. [Accessed 6 October 2020].

Ahmedzai, S., Balfour-Lynn, I. M., Bewick, T., et al. (2011). Managing passengers with stable respiratory disease planning air travel: British Thoracic Society recommendations. *Thorax, 66,* i1–i30.

Pulmonary Embolism

Howard, L. (2018). BTS guidelines for the initial outpatient management of pulmonary embolism: There's no place like home. *Thorax, 73,* 607–608.

Howard, L., Barden, S., Condliffe, R., Connolly, V., Davies, C., Donaldson, J., et al. (2018). British Thoracic Society Guideline for the initial outpatient management of pulmonary embolism (PE). *Thorax, 73,* ii1–ii29.

NICE. (2020). *CKS: Pulmonary embolism.* http://www.cks.nice.org.uk. [Accessed 8 October 2020].

British Thoracic Society Standards of Care Committee Pulmonary Embolism Guideline Development Group. (2003). British Thoracic Society guidelines for the management of suspected acute pulmonary embolism. *Thorax, 58,* 470–483.

Cardiovascular
Cardiac Arrest

Resuscitation Council UK. (2020). *Guidelines: Adult advanced life support.* http://www.resus.org.uk. [Accessed 2 October 2020].

Major Haemorrhage

Joint United Kingdom Blood Transfusion and Tissue Transplantation Services Professional Advisory Committee. (2014). *Transfusion handbook.* http://www.resus.org.uk. [Accessed 10 October 2020].

British Society for Haematology. (2017). *Haematological management of major haemorrhage.* http://www.b-s-h.org.uk. [Accessed 10 October 2020].

Sepsis

NICE. (2017). *NG51: Sepsis: Recognition, diagnosis and early management.* [www.nice.org.uk - Accessed February 2022].

HEE, e-LFH. (2020). *Anaesthesia eLA, core training, Sepsis.* http://portal.e-lfh.org.uk. [Accessed 18 November 2020].

HEE, e-LFH. (2020). *Anaesthesia eLA, core training, Assessment and differential diagnosis of sepsis.* http://portal.e-lfh.org.uk. [Accessed 18 November 2020].

Neurological
Convulsive Status Epilepticus

Best Practice, B. M. J. (2020). *Status epilepticus.* http://www.bestpractice.bmj.com. [Accessed 18 September 2020].

BNF. (2020). *Epilepsy | Treatment summary.* http://bnf.nice.org.uk. [Accessed 18 June 2020].

Nardone, R., Brigo, F., & Trinka, E. (2016). Acute symptomatic seizures caused by electrolyte disturbances. *Journal of Clinical Neurology, 12,* 21.

NICE. (2020). *Epilepsy - NICE Pathways.* http://www.pathways.nice.org.uk. [Accessed 18 June 2020].

Tidy, C. (2020). *Status epilepticus management information page.* Patient info. http://www.patient.info. [Accessed 20 June 2020].

Wyatt, J., Taylor, R., Wit, K., & Hotton, E. (2020). *Oxford handbook of emergency medicine* (5th ed.). Oxford University Press.

Acute Alcohol Withdrawal

Best Practice, B. M. J. (2020). *Alcohol withdrawal.* http://www.bestpractice.bmj.com. [Accessed 10 November 2020].

NICE. (2017). *Alcohol use disorders: Diagnosis and clinical management of alcohol-related physical complications.* http://www.nice.org.uk. [Accessed 11 November 2020].

Wyatt, J., Taylor, R., Wit, K., & Hotton, E. (2020). *Oxford handbook of emergency medicine* (5th ed.). Oxford University Press.

Wernicke's Encephalopathy & Korsakoff Syndrome

Best Practice, B. M. J. (2020). *Wernicke's encephalopathy.* http://www.bestpractice.bmj.com. [Accessed 14 November 2020].

NICE. (2017). *Alcohol use disorders: Diagnosis and clinical management of alcohol-related physical complications.* http://www.nice.org.uk. [Accessed 11 November 2020].

Wyatt, J., Taylor, R., Wit, K., & Hotton, E. (2020). *Oxford handbook of emergency medicine* (5th ed.). Oxford University Press.

Gastrointestinal
Upper GI Bleed

Best Practice, B. M. J. (2020). *Oesophageal varices.* http://www.bestpractice.bmj.com. [Accessed 27 August 2020].

Henderson, R. (2020). *Upper gastrointestinal bleeding (UGIB bleeding) Rockall Score*. Patient info. http://www.patient. info. [Accessed 10 July 2020].

NICE. (2016). *Overview | Acute upper gastrointestinal bleeding in over 16s: Management*. http://www.nice.org.uk. [Accessed 15 July 2020].

Endocrine
Hypoglycaemia
Best Practice, B. M. J. (2020). *Non-diabetic hypoglycaemia*. http://www.bestpractice.bmj.com. [Accessed 30 September 2020].

Diabetes. (2020). *Diabetes and hypoglycaemia*. http://www. diabetes.co.uk. [Accessed 30 September 2020].

BNF. (2020). *Medical emergencies in the community*. http:// www.bnf.nice.org.uk. [Accessed 28 September 2020].

NICE. (2020). *Type 1 diabetes in adults: Diagnosis and management*. http://www.nice.org.uk. [Accessed 28 September 2020].

Diabetic Ketoacidosis
NICE. (2020). *CKS: When to suspect diabetic ketoacidosis*. http://www.cks.nice.org.uk. [Accessed 17 September 2020].

Dhatariya, K., & Savage, M. (2013). *The management of diabetic ketoacidosis in adults* (2nd ed.). Joint British Diabetes Societies Inpatient Care Group. http://www.diabetes.org. uk. [Accessed 2 November 2020].

BNF. (2020). *Diabetic ketoacidosis*. http://www.bnf.nice.org. uk. [Accessed 17 September 2020].

HHS
Best Practice, B. M. J. (2020). *Hyperosmolar hyperglycaemic state*. http://www.bestpractice.bmj.com. [Accessed 13 April 2021].

Tidy, C. (2020). *Hyperosmolar hyperglycaemic state*. Patient info. http://www.patient.info. [Accessed 13 July 2020].

Scott, A., & Claydon, A. (2012). *The management of the hyperosmolar hyperglycaemic state (HHS) in adults with diabetes* (1st ed.). Joint British Diabetes Societies Inpatient Care Group. https://diabetes-resources-production.s3-eu-west-1.amazonaws.com/diabetes-storage/migration/pdf/JBDS-IP-HHS-Adults.pdf. [Accessed 13 July 2020].

Adrenal Crisis
NICE. (2020). *CKS: Addison's disease*. http://www.cks.nice. org.uk. [Accessed 12 December 2020].

Society for Endocrinology. n.d. *Management of adrenal crisis summary*. http://www.endocrinology.org. Accessed 3 April 2021.

Willacy, H. (2020). *Adrenal crisis. Information about adrenal/ Addisonian crisis*. Patient info. http://www.patient.info. [Accessed 17 July 2020].

Wyatt, J., Taylor, R., Wit, K., & Hotton, E. (2020). *Oxford handbook of emergency medicine* (5th ed.). Oxford University Press.

Hyperthyroid Crisis (Thyrotoxic Storm)
Carroll, R., & Matfin, G. (2010). Review: Endocrine and metabolic emergencies: Thyroid storm. *Therapeutic Advances in Endocrinology and Metabolism*, 1, 139–145.

NICE. (2020). *CKS: Hyperthyroidism*. http://www.cks.nice. org.uk. [Accessed 23 July 2020].

BNF. (2020). *Hyperthyroidism | Treatment summary*. http:// www.bnf.nice.org.uk. [Accessed 5 December 2020].

Willacy, H. (2020). *Hyperthyroid crisis (thyrotoxic storm) Medical information*. Patient info. http://www.patient.info. com. [Accessed 23 July 2020].

Poisoning

Paracetamol Overdose
NICE. (2017). *CKS: Poisoning or overdose*. http://www.cks. nice.org.uk. [Accessed 4 August 2020].

BNF. (2020). *Poisoning, emergency treatment*. http://www.bnf. nice.org.uk. [Accessed 4 August 2020].

TOXBASE – poisons information database for clinical toxicology advice. (2020). https://www.toxbase.org/. Accessed 7 December 2020.

Lithium Toxicity
BNF. (2020). *Poisoning, emergency treatment*. http://www.bnf. nice.org.uk. [Accessed 18 July 2020].

Hedya, S., Avula, A., & Swoboda, H. (2021). *Lithium toxicity*. StatPearls. http://www.ncbi.nlm.nih.gov. [Accessed 18 February 2021].

Stringer, S., Church, L., Davison, S., Lipsedge, M., Muenchrath, D., Potschisvili, H., et al. (2009). *Psychiatry P. R. N.* Oxford University Press.

TOXBASE – poisons information database for clinical toxicology advice. (2020). https://www.toxbase.org/. [Accessed 9 December 2020]

Willacy, H. (2020). *Lithium*. Patient info. http://www.patient. info. [Accessed 18 July 2020].

Serotonin Syndrome
Dunkley, E., Isbister, G., Sibbritt, D., Dawson, A., & Whyte, I. (2003). The Hunter Serotonin Toxicity Criteria: Simple and accurate diagnostic decision rules for serotonin toxicity. *QJM*, 96, 635–642.

BNF. (2020). *Antidepressant drugs*. http://www.bnf.nice.org. uk. [Accessed 24 July 2020].

Imm, N. (2020). *Serotonin syndrome. What is serotonin syndrome? Symptoms*. Patient info. http://www.patient.info. [Accessed 26 July 2020].

Neuroleptic Malignant Syndrome
BNF. (2020). *Psychoses and related disorders*. hhtp://www.bnf. nice.org.uk. [Accessed 26 July 2020].

Knott, L. (2020). *Neuroleptic malignant syndrome. NMS information*. Patient info. http://www.patient.info. [Accessed 26 July 2020].

National Organization for Rare Disorders. (2020). *Neuroleptic malignant syndrome – NORD (National Organization for Rare Disorders)*. http://www.rarediseases.org. [Accessed 27 December 2020].

TOXBASE – poisons information database for clinical toxicology advice. (2020). https://www.toxbase.org/. [Accessed 9 December 2020].

Poisoning of Unknown Origin & Common Toxidromes

BNF. (2020). *Poisoning, emergency treatment*. http://www.bnf.nice.org.uk. [Accessed 4 August 2020].

TOXBASE – poisons information database for clinical toxicology advice. (2020). https://www.toxbase.org/. [Accessed 9 December 2020].

Wyatt, J., Taylor, R., Wit, K., & Hotton, E. (2020). *Oxford handbook of emergency medicine* (5th ed.). Oxford University Press.

Other emergencies
Hyperthermia (Heat Stroke)

Best Practice, B. M. J. (2020). *Heat stroke in adults*. http://www.bestpractice.bmj.com. [Accessed 18 November 2020].

Newson, L. (2020). *Heat-related illness. Heat stroke information*. Patient info. http://www.patient.info. [Accessed 18 November 2020].

Wyatt, J., Taylor, R., Wit, K., & Hotton, E. (2020). *Oxford handbook of emergency medicine* (5th ed.). Oxford University Press.

Hypothermia

Best Practice, B. M. J. (2020). *Hypothermia*. www.bestpractice.bmj.com. [Accessed 3 December 2020].

Wyatt, J., Taylor, R., Wit, K., & Hotton, E. (2020). *Oxford handbook of emergency medicine* (5th ed.). Oxford University Press.

Dehydration

Taylor, K., & Jones, E. (2021). *Adult Dehydration*. StatPearls. http://www.ncbi.nlm.nih.gov. [Accessed 5 April 2021].

Bites

NICE. (2020). *CKS: Scenario: Managing a cat or dog bite*. http://www.cks.nice.org.uk. [Accessed 3 December 2020].

Wyatt, J., Taylor, R., Wit, K., & Hotton, E. (2020). *Oxford handbook of emergency medicine* (5th ed.). Oxford University Press.

Plastics emergencies
Burns

NICE. (2020). *CKS: Burns and scalds*. http://www.cks.nice.org.uk. [Accessed December 2020].

American College Of Surgeons. Committee On Trauma (2018). *Advanced trauma life support : student course manual*. Chicago. Tenth Edition.

Best Practice, B. M. J. (2018). *Burns*. http://www.bestpractice.bmj.com. [Accessed December 2020].

Frostbite

Patient info. (2016). *Cold injury*. [https://patient.info/doctor/cold-injury - Accessed February 2022]

Patient info. (2014). *Hypothermia*. [https://patient.info/doctor/hypothermia-pro - Accessed February 2022]

American College Of Surgeons. Committee On Trauma (2018). *Advanced trauma life support : student course manual*. Chicago. Tenth Edition.

NICE. (2016). *CG65: Hypothermia: prevention and management in adults having surgery*. [www.nice.org.uk - Accessed February 2022]

Crush Injuries

Patient info. (2015). *Crush syndrome*. http://www.patient.info. [Accessed December 2020].

American College Of Surgeons. Committee On Trauma (2018). *Advanced trauma life support : student course manual*. Chicago. Tenth Edition.

Best Practice, B. M. J. (2018). *Rhabdomyolysis*. http://www.bestpractice.bmj.com. [Accessed December 2020].

Necrotising Fasciitis

Pejman Davoudian, FRCA EDIC FFICM, Neil J Flint, FRCA EDIC, Necrotizing fasciitis, *Continuing Education in Anaesthesia Critical Care & Pain*, Volume 12, Issue 5, October 2012, Pages 245–250, https://doi.org/10.1093/bjaceaccp/mks033.

Best Practice, B. M. J. (2020). *Necrotising fasciitis*. http://www.bestpractice.bmj.com. [Accessed December 2020].

DermNet, N. Z. (2016). *Necrotising fasciitis*. http://www.dermnetnz.org. [Accessed December 2020].

Patient info. (2015). *Necrotising fasciitis*. http://www.patient.info. [Accessed December 2020].

Compartment Syndrome

Best Practice, B. M. J. (2019). *Compartment syndrome of extremities*. http:// www.bestpractice.bmj.com. [Accessed December 2020].

Patient info (2015). *Compartment syndrome*. http://www.patient.info. [Accessed December 2020].

8

Endocrinology in an Hour

Berenice Aguirrezabala Armbruster and Judith Fox

GROWTH HORMONE DISORDERS

Growth Hormone Axis (see Fig 8.1)

Mechanism of growth hormone release:
- Somatostatin inhibits growth hormone (GH) release from the anterior pituitary gland
- Growth hormone–releasing hormone (GHRH) stimulates GH release from the anterior pituitary gland

Action of growth hormone:
- GH stimulates insulin-like growth factor 1 (IGF-1) release from the liver
- IGF-1 stimulates fat breakdown, glucose release from the liver, cell division, protein synthesis and increased bone density and strength

Acromegaly

Definition: excess growth hormone in adults (acromegaly) or children (gigantism) due to a pituitary adenoma (most cases) or ectopic production of the hormones involved in the growth hormone axis

Buzzwords:
- **Risk factors:** multiple endocrine neoplasia 1 (MEN1)
- **Presentation:** bitemporal hemianopia; large physical features – large tongue (macroglossia), jaw (prognathism) and forehead (frontal bossing); organ dysfunction (heart failure (HF), hypertension (HTN), type 2 diabetes mellitus (T2DM), colorectal cancer)

Investigations:
- **Bloods:** IGF-1 levels increased
- **Oral glucose tolerance test:** glucose normally suppresses GH. However, in acromegaly, there is no GH suppression 2 h after 75 g of glucose is taken
- **MRI pituitary and hypothalamus:** may show a tumour

Differentials: familial tall stature, obesity

Management:
1. Transsphenoidal surgery
2. Medical treatment if surgery is not suitable:
- Somatostatin analogues (e.g., octreotide)
- GH-receptor antagonists (e.g., pegvisomant)
- Dopamine agonists (e.g., bromocriptine)

Growth Hormone Deficiency

Definition: insufficient GH

Buzzwords:
- **Risk factors:** brain injury, tumour, radiation
- **Presentation:** small physical features, energy levels reduced, short stature (<2nd percentile in childhood)

Investigations:
- **Bloods:** IGF-1 level decreased
- **X-ray wrist:** to assess bone age
- **GH provocation test:** IV arginine is administrated, which should raise the GH level. However, in patients with a GH deficiency, the GH level remains low

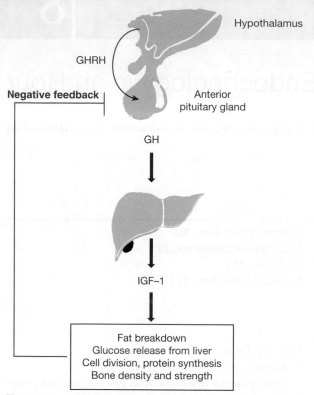

Fig 8.1 Growth Hormone Axis. (Illustrated by Dr Hollie Blaber.)

- **MRI pituitary:** may show a tumour
Differentials: hypothyroidism
Management: daily injections of recombinant human growth hormone

ANTIDIURETIC HORMONE DISORDERS

Antidiuretic Hormone Axis (see Fig 8.2 and Fig 8.3)

Mechanism of antidiuretic hormone (ADH) release:
- Low serum osmolality inhibits ADH release from the hypothalamus
- High serum osmolality stimulates ADH secretion from the hypothalamus. ADH is then transported to the posterior pituitary and secreted into the circulation

Action of ADH: ADH acts at two sites:
- **Adrenal glands:** ADH stimulates the adrenal glands to secrete **aldosterone.** Aldosterone causes sodium and water reabsorption from the collecting ducts of the kidneys
- **Blood vessels:** ADH stimulates **vasoconstriction**

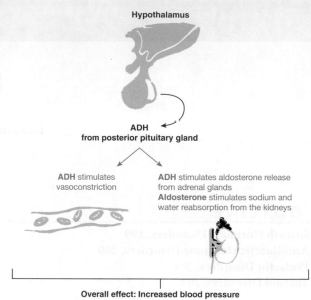

Fig 8.2 Antidiuretic Hormone Axis. (Illustrated by Hollie Blaber.)

Syndrome of Inappropriate ADH Secretion (SIADH)

Definition: also known as syndrome of antidiuresis (SIAD). Often caused by excess ADH (a.k.a., vasopressin), causing water retention, hyponatraemia (due to dilution of sodium in blood) and concentrated urine.

Causes (mnemonic SIADH):
- Small cell lung tumour producing ectopic ADH
- Intracranial infection (meningitis)
- Alveolar infection (tuberculosis (TB))
- Drugs (antidepressants, anticonvulsants, antipsychotics, cytotoxic agents, analgesics)
- Head injury/surgery

Buzzwords:
- **Risk factors:** depends on cause (see above)
- **Presentation:** euvolaemic hyponatraemia (normal fluid status and low serum sodium), confusion, drowsiness, reduced Glasgow Coma Scale (GCS) score, seizures

Investigations:
- A **diagnosis of exclusion** once other causes of hyponatraemia have been addressed (see Renal Medicine and Chemical Pathology in an Hour)
- **Bloods:** U&E (hyponatraemia), serum osmolality (hypoosmolality)

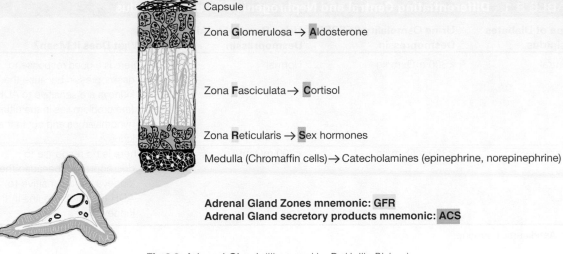

Capsule

Zona **G**lomerulosa → **A**ldosterone

Zona **F**asciculata → **C**ortisol

Zona **R**eticularis → **S**ex hormones

Medulla (Chromaffin cells) → Catecholamines (epinephrine, norepinephrine)

Adrenal Gland Zones mnemonic: GFR
Adrenal Gland secretory products mnemonic: ACS

Fig 8.3 **Adrenal Gland.** (Illustrated by Dr Hollie Blaber.)

- **Urine:** high urine osmolality, high urine sodium (>40 mmol/L)
- **Investigations for potential cause:** chest X-ray (CXR), CT head/chest, drug review

Differentials: other causes of hyponatraemia (see Renal Medicine and Chemical Pathology in an Hour)

Management:
- Fluid restriction between 500 mL and 1 L depending on severity and other factors such as renal failure
- Correct sodium slowly (10 mmol/L per 24 h) to avoid **central pontine myelinolysis**
- Treat underlying cause

Diabetes Insipidus (DI)

Definition: lack of production or loss of sensitivity to ADH. Two main types:
- **Central DI ('low level of ADH'):** not enough ADH is produced due to posterior pituitary damage or damage to the hypothalamus
- **Nephrogenic DI ('insensitivity to ADH'):** kidneys do not respond to ADH due to kidney damage or genetic mutations

Buzzwords:
- **Risk factors:**
  - **Central DI:** trauma, surgery
  - **Nephrogenic DI:** lithium toxicity, hypertension, inherited

- **Presentation:** polydipsia, polyuria (>3 L/day), nocturia, dilute urine, dehydration, hypernatremia

Investigations:
1. **Urinalysis:** low urinary osmolality (<300 mOsm/kg)
2. **Bloods:** U&E (hypernatremia)
3. **Water deprivation test:** No water for 8 h. Desmopressin (synthetic ADH) is given after water deprivation, and the urine osmolality is measured before and after desmopressin is given. For results interpretation, see Table 8.1

Differentials: diabetes mellitus (DM), primary polydipsia, hypercalcaemia

Management:
- **Central DI:** desmopressin
- **Nephrogenic DI:** treat underlying cause, consider thiazide diuretics

PROLACTIN DISORDERS

Prolactin Axis (see Fig 8.4)

Mechanism of prolactin release:
- Dopamine inhibits prolactin secretion, and thyrotropin-releasing hormone (TRH) stimulates prolactin secretion
- Dopamine is continuously secreted and, in the absence of pregnancy, it will inhibit prolactin secretion. Note: medications that inhibit dopamine

TABLE 8.1   Differentiating Central and Nephrogenic Diabetes Insipidus

Type of Diabetes Insipidus	Urine Osmolality BEFORE Desmopressin	Urine Osmolality AFTER Desmopressin	What Does it Mean?
Central	<300 mOsm/kg	Normal	There is a good response to desmopressin because the kidneys are sensitive to ADH (the problem lies in the pituitary/ hypothalamus and not in the kidneys)
Nephrogenic	<300 mOsm/kg	<300 mOsm/kg	There is no response to desmopressin because the kidneys are insensitive to ADH (the problem lies in the kidneys)

ADH, Antidiuretic hormone.

secretion (e.g., antipsychotics) will lead to prolactin secretion

- During pregnancy there are high levels of oestrogen, which promote mammary gland growth and prolactin secretion (minimal effect). Suckling or nipple stimulation has the greatest effect on prolactin secretion as it inhibits dopamine secretion

Actions of prolactin:
- Prolactin stimulates milk production
- Prolactin inhibits gonadotropin-releasing hormone (GnRH) release from the hypothalamus, thus inhibiting follicle-stimulating hormone (FSH) and luteinising hormone (LH) release from the anterior pituitary gland. FSH and LH regulate menstruation. Therefore, during lactation a period of amenorrhoea will take place, which may act as a natural contraceptive. After 1–2 weeks without breast feeding, however, prolactin levels will fall to pre-pregnancy levels, and GnRH will no longer be inhibited

Actions of oxytocin:
- Oxytocin levels increase during pregnancy
- Oxytocin inhibits dopamine, thereby promoting prolactin production

Prolactinoma

Definition: a prolactinoma is a pituitary adenoma (benign tumour) secreting prolactin.
Buzzwords:
- **Males:** gynaecomastia, impotence, loss of libido, galactorrhoea

- **Females:** amenorrhoea, galactorrhoea, infertility
Investigations:
1. **Bloods:** high prolactin (>5000 mU/L). If mildly raised (400–1000 mU/L), repeat test
2. **MRI pituitary:** may show tumour
Differentials: pregnancy, liver disease, antipsychotic use
Management:
If asymptomatic, no treatment. If symptomatic, treat:
1. **Medical:** dopamine agonists (e.g., cabergoline or bromocriptine) for both microprolactinomas (<1 cm) and macroprolactinomas (>1 cm)
2. **Surgery (only if medical treatment fails):** transsphenoidal surgery

THYROID DISORDERS

Thyroid Axis (see Fig 8.5)

Mechanism of thyroid hormone release:
- Hypothalamus secretes TRH
- TRH stimulates the anterior pituitary to secrete thyroid-stimulating hormone (TSH)
- TSH stimulates the thyroid gland to secrete T3, T4 and calcitonin
- When enough T3 and T4 is secreted, it is sensed by the hypothalamus and anterior pituitary, and TRH and TSH secretion is inhibited (negative feedback)
Actions of thyroid hormones:
- T3 and T4 regulate the rate of metabolism in many tissues of the body
- Calcitonin is involved in calcium homeostasis

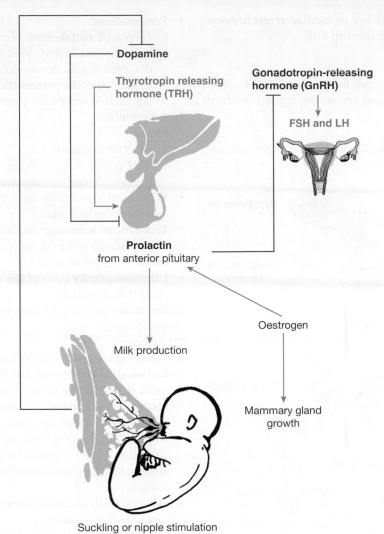

Dopamine

Thyrotropin releasing hormone (TRH)

Gonadotropin-releasing hormone (GnRH)

FSH and LH

Prolactin
from anterior pituitary

Oestrogen

Milk production

Mammary gland growth

Suckling or nipple stimulation

Fig 8.4 Prolactin Axis. *FSH,* Follicle-stimulating hormone. (Illustrated by Dr Hollie Blaber.)

Hypothyroidism

Definition: not enough T3/T4 hormones. Two causes: primary and secondary hypothyroidism (see Table 8.2)

Buzzwords:

- **Risk factors:** thyroid damage (e.g., surgery, radiation), family history, elderly, pregnancy, iodine deficiency
- **Presentation:**
  - **Decreased metabolism** of multiple tissues in the body: EVERYTHING SLOWS DOWN (e.g., fatigue, cold, bradycardia, constipation, fluid retention, menstrual irregularities)
  - **Myxoedema facies:** dry, cold, puffy skin (peaches and cream); thin eyebrows; eyelid oedema; goitre

Investigations:

1 **Bloods:**
- TFTs for diagnosis
- Lipid levels (at risk of hyperlipidaemia)
- Thyroid antibodies, including anti-thyroglobulin and anti-thyroid peroxidase

2 **Electrocardiogram (ECG)** (risk of arrhythmias in elderly)

Differentials: depression, anaemia, Alzheimer's disease

Management:

- **Adults 18–49 years of age:** levothyroxine 50–100 micrograms OD. Titrate to symptoms/TSH

- **Adults >50 years of age or cardiac arrest history:** levothyroxine 25 micrograms OD

Hyperthyroidism

Definition: excess thyroid hormones (T3, T4). Two main types: primary and secondary hyperthyroidism (see Table 8.3)

Buzzwords:

- **Risk factors:** female, family history, other autoimmune conditions

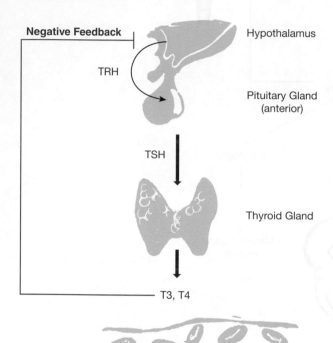

Fig 8.5 Thyroid Axis. *TRH,* Thyroid-releasing hormone; *TSH,* thyroid-stimulating hormone. (Illustrated by Hollie Blaber.)

- **Presentation:**
  - **Increased metabolism** of multiple tissues in the body: EVERYTHING SPEEDS UP (e.g., tachycardia, loose stools, sweaty, hot, lid retraction)
  - **Graves'-specific presentation:** exophthalmos, lid lag, thyroid acropachy, pretibial myxoedema

Investigations:

- **Bloods:**
  - TFTs for diagnosis
  - TSH-receptor antibodies (TR-Ab): positive (Graves' disease) or negative (toxic adenoma)
- **ECG:** most commonly sinus tachycardia, at risk of other tachyarrhythmias
- **Technetium scanning:** uniformly hot (Graves' disease), multiple hot nodules (toxic adenoma) or cold nodules (malignancy)
- **Ultrasonography (US) of the neck:** consider if palpable thyroid nodule

Differentials: generalized anxiety, menopause, phaeochromocytoma

Management:

1. **Symptom control:** beta blockers
2. **Radioiodine (I^{131}):** offer first line in most instances, medical Tx first line for mild/uncomplicated Graves'
3. **Medical:** carbimazole (drug warning: risk of neutropenia, agranulocytosis, congenital malformations). In the first trimester of pregnancy propylthiouracil (PTU) is used (at the smallest effective dose; can cross placenta and cause foetal hypothyroidism)
4. **Surgery:** total or subtotal thyroidectomy, especially if concern of malignancy
5. **Exophthalmos:** steroids, radiotherapy, surgical decompression

TABLE 8.2	Hypothyroidism				
Hypothyroidism	**Pathology**	**Disorder**	**TSH**	**T3 and T4**	
Primary hypothyroidism	Thyroid does not produce enough T3/T4. Low T3/T4 stimulates the pituitary gland to produce TSH	Hashimoto's thyroiditis Treatment-induced iodine deficiency	High	Low	
Secondary hypothyroidism	Pituitary does not produce enough TSH	Pituitary tumour Pituitary damage Sheehan's syndrome	Low	Low	

TSH, Thyroid-stimulating hormone.

TABLE 8.3 **Hyperthyroidism**

Hyperthyroidism	Site of Pathology	Disorder	TSH	T3 and T4
Subclinical			Low	Normal
Primary hyperthyroidism	Thyroid produces too much T3/T4, suppressing TSH production from pituitary (negative feedback)	Graves' disease Toxic nodular goitre Toxic multinodular goitre Iodine-rich drug	Low	High
Secondary hyperthyroidism	Excess TSH from pituitary drives T3/T4 levels up	Pituitary tumour High level of hCG	High	High

hCG, Human chorionic gonadotropin; TSH, thyroid-stimulating hormone.

ADRENAL DISORDERS

Renin-Angiotensin-Aldosterone System (see Fig 8.6)

Mechanism of angiotensin II release:

- Low blood pressure (BP) is sensed by juxtaglomerular cells in the afferent arterioles of the kidneys, which stimulates renin secretion
- Renin converts angiotensinogen (secreted by the liver) to angiotensin I
- Angiotensin-converting enzyme (ACE) (released by the lungs) converts angiotensin I to angiotensin II

Action of angiotensin II: angiotensin II stimulates thirst, vasoconstriction, ADH secretion from the pituitary gland and aldosterone secretion from the adrenal glands

Action of aldosterone: aldosterone acts on the kidneys and causes:

- Increased sodium (and water) reabsorption from the distal tubules, which, in turn, increases the blood pressure
- Increased potassium secretion from the distal tubules
- Increased hydrogen secretion from the collecting ducts
  Tip: aldosterone moves salts to correct fluids, and ADH moves fluids to correct salts

Adrenal Axis (see Fig 8.7)

Mechanism of glucocorticoid release:

- Stress and time of day (morning) stimulates the hypothalamus to secrete corticotropin-releasing hormone (CRH)
- CRH stimulates the anterior pituitary to secrete adrenocorticotropic hormone (ACTH)
- ACTH stimulates the adrenal gland to secrete glucocorticoids (cortisol, corticosterone, cortisone)

Action of cortisol: cortisol has the following functions:

- Stimulates the metabolic rate, increases alertness, increases sodium/water retention and increases blood glucose levels
- Inhibits the immune system, protein synthesis and bone formation

Adrenal Insufficiency

Definition: underproduction of adrenal cortex hormones, including the mineralocorticoids (aldosterone) and glucocorticoids (cortisol, corticosterone, cortisone). There are three types of adrenal insufficiency (see Table 8.4):

- **Primary adrenal insufficiency:** not enough adrenal cortex hormones are produced due to damage to the adrenal glands
- **Secondary adrenal insufficiency:** not enough adrenal cortex hormones are produced due to damage to the pituitary gland
- **Tertiary adrenal insufficiency:** not enough adrenal cortex hormones are produced due to hypothalamic damage/downregulation

Buzzwords:

- **Risk factors:** other autoimmune diseases, adrenal damage (e.g., metastasis, haemorrhage, infection, trauma), prolonged steroid use
- **Presentation:** low levels of different adrenal cortex hormones lead to various presentations depending on which site of the adrenal cortex is affected most:
  - **Low aldosterone:** postural hypotension, hyponatraemia, hyperkalaemia, hypoglycaemia
  - **Low cortisol:** fatigue, exhaustion, depression
  - **Low aldosterone and cortisol:** bronze hyperpigmentation

Investigations:

1. **Short Synacthen test to confirm adrenal insufficiency:** measure baseline serum cortisol, give Synacthen injection (synthetic ACTH) and measure serum cortisol 30-min post-Synacthen injection (see Table 8.5)
2. **ACTH test** to confirm the type of adrenal insufficiency. The test involves taking a blood sample, usually in the morning, to measure ACTH levels. (see Table 8.5)

3. **Pathology-specific investigations:** adrenal gland autoantibodies (Addison's disease), head MRI (pituitary/hypothalamic tumour)

Differentials: hypothyroid, intense diuretic use, depression, anorexia nervosa

Management:

1. Cortisol replacement therapy with hydrocortisone (glucocorticoid)
2. Aldosterone replacement therapy with fludrocortisone (mineralocorticoid)
3. Sick day rules: if acutely unwell, increased steroid doses are required: often *doubled* glucocorticoid

Cushing's Syndrome and Cushing's Disease

Definition: Cushing's syndrome refers to the collective signs and symptoms caused by a high blood cortisol level. Cushing's syndrome may be caused by:

- Use of long-term glucocorticoids (*most common cause*)
- Cushing's disease: pituitary adenoma secreting too much ACTH, stimulating excess cortisol production
- Adrenal adenoma secreting too much cortisol
- Ectopic secretion of ACTH (e.g., small cell lung cancer)

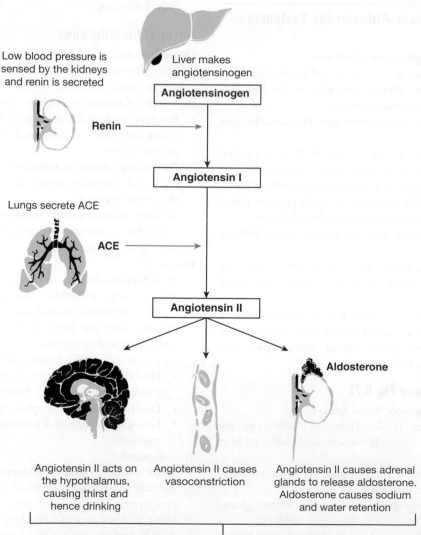

Low blood pressure is sensed by the kidneys and renin is secreted

Liver makes angiotensinogen

Angiotensinogen

Renin →

Angiotensin I

Lungs secrete ACE

ACE →

Angiotensin II

Aldosterone

Angiotensin II acts on the hypothalamus, causing thirst and hence drinking

Angiotensin II causes vasoconstriction

Angiotensin II causes adrenal glands to release aldosterone. Aldosterone causes sodium and water retention

All this leads to an increase in blood pressure

Fig 8.6 Renin-Angiotensin-Aldosterone Axis. *ACE,* Angiotensin-converting enzyme. (Illustrated by Hollie Blaber.)

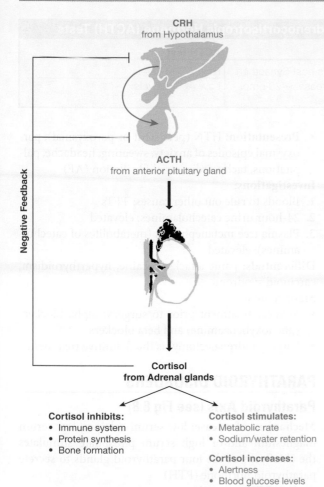

CRH
from Hypothalamus

Negative Feedback

ACTH
from anterior pituitary gland

Cortisol
from Adrenal glands

Cortisol inhibits:
• Immune system
• Protein synthesis
• Bone formation

Cortisol stimulates:
• Metabolic rate
• Sodium/water retention

Cortisol increases:
• Alertness
• Blood glucose levels

Fig 8.7 Adrenal Axis. *ACTH,* Adrenocorticotropic hormone; *CRH,* corticotropin-releasing hormone. (Illustrated by Hollie Blaber.)

Buzzwords:
• **Risk factors:** female between 25–40 years of age (pituitary/adrenal adenoma), steroid use

• **Presentation:** round moon facies, central obesity, abdominal striae, buffalo hump (fat pad on upper back), proximal limb muscle wasting, hypertension, cardiac hypertrophy, hyperglycaemia (T2DM), depression, insomnia, osteoporosis, easy bruising, poor skin healing
  • Cortisol has some mineralocorticoid activity and will cause electrolyte derangement – see Hyperaldosteronism

Investigations:
1. **Low-dose dexamethasone suppression test to confirm Cushing's syndrome:** give low-dose dexamethasone (1 mg) at night and measure ACTH and cortisol in the morning. Dexamethasone normally suppresses the cortisol level (<100 nmol/L). Failure to suppress confirms Cushing's syndrome of any aetiology
2. **High-dose dexamethasone suppression test to determine cause of Cushing's syndrome:** give high-dose dexamethasone (8 mg) at night and measure ACTH and cortisol levels in the morning (see Table 8.6)
3. **Pathology-specific investigations:** MRI, CT thorax and abdomen

Differentials: obesity, alcohol use disorder, polycystic ovarian syndrome

Management:
• **Cushing's disease (pituitary adenoma):** transsphenoidal surgical resection and steroid replacement postoperatively
• **Adrenal adenoma:** surgical adrenalectomy and steroid replacement postoperatively

Hyperaldosteronism

Definition: excess aldosterone secretion. Two types:
• **Primary hyperaldosteronism:** adrenal glands produce excess aldosterone, increasing the BP, which

TABLE 8.4	Adrenal Insufficiency	
Types	**Pathology Site**	**Causes**
Primary adrenal insufficiency	Adrenal gland	Addison's disease (adrenal autoantibodies)
		Adrenal gland injury by infection, surgery or malignancy
		Waterhouse-Friderichsen syndrome: bleeding into adrenal glands, typically secondary to *Neisseria meningitidis*
Secondary adrenal insufficiency	Pituitary gland	Pituitary adenoma (benign tumour)
		Sheehan's syndrome (postpartum pituitary gland necrosis due to hypovolaemia)
		Pituitary gland injury by infection, surgery or malignancy
Tertiary adrenal insufficiency	Hypothalamus	Cessation of long-term (>3 months) steroid use

TABLE 8.5	Interpretation of Synacthen and Adrenocorticotropic Hormone (ACTH) Tests	
	Synacthen test	**ACTH test**
Primary adrenal insufficiency	Serum Cortisol levels post-Synacthen injection fail to increase >420 nmol (or less than double)	High ACTH levels
Secondary adrenal insufficiency		Low ACTH levels

reduces renin production. Causes include anything that will affect the **adrenal glands** directly:
- Conn syndrome (most cases): an adrenal adenoma that secretes too much aldosterone
- Bilateral adrenal hyperplasia
- Familial hyperaldosteronism type 1 and type 2 (rare)
- Adrenal carcinoma (rare)
- Isolated glucocorticoid deficiency
- Idiopathic
- **Secondary hyperaldosteronism:** kidneys produce excess renin, leading to increased aldosterone levels. Causes include anything that will **reduce the blood flow** to the kidneys, including renal artery stenosis, a renal artery obstruction and heart failure

Buzzwords:
- **Risk factors:** family history of early HTN or early stroke
- **Presentation:** generally asymptomatic, treatment-resistant HTN, HTN <20 years of age, hypokalaemia, adrenal 'incidentaloma' on CT with HTN

Investigations:
1. **Aldosterone-renin ratio** to determine if it is a primary or secondary hyperaldosteronism (see Table 8.7)
2. **Pathology-specific investigations:** renal ultrasound scan, CT renal angiogram (stenosis)
3. **Investigations for complications:** U&E (hypokalaemia), VBG (alkalosis), BP (HTN)

Differentials: Cushing's, Liddle's syndrome, renovascular disease, excessive liquorice ingestion

Management:
1. Aldosterone-antagonist therapy (e.g., eplerenone, spironolactone)
2. Treat underlying cause (e.g., surgical removal of adenoma, percutaneous renal artery angioplasty)

Phaeochromocytoma

Definition: chromaffin cell tumour of the adrenal gland that produces excess adrenaline

Buzzwords:
- **Risk factors:** MEN2, Von Hippel-Lindau

- **Presentation:** HTN (persistent or paroxysmal); paroxysmal episodes of anxiety, sweating, headache, palpitations, tachycardia, atrial fibrillation (AF)

Investigations:
1. Bloods to rule out other causes: TFTs
2. 24-hour urine catecholamines: elevated
3. Plasma free metanephrines (metabolites of catecholamines): elevated

Differentials: panic attacks, cocaine, hyperthyroidism, carcinoid syndrome

Management:
- Medical treatment prior to surgery: alpha blockers (phenoxybenzamine) and beta blockers
- Surgery (adrenalectomy) is the definitive treatment

PARATHYROID DISORDERS

Parathyroid Axis (see Fig 8.8)

Mechanism of release: low serum calcium, low serum magnesium and/or high serum phosphate stimulates the chief cells of the four parathyroid glands to secrete parathyroid hormone (PTH)

Action: PTH acts at three main sites:
- **Bone:** PTH stimulates bone reabsorption by increasing osteoclast numbers and activity. Normal levels of vitamin D needed for this action.
- **Kidneys:** PTH **increases calcium reabsorption** and **decreases phosphate reabsorption** from the kidneys. It also stimulates the **formation of active Vitamin D** (Calcitriol and Ercalcitriol). Vitamin D3 (a.k.a. Cholecalciferol) comes from dietary animal products or it can be produced in the skin from 7-dehydrocholesterol upon sun exposure. Vitamin D2 (a.k.a. Ergocalciferol) comes from dietary plant products. Both Vitamin D3 and D2 are biologically inactive and need to be converted into their active forms by two steps. First, **in the liver**, Vitamin D3 is converted into **Calcifediol** (a.k.a. 25-hydroxy-cholecalciferol) and Vitamin D2 into **Ercalcidiol** (a.k.a. 25-hydroxyergocalciferol). Then, **in the kidneys**, PTH stimulates the conversion of Calcifediol

TABLE 8.6   **Dexamethasone Test**

	ACTH	CORTISOL	INTERPRETATION
Low-dose dexamethasone test (1 mg)	Low	Low	Normal
	High	High	Cushing's syndrome (of any aetiology): ACTH cannot be suppressed by low-dose dexamethasone
High-dose dexamethasone test (8 mg)	Low	Low	Cushing's disease (pituitary adenoma): high-dose dexamethasone can suppress ACTH (and hence cortisol)
	Low	High	Adrenal pathology (e.g., adrenal adenoma): dexamethasone suppresses ACTH, but cortisol is produced independently of ACTH levels
	High	High	Ectopic ACTH (e.g., small-cell lung tumour): ACTH is produced independently of the adrenal axis

ACTH, Adrenocorticotropic hormone.

TABLE 8.7   **Investigations to Determine the Type of Hyperaldosteronism (Primary vs Secondary)**

	Renin	Aldosterone	Aldosterone-Renin Ratio
Primary hyperaldosteronism (e.g., Conn syndrome)	Low	High	High
Secondary hyperaldosteronism (e.g., renal artery stenosis)	High	High	Low

and Ercalcidiol into their biologically active forms: **Calcitriol** (a.k.a. 1,25-dihydroxycholecalciferol) and **Ercalcitriol** (a.k.a. 1,25-dihydroxyergocalciferol) respectively. Both known as **active Vitamin D**.

- **Small bowel:** PTH stimulates calcium reabsorption
Net effect of PTH: serum calcium levels increase, and serum phosphate levels decrease

When the serum calcium level is high, the release of PTH is suppressed (via **negative feedback**), helping to reduce the serum calcium level.

Hyperparathyroidism

Definition: excess PTH production. There are three types of hyperparathyroidism:

- **Primary hyperparathyroidism:** a problem in the parathyroid glands leads to excess PTH secretion (e.g., parathyroid adenoma, parathyroid hyperplasia)
- **Secondary hyperparathyroidism:** caused by a problem in a target tissue (e.g., chronic kidney disease (CKD)) or if there are insufficient levels of vitamin D, which is needed for calcium reabsorption. PTH is produced in excess to try to compensate for these abnormalities
- **Tertiary hyperparathyroidism:** long-standing secondary hyperparathyroidism leads to parathyroid

gland hyperplasia and the secretion of excess PTH, even after correction of the cause of secondary hyperparathyroidism

Buzzwords:

- **Risk factors:** MEN 1/2
- **Presentation:** hypercalcaemia symptoms
  - **Bone:** pain, deformities, osteoporosis, fragility fractures, pathological fractures in context of malignancy
  - **Renal:** renal stones, nephrogenic DI, renal impairment
  - **Gastrointestinal:** abdominal pain, constipation, nausea, vomiting
  - **Psychiatric and neurological:** depression, lethargy, seizures
  - **Cardiac:** arrhythmias, ECG changes, hypotension

Investigations:

1. **Bloods:** PTH, calcium, phosphate, alkaline phosphatase level (ALP) (see Table 8.8)
2. **Urine calcium:** familial hypocalciuric hypercalcaemia presents as a primary hyperparathyroidism but with low urine calcium levels

Differentials: hypercalcaemia of malignancy, milk-alkali syndrome, familial hypocalciuric hypercalcaemia

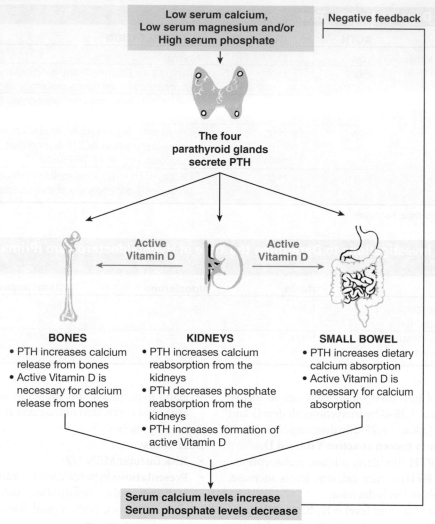

Low serum calcium,
Low serum magnesium and/or
High serum phosphate

Negative feedback

The four
parathyroid glands
secrete PTH

Active
Vitamin D

Active
Vitamin D

BONES
- PTH increases calcium release from bones
- Active Vitamin D is necessary for calcium release from bones

KIDNEYS
- PTH increases calcium reabsorption from the kidneys
- PTH decreases phosphate reabsorption from the kidneys
- PTH increases formation of active Vitamin D

SMALL BOWEL
- PTH increases dietary calcium absorption
- Active Vitamin D is necessary for calcium absorption

Serum calcium levels increase
Serum phosphate levels decrease

Fig 8.8 Parathyroid Axis. (Illustrated by Hollie Blaber.)

TABLE 8.8 Hyperparathyroidism Investigations

	Pathology	Parathyroid Hormone	Calcium	Phosphate	Alkaline Phosphatase
Primary	Parathyroid gland pathology	High	High	Low	High
Secondary	Target tissue pathology Vitamin D deficiency	High	Normal (or even low)	High	High
Tertiary	Long-standing secondary hyperparathyroidism	Very high	Very high	High	High

TABLE 8.9	Multiple Endocrine Neoplasia (MEN) Syndrome Buzzwords		
MEN Subtype	**Tissue affected**	**Gene Mutation**	**Chromosome**
MEN 1	Pancreas Pituitary Parathyroid	MEN 1	11q13
MEN 2A	Parathyroid Pheochromocytoma Medullary thyroid	*RET* proto-oncogene	10
MEN 2B	Pheochromocytoma Medullary thyroid Marfanoid habitus Neuromas	*RET* proto-oncogene	10

Management:
- **Primary and tertiary:** surgery. If unsuitable, medical treatment with Cinacalcet
- **Secondary:** manage CKD and/or vitamin D deficiency

Multiple Endocrine Neoplasia Syndromes

Definition: autosomal-dominant disorders causing different endocrine glands to grow benign, malignant or noncancerous growths.

Buzzwords: (see Table 8.9)

Investigations:

1 Screening of first- and second-degree relatives:
- MEN 1: full gut hormone screen, serum calcium, serum prolactin, genetic mutations
- MEN 2A/B: screen for associated conditions (see ENT and Ophthalmology in an Hour for thyroid cancer), genetic mutations

2 Imaging of relevant organ:
- MRI pituitary
- MRI abdomen
- Thyroid US and fine-needle biopsy

Differentials: other MEN disorders, other conditions affecting the organs involved in MEN syndromes

Management: genetic counselling and surgery to remove affected tissue.

Hypoparathyroidism

Definition: underproduction of PTH by parathyroid glands, which leads to hypocalcaemia and hyperphosphatemia. Causes include:
- **Acquired hypoparathyroidism:** damage to the parathyroid glands (e.g., by surgery, radiation, infection, autoimmune disease) leads to low PTH levels

- **Congenital hypoparathyroidism:** the parathyroid gland does not fully develop, leading to low PTH levels. This condition may be associated with certain congenital conditions (e.g., DiGeorge syndrome)
- **Physiological hypoparathyroidism:** PTH production is suppressed by physiological factors (e.g., high calcium and/or low magnesium)
- **Pseudohypoparathyroidism** (rare inherited disorder): PTH is present, but the body is unable to respond to it due to genetic mutations in PTH receptors (G-protein mutation)

Note: Sometimes, hypoparathyroidism is classified as:
- **Primary hypoparathyroidism:** consists of acquired and congenital causes
- **Secondary hypoparathyroidism:** consists of physiological causes
- **Pseudohypoparathyroidism**

Buzzwords:
- **Signs:** Trousseau's sign (carpopedal spasm caused by BP cuff) and Chvostek's sign (facial contraction caused by tapping facial nerve) – both due to hypocalcaemia
- **Symptoms:** muscle cramps, muscle pain, twitching, paraesthesia, confusion, fatigue

Investigations:

1. Bloods to diagnose hypoparathyroidism: PTH, calcium, phosphate, ALP
2. Tests for suspected underlying cause: auto-antibodies, infection screen, genetic studies
3. Tests for complications: ECG (prolonged QT with hypocalcaemia)

Differentials: hypomagnesaemia, vitamin D deficiency, tetanus, Parkinson's disease

TABLE 8.10 Hypoparathyroidism Investigations

	PTH	Calcium	Phosphate	ALP
Acquired and congenital hypoparathy-roidism (primary hypoparathyroidism)	Low	Low	High	Normal
Physiological hypoparathyroidism (secondary hypoparathyroidism)	Low	High	High	Normal
Pseudohypoparathyroidism	High	Low	Low	Normal

ALP, Alkaline phosphatase; PTH, parathyroid hormone.

Management:
- Treat underlying cause if possible
- **Hypomagnaesemia:** Consult local guidelines. In mild cases, PO Magnesium glycerophosphate. In severe cases, IV Magnesium sulfate
- **Vitamin D deficiency:** Loading regimen of PO Vitamin D 300'000 IU as separate weekly or daily doses over 6-10 weeks (e.g. 50'000 IU once weekly for 6 weeks). Maintenance regimen of 800-2000 IU daily.
- **Acute Hypocalcaemia:** Consult local guidelines. In mild cases, PO calcium supplementation (e.g. Adcal D3). In severe cases, give 10-20ml 10% Calcium Gluconate in 50-100 mL of 5% Glucose IV over 5 to 10 minutes with ECG monitoring. Repeat if necessary, with senior input. In exceptional cases a continuous calcium infusion may be required. If infusion is required, dilute 100mL of 10% calcium gluconate (10 x 10ml ampoules) in 1L of 0.9% NaCl or 5% Glucose and infuse at a rate of 50-100 ml/hour. Note: Calcium chloride injections are available but are more irritant.
- **Persistent hypocalcaemia:** PO calcium supplements + Vitamin D analogue (Alfacalcidol or Calcitriol) for hypoparathyroidism and pseudohypoparathyroidism or natural vitamin D (calciferol) if due to vitamin D deficiency. For long-term use monitor plasma and urinary calcium.

DIABETES

Blood Sugar Control (See Fig 8.9)

Type 1 Diabetes Mellitus

Definition: autoimmune destruction of beta cells (insulin producing) in the pancreas, leading to low/no insulin production and high blood glucose. The onset of symptoms is often in childhood.

Buzzwords:
- **Risk factors:** family history, autoimmune conditions

- **Presentation:** fatigue, polydipsia, nocturia, polyuria. May present with ketoacidosis, abdominal pain or rapid weight loss

Investigations:
- Diagnosis of T1DM often made on clinical grounds
- Secondary care may test for C-peptide/diabetes-specific autoantibodies
- HbA1c every 3–6 months to assess glucose control once being treated

Differentials: T2DM, maturity-onset diabetes of the young (MODY), DI

Management:
1. Immediate referral to secondary care to establish diagnosis
2. Insulin regimen
3. Manage complications
4. Diabetic screening for microvascular and macrovascular complications (e.g., eye screening, foot screening, renal screening)

Insulin types:
- **Rapid acting:** Actrapid, Humalog, Novorapid
- **Short acting:** Actrapid, Humulin S, Insuman rapid
- **Intermediate acting:** Humulin I, Insulatard, Insuman Basal
- **Long acting:** Lantus, Levemir, Tresiba

Type 2 Diabetes Mellitus

Definition:
- Insensitivity to insulin and a relative insufficiency of insulin leading to raised blood glucose levels
- In prediabetes, there is a decreased responsiveness to insulin, leading to high blood glucose levels. Prediabetes can be divided into:
  - Impaired fasting glucose (IFG): glucose levels are high during fasting
  - Impaired glucose tolerance (IGT): glucose levels are high during fasting AND after a 75g glucose challenge

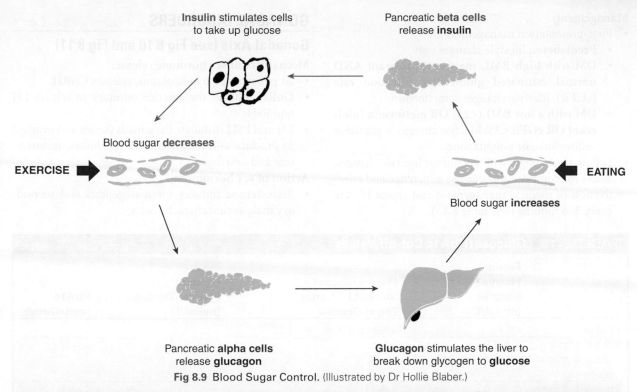

Insulin stimulates cells to take up glucose

Pancreatic **beta cells** release **insulin**

Blood sugar **decreases**

EXERCISE ➡

⬅ EATING

Blood sugar **increases**

Pancreatic **alpha cells** release **glucagon**

Glucagon stimulates the liver to break down glycogen to **glucose**

Fig 8.9 Blood Sugar Control. (Illustrated by Dr Hollie Blaber.)

TABLE 8.11 **Various Insulin Regimes**

Insulin Regimen	Indication	Components
Once daily	T2DM	Single injection of long-acting insulin given at night
Basal bolus	T1DM	Single injection of long-acting insulin given at night AND short-acting injections before each mealtime
Twice daily	T1DM or T2DM	Injection containing both short- and long-acting insulin given in the morning and evening
Continuous subcutaneous infusion or pump	T1DM	Rapid/short-acting insulin given subcutaneously via a pump – reduces the number of injections and can be programmed to deliver regular insulin/boluses at mealtimes
Insulin infusions	T1DM or T2DM	Variable: used in IDDM when Nil by mouth (NBM) Fixed rate (e.g., 0.1 units/kg/hr) – used in diabetic ketoacidosis

T1DM, Type 1 diabetes mellitus; T2DM, type 2 diabetes mellitus.

Buzzwords:
- **Risk factors:** obesity, family history, increasing age
- **Presentation:** symptom onset usually in adulthood, asymptomatic, tiredness, polydipsia, nocturia, polyuria

Investigations: (see Table 8.12)
- **HbA1c:** primary test to diagnose T2DM. Reflects blood glucose levels over the previous 8–12 weeks
  - If *asymptomatic*: two positive tests required (i.e., HbA1c >48 on two different occasions)

- If *symptomatic*: one positive test required
- Do not use HbA1c for diagnosis in the following patient groups: pregnant, acutely unwell, red blood cell (RBC) disorders, CKD
  - In these patients, the fasting plasma glucose/oral GTT is more useful
  - Fasting plasma glucose can be used to *assess risk* of progression to T2DM/presence of IFG

Differentials: MODY, hypothyroid, hypercalcaemia, Cushing's

Management:

- First-presentation management:
  - **Prediabetes:** lifestyle changes only
  - **DM with high BMI, metformin tolerant AND normal estimated glomerular filtration rate (eGFR):** lifestyle changes + metformin
  - **DM with a low BMI (<25) OR metformin intolerant OR eGFR <35:** lifestyle changes + gliptin or sulfonylurea or pioglitazone
- Follow-up management: encourage lifestyle changes, assess for complications, assess adherence and effectiveness of medical management and repeat HbA1c every 3–6 months (see Table 8.13)

GONADAL DISORDERS

Gonadal Axis (see Fig 8.10 and Fig 8.11)

Mechanism of sex hormone release:

- At puberty, the hypothalamus releases GnRH
- GnRH induces the anterior pituitary to release LH and FSH
- LH and FSH stimulate the gonads (testes and ovaries) to produce and release the sex hormones, testosterone and oestrogen

Action of sex hormones:

- Testosterone induces spermatogenesis and secondary male sexual characteristics

TABLE 8.12 Glucose/HbA1c Cut-off Values

	Fasting Plasma Glucose (mmol/L)		Plasma Glucose (mmol/L) 2 h after 75g of Glucose		Random Plasma Glucose (mmol/L)		HbA1c (mmol/mol)
Normal	<6.1		<7.8				
Impaired fasting glucose prediabetes	6.1–6.9	and	<7.8			or	42–47
Impaired glucose tolerance prediabetes	6.1–6.9	and	7.8–11			or	42–47
Diabetes mellitus	≥7	or	>11.1	or	>11.1	or	>48

TABLE 8.13 Management Based on Follow-up HbA1c

HbA1c at Follow-up (mmol/mol)	Management of Patient with High BMI, Metformin Tolerant and Normal eGFR (>60 mL/min/1.73m²)	Management of patient with a Low BMI (<25) or Metformin Intolerant or eGFR (<35 mL/min/1.73m²)
48–57	Intensify current monotherapy (e.g., prescribe drug TDS instead of BD)	
>58	Prescribe dual therapy. Options include: Metformin + Gliptin Metformin + Sulfonylurea Metformin + Pioglitazone Metformin + SGLT-2 inhibitor	Prescribe dual therapy. Options include: Sulfonylurea + Gliptin Sulfonylurea + Pioglitazone Gliptin + Pioglitazone
>58 despite dual therapy	Prescribe triple therapy. Options include: Metformin + Sulfonylurea + Gliptin Metformin + Sulfonylurea + Pioglitazone Metformin + Sulfonylurea + SGLT-2 Metformin + SGLT-2 + Pioglitazone	Prescribe insulin regimen
>58 despite triple therapy	Metformin + Sulfonylurea + GLP-1 mimetic	

- Oestrogen induces the formation of follicles and secondary female sexual characteristics

Hypogonadism

Definition: decreased secretion of sex hormones (testosterone and oestrogen) by gonads (testis and ovaries). Two types:

- **Primary hypogonadism** (a.k.a., hypergonadotropic hypogonadism): gonads do not respond to LH or FSH (e.g., testicular or ovarian failure). Causes include:
  - Genetic disorders (e.g., Klinefelter syndrome, Turner syndrome)
  - Damage to gonads (e.g., trauma, surgery, infection)
- **Secondary hypogonadism** (a.k.a., hypogonadotropic hypogonadism): low levels of gonadotrophins. The hypothalamus does not produce enough GnRH or the pituitary does not produce enough LH and/or FSH. Causes include:
  - Genetic disorders (e.g., Kallman syndrome)
  - Damage to hypothalamus/pituitary (e.g., trauma, surgery, infection)

Buzzwords:

- **Risk factors:** damage to gonads or hypothalamus/pituitary, family history, chronic renal/cardiac/hepatic disease, haemochromatosis, sickle cell, alcohol use disorder
- **Presentation:** delayed puberty, absent secondary sexual characteristics, osteoporosis, small testes

Investigations: if puberty does not develop by age 13 in females and 14 in males, request the following tests:

1. Tests to rule out other causes: FBC, U&E, TFTs
2. Test to confirm hypogonadism: FSH, LH, testosterone, oestrogen (see Table 8.14)
3. Wrist X-ray to assess for constitutional delay
4. Consider Brain MRI: assess hypothalamus/pituitary for damage or mass

Differentials: various congenital/genetic (see definition), cryptorchidism, orchitis in childhood, polycystic ovarian syndrome

Management:

- Constitutional delay: reassurance and observation
- Nonconstitutional delay: treat underlying condition. Consider replacing sex hormones

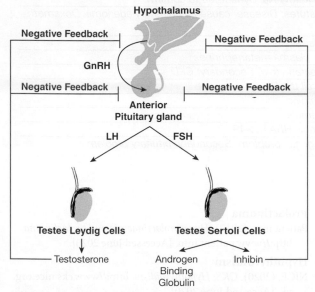

Fig 8.10 Male Gonadal Axis. (Illustrated by Dr Hollie Blaber.)

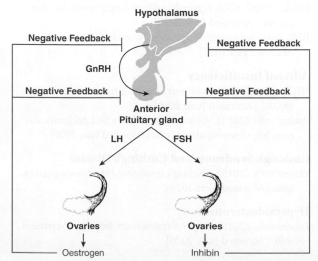

Fig 8.11 Female Gonadal Axis. (Illustrated by Dr Hollie Blaber.)

TABLE 8.14	**Hypogonadism**	
	LH and FSH	**Sex Hormones (Testosterone and Oestrogen)**
Primary hypogonadism (hypergonadotropic hypogonadism)	High	Low
Secondary hypogonadism (hypogonadotropic hypogonadism)	Low	Low

FSH, Follicle-stimulating hormone; LH, luteinising hormone.

THE ONE-LINE ROUND-UP!

Here are some key words to help you remember each condition/concept.

Condition	One-line Description
Acromegaly	GH not suppressed by glucose, bitemporal hemianopia
GH deficiency	Small child, post-brain injury
SIADH	Euvolemic, small-cell lung cancer
Diabetes insipidus	Central vs nephrogenic, low urine osmolarity
Prolactinoma	Men: gynaecomastia; Women: amenorrhoea; Both: galactorrhoea
Hypothyroidism	Everything slows down, consider depression
Hyperthyroidism	Everything speeds up, Graves' most common
Adrenal insufficiency	Postural hypotension, high K, low Na: Synacthen to confirm
Cushing's	Syndrome: collection of features; Disease: caused by pituitary adenoma. Dexamethasone to confirm
Hyperaldosteronism	Resistant HTN with low K/alkalosis
Phaeochromocytoma	Episodic symptoms, check plasma metanephrines
Hyperparathyroidism	Hypercalcaemia. Primary: parathyroid, Secondary: CKD
MEN syndromes	Family history, MEN 1 has all the Ps
Hypoparathyroidism	Low Ca, paraesthesia, twitching
T1DM	Autoimmune beta-cell destruction
T2DM	Insulin insensitivity/deficiency. HBA1c >48
Hypogonadism	Delayed puberty. Primary: gonad problem; Secondary: pituitary problem

READING LIST: ENDOCRINOLOGY IN AN HOUR

Acromegaly
Patient info. (2016). *Acromegaly*. http://www.patient.info. [Accessed April 2020].

BMJ Best Practice. (2020). *Acromegaly*. http://www.bestpractice.bmj.com. [Accessed January 2021].

Growth Hormone Deficiency
Hormone Health Network. (2017). *Growth hormone deficiency*. http://www.hormone.org. [Accessed June 2020].

Syndrome of Inappropriate ADH Secretion
NICE. (2015). *CKS: Hyponatraemia*. [https://cks.nice.org.uk/topics/hyponatraemia/ - Accessed Feb 2022].

Diabetes Insipidus
Patient info. (2015). *Diabetes insipidus*. http://www.patient.info. [Accessed June 2020].

Prolactin Axis
Al-Chalabi, M., Bass, A. N., & Alsalman, I. (2021). *Physiology, prolactin*. StatPearls. StatPearls Publishing. https://www.ncbi.nlm.nih.gov/books/NBK507829.

Prolactinoma
Patient info. (2017). *Hyperprolactinaemia and prolactinoma*. http://www.patient.info. [Accessed June 2020].

Hypothyroidism
NICE. (2020). *CKS: Hypothyroidism*. http://www.cks.nice.org.uk. [Accessed June 2020].

Hyperthyroidism
NICE. (2020). *CKS: Hyperthyroidism*. http://www.cks.nice.org.uk. [Accessed June 2020].

BNF. *Propylthiouracil: Pregnancy*. [www.bnf.nice.org.uk - Accessed Feb 2022].

Adrenal Insufficiency
NICE. (2016). *CKS: Addison's disease*. http://www.cks.nice.org.uk. [Accessed June 2020].

Patient info. (2015). *Adrenal insufficiency and Addison's disease*. http://www.patient.info. [Accessed June 2020].

Cushing's Syndrome and Cushing's Disease
Patient info. (2015). *Cushing's syndrome*. http://www.patient.info. [Accessed June 2020].

Hyperaldosteronism
Patient info. (2015). *Hyperaldosteronism*. http://www.patient.info. [Accessed June 2020].

Fay, K., & Cohen, D. (2021). Aldosteronism (hyperaldosteronism, primary). In *Ferri's clinical advisor* (pp. 94–95.e1). Elsevier.

Phaeochromocytoma

Patient info. (2016). *Pheochromocytoma*. http://www.patient. info. [Accessed June 2020].

Patrick, B., Brady, M., & Ferri, F. (2021). Pheochromocytoma. In *Ferri's clinical advisor* (pp. 94–95.e1).

Parathyroid axis

Bikle, D. D. (2000). Vitamin D: Production, metabolism and mechanisms of action. [Updated 2021 Dec 31]. In K. R. Feingold, B. Anawalt, A. Boyce, et al., (Eds.). *Endotext [Internet]*. South Dartmouth (MA): MDText.com, Inc. Available from: https://www.ncbi.nlm.nih.gov/books/ NBK278935/ [Accessed Feb 2022].

Khan, M., Jose, A., & Sharma, S. (2022). Physiology, Para-thyroid Hormone. [Updated 2021 Dec 28]. In *StatPearls [Internet]*. Treasure Island (FL): StatPearls Publishing. Available from: https://www.ncbi.nlm.nih.gov/books/ NBK499940/ [Accessed Feb 2022].

Hyperparathyroidism

Patient info. (2016). *Hyperparathyroidism*. http://www.pa-tient.info. [Accessed June 2020].

NICE. (2019). *CKS: Hypercalcaemia*. http://www.cks.nice.org. uk. [Accessed June 2020].

Multiple Endocrine Neoplasia Syndromes

Patient info. (2016). *Multiple endocrine neoplasia 1*. http:// www.patient.info. [Accessed June 2020].

Patient info. (2016). *Multiple endocrine neoplasia 2*. http:// www.patient.info. [Accessed June 2020].

Hypoparathyroidism

BNF: Calcium imbalance [www.bnf.nice.org.uk - Accessed February 2022].

BNF: Magnesium imbalance [www.bnf.nice.org.uk - Accessed February 2022].

NICE CKS: Vitamin D Deficiency in adults [www.cks.nice. org.uk - Accessed February 2022].

Management of Hypocalcaemia [https://handbook.ggc-medicines.org.uk/guidelines/electrolyte-disturbances/ management-of-hypocalcaemia/ - Accessed February 2022].

Patient info. (2015). *Hypocalcaemia*. http://www.patient.info. [Accessed June 2020].

Resuscitation Council. (2018). *Advanced life support guidelines*. http://www.resus.org.uk. [Accessed June 2020].

Patient info. (2014). *Hypoparathyroidism*. http://www.patient. info. [Accessed June 2020].

Medscape. (2018). *Hypoparathyroidism*. http://www.emedi-cine.medscape.com. [Accessed June 2020].

Type 1 Diabetes Mellitus

NICE. (2016). *CKS: Diabetes – type 1*. http://www.cks.nice. org.uk. [Accessed June 2020].

Patient info. (2016). *Diabetes mellitus*. http://www.patient. info. [Accessed June 2020].

Patient info. (2017). *Type 1 diabetes*. http://www.patient.info. [Accessed June 2020].

Type 2 Diabetes Mellitus

NICE. (2019). *CKS: Diabetes – type 2*. http://www.cks.nice. org.uk. [Accessed June 2020].

Patient info. (2016). *Diabetes mellitus*. http://www.patient. info. [Accessed June 2020].

Patient info. (2020). *Type 2 diabetes*. http://www.patient.info. [Accessed June 2020].

Hypogonadism

Patient info. (2015). *Delayed puberty*. http://www.patient.info. [Accessed June 2020].

Medscape. (2019). *Hypogonadism*. http://www.emedicine. medscape.com. [Accessed June 2020].

Tucci, J. (2021). Hypogonadism. In *Ferri's clinical advisor 2021* (pp. 94–95.e1). Elsevier.

9

General Surgery in an Hour

Ruth Perkins, Berenice Aguirrezabala Armbruster, Nagarjun Konda and Jonathan Rees

OUTLINE

UPPER GASTROINTESTINAL SURGERY

Achalasia

Definition: a dysmotility disorder characterised by a failure of the lower oesophageal sphincter to relax, resulting in an oesophageal stricture. Pseudoachalasia is when symptoms of achalasia are present, but manometry results are normal. Pseudoachalasia may be caused by a malignancy.

Buzzwords:

- **Risk factors:** underlying oesophageal disorder, underlying autoimmune disorder
- **Presentation:** progressive dysphagia for both solids and liquids (solids>liquids), reflux symptoms

Investigations:

- **Chest x-ray (CXR):** widened mediastinum due to a dilated oesophagus
- **Barium swallow:** 'bird's beak' appearance. Also used to rule out a malignancy before manometry is performed
- ***Manometry (gold standard for diagnosis)*:** shows a high resting pressure in the lower oesophageal sphincter
- **Consider endoscopy and biopsy** if manometry results are normal (i.e., suspected pseudoachalasia)

Differentials: gastrooesophageal reflux disease (GORD), oesophageal cancer, oesophageal stricture

Management:

- Surgical management with a Heller myotomy (if fit) or an endoscopic pneumatic dilatation (if elderly with comorbidities)
- Medical management (if unsuitable for surgery) with nitrates and calcium-channel blockers (CCBs) (e.g., nifedipine)

Diffuse Oeophageal Spasm

Definition: a dysmotility disorder of the oesophagus characterised by uncoordinated oesophageal contractions

Buzzwords:

- **Risk factors:** >50 years of age
- **Presentation:** intermittent dysphagia for both solids and liquids, reflux symptoms

Investigations:

- **Barium swallow:** corkscrew or 'rosary bead' appearance. Also used to rule out a malignancy before manometry is performed
- ***Manometry (gold standard for diagnosis)*:** shows uncoordinated contractions

Differentials: GORD, achalasia, acute coronary syndrome

Management:

- Manage reflux
- Medical management with nitrates and CCBs (e.g., nifedipine)

- Surgery (last resort) with a Heller myotomy (if fit) or an endoscopic pneumatic dilatation (if elderly with comorbidities)

Pharyngeal Pouch (A.K.A., Zenker's Diverticulum)

Definition: a herniation of the pharyngeal lining through the pharyngeal wall muscle
Buzzwords:
- **Risk factors:** Northern European, male, >70 years of age
- **Presentation:** dysphagia, food regurgitation, cough, halitosis, neck lump

Investigations: barium swallow shows a pharyngeal pouch
Differentials: oesophageal carcinoma, oesophageal stricture
Management: surgery (diverticulectomy for larger lesions or Dohlman's procedure for smaller lesions)

Oesophageal Cancer

Definition: There are two main types of oesophageal cancer:
- **Adenocarcinoma:** originates in the lower oesophagus
- **Squamous cell carcinoma (SCC):** originates in first two-thirds of the oesophagus

Buzzwords:
- **Risk factors for Adenocarcinoma:** Barrett's oesophagus (due to persistent reflux), an increased body mass index (BMI)
- **Risk factors for SCC:** smoking, alcohol
- **Presentation:** progressive dysphagia (solids then liquids), odynophagia (painful swallowing), hoarseness of the voice (if mediastinal invasion), upper gastrointestinal (GI) bleeding, anaemia, weight loss, lymphadenopathy

Investigations:
- **Bloods:** FBC (anaemia), coagulation, U&E, LFTs (deranged if metastasis)
- **Oesophagogastroduodenoscopy (OGD)** and biopsy for diagnosis
- **Staging:** CT of thorax, abdomen, and pelvis (CT TAP), and CT-PET for distant staging, endoscopic ultrasound scan (USS) for local staging and laparoscopy for TNM staging of lower oesophageal tumours

Differentials: oesophageal stricture, achalasia, external mass compressing the oesophagus (e.g., lymph nodes)
Management:
- **Palliative care (most cases):** chemo/radiotherapy and oesophageal stenting
- **Curative aim:** oesophagectomy using the Ivor-Lewis procedure +/- neoadjuvant chemo/ radiotherapy

Zollinger–Ellison Syndrome

Definition: a gastrin-secreting tumour of the head of pancreas or proximal duodenum causing recurrent peptic ulcers. Tumours are often called gastrinomas and are typically situated in the regions mentioned above, which is sometimes called the gastrinoma triangle
Buzzwords:
- **Risk factors:** multiple endocrine neoplasia type 1 (MEN1)
- **Presentation:** recurrent peptic ulcers

Investigations: fasting serum gastrin levels (>1000 pg/mL)
Differentials: GORD, peptic ulcer disease, atrophic gastritis
Management:
1. Manage peptic ulcers with high-dose proton-pump inhibitors (PPIs)
2. Surgical resection if the tumour is localized
3. Somatostatin analogues (e.g., octreotide) and chemotherapy if metastasised

Gastric Cancer

Definition: a malignancy of the stomach. The most common type is adenocarcinoma, although this type is becoming less common, perhaps because of *Heliobacter pylori* treatment and dietary changes. The incidence varies significantly in different parts of the world and is particularly high in the Far East.
Buzzwords:
- **Risk factors:** male, increasing age
- **Presentation:** vague presentation initially (e.g., reflux, epigastric pain after eating)
  - **Malignancy symptoms (late):** anaemia, weight loss, anorexia
  - **Metastasis signs:** Troisier sign (palpable Virchow's node), acanthosis nigricans, Sister Joseph nodules (umbilicus), ascites, hepatomegaly, jaundice

Investigations:
- **Bloods:** FBC (anaemia), LFTs (deranged if metastasis)

- **Gastroscopy and biopsy:** for diagnosis
- **CT TAP:** for staging
- **Laparoscopy:** for peritoneal disease
- **MRI** (if CT suggests lesions that need better characterisation): for metastasis (particularly in the liver)

Differentials: peptic ulcer disease, benign oesophageal stricture and achalasia for gastroesophageal junction tumours

Management:

- **Curative aim:** surgery to remove the tumour followed by a reconstruction of the GI system using the Roux-en-Y reconstruction method. The surgical method depends on the tumour location:
  - Total gastrectomy for proximal cancers
  - Subtotal gastrectomy for distal cancers
  - Endoscopic mucosal resection for early tumours (e.g., T1a)
- **Palliative care (many cases):** chemotherapy and surgery for symptomatic relief (e.g., stenting for gastric outlet obstruction)

Complications after surgery: dumping syndrome (food passing too quickly through the GI tract leading to hypoglycaemia), vitamin B12 deficiency

Oesophageal Narrowing

Definition: refers to a decreased diameter of the oesophagus caused by one of the following factors:

- **Strictures:** caused by benign or malignant oesophageal disease
- **Webs:** caused by changes in the mucosa and submucosa only. The most common cause is

Plummer-Vinson syndrome (an iron-deficiency anaemia associated with post-cricoid webs)

- **Rings:** caused by changes in the mucosa, submucosa and muscle
- **External compression:** caused by benign or malignant disease

Buzzwords:

- **Risk factors:** history of persistent reflux, underlying cancer, previous oesophageal surgery, iron-deficiency anaemia, hiatus hernia
- **Presentation:** heartburn, dysphagia, food impaction, weight loss, chest pain

Investigations:

- **CXR:** to rule out external compression
- **Barium swallow:** to identify the cause and extent of the stricture and to determine if it is safe to perform an endoscopy
- ***Endoscopy*:** gold standard for diagnosis

Differentials: oesophageal cancer, achalasia, GORD

Management: treat the underlying diagnosis

Hiatus Hernia

Definition: there are two types of hiatus hernias (see Fig 9.1):

- **Sliding (most cases):** occurs when the gastrooesophageal junction slides up into the thoracic cavity
- **Rolling (a.k.a., paraoesophageal):** occurs when the gastrooesophageal junction remains in place but part of the stomach slides into the thoracic cavity

Buzzwords:

- **Risk factors:** obesity, pregnancy, ascites, advanced age, previous GI surgery

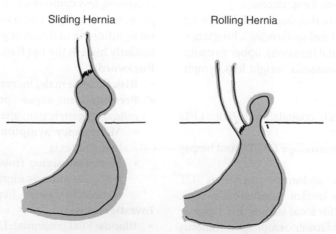

Sliding Hernia   Rolling Hernia

Fig 9.1 Sliding Versus Rolling Hernias. (Illustrated by Hollie Blaber.)

- **Presentation:** reflux worst when lying down

Investigations:
- **OGD:** to visualise the hernia
- **Contrast swallow and contrast meals:** can help to delineate the anatomy
- **CT chest and abdomen:** to determine the structural anatomy if surgery is being considered

Differentials: GORD, oesophageal dysmotility disorders, angina (particularly if there is oesophageal spasm)

Management:
- **Sliding hernia:** conservative (e.g., PPI, weight loss, reduced alcohol intake, smoking cessation). Surgery is a second-line approach
- **Rolling hernia:** surgery always (Nissen fundoplication surgery)

Obesity

Definition: NICE uses the BMI to assess weight and define obesity. A BMI of ≥ 30 kg/m^2 is considered obese, while a BMI of ≥ 40 kg/m^2 is considered morbidly obese. The BMI may be used in conjunction with the waist circumference. Obesity raises the risks associated with surgery, particularly with general anaesthesia.

Buzzwords:
- **Risk factors:** metabolic dysfunction, hypothyroidism, polycystic ovarian syndrome, dietary factors, inactivity, medication (e.g., steroids)
- **Presentation:** raised BMI, +/- type 2 diabetes mellitus (T2DM), hypertension, metabolic syndrome, cardiovascular disease, obstructive sleep apnoea

Investigations:
- BMI and waist circumference measurements
- **Bloods:** ↑ lipids, ↑ capillary blood glucose (CBG), thyroid function tests (TFTs) (may show hypothyroidism)

Management:
- **Dietary and lifestyle advice:** education regarding risks, dietary input, exercise advice
- **Risk stratification:** if appropriate: statins for hyperlipidaemia, antihypertensives, diabetic medications
- **Medication:** consider when initial diet and lifestyle interventions have failed and if a patient meets specific BMI/comorbidity criteria
    - Orlistat (the only medication currently licensed in the United Kingdom) may be used as an adjunct treatment in those with a BMI of ≥ 30 kg/m^2 or in those with a BMI of ≥ 28 kg/m^2 AND additional risk factors

- Treatment with orlistat should be reviewed after 12 weeks and discontinued if $\geq 5\%$ weight loss has not been achieved.
- **Surgery:** consider bariatric surgery for people who meet all the following NICE criteria:
    - BMI >40 kg/m^2 or BMI >35 kg/m^2 with significant comorbidities that could be improved with weight loss
    - All nonsurgical options have been tried without adequate success
    - The patient is under a specialist management service, is fit for surgery and is able to commit to ongoing follow-up and management
    - Procedures commonly performed in the United Kingdom include:

Adjustable gastric banding: a band is placed around the upper part of the stomach, creating a small stomach pouch situated above the band. This band creates a narrowing in the stomach, with the ability to adjust the degree of stomach compression by altering the degree of narrowing. Therefore, the amount of food held up in the stomach pouch as a result of band narrowing can be altered in response to the degree of weight loss. These bands are typically placed laparoscopically

Sleeve gastrectomy: the majority of the body of the stomach is removed to create a more cylindrical structure with a lower capacity

Gastric bypass: a small gastric pouch is created by stapling across the upper part of the stomach. A loop of jejunum is then anastomosed directly to this pouch. This anatomy bypasses a length of the jejunum, reducing the length of small bowel available for food absorption

HEPATOBILLIARY SURGERY

Hepatocellular Carcinoma

Definition: the most common type of primary liver cancer. Secondary liver cancer is far more common than primary liver cancer

Buzzwords:
- **Risk factors:** male, >45 years of age, cirrhosis, hepatitis B/C infection, alcohol, nonalcoholic fatty liver disease, other chronic liver conditions
- **Presentation:** initially asymptomatic, followed by vague symptoms (presenting late), including fatigue, loss of appetite, nausea, vomiting, weight loss, right

upper quadrant (RUQ) discomfort, jaundice, dark urine, pale faeces, pruritus (itchy skin)

Investigations:

- **Bloods:** LFTs (deranged), U&E, clotting (deranged), ↑ alpha-fetoprotein (AFP) tumour marker (NB: may also be elevated with ovarian and testicular malignancies, pregnancy and choriocarcinoma. If the AFP is negative, it does not exclude hepatocellular carcinoma (HCC))
- **Imaging:** abdominal ultrasound, CT scan with contrast, MRI scan with liver-specific contrast to show HCC
- **Biopsy** if the diagnosis is still unclear

Differentials: cholangiocarcinoma (primary bile duct cancer), hepatic adenoma, benign hepatic lesions (e.g., focal nodule hyperplasia), metastatic disease

Management:

1. Treat any complications of cirrhosis (e.g., ascites, hepatic encephalopathy, spontaneous bacterial peritonitis, oesophageal varices)
2. Use a scoring system to guide your treatment:
   - **Child-Pugh score:** estimates cirrhosis severity
   - **Model for End-stage Liver Disease (MELD) score:** stratifies the severity of end-stage liver disease
   - **Barcelona Clinic Liver Cancer (BCLC) score:** for staging
3. Consider the following factors when determining if a patient is suitable for surgery: tumour size, location, spread, degree of cirrhosis and other health conditions. Surgical options include a **resection** (small part of the liver removed) or **transplantation**
4. If unsuitable for surgery, consider nonsurgical options (e.g., ablative therapies, embolisation, targeted cancer drugs (e.g., sorafenib, regorafenib)). HCC tends to be resistant to chemotherapy and radiotherapy

Prognosis: median survival is 6 months. With a surgical intervention, the 5-year survival is between 50%–70%

Cholangiocarcinoma

Definition: biliary tree tumour involving intrahepatic, perihilar (most common) and/or extrahepatic lesions (see Table 9.1 and Fig 9.2). Cholangiocarcinoma is the second most common type of liver tumour after HCC.

Buzzwords:

- **Risk factors:** primary sclerosing cholangitis, age >65 years, bile duct cysts, bile duct stones, parasitic infection with liver flukes (e.g., *Opisthorchis viverrini* and *Clornorchis sinensis*), toxin exposure

- **Presentation:** initially asymptomatic. Presentation tends to be late with vague symptoms like fatigue, loss of appetite, nausea, vomiting, weight loss, RUQ discomfort, jaundice, dark urine, pale faeces and pruritus (itchy skin). Jaundice can be the predominant sign of perihilar and extrahepatic cholangiocarcinomas. **Courvoisier's law** states that, in the presence of a painless palpably enlarged gallbladder and mild jaundice, the cause is unlikely to be gallstones

Investigations:

- **Bloods:** ↑ alkaline phosphatase (ALP), ↑ bilirubin, ↑ gamma glutamyl transferase (GGT), clotting deranged, baseline U&Es
- **Serum tumour markers:**
  - **CA-19:** elevated in 85% of patients. Measured after decompression. Low sensitivity and low specificity.

TABLE 9.1 World Health Organization Classification of Biliary Malignancies

INTRAHEPATIC CHOLANGIOCARCINOMA	
Benign	Bile duct adenoma
	Microcystic adenoma
	Biliary adenofibroma
Premalignant	Biliary intraepithelial neoplasia
	Intraductal papillary neoplasm
	Mucinous cystic neoplasm
Malignant	Intrahepatic cholangiocarcinoma
	Intraductal papillary neoplasm with associated invasive neoplasia
	Mucinous cystic neoplasm with associated invasive neoplasia
EXTRAHEPATIC CHOLANGIOCARCINOMA	
Premalignant	Adenoma
	Biliary intrahepatic neoplasia
	Intracystic (gall bladder) or intraductal (bile duct) papillary neoplasm
	Mucinous cystic neoplasm
Carcinoma	Adenocarcinoma
	Adenosquamous carcinoma
	Intracystic (gall bladder) or intraductal (bile duct) papillary neoplasm with associated invasive neoplasia
	Squamous cell carcinoma
	Undifferentiated carcinoma

Adapted from Khan, S.A., Davidson, B.R., Goldin, R.D., et al. (2012). Guidelines for the diagnosis and treatment of cholangiocarcinoma: An update. *Gut*, *61*,1657–1669.

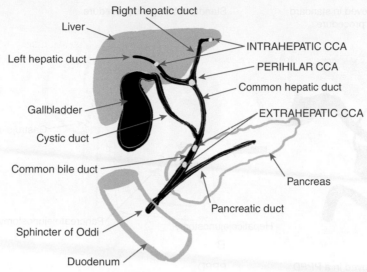

Fig 9.2 Cholangiocarcinoma Tumour Sites. *CCA*, Cholangiocarcinoma. (Illustrated by Hollie Blaber.)

Not useful for diagnosis but useful for monitoring if the CA19-9 level is high prior to treatment

- **CA-125:** elevated in 65% of patients. Low sensitivity and low specificity. Not used for monitoring
- **USS:** may show biliary duct dilatation
- **CT TAP** and triple phase of liver
- ***Magnetic resonance cholangiopancreatography (MRCP)*** +/- **MRI liver** are the principal diagnostic tests for identifying biliary anatomy, particularly for perihilar and intrahepatic lesions
- **CT:** for staging
- **Endoscopic retrograde cholangiopancreatography (ERCP)** +/- **ERCP spyglass** (a microcamera deployed to view the inside of the bile ducts and to take more targeted biopsies) is used to achieve biliary drainage (if indicated), to obtain samples for diagnosis and, if indicated, for histology/cytology and tumour grading
  - **Grade 1 (low grade):** slow-growing cancer cells that look similar to bile duct cells
  - **Grade 2 (intermediate grade):** fast-growing cancer cells that look slightly different to bile duct cells
  - **Grade 3 (high grade):** very fast-growing cancer cells that look very different to bile duct cells

Differentials: pancreatic carcinoma, cholecystitis/choledocholithiasis, HCC (although jaundice may occur, pain is uncommon)

Management: resectable tumours may be treated with surgery and adjuvant therapy (e.g., postsurgical chemo/radiotherapy). Surgical options include:

- **Bile duct removal:** removal of the area of bile duct containing the tumour as well as nearby lymph nodes. Indicated for tumours localised to the **extrahepatic bile duct only**
- **Partial hepatectomy:** removal of part of the liver (either a wedge of tissue, a liver lobe or a larger section). Indicated for **intrahepatic tumours** involving the liver
- **Extended hepatectomy:** removal of a much larger part of the liver and bile ducts down to the tip of the head of the pancreas with attachment of the jejunum to the remaining bile duct just as it leaves the liver portion that remains. Indicated for **perihilar tumours**
- **Whipple procedure:** removal of the bile ducts, head of the pancreas, gallbladder and parts of the stomach and small intestines. Indicated for **extrahepatic tumours** situated within the **head of the pancreas** (see Fig 9.3)

Palliative treatment: may involve surgery for symptomatic relief and/or medical treatment using chemo-/radio-/immuno-targeted therapy. Palliative surgical options include:

- **Biliary bypass:** using the **patient's bile duct** to form a bypass by either attaching the preblocked bile duct to the postblocked bile duct or by directly attaching the preblocked bile duct to the small intestine
- **Endoscopic stent placement:** a stent (small tube) is inserted endoscopically to bypass the blocked area
- **Percutaneous transhepatic biliary drainage:** insertion of contrast material through the skin into the

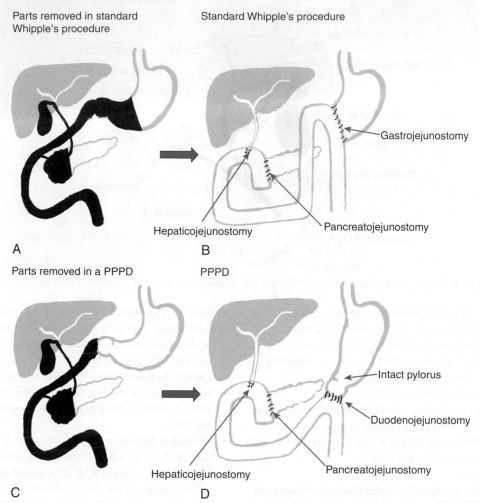

Parts removed in standard
Whipple's procedure

Standard Whipple's procedure

Gastrojejunostomy

Hepaticojejunostomy

Pancreatojejunostomy

A

B

Parts removed in a PPPD

PPPD

Intact pylorus

Duodenojejunostomy

Hepaticojejunostomy

Pancreatojejunostomy

C

D

Fig 9.3 Standard Whipple Procedure vs a Pylorus-Preserving Pancreatoduodectomy (*PPPD*) (Illustrated by Hollie Blaber.)

biliary tree to perform an X-ray of the biliary tree with contrast. If a blockage is present, a stent is used to drain bile from the liver to the small intestines

Prognosis (percentage survival for ≥5 years after diagnosis):

- **Intrahepatic:** localised (15%), regional (5%), distant (2%)
- **Extrahepatic:** localised (30%), regional (25%), distant (2%)

Pancreatic Cancer

Definition: a cancer affecting any area of the pancreas

Buzzwords:

- **Risk factors:** family history, cigarette smoke, obesity, chronic pancreatitis, other cancers/syndromes (e.g.,

Peutz-Jeghers syndrome (PJS), familial atypical multiple mole melanoma syndrome, Lynch syndrome/hereditary nonpolyposis colorectal cancer (HNPCC), BRAC1/BRAC2 breast cancer)

- **Presentation:** late presentation with jaundice, pale stools, dark urine, nonspecific cancer symptoms (e.g., fatigue, weight loss, loss of appetite), **Courvoisier's law**

Investigations:

- **Bloods:** U&E, LFTs (↑ ALP and ↑ bilirubin if obstructive), ↑ GGT (if obstructive), clotting (prolonged prothrombin time (PT) if liver dysfunction)
- **Abdominal USS:** may show biliary duct dilatation demonstrating obstruction

- **CT TAP and pancreas:** for staging (e.g., to identify spread) and to highlight the relationship of the tumour to key vascular structures
- **CT-PET:** for distant staging
- **MRI liver** (if CT or CT-PET raises suspicions): for liver metastasis
- **Serum tumour markers including CA 19-9 and CEA** can support the diagnosis in conjunction with other tests; however, they can also be elevated in nonmalignant conditions
- Regular blood tests to monitor disease progression or new complications

Differentials: cholelithiasis, chronic pancreatitis, cholangiocarcinoma

Management:
- Analgesia +/- coeliac plexus block, pancreatic enzyme supplements (e.g., Creon or Pancrease)
- **Resectable pancreatic cancer (minority):**
  - Neoadjuvant chemotherapy (in clinical trials only)
  - Surgery: a pylorus-preserving pancreatoduodectomy is the first-line procedure. The Whipple procedure is the second-line procedure (see Fig 9.3)
  - Adjuvant chemotherapy: gemcitabine with capecitabine (GemCap)
- **Borderline resectable pancreatic cancer:** refers to tumours growing near large blood vessels (i.e., the portal vein, superior mesenteric artery). In these cases, chemotherapy is often offered, and the patient is then reassessed
- **Unresectable tumours (majority)**
  - **Locally advanced** (cancer has spread to local organs/vessels): chemotherapy and/or radiotherapy
  - **Metastatic:** chemotherapy

Gallstones

Definition: gallstones (cholelithiasis) is a general term used to describe the formation of gallstones either in the gallbladder or biliary tree. Different terms are used to describe gallstones in different locations:
- Chole**cysto**lithiasis: gallstones in the gallbladder
- Chole**docho**lithiasis: gallstones in the common bile duct

Classification by stone composition:
- **Old classification (three types):** cholesterol (most common), pigmented and mixed stones

- **New classification (eight types):** cholesterol (most common), pigment, calcium carbonate, phosphate, calcium stearate, protein, cystine, and mixed stones

Buzzwords:
- **Risk factors:** 5 Fs (**F**at, **F**emale, **F**ertile, **F**orty, **F**amily history), 3 Ds (**D**iabetes, **D**iet, **D**rugs (e.g., hormone replacement therapy, somatostatin analogue octreotide, glucagon-like peptide-1 analogues, ceftriaxone)), Crohn's disease
- **Presentation:** asymptomatic in most cases (80%). Symptoms appear if a complication arises (see Table 9.2 and Fig 9.4)

Investigations:
- **Bloods:** blood test results depend on the location of the stone and any associated complications. For example:
  - Gallstones causing an obstruction: ↑ ALP, ↑ GGT, ↑ bilirubin. Alanine aminotransferase (ALT)/aspartate aminotransferase (AST) may also be raised but to a lesser extent
  - Ascending cholangitis: ↑ WCC, ↑ neutrophils, ↑ CRP
- ***USS*** **is the principal diagnostic test:** detects stones in the gallbladder and/or may show biliary duct dilatation if a stone is in the common bile duct
- **MRCP** if a USS does not detect stones but gallstones are still suspected. May detect stones in the gallbladder or common bile duct
- **Endoscopic ultrasound (EUS)** is used if USS and MRCP have failed to detect stones but gallstones are still suspected. Can detect stones in the common bile duct

Differentials: peptic ulcer disease, acute pancreatitis

Management:
- **Asymptomatic gallbladder stones:** reassurance
- **Asymptomatic common bile duct stones:** consider clearance of the duct by ERCP or a laparoscopic cholecystectomy and bile duct exploration. Monitoring if an intervention represents a greater risk than leaving the stones
- **Symptomatic gallbladder stones:** laparoscopic cholecystectomy
- **Symptomatic common bile duct stones:** ERCP and laparoscopic cholecystectomy or laparoscopic cholecystectomy and bile duct exploration
- **Symptomatic gallstone empyema:** percutaneous cholecystostomy

TABLE 9.2   Gallstone Complications

Complications of Cystic Duct Stones	Present	Not Present
Biliary colic (stone in cystic duct lodging and dislodging)	Colicky RUQ/epigastric pain after meals which lasts 30 min to 8 h	Cholestasis signs (jaundice + dark urine + pale stools) Fever Murphy's sign[a]
Acute cholecystitis (stone stuck in the cystic duct causing gallbladder inflammation)	Constant RUQ/epigastric pain Fever Murphy's sign[a]	Cholestasis signs (jaundice + dark urine + pale stools)
Gallbladder empyema (stone stuck in the cystic duct causing gallbladder inflammation and infection (pus))	Constant RUQ/epigastric pain Fever Murphy's sign[a]	Cholestasis signs (jaundice + dark urine + pale stools)
Mirizzi's syndrome (stone stuck in the cystic duct but also compressing the common bile duct)	Constant RUQ/epigastric pain Fever Murphy's sign[a] Cholestasis signs (jaundice + dark urine + pale stools)	
Fistula formation (acute cholecystitis causing fistula formation between the gallbladder and small bowel)	Gallstone ileus (stone gets stuck in the terminal ileum causing a small bowel obstruction) or Bouveret's syndrome (stone stuck in the duodenum causing gastric outlet obstruction)	
Complications of Common Bile Duct Stones	**Present**	**Not Present**
Cholelithiasis (stone stuck in the common bile duct)	Constant RUQ/epigastric pain Cholestasis signs (jaundice + dark urine + pale stools)	Fever Murphy's sign[a]
Ascending cholangitis (stone stuck in the common bile duct causing inflammation and infection)	Charcot's triad (RUQ pain + fever + jaundice) or Reynold's pentad (RUQ pain + fever + jaundice + shock + altered mental status)	Murphy's sign[a]
Complications of Common Hepatopancreatic Duct Stones	**Present**	**Not Present**
Pancreatitis	See Pancreatitis section	

[a]*Murphy's sign* is pain on inspiration when palpating the right subcostal area due to an inflamed gallbladder coming into contact with the examiner's hand.
RUQ, Right upper quadrant.

Ascending Cholangitis (A.K.A., Acute Cholangitis)

Definition: infection of the biliary tract, most often secondary to an obstruction. Characterised by the presence of Charcot's triad: fever, jaundice and RUQ pain. Severe cases can progress to sepsis, typically with Gram-negative organisms
Buzzwords:

- **Risk factors:** presence of gallstones (by extension, risk factors for gallstone disease), strictures of the biliary tract, malignancy of the biliary tract
- **Presentation:** Charcot's triad, features of sepsis
Investigations:
- **Bloods:** ↑ LFTs, ↑ inflammatory markers, U&Es (may show evidence of acute kidney injury)
- **Bloods cultures:** to identify organism

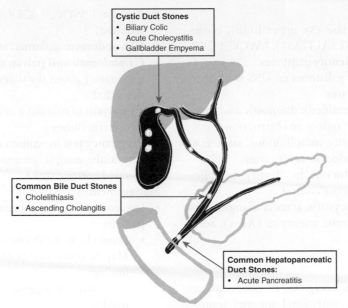

Cystic Duct Stones
- Biliary Colic
- Acute Cholecystitis
- Gallbladder Empyema

Common Bile Duct Stones
- Cholelithiasis
- Ascending Cholangitis

Common Hepatopancreatic Duct Stones:
- Acute Pancreatitis

Fig 9.4 Complications of Gallstones. (Illustrated by Hollie Blaber.)

- **USS abdomen:** presence of gallstones, dilated bile ducts +/- a thickened gallbladder if concurrent cholecystitis
- **MRCP:** presence of an obstructing gallstone or stricture
- **CT abdomen** may be indicated if the cause isn't gallstones (CT imaging is less effective for identifying gallstones)

Differentials: acute cholecystitis, peptic ulcer disease, acute pancreatitis

Management:
- **Antibiotics:** usually broad spectrum with coverage for Gram-negative bacteria
- Treat any associated consequences of sepsis
- **ERCP:** if USS or MRCP show evidence of gallstones in the common hepatic or common bile ducts, an ERCP may be beneficial for removing the obstruction. If the patient is very unwell, an ERCP can be performed to place a stent to drain the bile duct. A second ERCP can then be undertaken later to remove the stones and the previously placed stent
- Lifestyle modifications to address underlying risk factors
- If known gallstones, consider a referral for a cholecystectomy

Pancreatitis

Definition: an inflammation of the pancreas that can lead to local and widespread effects depending on the severity. Acute pancreatitis is characterised by an exocrine insufficiency, and chronic pancreatitis is characterised by both endocrine and exocrine insufficiencies.

Buzzwords:
- **Causes:** mnemonic 'I GET SMASHED' - Idiopathic, Gallstones (**most common**), Ethanol (**most common**), Trauma, Steroid use, Mumps and other infections/Malignancy, Autoimmune, Scorpion sting, Hyperlipidaemia/Hypercalcaemia, ERCP, Drugs (e.g., thiazide diuretics, azathioprine, tetracyclines, oestrogens, valproic acid and dipeptidylpeptidase-4 inhibitors, such as sitagliptin and vildagliptin)
- **Presentation:**
  - **Acute:** sudden-onset abdominal pain, nausea, vomiting. Risk stratification is carried out using the Glasgow pancreatitis score
  - **Chronic:** chronic or recurrent abdominal pain that may radiate to the back, is relieved by sitting forward, and may be accompanied by nausea, vomiting, bloating, weight loss, steatorrhea

Investigations:

- **Bloods:** ↑↑ lipase/amylase (3× upper limit), cholestatic picture (ALP/GGT>ALT/AST), ↑ WCC, ↑ CRP
- **Abdominal USS:** to identify gallstones
- **MRCP** (if evidence of gallstones on USS is unclear): to visualise the biliary tree
- **ERCP** (if gallstones identified): diagnostic and therapeutic, to visualise and relieve an obstruction
- **CT abdomen:** to identify complications, such as an abscess, necrosis, pseudocyst, calcification
- **Blood glucose monitoring:** to identify complications, such as poor glucose control

Differentials: acute cholecystitis, acute cholangitis, gastroenteritis, abdominal aortic aneurysm (AAA), aortic dissection

Management:

- **Acute pancreatitis:**
  - Hospital admission, analgesia, IV fluids, oxygen (only if required), nutritional support (enteral feeding is preferred over parenteral feeding)
  - Treat underlying cause
  - ITU support if severe pancreatitis
  - Antibiotics only indicated if evidence of pancreatic necrosis
- **Chronic pancreatitis:** alcohol cessation, long-term pancreatic enzyme replacement therapy, fat-soluble vitamin supplementation, dietary advice (low-fat, high-protein, high-caloric diet), diabetic control. Pancreatic cancer monitoring every 12 months and DEXA scanning every 2 years

LOWER GASTROINTESTINAL SURGERY

Appendicitis

Definition: inflammation and then infection of the appendix as a result of a luminal obstruction created by a faecolith, stool or, rarely, cellular hypertrophy

Buzzwords:

- **Risk factors:** teens to 40s, mild increase in the lifetime risk of males
- **Presentation:** migratory abdominal pain that starts centrally and then migrates to the right iliac fossa, loss of appetite, nausea, vomiting, possible change in bowel habits. Note: atypical presentations can occur because of a retrocaecal appendix, leading to pain presenting in the flank
- **Complications:** perforation, abscess

Investigations:

- **Bloods:** ↑ WCC, ↑ CRP (preoperative blood tests required)
- **USS abdomen:** inflamed and thickened appendix
- **CT abdomen and pelvis:** may be indicated if there is uncertainty about the diagnosis or complications are suspected
- **Urinalysis:** to rule out a urinary tract infection (UTI) or ureteric stones
- **Pregnancy test** in women of childbearing age

Differentials: ectopic pregnancy, gastroenteritis, UTI, right-sided ureteric stone

Management:

- **Laparoscopic appendicectomy:** indicated for most patients
  - Prophylactic antibiotics in the preoperative period May be continued postoperatively depending on findings
  - Adequate analgesia, fluid resuscitation as needed
  - Maintenance fluids while waiting for surgery
- For patients who are unfit for/don't want surgery, conservative management with antibiotics: 30% recurrence rate

Diverticular Conditions

Definition:

- **Diverticula:** outpouching of the colon
- **Diverticulosis:** diverticula without symptoms
- **Diverticular disease** (may be called painful diverticular disease): diverticula with symptoms and WITHOUT inflammation/infection
- **Diverticulitis:** diverticula with symptoms and WITH inflammation/infection
  - Uncomplicated diverticulitis: localised diverticulitis
  - Complicated diverticulitis: diverticulitis with complications (e.g., fistula, obstruction, perforation, abscess)

Buzzwords:

- **Risk factors:** genetics, increasing age, low-fibre diet, obesity, smoking, drugs (e.g., NSAIDS, opioids, corticosteroids)
- **Presentation:**
  - **Diverticular disease:** intermittent left lower quadrant (LLQ) pain (in most cases, but can also be a right lower quadrant (RLQ) pain) that is worst with eating and is relieved by flatus/stool passage. Accompanied by constipation, diarrhoea, bloating, passage of mucus, per rectum (PR) bleeding

- **Diverticulitis:** a constant hypogastric pain that then becomes localised to the LLQ (most cases, but can also be RLQ) with fever, nausea, vomiting, diarrhoea, constipation, bloating, passage of mucus, PR blood

Investigations:

- **Bloods:** ↑ WCC, ↑ CRP (in diverticulitis)
- **CT abdomen and pelvis:** presence of diverticula and/or inflammation
- **Colonoscopy/flexible sigmoidoscopy:** to identify the presence of diverticula and to rule out an underlying malignancy. Rarely performed during periods of acute inflammation, instead 6–8 weeks later once the inflammation has decreased

Differentials: inflammatory bowel disease (IBD), colorectal cancer, irritable bowel syndrome (IBS), acute gynaecological conditions

Management:

- Asymptomatic diverticular disease: surveillance and dietary and lifestyle advice
- Diverticulitis: analgesia as required, may require hospitalisation for fluids
- Antibiotic therapy for complicated diverticulitis
- Surgery: acutely indicated if concerns about perforation, may be considered electively for patients with multiple episodes

Adenomas

Definition:

- **Hyperplastic polyp:** bowel epithelial hyperplasia of no concern. These growths do not lead to adenomatous polyps
- **Adenomatous polyp:** bowel epithelial hyperplasia with a potential cancer risk

Buzzwords:

- **Risk factors:** increasing age, family history, male, genetics (see familial adenomatous polyposis (FAP) and Lynch syndrome)
- **Presentation:** often asymptomatic and may be picked up on a routine bowel screening. If a polyp is large, it may present with rectal bleeding, mucus and tenesmus

Investigations: to rule out an established bowel cancer and to permit the early identification of adenomas that may progress to adenocarcinoma

- **Colonoscopy:** to identify the presence of adenomas and to remove them on sight for histological testing
- **CT colonography** (also called CT colonoscopy)
- **Blood:** anaemia

Differentials: hamartomatous polyp, hyperplastic polyps, malignancy

Management:

- Definitive treatment involves the removal of adenomas during colonoscopy
- Ongoing surveillance is offered to those who are found to have intermediate- or high-grade adenomas
- If there are signs of cancer on histology, referral for treatment

Familial Adenomatous Polyposis

Definition: a hereditary condition in which hundreds to thousands of adenomas form in the small and large bowels, increasing the risk of colorectal cancer. Retroperitoneal desmoid tumours (e.g., tumours of connective tissue) can also form. Occurs as a result of mutations in the adenomatous polyposis coli (*APC*) gene. Incidence is 1 in 10,000, of which 30% are thought to be de novo mutations. Accounts for 1% of colorectal cancers. Classification:

- **Classic FAP:** autosomal-dominant inheritance, hundreds to thousands of polyps in the bowel. Carries the highest risk of cancer, with almost 100% of individuals diagnosed with cancer by the age of 40 years. Cancers are usually found in the descending/sigmoid colon and rectum
- **Attenuated FAP:** autosomal-dominant inheritance, up to hundreds of polyps in the bowel. Carries a slightly lower risk of cancer, with approximately 80% of individuals diagnosed with cancer by the age of 60 years. Cancers are usually found in the ascending colon

Buzzwords:

- **Risk factors:** family history
- **Presentation:** unless previously known to have FAP, the presentation usually involves symptoms suggestive of colorectal cancer (see section below). Features suggestive of FAP include an early age of onset, multiple adenomas on endoscopy and bilateral pigmentation of the retina.

Investigations:

- **Colonoscopy:** presence of a large number of polyps throughout the colon
- **Extended side–viewing OGD:** gastric or duodenal polyps
- **Genetic testing:** mutations of the *APC* gene
- **Consider CT abdomen and pelvis:** presence of desmoid tumours

Differentials: juvenile polyposis syndrome (JPS), PJS

Management:
- Total proctocolectomy with the formation of an ileo-anal pouch anastomosis or ileostomy
- Screening of first-degree family members, usually starting in the teenage years
- Consider genetic screening of first-degree family members

Hereditary Nonpolyposis Colorectal Cancer

Definition: an autosomal-dominant condition involving mutations in DNA mismatch repair genes. Accounts for 3%–4% of colorectal cancers. An individual's lifetime risk of colorectal cancer depends on which mutation is present. Previously known as Lynch syndrome.

Buzzwords:
- **Risk factors:** family history
- **Presentation:** symptoms of colorectal cancer (see later) in patients <40 years of age. Associated cancers include endometrial, uterine, hepatobiliary and upper GI cancers

Investigations:
- **Colonoscopy + biopsy:** presence of colorectal lesions that are most commonly flat but can also be polypoid. Note: all resected colorectal cancers should be tested for HNPCC
- Consider **CT imaging** for extra-gastrointestinal manifestations
- **Genetic testing**

Differentials: colorectal cancer

Management:
- Colectomy is the most common treatment option
- Regular colonoscopic surveillance of those with known or suspected HNPCC
- Prophylactic daily aspirin
- Referral to familial cancer services

Peutz-Jeghers Syndrome

Definition: an autosomal-dominant syndrome characterised by the formation of hamartomatous polyps in the GI tract. While less common in the general population, hamartomas are the most common polyp found in children. This condition carries a high lifetime risk (70%–80%) of developing colorectal cancer. There is also an increased lifetime risk of breast cancer in females and, to a lesser degree, of pancreatic cancer in both males and females. For diagnosis, one of the following **diagnostic criteria** must be met:

- 2 or more Peutz-Jegher polyps (confirmed on histology)
- 1 or more Peutz-Jegher polyps and a family history of PJS
- Characteristic mucosal pigmentation with a family history of PJS

Buzzwords:
- **Risk factors:** family history, more common in children
- **Presentation:** associated with **pigmentation** of the mucosal membranes (e.g., lips, oral mucosa), rectal bleeding, change in bowel habits, intussusception in young children

Investigations:
- **Colonoscopy:** colonic polyps
- **OGD:** gastric polyps
- Consider **capsule endoscopy** for small bowel polyps
- **Genetic testing**

Differentials: FAP, JPS

Management:
- Regular (surveillance) colonoscopies
- Polypectomy
- Consider resection if polyps are larger in size
- Genetic/family counselling

Juvenile Polyposis Syndrome

Definition: an autosomal-dominant condition characterised by the presence of multiple juvenile polyps (a form of hamartomatous polyp) in the GI tract, most commonly in the large bowel but may also be found in the small bowel and stomach. While this condition increases an individual's lifetime risk of colorectal cancer, the risk is approximately half that of PJS. For diagnosis, one or more of the following **diagnostic criteria** must be met:

- Greater than five juvenile polyps in the colon
- Multiple juvenile polyps in the wider GI tract
- Presence of juvenile polyps with a family history of JPS

Buzzwords:
- **Risk factors:** family history, more common in children
- **Presentation:** rectal bleeding, change in bowel habits, abdominal pain, fatigue secondary to anaemia, some phenotypes are associated with hereditary haemorrhagic telangiectasia

Investigations:
- **Colonoscopy:** presence of polyps and/or colorectal cancer depending on the timing of presentation
- **OGD:** gastric or duodenal polyps

- **Genetic testing**

Differentials: PJS, FAP

Management:

- Regular (surveillance) colonoscopies
- Surgery: polypectomies. May require a bowel resection if cancer is present
- Genetic/family counselling

Colorectal Cancer

Definition: colorectal cancer, one of the most common cancers in the United Kingdom, results from a build-up of sporadic mutations leading to the progression of an adenoma to an adenocarcinoma. A small proportion (2%–5%) are familial and due to germline mutations

Buzzwords:

- **Risk factors:** increasing age, family history, obesity, sedentary lifestyle, diet high in red meat and low in fibre
- **Presentation** (can vary and may be nonspecific): weight loss, rectal bleeding, fatigue (due to iron-deficiency anaemia), change in bowel habits, abdominal pain. May present acutely with a bowel obstruction or perforation.

Investigations:

- **Bloods:** ↓ Hb, ↓ MCV, ↓ ferritin, CEA (may be raised – not a diagnostic test but can be indicative of the underlying process and can be used for monitoring), U&E (baseline), LFTs (baseline)
- **Colonoscopy:** favoured over a flexible sigmoidoscopy because it gives better coverage of the bowel (see Fig 9.5). This procedure can identify any lesions or at-risk polyps, and biopsies can be taken at the same time
- **CT TAP:** to stage cancer and identify the extent of spread
- **MRI pelvis:** better local staging than CT for rectal tumours

Classification, staging and grading:

- **Duke's classification**
  - A: Tumour is limited to the bowel wall
  - B: Tumour has passed through the bowel wall and is invading the muscle
  - C: Spread to local lymph nodes
  - D: Spread to distant organs such as the liver
- **TNM staging system:** accounts for tumour invasion (see Table 9.3 and Fig 9.6), involvement of nodes and metastases (see Table 9.3)
- **Grading** is based on cell differentiation:
  - Grade 1: Cells remain well differentiated (cancer is low grade)
  - Grade 2: Cells remain moderately differentiated (cancer is moderate grade)
  - Grade 3: Cells are poorly differentiated (cancer is high grade)

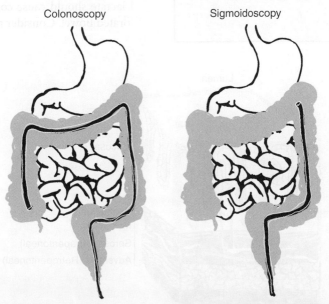

Colonoscopy   Sigmoidoscopy

Fig 9.5 Colonoscopy Versus Sigmoidoscopy. (Illustrated by Hollie Blaber.)

Differentials: IBS, IBD, diverticular disease
Management:
- **Preoperative:** neoadjuvant radiotherapy may be offered to downsize tumours that have not spread, and neoadjuvant chemotherapy may be offered to patients with disease spread. Chemotherapy regimens often involve one or more of fluorouracil, capecitabine and oxaliplatin
- **Surgical resection:** type of surgery depends on the location and spread (see Table 9.4 and Fig 9.7)
- **Postoperative:** adjuvant chemotherapy may be considered in patients with disease spread
- **Symptom control:**
  - Analgesia, laxatives, iron supplementation

TABLE 9.3		**TNM Staging**			
T	**Tumour**	**N**	**Nodes**	**M**	**Metastasis**
Tx	Cannot be assessed	Nx	Cannot be assessed	Mx	Cannot be assessed
T0	No evidence	N0	No evidence	M0	No evidence
T1	Invades submucosa	N1	1–3 regional nodes	M1	Distant metastasis
T2	Invades muscularis propria	N2	4 or more regional nodes		
T3	Invades subserosa				
T4	Invades other tissues				

- Stenting may be considered for patients with obstructing rectal or sigmoid tumours
- Defunctioning stomas may also be considered for patients with recurrent obstructions

Bowel Obstruction

Definition: a mechanical obstruction of the bowel lumen that may be partial or complete. Typically categorised into a small bowel obstruction (SBO) or a large bowel obstruction (LBO) because the level of the obstruction influences the symptoms.
Buzzwords:
- **Risk factors:** previous surgery and presence of **adhesions**, intra-abdominal malignancy, hernias, IBD, volvulus
- **Presentation:** absolute constipation, nausea, vomiting, colicky abdominal pain, abdominal distention, loss of appetite, bowels sounds are typically active and may be described as 'tinkling'
  - SBO: nausea and vomiting occur early, while absolute constipation (no flatus) occurs later
  - LBO: absolute constipation (no flatus) occurs early, while nausea and vomiting occur later
- **Complications:** if the patient is in pain out of proportion to the presentation, consider a perforation/ischaemia
Investigations:
- **Bloods:** may be normal. ↑ inflammatory markers and ↑ lactate should cause concern for strangulated/perforated bowel. Consider pre-operative bloods

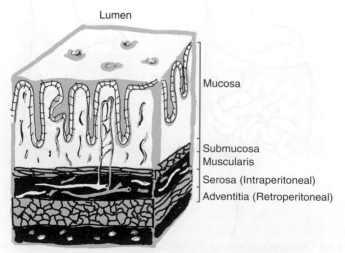

Lumen

Mucosa

Submucosa
Muscularis

Serosa (Intraperitoneal)

Adventitia (Retroperitoneal)

Fig 9.6 Lumen of the Colon. (Illustrated by Dr Hollie Blaber.)

TABLE 9.4   Surgical Procedures for Colon Cancer

Surgery	Procedure	Indications
Right hemicolectomy	Surgical resection from terminal ileum to hepatic flexure. Bowel ends are then joined (anastomosis) and, in rare cases, a temporary stoma is created. Reversal of the stoma may occur at a later stage.	Caecal tumours, ascending colon tumours and some transverse colon tumours (if transverse colon is resected, the surgical procedure is called an extended right hemicolectomy)
Extended right hemicolectomy	Surgical resection from the terminal ileum to the proximal part of the descending colon. Bowel ends are then joined (anastomosis), and, in rare cases, a temporary stoma is created. Reversal of the stoma may occur at a later stage.	
Left hemicolectomy	Surgical resection of the descending colon. Bowel ends are then joined (anastomosis), and, in rare cases, a temporary stoma is created. Reversal of the stoma may occur at a later stage.	Descending colon tumours
Hartmann's procedure	Emergency surgical resection of the sigmoid colon and upper rectum. An end colostomy (colonic stoma) is created, and a rectal stump is left.	Sigmoid colon tumours
Anterior resection of the rectum	Surgical resection of the upper rectum, mesorectum and regional lymphatics via the anterior abdominal wall. Bowel ends are then joined (anastomosis). A defunctioning loop ileostomy may be performed to allow for healing of the anastomosis.	High rectal tumours **without** invasion of the anal sphincter
Abdominoperineal resection	Surgical resection of the sigmoid colon, rectum and anus. After surgical resection, a permanent end colostomy is formed	Low rectal tumours **with** invasion of the anal sphincter

- **Abdominal X-ray (AXR):** evidence of dilated bowel loops (see Radiology in an Hour)
  - SBO: continuous valvulae conniventes across the lumen, may be centrally located
  - LBO: haustra do not cross the width of the lumen, may be more peripheral
- **Erect CXR:** presence of air under the diaphragm with perforations
- **CT abdomen and pelvis:** level of obstruction (used increasingly early in current UK practice)

Differentials: ileus, toxic megacolon, gastroenteritis, ischaemic bowel

Management:
- 'Drip and suck': maintenance IV fluids ('drip'), nil by mouth (NBM) and NG tube insertion ('suck')
- Correct electrolyte imbalances and fluid resuscitate
- Surgery may be indicated, especially if there is suspicion of a perforation or a failure of conservative measures to resolve. Can often be avoided in patients in

whom an obstruction (typically of the small bowel) is caused by adhesions from previous surgery, as most improve with conservative therapy
- For patients with malignancies, stenting may be indicated or, if not possible, surgical defunctioning (i.e., forming a stoma with a loop of bowel that is above the site of obstruction) may be indicated

Volvulus

Definition: rotation of the gut on its mesentery (the length of which increases with age, particularly for the sigmoid colonic mesentery), typically occurring in the sigmoid or caecum. A sigmoid volvulus is more common than a caecal volvulus

Buzzwords:
- **Risk factors:** elderly, chronic constipation, an unusually mobile colon, presence of psychiatric illness, neurological disorders (e.g., Parkinson's disease)
- **Presentation:** as with an obstruction

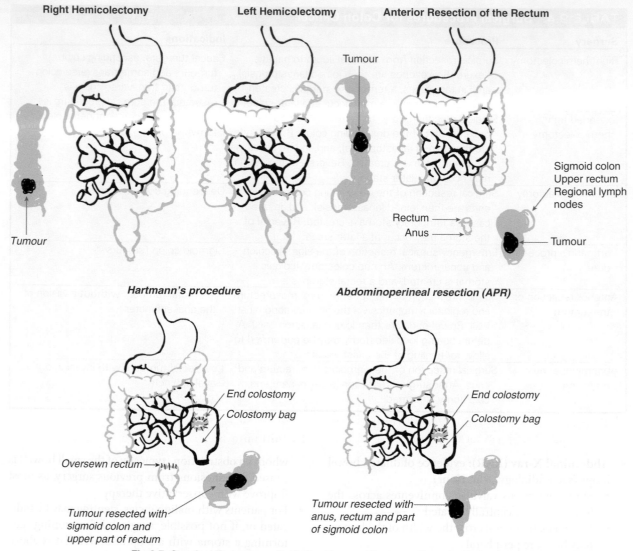

Fig 9.7 Surgical Procedures for Colon Cancer. (Illustrated by Hollie Blaber.)

Investigations:
- **AXR:** dilated large bowel loops (see Radiology in an Hour). Sigmoid volvulus: 'coffee bean' sign
- **Bloods and VBG:** ↑ inflammatory markers, ↑ lactate
- **CT abdomen and pelvis:** level of rotation, presence of whirlpool sign

Differentials: ileus, other causes of obstruction

Management:
- NG tube insertion, fluid and electrolyte replacement +/- urinary catheter for monitoring

- **Sigmoid volvulus:** rigid or flexible sigmoidoscopy +/- flatus tube insertion is usually successful at decompression. If this fails or if there is a suspicion of perforation or ischaemia, surgery should be considered
- **Caecal volvulus:** surgery by a limited right hemicolectomy is typically indicated, although a colonoscopy may rarely help
- Elective surgery may be considered to prevent a recurrence of a sigmoid volvulus

Ileus

Definition: a functional obstruction, i.e., no structural blockage (as opposed to a mechanical blockage), caused by a lack of coordinated peristaltic movements within the bowel, preventing its functioning. In the context of a recent surgery, the term ileus or paralytic ileus is used. In those who haven't had a surgery but have developed an 'ileus', the term pseudo-obstruction can be used. Causes include an electrolyte imbalance, severe infection and spinal fractures.

Buzzwords:

- **Risk factors:** abdominal surgery, sepsis, electrolyte derangements, acute illness
- **Presentation:** absolute constipation, typically less associated with pain (as opposed to a mechanical obstruction), abdominal distension, nausea, vomiting, quiet or absent bowel sounds

Investigations:

- **Bloods:** ↑/↔ inflammatory markers, serum electrolytes and micronutrients may be deranged
- **AXR:** nonspecific bowel gas/fluid or appearance of a dilated small or large bowel
- **CT:** No mechanical obstruction

Differentials: obstruction, gastroenteritis

Management:

- **'Drip and suck':** maintenance IV fluids ('drip'), NBM and NG tube insertion ('suck')
- Treat underlying condition (e.g., sepsis, electrolyte disturbances)
- Good analgesia with judicious use of opiates (some evidence that these agents may make an ileus worse, but pain control is most important)

Haemorrhoids

Definition: occurs due to a combination of connective tissue degeneration and vascular congestion, leading to the protrusion of the highly vascular anal cushions into the anal canal. Haemorrhoids are found at positions 3, 7 and 11 around the anus

They are classified based on their relation to the dentate line:

- External haemorrhoids arise **below** the dentate line
- Internal haemorrhoids arise **above** the dentate line and can be further classified by the degree of prolapse, from 1st degree (into the anal canal) to 4th degree (prolapsed and incarcerated)

Buzzwords:

- **Risk factors:** increasing age, constipation, straining to pass stool, heavy lifting, increased intra-abdominal pressure (e.g., chronic cough, pregnancy)
- **Presentation:** blood on wiping, pruritis ani, fresh rectal bleeding that is painless, a sense of incomplete bowel evacuation, pain if a haemorrhoid becomes strangulated

Investigations:

- Clinical diagnosis based on the results of an external and digital rectal examination
- **Bloods:** ↓/↔ Hb
- **Flexible sigmoidoscopy:** to rule out rectal disease

Differentials: anal fissure, proctitis, anorectal abscess

Management:

- Treat constipation with laxatives
- Lifestyle advice: maintaining good hygiene, avoiding straining
- Symptom control: topical preparations (such as steroids) and analgesia
- For prolapsing haemorrhoids: consider rubber band ligation or sclerotherapy
- Haemorrhoidectomy may be considered for grade 4 haemorrhoids

Anal Fissure

Definition: a break in the rectal mucosa associated with severe pain when passing stool and fresh rectal bleeding.

Classification:

- Duration: acute (<6 weeks) or chronic (>6 weeks)
- Cause: primary (no underlying cause) or secondary (an underlying cause, such as constipation, IBD, sexually transmitted infections or rectal cancer)

Buzzwords:

- **Risk factors:** constipation or hard stool, use of opioids, pregnancy, an underlying pathology, such as IBD, HIV or rectal cancer
- **Presentation:** severe pain on passing stool, red blood noted on wiping, a proportion of patients report an intermittent nature to their symptoms. **In children presenting with an anal fissure, always consider abuse**

Investigations:

- Clinical diagnosis based on external examination – no further investigations are usually required

- If an underlying cause is suspected, further investigations may be carried out based on the likely diagnosis

Differentials: haemorrhoids, anorectal abscess, proctitis

Management:

- Symptom control: oral analgesia if pain is prolonged, regular shallow warm baths, and topical lidocaine, GTN or diltiazem ointment may be considered
- Laxatives
- Lifestyle advice: good anal hygiene, avoiding straining, good fluid and fibre intake to encourage soft stools

Perianal Abscess and Fistulae

Definition: a perianal abscess is the term commonly used to describe a group of anatomically distinct locations in which abscesses can form. Perianal, intersphincteric, ischiorectal and supralevator abscesses are typically the result of blocked glands in the anus. The presence of an abscess can increase the risk of fistula formation. Fistulas may also form spontaneously, in the presence of IBD or following a local surgery.

Buzzwords:

- **Risk factors:** DM, smoking, trauma to the area
- **Presentation:** painful swelling and erythema, may see systemic symptoms of infection, such as fever, rigors, tachycardia and general malaise

Investigations:

- Clinical diagnosis based on history and examination
- **Bloods:** ↑ /↔ WCC, ↑ /↔ neutrophils, ↑ /↔ CRP
- **MRI:** may be beneficial to define the anatomy of the abscess or, more commonly, any associated fistulas
- **Rigid sigmoidoscopy** may show the presence of an internal disease (e.g., Crohn's disease) or fistulas

Differentials: perineal abscess, Crohn's disease

Management:

- Analgesia and consider antibiotics for systemic symptoms of infection
- Incision and drainage of abscess
- Fistulas: setons may be used to encourage tract closure
- Good perianal hygiene to prevent reinfection following an incision and drainage

Hernias

Definition: hernias occur when internal structures, usually abdominal contents, protrude through layers of connective tissue or muscle. Hernias can be classified according to whether they can return through their origin (reducible) or not (irreducible). Irreducible hernias may have a restricted blood supply, known as strangulation.

Types of hernia include:

- **Inguinal hernias:** found superolateral to the pubic tubercle and classified as direct or indirect depending on their relationship to the inguinal canal. **Direct hernias** originate **inferomedial** to the inferior epigastric vessels (superficial ring), while **indirect hernias** originate **superolateral** to them (deep ring). Inguinal hernias are the most common type of hernia and are more common in males than females
- **Femoral hernias:** arise in the femoral triangle, adjacent to the femoral vessels and inferior to the inguinal ligament. More common in females than males and carry a higher risk of strangulation than inguinal hernias (NB: the most common type of hernia in women is inguinal due to the overall higher incidence)
- **Umbilical hernias:** can be congenital (embryonic or foetal, also called omphaloceles) or acquired, which are termed paraumbilical
- **Incisional hernias:** surgical incisions introduce a point of weakness into the muscle wall/tissue layers, which allows abdominal contents to protrude through
- **Hiatus hernia:** a protrusion of the stomach through the diaphragm into the thorax

Buzzwords:

- **Risk factors:** increasing age, previous surgery, increased intra-abdominal pressure (e.g., in pregnancy), strenuous lifting
- **Presentation:** lump on the abdominal wall or groin, may be associated with a positive cough impulse, pain if strangulated. If bowel is involved, may cause features of a bowel obstruction

Investigations:

- Diagnosis is typically clinical and based on the history and examination
- **USS or CT** (if there are concerns about hernia contents): may show bowel loops being trapped or obstructed if inside the hernia

Differentials: lymphadenopathy, undescended testis, scrotal pathology (e.g., hydrocele), sebaceous cyst

Management:

- Conservative treatment/watchful waiting for small and reducible hernias that are asymptomatic
- Surgery: typically involves placing a mesh or reinforcing the abdominal wall. The urgency of the situation depends on the size of the hernia and if there's associated pain or signs of strangulation

Peritonitis

Definition: a common feature of an 'acute abdomen', peritonitis occurs when the visceral or parietal peritoneum becomes inflamed. Peritonitis can be primary (occurs spontaneously) or secondary to trauma/iatrogenic insult (e.g., following surgery) or an internal pathology (e.g., perforated diverticulum or appendix).

Buzzwords:

- **Risk factors:** recent surgery, known diverticular disease, IBD, known gallstones, history of peptic ulcer disease
- **Presentation:** tense and painful abdomen, may be distended, may show involuntary guarding.
  - **Systemic features:** tachycardia, fever, shock

Investigations:

- **Bloods:** ↑ WCC, ↑ CRP
- **Venous Blood gas:** ↑ lactate may indicate underlying ischaemia
- **CT abdomen and pelvis:** may identify an underlying pathology

Differentials: acute appendicitis, acute diverticulitis, acute cholecystitis, any acute intra-abdominal pathology

Management: treat the underlying cause

GI Perforation

Definition: a perforation of the GI tract can occur at any point. Common examples include a perforated appendicitis, perforated diverticulum, perforated peptic ulcer, ischaemic colitis or a perforated gallbladder.

Buzzwords:

- **Risk factors:** underlying condition (e.g., diverticulitis, acute appendicitis, peptic ulcer disease, IBD), chronic NSAID use, recent surgery, malignancy, endoscopy, ischaemic colitis, bowel obstruction, foreign body
- **Presentation:** abdominal pain, may be associated with vomiting, peritonitis, guarding. May have associated signs of sepsis (e.g., fevers, rigors, shock)

Investigations:

- **Bloods:** ↑ WCC, ↑ CRP
- **VBG:** an elevated lactate may indicate underlying sepsis/septic shock, leading to hypoperfusion of tissue and a switch to anaerobic metabolism and lactic acid production
- **CT abdomen and pelvis:** to identify the point of perforation and any associated pathologies

Differentials: acute appendicitis, acute diverticulitis, acute cholecystitis, any acute intra-abdominal pathology (e.g., SBO – rare as a spontaneous cause)

Management:

- Analgesia and antibiotics
- Localised perforation: some perforations may be localised by the omentum/location within the abdomen. These can sometimes be monitored and may be treated with antibiotics
- Surgery: the perforated segment of bowel is typically removed, with the location of the perforation dictating the type of procedure. May involve stoma formation (potentially with a goal of reversing the stoma in the future)

Ischaemic Colitis

Definition: a reduction in the blood supply to a segment of the intestine, leading to inflammation and ulceration of the mucosa. The degree of injury depends on the duration of the period of hypoperfusion. Watershed areas within the bowel are particularly susceptible (e.g., the splenic flexure (place of overlap between superior and inferior mesenteric arteries)).

Buzzwords:

- **Risk factors:** embolic disease (e.g., atrial fibrillation (AF)), atherosclerosis, conditions with a reduced cardiac output, surgeries such as aortic aneurysm repair, hypovolaemia, lifestyle factors (e.g., smoking, hypercholesterolaemia)
- **Presentation:** pain, usually colicky in nature, and associated with diarrhoea and rectal bleeding. On examination, there may be guarding in the affected region. Onset is gradual (hours) as opposed to mesenteric ischaemia (sudden onset). Systemic features can include tachycardia, hypotension, shortness of breath.

Investigations:
- **Bloods:** ↑ WCC, ↑ CRP
- **VBG:** an elevated lactate can indicate underlying ischaemia with a metabolic acidosis
- **CT with contrast:** may show areas of inflammation and mucosal thickening. May see reduced contrast enhancement (if hypoperfusion is ongoing) or the site of vascular obstruction
- **Colonoscopy:** mucosal inflammation +/- ulceration. Areas of haemorrhage may be present
- **ECG:** may show AF

Differentials: AAA, mesenteric angina, acute abdominal pathology

Management:
- Treat underlying cause
- **Surgery:** indicated in patients with peritonitis or an ongoing haemorrhage who are unlikely to respond to conservative management. Typically involves resection and stoma formation.
- **Conservative management:** antibiotic therapy, nutritional support (patients may be kept NBM)

Acute Mesenteric Ischaemia

Definition: a sudden decrease in the blood flow to the intestines leading to tissue death and a systemic inflammatory response. Includes:
- Arterial embolus/thrombus: may be seen with AF and valvular endocarditis
- Mesenteric venous thrombosis: caused by hypercoagulable states, malignancy, intra-abdominal infection
- Non-occlusive mesenteric ischaemia: caused by hypotension (hypovolaemic and cardiogenic shock), digitalis, cocaine

Buzzwords:
- **Risk factors:** atherosclerosis, AF, myocardial infarction, infective endocarditis, increasing age, smoking, structural heart defects
- **Presentation:** diffuse, severe, colicky or constant, poorly localised pain. Later signs include rebound tenderness and guarding. Other signs include melaena, haematochezia (PR blood) and diarrhoea. Pain out of proportion to clinical findings is a characteristic of acute mesenteric ischaemia (AMI). A real challenge is that the signs aren't specific and are often variable in their severity over time. This condition

should be actively considered because it is readily missed

Investigations:
- **VBG:** metabolic acidosis, ↑ lactate
- **Bloods:** ↑ WCC, amylase/lipase (to rule out pancreatitis)
- **AXR:** thumb-printing sign (mucosal oedema)
- **Erect CXR:** to assess for pneumoperitoneum (see Radiology in an Hour)
- ***CT angiogram*:** thrombus/embolus

Differentials: appendicitis, ascending cholangitis/acute cholecystitis, AAA, pancreatitis, diverticulitis, ruptured ectopic pregnancy, testicular torsion, perforated viscus, IBD

Management:
1. A–E management with fluid replacement, NG tube (catheterise, keep NBM) and IV broad-spectrum antibiotics. IV unfractionated heparin unless contraindicated may be considered – a senior doctor decision
2. Diagnostic laparoscopy may help. If ischaemia is seen during an exploratory laparotomy, resection of non-viable bowel +/- revascularisation of bowel if appropriate

Prognosis: mortality is between 60%–100% for AMI. A missed diagnosis results in a mortality rate of 90%

Short Bowel Syndrome

Definition: a malabsorption disorder that occurs due to a small bowel resection, damage or poor motility. Absorption of different nutrients and vitamins occurs at different sites in the small bowel:
- Duodenum: absorption of iron and minerals
- Jejunum: absorption of carbohydrates, proteins, fat and most vitamins
- Ileum: absorption of bile acids and vitamin B12

Buzzwords:
- **Risk factors:** necrotising enterocolitis, Crohn's disease, malignancy
- **Presentation:** diarrhoea, complications of malnutrition (e.g., peripheral neuropathy in a vitamin B12 deficiency)

Investigations:
- **Bloods:** nutritional deficiencies, electrolyte imbalances
- **Stool sample:** faecal fat test shows excess faecal fat (steatorrhoea)

- **CT abdomen:** short bowel

Differentials: malabsorption disorders (e.g., coeliac disease), poor oral intake (e.g., anorexia nervosa)

Management:

1. Nutritional support
2. Medications:
   - To slow down bowel transit (antimotility drugs): loperamide hydrochloride or codeine phosphate
   - To reduce diarrhoea by binding to unabsorbed bile salts: cholestyramine
   - To reduce gastric acid secretion: omeprazole
   - To promote mucosal growth: teduglutide (GLP-2 analogue)

Vitamin B12 and/or Folate Deficiency

Definition: vitamin B12 and folate are essential elements of haematopoiesis, and deficiencies can manifest as a macrocytic anaemia. Vitamin B12 is absorbed in the ileum, while folate is absorbed in the jejunum. Diseases affecting the small bowel or the production of binding proteins (e.g., intrinsic factor) can affect absorption. Pernicious anaemia, the most common severe cause of a vitamin B12 deficiency, results from autoimmune destruction of parietal cells and reduced intrinsic factor production.

Buzzwords:

- **Risk factors:** pernicious anaemia, Crohn's disease, coeliac disease, terminal ileum resection, medications (e.g., disease-modifying antirheumatic drugs, such as methotrexate, antiepileptics), malnutrition
- **Presentation:** fatigue, pale conjunctiva, confusion, shortness of breath. If the deficiency is severe, symptoms of neuropathy may be present (see Neurology in an Hour)

Investigations:

- **Bloods:** ↓ Hb, ↑ MCV, ↓ vitamin B12/folate
- **Serum anti-intrinsic factor:** may show presence of antibodies indicating pernicious anaemia

Differentials: iron-deficiency anaemia

Management: folic acid for folate deficiency.

Vitamin B12 deficiency management depends on the cause:

- If dietary related, offer dietary advice (sources of vitamin B12 include eggs, meat, dairy, fortified cereals)
- If malabsorption related (i.e., Crohn's, pernicious anaemia), offer regular **hydroxocobalamin injections**

THE ONE-LINE ROUND-UP!

Here are some key words to help you remember each condition/concept.

Upper GI Condition

Achalasia	Progressive dysphagia, manometry
Diffuse oesophageal spasm	Intermittent dysphagia, manometry
Pharyngeal pouch	Halitosis, regurgitation
Oesophageal cancer	Adenocarcinoma, Squamous Cell Carcinoma
Zollinger-Ellison syndrome	MEN1
Gastric cancer	Adenocarcinoma
Oesophageal narrowing	Endoscopy, dysphagia
Hiatus hernia	Rolling or sliding
Obesity	Raised BMI

Hepatobiliary surgery

Hepatocellular carcinoma	Most common primary liver cancer
Cholangiocarcinoma	Primary sclerosing cholangitis
Pancreatic cancer	Insidious-onset obstructive jaundice
Gallstones	5 F's, 3D's, Crohn's disease
Acute cholangitis	Charcot's triad

Lower GI surgery

Appendicitis	Migratory umbilical to RIF pain
Diverticular disease	LIF pain in older people, low-fibre diet
Adenoma	Precancerous lesions
Familial adenomatous polyposis	Hundreds to thousands of polyps
HNPCC	Early-onset colorectal cancer, family history
Peutz-Jeghers syndrome	Paediatric colorectal cancer – hamartomatous polyps with mucosal pigmentation
Juvenile polyposis syndrome	Paediatric colorectal cancer – hamartomatous polyps
Colorectal cancer	Rectal bleeding, weight loss, Duke's classification
Bowel obstruction	Absolute constipation with bowel sounds
Volvulus	Coffee bean sign in sigmoid volvulus
Ileus	Absolute constipation with absent bowel sound
Haemorrhoids	Fresh blood on wiping
Anal fissure	Severe, sharp pain on defecating

Continued

THE ONE-LINE ROUND-UP!—Cont'd

Perineal abscess and fistulae	Incision and drainage
Hernias	Reducible, irreducible or strangulated
Peritonitis	Acute abdomen
GI perforation	Peritonitic, septic
Ischaemic colitis	Hypoperfusion, inflammation
Acute mesenteric ischaemia	Pain out of proportion
Short bowel syndrome	Malabsorption
Vitamin B12/folate deficiency	Fatigue, supplementation, malabsorption

READING LIST: GENERAL SURGERY IN AN HOUR

Upper GI Surgery
Achalasia
Patient info. (2016). *Achalasia*. http://www.patient.info. [Accessed February 2021].

BMJ Best Practice. *Achalasia*. http://www.bestpractice.bmj.com. [Accessed February 2021].

Diffuse Oesophageal Spasm
Patient info. (2014). *Oesophageal spasm*. http://www.patient.info. [Accessed February 2021].

Pharyngeal Pouch
Patient info. (2019). *Pharyngeal pouch*. http://www.patient.info. [Accessed July 2021].

NICE. (2003). *IPG22: Endoscopic stapling of pharyngeal pouch*. http://www.nice.org.uk. [Accessed July 2020].

Oesophageal Cancer
NICE. (2020). *Oesophago-gastric cancer: assessment and management in adults*. https://www.nice.org.uk/guidance/ng83. [Accessed April 2021].

Patient info. Oesophageal cancer. http://www.patient.info. [Accessed February 2021].

Zollinger-Ellison Syndrome
Patient info. (2014). *Zollinger-Ellison syndrome*. http://www.patient.info. [Accessed July 2020].

BMJ Best Practice. (2020). *Zollinger-Ellison syndrome*. http://www.bestpractice.bmj.com. [Accessed February 2021].

Gastric Cancer
Patient info. (2017). *Gastric cancer*. http://www.patient.info. [Accessed February 2021].

BMJ Best Practice. (2020). *Stomach cancer*. http://www.bestpractice.bmj.com. [Accessed February 2021].

Oesophageal Narrowing
Patient info. (2017). *Oesophageal strictures, rings and webs*. http://www.patient.info. [Accessed February 2021].

Hiatus Hernia
Patient info. (2020). *Hiatus hernia*. http://www.patient.info. [Accessed July 2020].

BMJ Best Practice. *Hiatus hernia*. http://www.bestpractice.bmj.com. [Accessed February 2021].

Obesity
NICE Guidelines. (2014). *CG189: Obesity: Identification, assessment and management*. https://www.nice.org.uk/guidance/cg189. [Accessed March 2021].

Patient info. (2015). *Obesity in adults*. http://www.patient.info. [Accessed March 2021].

Patient info. (2015). *Bariatric surgery*. http://www.patient.info. [Accessed March 2021].

Hepatobiliary Surgery
Hepatocellular Carcinoma
British Society of Gastroenterology. (2003). *Guidelines for the diagnosis and treatment of hepatocellular carcinoma (HCC) in adults*. http://www.bsg.org.uk. [Accessed July 2020].

Patient info. (2015). *Primary liver cancer*. http://www.patient.info. [Accessed July 2020].

British Liver Trust. *Liver cancer*. http://www.britishlivertrust.org.uk. [Accessed July 2020].

MD Calc. *Child-Pugh score for cirrhosis mortality*. http://www.mdcalc.com. [Accessed July 2020].

MC Calc. *MELD score (model for end-stage liver disease) (12 and older)*. http://www.mdcalc.com. [Accessed July 2020].

BMJ Best Practice. *Hepatocellular carcinoma*. http://www.bestpractice.bmj.com. [Accessed February 2021].

Cholangiocarcinoma
Khan, S. A., Davidson, B. R., Goldin, R. D., et al. (2012). Guidelines for the diagnosis and treatment of cholangiocarcinoma: An update. *Gut, 61*, 1657–1669.

National Cancer Institute. *Bile duct cancer (cholangiocarcinoma) treatment (PDQ®)*. http://www.cancer.gov. [Accessed Oct 2020].

Cancer Research. *Bile duct cancer*. http://www.cancerresearchuk.org. [Accessed Oct 2020].

BMJ Best Practice. *Cholangiocarcinoma*. http://www.bestpractice.bmj.com. [Accessed February 2021].

Pancreatic Cancer
NICE Guidelines. *Pancreatic cancer in adults*. http://www.nice.org.uk. [Accessed Oct 2020].

BMJ Best Practice. (2021). *Pancreatic cancer*. http://www.bestpractice.bmj.com. [Accessed February 2021].

Gallstones

NICE. (2019). *CKS: Gallstones*. http://www.nice.cks.uk. [Accessed October 2020].

BMJ Best Practice. (2021). *Cholelithiasis (gallstones)*. http://www.bestpractice.bmj.com. [Accessed February 2021].

Acute Cholangitis

BMJ Best Practice. (2020). *Acute cholangitis*. http://www.bestpractice.bmj.com. [Accessed March 2021].

Pancreatitis

NICE. (2016). *CKS: Pancreatitis – Acute*. http://www.cks.nice.org.uk. [Accessed March 2021].

NICE Guidelines. (2018). *NG104: Pancreatitis*. http://www.nice.org.uk. [Accessed March 2021].

Goodchild, G., Chouhan, M., & Johnson, G. J. (2019). Practical guide to the management of acute pancreatitis. *Frontline Gastroenterology*, *10*, 292–299. [Accessed March 2021].

Jalal, M., Campbell, J. A., & Hopper, A. D. (2019). Practical guide to the management of chronic pancreatitis. *Frontline Gastroenterology*, *10*, 253–260. [Accessed March 2021].

Lower GI Surgery
Appendicitis

BMJ Best Practice. (2020). *Acute appendicitis*. http://www.bestpractice.bmj.com. [Accessed March 2021].

Patient info. (2019). *Appendicitis*. http://www.patient.info. [Accessed March 2021].

Diverticular Disease

Patient info. (2020). *Diverticular disease*. http://www.patient.info. [Accessed February 2021].

BMJ Best Practice. (2021). *Diverticular disease*. http://www.bestpractice.bmj.com. [Accessed February 2021].

Adenomas

BMJ Best Practice. *Colonic polyps*. http://www.bestpractice.bmj.com. [Accessed February 2021].

NICE. *CKS: Bowel screening*. http://www.cks.nice.org.uk. [Accessed February 2021].

Familial Adenomatous Polyposis

BMJ Best Practice. *Familial adenomatous polyposis syndromes*. http://www.bestpractice.bmj.com. [Accessed 2021].

Online Mendelian Inheritance in Man (OMIM). *Familial adenomatous polyposis 1, FAP1*. http://www.omin.org. [Accessed February 2021].

Patient info. *Bowel (colonic) polyps*. http://www.patient.info. [Accessed February 2021].

Hereditary Nonpolyposis Colorectal Cancer (HNPCC)

Genetic and Rare Disease Information Centre (GARD). (2020). *Lynch syndrome*. http://www.rarediseases.info.nih.gov. [Accessed February 2021].

British Society of Gastroenterology. *A brief guide to the management of Lynch syndrome*. http://www.bsg.org.uk. [Accessed February 2021].

Guidelines for the management of hereditary colorectal cancer from the British Society of Gastroenterology (BSG)/Association of Coloproctology of Great Britain and Ireland (ACPGBI)/United Kingdom Cancer Genetics Group (UKCGG). http://gut.bmj.com.

NICE Guidelines. *NG151: Colorectal cancer*. http://www.nice.org.uk. [Accessed February 2021].

Peutz-Jeghers Syndrome

Rare Diseases. *Peutz-Jeghers syndrome*. http://www.rarediseases.org. [Accessed February 2021].

Guidelines for the management of hereditary colorectal cancer from the British Society of Gastroenterology (BSG)/Association of Coloproctology of Great Britain and Ireland (ACPGBI)/United Kingdom Cancer Genetics Group (UKCGG). http://gut.bmj.com.

Jasperson, K., Tuohy, T., Neklason, D., & Burt, R. (2010). Hereditary and familial colon cancer. *Gastroenterology*, *138*, 2044–2058.

Jelsig, A., Qvist, N., Brusgaard, K., Nielsen, C., Hansen, T., & Ousager, L. (2014). Hamartomatous polyposis syndromes: A review. *Orphanet Journal of Rare Diseases*, *9*, 101.

Juvenile Polyposis Syndrome

Jelsig, A., Qvist, N., Brusgaard, K., Nielsen, C., Hansen, T., & Ousager, L. (2014). Hamartomatous polyposis syndromes: A review. *Orphanet Journal of Rare Diseases*, *9*, 101.

Guidelines for the management of hereditary colorectal cancer from the British Society of Gastroenterology (BSG)/Association of Coloproctology of Great Britain and Ireland (ACPGBI)/United Kingdom Cancer Genetics Group (UKCGG). http://gut.bmj.com

Colorectal Cancer

NICE Guidelines. NG151: Colorectal cancer. https://www.nice.org.uk/guidance/ng151. [Accessed March 2021].

Patient info. (2020). *Colorectal cancer*. http://www.patient.info. [Accessed February 2021].

BMJ Best Practice. (2021). *Colorectal cancer*. http://www.bestpractice.bmj.com. [Accessed February 2021].

Cancer Research. Bowel cancer. http://www.cancerresearchuk.org/about-cancer/bowel-cancer. [Accessed February 2021].

Mason, K., Rogers, G., Gimzewska, M., & Qureshi, Z. (2019). *The unofficial guide to surgery: Core operations*.

Bowel Obstruction

Patient info. (2020). *Intestinal obstruction and ileus*. http://www.patient.info. [Accessed March 2021].

Teach Me Surgery. (2020). *Bowel obstruction*. http://www.teachmesurgery.com. [Accessed March 2021].

BMJ Best Practice. (2020). *Small bowel obstruction*. http://www.bestpractice.bmj.com. [Accessed March 2021].

BMJ Best Practice. (2021). *Large bowel obstruction*. http://www.bestpractice.bmj.com. [Accessed March 2021].

Volvulus

Patient info. (2020). *Intestinal obstruction and ileus*. http://www.patient.info. [Accessed March 2021]

Patient info. (2015). *Volvulus and midgut malrotations*. http://www.patient.info. [Accessed March 2021].

BMJ Best Practice. (2021). *Large bowel obstruction*. http://www.bestpractice.bmj.com. [Accessed March 2021].

Teach Me Surgery. (2021). *Volvulus*. http://www.teachmesurgery.com. [Accessed March 2021].

Ileus

Patient info. (2020). *Intestinal obstruction and ileus*. http://www.patient.info. [Accessed March 2021].

BMJ Best Practice. (2019). *Ileus*. http://www.bestpractice.bmj.com. [Accessed March 2021].

Haemorrhoids

NICE. *CKS: Haemorrhoids*. http://www.cks.nice.org.yk. [Accessed February 2021].

BMJ Best Practice. *Haemorrhoids*. http://www.bestpractice.bmj.com. [Accessed February 2021].

Anal Fissure

NICE. *CKS: Anal fissure*. http://www.cks.nice.org.uk. [Accessed February 2021].

BMJ Best Practice. *Anal fissure*. http://www.bestpractice.bmj.com. [Accessed February 2021].

Patient info. (2017). *Anal fissure*. http://www.patient.info. [Accessed February 2021].

Perineal Abscess and Fistulae

Teach Me Surgery. (2020). *Anorectal abscess*. http://www.teachmesurgery.com. [Accessed February 2021].

Sahnan, K., Adegbola, S., Tozer, P., Watfah, J., & Phillips, R. (2017). Perianal abscess. *BMJ, 356*, j475.

Hernias

Patient info. *Femoral hernias*. http://www.patient.info. [Accessed February 2021].

Patient info. *Inguinal hernias*. http://www.patient.info. [Accessed February 2021].

Patient info. *Abdominal wall hernias*. http://www.patient.info. [Accessed February 2021].

BMJ Best Practice. *Inguinal hernia in adults*. http://www.bestpractice.bmj.com. [Accessed February 2021].

Peritonitis

NHS UK. *Peritonitis*. http://www.nhs.uk. [Accessed February 2021].

Medscape. (2021). *Peritonitis and abdominal sepsis*. http://www.emedicine.medscape.com. [Accessed February 2021].

Parsons, P., Wiener-Kronish, J., Berra, L., & Stapleton, R. (2013). *Critical care secrets E-book* (5th ed.). Elsevier, 352–357.

GI Perforation

Parsons, P., Wiener-Kronish, J., Berra, L., & Stapleton, R. (2013). *Critical care secrets E-book* (5th ed.). Elsevier, 352–357.

Medscape. (2020). *Intestinal perforation*. http://www.emedicine.medscape.com. [Accessed February 2021].

Ischaemic Colitis

Parsons, P., Wiener-Kronish, J., Berra, L., & Stapleton, R. (2013). *Critical care secrets E-book* (5th ed.). Elsevier, 352–357.

Trotter, J., Hunt, L., & Peter, M. (2016). Ischaemic colitis. *BMJ, 355*, j6600.

Acute Mesenteric Ischaemia

BMJ Best Practice. (2020). *Ischaemic bowel disease*. https://bestpractice.bmj.com/topics/en-gb/3000223. [Accessed March 2021].

Patient info. (2019). *Bowel ischaemia*. https://patient.info/doctor/bowel-ischaemia. [Accessed March 2021].

Short Bowel Syndrome

National Institute of Diabetes and Digestive and Kidney Diseases (NIDDK). (2015). *Short bowel syndrome*. http://www.niddk.nih.gov. [Accessed November 2020].

BNF. *Short bowel syndrome*. www.bnf.nice.org.uk. [Accessed November 2020].

Nightingale J, Woodward JM; Small Bowel and Nutrition Committee of the British Society of Gastroenterology. Guidelines for management of patients with a short bowel. *Gut*. 2006;55 (Suppl. 4):iv1-iv12. https://doi.org/10.1136/gut.2006.091108. [Accessed November 2020].

Vitamin B12 and/or Folate Deficiency

NICE. *CKS: Anaemia: B12 and folate deficiency*. http://www.cks.nice.org.uk. [Accessed February 2021].

10

Gastroenterology in an Hour

*Berenice Aguirrezabala Armbruster, Luke Rutter,
Ruth Perkins and Jonathan Tyrrell-Price*

OUTLINE

ORAL DISORDERS

Oral Hairy Leucoplakia

Definition: mucosal membrane disorder characterised by the formation of white patches on the tongue border
Buzzwords:
* **Risk factors:** immunosuppressed, Epstein-Barr virus (EBV) infection
* **Presentation:** painless, white plaques on the side of the tongue that **cannot be scraped off** with a tongue blade (see Fig 10.1)
Investigations: clinical diagnosis
Differentials: traumatic (frictional keratosis), oral candidiasis, oral lichen planus, oral leucoplakia, malignancy
Management: spontaneous resolution in most cases (consider why patient is immunosuppressed if no known condition)
* If treatment considered: topical antivirals or topical podophyllin resin 25% solution or topical retinoic acid

Aphthous Ulcers

Definition: mucosal membrane disorder characterised by recurrent small, round, red ulcers
Buzzwords:
* **Risk factors:** female, non-smoker, high socioeconomic status, age <40 years, inflammatory bowel disease ((IBD) Crohn's), vitamin B12 deficiency
* **Presentation:** painful, round ulcer with a halo around it located anywhere in the mouth (see Fig 10.2)
Investigations: clinical diagnosis

Differentials: primary herpetic gingivostomatitis, traumatic ulcer, malignant ulcer
Management:
1. Avoid triggers, such as coffee, chocolate, peanuts, gluten-containing foods
2. If interfering with daily activities, consider topical corticosteroids +/- topical anaesthetics/antiinflammatories/antimicrobials

Oral Candidiasis

Definition: an oral overgrowth of the normal commensal *Candida*
Buzzwords:
* **Risk factors:** age extremes, immunosuppression, drugs (e.g., antibiotics, corticosteroids), underlying endocrine disorder (e.g., diabetes mellitus (DM), hypothyroidism, Addison's disease), poor dental hygiene, trauma, smoking, malnutrition
* **Presentation:** painless, white/yellow plaques located anywhere in the mouth that **can be scraped off** (see Fig 10.3)
Investigations: clinical diagnosis
Differentials: oral hairy leucoplakia, oral lichen planus
Management: topical antifungal treatment for 7 days
* Children and adults: miconazole PO
* HIV positive: fluconazole PO

Oral Lichen Planus

Definition: inflammation of the oral mucosa of unknown cause

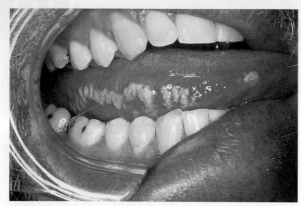

Fig 10.1 Oral Hairy Leucoplakia. (With permission from Callen J.P., et al. (2017). *Dermatological signs of systemic disease* (5th ed.). Philadelphia: Elsevier.)

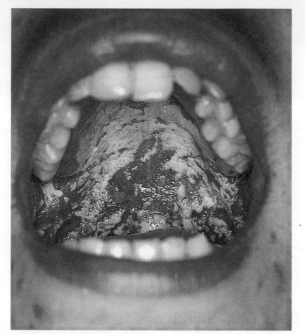

Fig 10.3 Oral Candidiasis. (With permission from Swash, M., & Glynn, M (2007). *Hutchison's clinical methods* (Fig. 27.8), (22nd ed.). Elsevier Ltd.)

- **Topical treatment for severe cases:** topical anaesthetics, topical steroids
- **Systemic treatment if no improvement:** oral corticosteroids

UPPER GASTROINTESTINAL DISORDERS

Gastrooesophageal Reflux Disease

Definition: excessive reflux of gastric contents into the oesophagus causing symptoms and/or complications

Buzzwords:
- **Risk factors:** increased intra-abdominal pressure (e.g., pregnancy, obesity), drugs (e.g., nonsteroidal antiinflammatory drugs (NSAIDs), steroids, bisphosphonates), smoking, alcohol, hiatus hernia
- **Presentation:** dyspepsia (upper abdominal pain or discomfort, heartburn, gastric reflux, nausea or vomiting)
  - Red-flag symptoms of an upper gastrointestinal (GI) malignancy (**ALARM mnemonic**): **A**naemia, **L**oss of weight, **A**norexia, **R**ecent progressive dysphagia, **M**elaena or haematemesis

Investigations:
- *Heliobacter pylori* test (if no ALARM symptoms present)

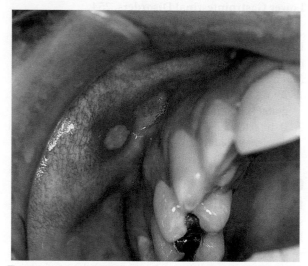

Fig 10.2 Aphthous Ulcers. (With permission from Bolognia, J., et al. (2018). *Dermatology* (4th ed.). Philadelphia: Elsevier.)

Buzzwords:
- **Risk factors:** chronic hepatitis C infection (rare), female >40 years of age
- **Presentation:** white, lacy pattern on the cheeks and tongue (see Fig 10.4). Asymptomatic (if mild) or a stinging sensation when eating

Investigations: clinical diagnosis

Differentials: traumatic (frictional keratosis), oral hairy leucoplakia, oral leucoplakia, oral candidiasis, lichenoid reaction

Management:
- **Mild cases:** no treatment required

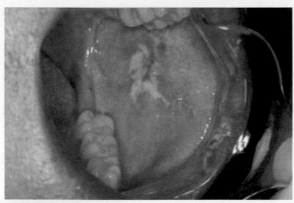

Fig 10.4 **Oral Lichen Planus**. (With permission from Olson, M. A., Rogers, R. S.,& Bruce, A. J. (2016). Oral lichen planus (Fig. 10.2). In *Clinics in dermatology*. Elsevier. © 2016 Elsevier Inc. All rights reserved.)

- **Endoscopy** (if ALARM symptoms present): findings are normal in 60% of cases (do NOT exclude GORD if normal), 30% show oesophagitis and 10% show Barrett's oesophagus. Speed of referral:
  - 2 week–wait (2WW) referral if there is dysphagia **OR** an upper abdominal mass consistent with cancer **OR** age is >55 years with weight loss and one of the following symptoms: upper abdominal pain, reflux or dyspepsia
  - Urgent referral if melaena or haematemesis
  - Nonurgent referral if anaemia or anorexia
- **Ambulatory reflux monitoring** (if endoscopy is normal): 24-hour pH catheter or a wireless pH capsule showing a low pH

Differentials: peptic ulcers, functional dyspepsia, Barrett's oesophagus

Management:
- **Noninvestigated dyspepsia:**
  1. One month of full-dose proton pump inhibitor (PPI) **or** *H. pylori* test and treat
  2. Switch to alternative strategy (e.g., *H. pylori* test and treat if 1 month of PPI has been tried)
  3. Reassess for any new ALARM symptoms and consider histamine 2–receptor antagonist (H$_2$RA)
  4. Step-down approach: prescribe PPI/H$_2$RA at lowest effective dose
  5. If symptoms improve, prescribe PPI at lowest effective dose and carry out annual reviews
- **Erosive GORD on endoscopy:**
  1. Two months of full-dose PPI. Do not arrange *H. pylori* test
  2. One further month of PPI at same dose or a doubled dose. Alternatively, add H$_2$RA

3. Step-down approach: use PPI/H$_2$RA at lowest effective dose
4. Step-up approach (8 weeks of high-dose PPI) or switch to alternative PPI for 8 weeks
5. If symptoms improve, prescribe PPI at lowest effective dose and carry out annual reviews
- **Nonerosive GORD on endoscopy:**
  1. One month of full-dose PPI
  2. Switch to H$_2$RA (e.g., ranitidine)
  3. Referral for a second opinion
  4. If symptoms improve, prescribe PPI at lowest effective dose and carry out annual reviews

Barrett's Oesophagus

Definition: premalignant lesion in which the **squamous epithelium** of the oesophagus is replaced by **columnar epithelium**. These lesions can progress to adenocarcinoma.

Buzzwords:
- **Risk factors:** chronic GORD, hiatus hernia, obesity, smoking, alcohol
- **Presentation:** dyspepsia symptoms

Investigations:
- **Endoscopy with multiple biopsies:** to visualise metaplasia and obtain histological confirmation

Differentials: GORD, peptic ulcers, functional dyspepsia

Management:
- **Low-grade dysplasia:** surveillance and biopsy every 6 months
- **Flat high-grade dysplasia:** endoscopic ablation (radiofrequency/photodynamic)
- **Localised high-grade dysplasia:** endoscopic mucosal resection
- **Diffuse high-grade dysplasia:** oesophagectomy

Peptic Ulcers

Definition: peptic ulcers refer to both gastric and duodenal ulcers confirmed by endoscopy.

Buzzwords:
- **Risk factors:**
  - **Gastric ulcers:** *H. pylori*, drugs (e.g., NSAIDs, aspirin, bisphosphonates, potassium supplements, steroids, selective serotonin reuptake inhibitors (SSRIs), crack cocaine)
  - **Duodenal ulcers:** *H. pylori* is a greater risk factor for duodenal ulcers than gastric ulcers
- **Presentation** (both): bleeding, pain, perforation
  - **Gastric ulcers:** pain is worst after eating – hint: think where acid is going to be at these times to cause pain
  - **Duodenal ulcers:** pain improves after eating and drinking milk

Investigations:

- ***H. pylori* test (if no ALARM symptoms):** urea ($_{13}$C) breath test **OR** stool *Helicobacter* antigen test (SAT). *H. pylori* test should **not** be performed within 2 weeks of PPI use or within 4 weeks of antibacterial treatment
- **Endoscopy (if ALARM symptoms):** to visualize the ulcer

Differentials: GORD, Barrett's oesophagus, functional dyspepsia

Management:

- ***H. pylori* positive:**
  - Regular treatment: 7 days of PPI + amoxicillin + clarithromycin or metronidazole
  - Penicillin allergy: 7 days of PPI + clarithromycin + metronidazole
  - Retesting for *H. pylori* is not usually performed unless there is an associated GI disorder (e.g., peptic ulcer or MALT lymphoma), persistent symptoms or poor compliance
- ***H. pylori* negative:** 4–8 weeks of full-dose PPI

HEPATOBILIARY DISORDERS

Jaundice

Definition: a yellow discoloration of the skin caused by bilirubin accumulation in tissues. Bilirubin is a byproduct created by the breakdown of haemoglobin in red blood cells. Normally, bilirubin is conjugated in the liver and then excreted via the common bile duct into the duodenum and ultimately excreted from the body via the faeces and urine (see Fig 10.5). Jaundice can be classified as:

- **Prehepatic jaundice:** haemolysis exceeds the ability of the liver to conjugate bilirubin
  - **Causes:** haemolytic anaemia, drugs, malaria, Gilbert's syndrome, Crigler-Najjar syndrome
- **Hepatic jaundice:** impaired conjugation **OR** impaired excretion of conjugated bilirubin because of a liver disease compressing the **intrahepatic** bile ducts
  - **Causes:** hepatitis (viral and autoimmune), alcohol misuse, liver malignancy, hereditary disorders leading to hepatitis (e.g., haemochromatosis, alpha-1 antitrypsin (AAT) deficiency, Wilson's disease), Dubin-Johnson syndrome, Rotor's syndrome, drugs (e.g., paracetamol, statins, antibiotics)
- **Posthepatic jaundice:** impaired excretion of conjugated bilirubin because of an extrahepatic biliary disease preventing the bilirubin from entering the duodenum
  - **Causes:** gallstones, pancreatic/bile duct malignancy, autoimmune (e.g., primary biliary cholangitis (PBC) and primary sclerosing cholangitis (PSC)), cholestatic drugs (e.g., antibiotics)

Abnormal Liver Function Test

Liver function tests (LFTs) include:

- **Alanine aminotransferase (ALT):** enzyme mainly found in the liver
- **Alkaline phosphatase (ALP):** enzyme found in the bile ducts, bone and placenta
- **Aspartate aminotransferase (AST):** enzyme found in the liver, heart and muscles

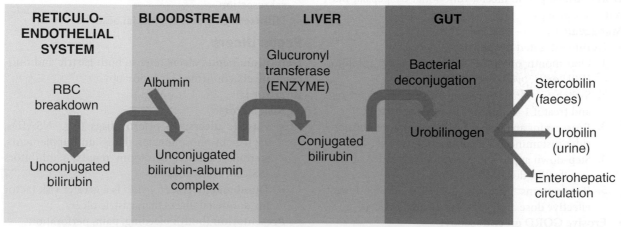

Fig 10.5 Bilirubin-processing Pathway. *RBC*, Red blood cell. (Adapted from Tsai, M.-T.; Tarng, D.-C. (2019). Beyond a measure of liver function – bilirubin acts as a potential cardiovascular protector in chronic kidney disease patients. *International Journal of Molecular Sciences, 20,* 117.)

- **Albumin:** most abundant protein found in the blood. Prevents fluid leakage from blood vessels. Decreased in liver disease, kidney disease and inflammatory conditions. Increased in dehydration
- **Total protein:** measures all proteins found in the blood. Decreased in liver diseases, bone marrow failure, kidney disease. Increased in malignancies or dehydration (if albumin is low and total protein is high, think multiple myeloma)
- **Total bilirubin:** measures both conjugated and unconjugated bilirubin
- **Unconjugated bilirubin:** distinguishes between pre- and posthepatic jaundice

Other useful blood tests to help differentiate between causes:

- **Gamma glutamyl transferase (GGT):** raised in liver and bile duct diseases but not bone diseases. Useful to request when the ALP is raised but the cause could be either a bone or bile duct disease
- **Alkaline phosphatase isoenzymes:** differs based on where the ALP is being produced
- **Creatinine kinase (CK):** useful to request when the AST is raised but the cause is unknown
  - CK-MB: enzyme found in heart muscle mainly
  - CK-BB: enzyme found in brain tissue mainly
  - CK-MM: enzyme found in skeletal muscle mainly
- **Troponin:** useful to request when the AST is raised but the cause is unknown. There are three types:
  - Skeletal muscle troponin C (TnC)
  - Cardiac troponin T (cTnT)
  - Cardiac troponin I (cTnI)

See Tables 10.1-10.3 for a summary of expected results in hepatobiliary disorders.

TABLE 10.2 Findings in Acute Hepatocellular Damage, Chronic Hepatocellular Damage and Cholestasis

Test	Acute Hepatocellular Damage	Chronic Hepatocellular Damage	Cholestasis
ALT	↑↑	Normal or ↑	Normal or ↑
ALP	Normal or ↑	Normal or ↑	↑↑
GGT	Normal or ↑	Normal or ↑	↑↑
Bilirubin	↑ or ↑↑	Normal or ↑	↑↑

ALP, Alkaline phosphatase; ALT, alanine aminotransferase; GGT, gamma glutamyl transferase.

TABLE 10.3 Key Tests for Hepatobiliary Disease

Test (+ Hx and Exam)	Disease
ALT>ALP, GGT, coagulation	Alcohol-related liver disease
LFTs +/- FibroScan/ enhanced liver fibrosis score/biopsy	Nonalcoholic fatty liver disease
Hepatitis serology-HBsAg	Hepatitis B
HCV/HAV Ab	Hepatitis C/A
Viral screen	Acute viral hepatitis
AMA, IgM	Primary biliary cholangitis
ASMA, ANA, A-LKM, IgG	Autoimmune hepatitis
P-ANCA	Primary sclerosing cholangitis
Alpha-1 antitrypsin	Alpha-1 antitrypsin deficiency
Ceruloplasmin	Wilson's disease
Ferritin	Haemochromatosis

A-LKM: Anti-liver kidney microsomal antibody; ALP, alkaline phosphatase; ALT, alanine aminotransferase; AMA, antimitochondrial antibody; ANA, antinuclear antibody; ASMA, antismooth muscle antibody; GGT, gamma glutamyl transferase; HAV, hepatitis A virus; HBsAG, hepatitis B surface antigen; HCV, hepatitis C virus; LFT, liver function test.

TABLE 10.1 Findings in Prehepatic, Hepatic and Posthepatic Jaundice.

	Prehepatic	Hepatic	Posthepatic
ALT or AST	Normal	↑↑	↑
ALP or GGT	Normal	↑	↑↑
Total bilirubin	↑	↑	↑
Unconjugated bilirubin	↑↑	Normal or ↑	Normal
Stool and urine	Normal	Normal stools Dark urine	Pale stools Dark urine

ALP, Alkaline phosphatase; ALT, alanine aminotransferase; AST, aspartate aminotransferase; GGT, gamma glutamyl transferase.

Hepatitis A

Definition: liver inflammation caused by the hepatitis A (HAV) RNA virus

- **Transmission:** faecal-oral route, ingestion of water/ food contaminated with faeces, oral-anal sex with infected individual
- **Incubation period:** 14–28 days
- **Vaccination:** available

Buzzwords:
- **Risk factors:** see transmission
- **Presentation:** fever, malaise, loss of appetite, diarrhoea, nausea, abdominal discomfort, dark-coloured urine, jaundice

Investigations:
- **Viral serology:** detects antibodies (IgM and IgG) against HAV (see Table 10.4)
  - HAV IgM antibodies are detectable 5 days after symptom onset and remain present for 60 days
  - HAV IgG antibodies are detectable 5–10 days after symptom onset and persist for life
- **Blood:** hepatic picture (ALT>ALP), prolonged prothrombin time (PT)

Differentials: other viral hepatitides, drug/alcohol-induced liver disease, autoimmune hepatitis

Management: HAV is a notifiable disease
- **Supportive:** painkillers (avoid paracetamol), antiemetics, chlorphenamine for pruritus
- **Monitor for complications:** relapses (15%), fulminant liver disease (0.4%)

Prognosis: full recovery in 6 months in most cases with lifelong immunity. HAV infection does not cause chronic liver disease

Hepatitis B

Definition: viral infection by the hepatitis B (HBV) DNA virus, which leads to liver inflammation

- **Transmission:** infected blood, bodily fluids, such as needle sharing, childbirth, sex
- **Incubation:** 75 days on average
- **Vaccination:** available

Buzzwords:
- **Risk factors:** see transmission
- **Presentation:** flu-like illness, malaise +/- jaundice

Investigations:
- **Viral serology:** detects antibodies against HBV and the presence of antigen (viral protein) (see Table 10.5)
  - **Hepatitis B surface antigen (HBsAg):** indicates infection. If present for <6 months, it indicates acute infection. If present for >6 months, it indicates chronic infection
  - **Antibodies against hepatitis B surface antigen (anti-HBs):** appear 3 months after an infection **or** after vaccination
  - **IgM antibodies against hepatitis B core antigen (anti-HBc IgM):** indicates acute infection
  - **IgG antibodies against hepatitis B core antigen (anti-HBc IgG):** made after IgM antibodies and indicates a previous or chronic infection
  - **Hepatitis B envelope antigen (HBeAg):** indicates a high level of replication and that an individual is highly infectious. HBeAg indicates active viral replication
  - **HBV DNA:** represents the viral load and is used to monitor treatment

Differentials: other viral hepatitides, drug/alcohol-induced liver disease, autoimmune hepatitis

Management: HBV is a notifiable disease
- **Acute infection:** supportive care
- **Chronic infection:** antivirals (e.g., tenofovir, entecavir)
- **Monitor for complications:** cirrhosis (8%–20% without treatment), hepatocellular carcinoma (HCC)

Hepatitis C

Definition: viral infection by the hepatitis C (HCV) RNA virus, which leads to liver inflammation. Classified

TABLE 10.4   Hepatitis A Virus (HAV) Serology

	ACTIVE INFECTION	PREVIOUS INFECTION	VACCINATED INDIVIDUAL
HAV IgM	Positive	Negative	Negative
HAV IgG	Positive	Positive	Positive

TABLE 10.5   Hepatitis B Serology

	ACUTE INFECTION	CHRONIC INFECTION	VACCINATED INDIVIDUAL	PREVIOUS INFECTION
HBsAg	Present	Present	Absent	Absent
Anti-HBs	Absent	Absent	Present	Present
Anti-HBc IgM	Present	Absent	Absent	Absent
Anti-HBc IgG	Absent	Present	Absent	Present

into an acute phase (symptoms <6 months) and chronic phase (symptoms >6 months)

- **Transmission:** main route is parenteral (e.g., infected blood, needlestick injury, sharing needles). Also, vertical transmission (from mother to child) and sexual transmission.
- **Incubation period:** 2 weeks to 6 months
- **Vaccine:** <u>NOT</u> available

Buzzwords:

- **Risk factors:** see transmission
- **Presentation:** asymptomatic (80%), fatigue, fever, decreased appetite, nausea and vomiting, abdominal pain, jaundice, dark urine, pale stools, joint pain

Investigations:

- **Hepatitis serology:** detects antibodies against hepatitis C (anti-HCV)
  - Presence of anti-HCV indicates a previous infection
  - A positive nucleic acid test for HCV RNA confirms a chronic infection

Differentials: other viral hepatitides, drug/alcohol-induced liver disease, autoimmune hepatitis

Management: HCV is a notifiable disease. Referral to Gastroenterology for further care

- **If treatment required:** direct-acting antiviral (DAA) treatment for 12–24 months
- **Monitoring of complications:** cirrhosis, HCC

Prognosis: spontaneous resolution occurs in 15%–45% of patients

Hepatitis D

Definition: only found in conjunction with HBV, as it requires HBV for its replication cycle. This infection can be acquired at the same time as HBV (coinfection) or later (superinfection). A coinfection is more likely to be cleared in immunocompetent individuals. More common in Western and Central areas of Africa

- **Transmission:** bloodborne virus
- **Incubation period:** 3–7 weeks
- **Vaccine:** no specific vaccine. (Vaccination against HBV protects against HDV by extension)

Buzzwords:

- **Risk factors:** unprotected sex with an infected partner, needle sharing, infected mother, not vaccinated against HBV
- **Presentation:** may be asymptomatic, fatigue, right upper quadrant (RUQ) pain, jaundice, nausea, vomiting. Infection with HDV often increases the rate at which people with HBV progress to liver failure

Investigations: hepatitis D antigen, hepatitis B serology

Differentials: other viral hepatitides, autoimmune hepatitis, drug-induced hepatitis

Management:

- Largely supportive
- Pegylated interferon alpha
- Liver transplantation if required
- Advise on precautions, such as safe sex, needle sharing, risk of transfer during birth (vertical transmission is uncommon). For partners, vaccination against HBV prevents HDV infection

Hepatitis E

Definition: liver inflammation caused by the hepatitis E (HEV) RNA virus

- **Transmission:** faecal-oral route, ingestion of contaminated water/food, consumption of undercooked meat or meat products (main reservoir in pigs), transfusion of infected blood, vertical transmission (from mother to child)
- **Incubation period:** 2–10 weeks
- **Vaccine:** <u>NOT</u> available

Buzzwords:

- **Risk factors:** second/third trimesters of **pregnancy** significantly increases the mortality rate (up to 25% death rate) from HEV, also see Transmission section
- **Presentation:** jaundice, dark urine, pale stools, nausea, vomiting, fatigue, abdominal pain

Investigations:

- **Hepatitis serology:** detects antibodies (IgM) against HEV. Anti-HEV IgM antibodies indicate **active** infection

Differentials: other viral hepatitides, drug/alcohol-induced liver disease, autoimmune hepatitis

Management: HEV is a notifiable disease

- **Provide reassurance:** self-limiting illness that resolves in 1–4 weeks
- **Monitor for complications** in immunocompromised and pregnant patients (mortality risk)

Nonalcoholic Fatty Liver Disease

Definition: this disorder results from fatty infiltration of the liver and is an increasingly common cause of chronic liver disease. This condition can only be diagnosed after exclusion of alcohol-related liver disease (ARLD). Inflammation with a history of nonalcoholic fatty liver disease (NAFLD) is known as nonalcoholic steatohepatitis (NASH), which is associated with an increased risk of progression to cirrhosis and potentially HCC.

- Exclusion of ARLD:
  - Males: <30 g (or 3.75 units)/day of alcohol
  - Females: <20 g (or 2.5 units)/day of alcohol
- Complications:
  - Cardiovascular disease: common cause of death in patients with NAFLD
  - Impaired glucose regulation
  - Cirrhosis leading to portal hypertension and the formation of varices and ascites
  - HCC

Buzzwords:
- **Risk factors:** metabolic syndrome (diabetes, hyperlipidaemia, hypertension, central obesity), metabolic conditions (e.g., polycystic ovarian syndrome), medications (e.g., steroids, amiodarone, methotrexate), refeeding syndrome, gastric bypass surgery
- **Presentation:** slow onset with fatigue, malaise, generalised abdominal discomfort. Hepatomegaly may be palpable (NB: in cirrhosis, the liver shrinks), and there may be signs of cirrhosis, including spider naevi, ascites and caput medusa

Investigations:
- **Bloods:** ↑↑ ALT
- **Ultrasound scan (USS) abdomen:** fatty infiltration of the liver
- **FibroTest:** reduced elasticity within the liver
- **Liver biopsy:** assesses the level of inflammation and fibrosis, excludes other conditions
- **Assessment scores:** NAFLD Fibrosis Score (NFS), Fibrosis-4 (FIB-4), Enhanced Liver Fibrosis (ELF)

Differentials: ARLD, viral hepatitis
Management:
- Aim is to limit progression. Lifestyle modification advice, including cardiovascular risk stratification, diet and alcohol advice and gradual weight loss. Monitor for development of complications
- Advanced fibrosis: consider off-licence treatments, such as pioglitazone and vitamin E (only for secondary care)
- Liver transplantation

Alcohol-related Liver Disease

Definition: liver damage as a result of long-term, excessive alcohol consumption. Disease progresses through three stages, from steatosis to hepatitis/inflammation to cirrhosis. ALD typically has a chronic onset. However, as the disease progresses, patients may present with episodes of acute decompensation.

Buzzwords:
- **Risk factors:** excessive alcohol consumption, female, concurrent HCV infection
- **Presentation:** generalised abdominal pain and fatigue, may have associated weight loss, hepatomegaly and other features of chronic liver disease (e.g., ascites, spider naevi, caput medusa)
  - **Acute decompensation:** jaundice, ascites, encephalopathy, sepsis, GI bleeding

Investigations:
- **Bloods:** ↑ AST/ALT, ↓ albumin/total protein, anaemia, associated infection, ↑ INR, deranged U&Es
- **Liver screen:** varies but typically includes hepatitis serology, iron studies, antimitochondrial antibody (AMA), antinuclear antibody (ANA), antismooth muscle antibody (ASMA), caeruloplasmin, AAT level
- **USS liver:** fatty infiltration or cirrhosis, direction of flow in the portal vein, presence of ascites
- **CT:** cirrhosis of the liver, presence of complications
- **Ascitic tap** (if ascites): to determine the serumascites albumin gradient (SAAG) (see Table 10.6)
- **Scoring systems:** Maddrey's discriminant function identifies patients with acute decompensation who may benefit from steroids

Differentials: NAFLD, viral hepatitis, cholecystitis
Management:
1. Alcohol cessation, nutritional support and multivitamins (often vitamin B and thiamine)
2. Immunisation: yearly flu vaccine and one-off pneumococcal vaccine
3. Acute management: Pabrinex if ongoing alcohol consumption/concerns about malnutrition, steroids (see Maddrey's score)
4. Treatment of complications: paracentesis for ascites, spontaneous bacterial peritonitis (SBP) prophylaxis
5. Liver transplantation

Liver Cirrhosis

Definition: cirrhosis is a histological diagnosis that represents the end stage of chronic liver disease. It is characterised by widespread hepatocellular fibrosis.
Buzzwords:
- **Risk factors:** chronic liver disease (e.g., NAFLD, ARLD, viral hepatitis)
- **Presentation:** features of portal hypertension, including spider naevi, caput medusa and ascites; features of impaired glucose regulation, such as sarcopenia

Investigations:

- **FibroScan** (transient elastography)
- **Screening for viral hepatitis serology**
- **Screening tools,** such as the ELF and Model of End-stage Liver Disease (MELD) scores
- **Oesophageogastroduodenoscopy (OGD):** screening for varices
- **USS +/- alpha fetoprotein levels:** monitor for HCC

Management:

- **Long term:** low-sodium diet +/- diuretics (e.g., spironolactone and furosemide), treat vitamin deficiencies/malnutrition
- **Acute decompensation:**
  - Lactulose if encephalopathic
  - Human albumin solution (HAS) if in acute kidney injury (AKI)
  - Antibiotics for suspected infections

Ascites

Definition: an accumulation of ascitic fluid in the abdomen. Causes include:

- Portal hypertension secondary to chronic liver disease
- Peritoneal pathologies, such as sarcoidosis, peritoneal mesothelioma, tuberculous peritonitis, GI/genitourinary (GU) malignancies

Buzzwords:

- **Risk factors:** liver cirrhosis, portal hypertension, malignancy, infection, heart/kidney failure, high-salt/low-protein intake can increase the rate of accumulation in those with chronic ascites
- **Presentation:** abdominal distention, discomfort, nausea, vomiting and, in severe cases, dyspnoea

Investigations:

- **Bloods:** FBC, U&E, LFTs, PT, serum albumin
- **Diagnostic paracentesis (i.e., ascitic tap):**
  - **Ascitic fluid albumin:** to calculate the SAAG, which allows for categorisation of the cause of ascites (see Table 10.6)
  - **Ascitic fluid neutrophil count:** to screen for SBP. A neutrophil count >250 cells/mm^3 (0.25×10^9/l) is diagnostic of SBP
  - **Ascitic fluid amylase:** to diagnose pancreatitis ascites. A high ascitic amylase is diagnostic of pancreatic ascites

Management:

1. Identify and treat cause
2. Dietary salt restriction: no added–salt diet of 90 mmol salt/day (5.2 g salt/day)

TABLE 10.6 **Serum-Ascites Albumin Gradient (SAAG)**

SAAG >11 g/L (High Gradient)	SAAG <11 g/L (Low Gradient)
Cirrhosis	Malignancy
Cardiac failure	Pancreatitis
Nephrotic syndrome	Tuberculosis

3. Spironolactone (100 mg/day initially to a dose of 400 mg/day)
4. If spironolactone is unsuccessful, add furosemide (160 mg/day)
5. Therapeutic paracentesis if large and symptomatic or if medical management with HAS replacement has been unsuccessful (typically 1 unit per 2 L drained)
6. Consider a transjugular intrahepatic portosystemic shunt in patients with refractory ascites who require very frequent paracenteses

Spontaneous Bacterial Peritonitis

Definition: an infection of ascitic fluid in the absence of an intra-abdominal or surgically treatable source. This condition is thought to result from haematogenous spread of bacteria into ascitic fluid. The pathogens are more commonly intestinal pathogens (such as *Escherichia coli*). Intestinal colonisation is thought to occur by translocation, a process made more likely by cirrhosis. Non-intestinal sources include respiratory and urinary tract infections

Some common pathogens include *E. coli* (most common), *Klebsiella pneumoniae*, *Staphylococcus aureus* and *Streptococcus pneumonia*.

Buzzwords:

- **Risk factors:** liver cirrhosis, infection, recent endoscopy, GI bleed, previous paracentesis
- **Presentation:** abdominal distention, fever, abdominal pain, nausea, vomiting, signs of encephalopathy or confusion

Investigations:

- **Blood:** ↑ WCC, ↑ CRP, monitor U&Es for hepatorenal syndrome in acute decompensation, monitor clotting/LFTs for liver function, cultures
- **Ascitic tap:** cytology (neutrophil count >250 cells/mm^3 is diagnostic), cultures and sensitivity (causative organism)

Differentials: peritonitis secondary to a pathology (e.g., perforation, bowel obstruction, acute cholecystitis). In patients with liver disease and large-volume ascites, SBP is the most likely cause

Management:

1. **IV antibiotics** are the mainstay of treatment (in accordance with local guidelines)
2. Treat any associated features of decompensated liver disease
3. Albumin may be indicated for patients with renal dysfunction
4. Consider a re-tap at 48 h if the patient is not responding to treatment

Long term: prophylactic antibiotics may be considered

Alpha-1 Antitrypsin Deficiency

Definition: genetic disorder characterised by a defective AAT enzyme. AAT is normally made in the liver and travels via the bloodstream to the lungs where it neutralises the enzyme, neutrophil elastase. A defective AAT enzyme is unable to leave the liver (causing liver damage) and is therefore unable to travel to the lungs to exert its actions on neutrophil elastase. When neutrophil elastase is not inhibited, lung inflammation occurs (i.e., paracinar emphysema). Therefore, this disorder is characterised by both liver AND lung damage.

- **Inheritance:** autosomal codominant (one allele is inherited from each parent, both alleles are expressed and slightly different proteins are made, which determines the characteristics of the condition)
- **Gene mutation:** *SERPINA-1* gene on Chromosome 14
- **Protein affected:** AAT enzyme

Buzzwords:

- **Risk factors:** family history
- **Presentation:**
  - **Paracinar emphysema (always present):** dyspnoea, wheezing at age 30–40 years (suspect in young adults with chronic obstructive pulmonary disease (COPD))
  - **Liver disease (late sign – not always present):** hepatitis, cirrhosis

Investigations:

- **Blood:** ↓ serum AAT (<10 micromol/L)
- **Spirometry:** obstructive picture
- **Chest X-ray (CXR) and high-resolution CT chest (more sensitive than CXR):** paracinar emphysema, basal predominance

- **Consider liver biopsy:** periodic acid-Schiff (PAS)-positive globules
- **Consider genetic testing**

Differentials: COPD, viral hepatitis, drug/alcohol-induced liver disease, autoimmune hepatitis

Management:

1. Smoking cessation
2. Treat COPD symptoms (see Respiratory Medicine in an Hour)
3. Monitor

Note: NICE does not recommend the use of IV recombinant AAT

Hereditary Haemochromatosis

Definition: genetic disorder characterised by an excessive absorption of iron from the diet due to a defective hepcidin hormone. Hepcidin normally controls iron absorption from the diet, and a defective hepcidin leads to iron overload. There is no biochemical pathway to rid the body of this excess iron except through blood loss

- **Inheritance:** autosomal recessive
- **Gene mutation:** *HFE* gene (C282Y and H63D) on Chromosome 6
- **Protein affected:** Hepcidin

Buzzwords:

- **Risk factors:** family history, northern European
- **Presentation: usually presents in males 30-40 years old**
  - Early symptoms: fatigue, abdominal pain, arthralgia, erectile dysfunction
  - Late symptoms: bronze pigmentation, type 1 DM (T1DM), hepatomegaly, cirrhosis, arrhythmias, cardiomyopathy, mood disturbances, memory impairment

Investigations:

- **Blood:** high serum iron concentration **AND** high transferrin saturation
- **Genetic testing**
- **Liver MRI:** reduced organ signal
- **Liver biopsy (rarely performed): Perls' Prussian blue**-positive deposits in the liver

Differentials: excessive dietary intake, blood transfusions, liver disease

Management:

1. Dietary advice: avoid an iron-rich diet, reduce alcohol intake
2. Regular venesection

3. Iron chelation therapy (desferrioxamine mesylate) if venesection is not possible
4. Genetic counselling
5. Consider liver transplantation for end-stage disease

Wilson's Disease

Definition: a genetic disorder characterised by abnormal copper deposition in organs due to a defective copper-transporting ATPase 2 protein, which is normally responsible for the elimination of copper from the body.

- **Inheritance:** autosomal recessive
- **Gene mutation:** *ATP7B* gene on Chromosome 13
- **Protein affected:** ATPase 2 protein

Buzzwords:
- **Risk factors:** family history
- **Presentation:** symptom onset between 6–45 years but most commonly during the teenage years. Mnemonic: **COPPER AAA**
  - **C**irrhosis
  - **O**steopenia
  - **P**arkinsonism (symmetrical)
  - **P**sychiatric disease: psychosis, hallucinations, personality changes
  - **E**yes: Kayser-Fleischer rings (see Fig 10.6), sunflower cataracts
  - **R**enal failure
  - **A**bdominal Pain, **A**rthritis, **A**scites
  - +/- Fanconi anaemia

Investigations:
- **Slit-lamp examination** (repeated annually): Kayser-Fleischer rings (present in 50% of cases)
- **Blood:** LFTs deranged
- **CT and MRI** to determine organ damage
- **Liver biopsy** to determine the level of copper in the liver
- Other tests mentioned in the literature that are not very specific for Wilson's disease include:
  - 24-hour urinary copper excretion. Usually present but not always
  - Low serum caeruloplasmin (<0.1 g/L). Serum caeruloplasmin is an acute-phase protein (like ferritin). Therefore, it will be elevated during inflammation

Differentials: liver disease (e.g., hepatitis, cirrhosis), psychiatric disease (e.g., psychosis), neurological disease (e.g., Parkinson's disease, dementia)

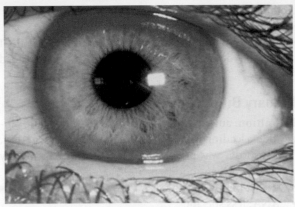

Management:
- Dietary advice: avoid foods that are high in copper content
- Lifelong penicillamine +/- zinc acetate
- Consider liver transplantation for severe liver disease

Autoimmune Hepatitis

Definition: Autoantibodies to the liver leading to chronic inflammation and cirrhosis if left untreated. This condition is caused by the combination of a genetic predisposition and environmental triggers (e.g., drugs, infection). However, most cases have no identifiable precipitant. There are two types of autoimmune hepatitis based on the autoantibodies present:
- **Type 1:** ANA or ASMA
- **Type 2:** liver kidney microsome 1 (LKM-1) or anti-liver cytosolic-1 (LC-1) antibodies

Buzzwords:
- **Risk factors:** female, other autoimmune disorders
- **Presentation:** fatigue, anorexia, weight loss, nausea, vomiting, joint pain, amenorrhoea. Type 2 presents with more severe disease than type 1

Investigations:
- **Blood:** hepatic picture (ALT or AST>ALP), autoantibodies present (e.g., ANA, ASMA, LKM-1 or LC-1)
- **Liver biopsy** to confirm diagnosis

Differentials: viral hepatitis

Management:
- Prednisolone +/- azathioprine
- If a decision is made to not treat, monitor the patient for the development of symptoms and deranged LFTs

Primary Biliary Cholangitis

Definition: autoantibodies against the intrahepatic biliary ducts leading to **intrahepatic bile duct destruction.** This disorder was previously known as primary biliary cirrhosis. Autoantibodies include:
- **AMA:** highly specific
- **ANA:** less specific

Buzzwords:
- **Risk factors:** female, age 50 years, other autoimmune conditions (especially coeliac, thyroid disease, Sjögren's syndrome)
- **Presentation:** fatigue, jaundice, pruritus, ascites, abdominal pain, xanthelasmas (yellow deposits around the eyes), xanthomas (yellow deposits under the skin)

Investigations:
- **Blood:** cholestatic picture (ALP or GGT>ALT or AST), AMA autoantibodies present (highly specific), ANA autoantibodies present (less specific)
- **Liver biopsy** (ONLY if bloods show cholestatic picture and no autoantibodies are present): granulomas
- **Abdominal USS +/- magnetic resonance cholangiopancreatography** (MRCP) to exclude gallstones

Differentials: gallstones, liver disease

Management:
- Lifelong ursodeoxycholic acid and follow-up
- If inadequate response to ursodeoxycholic acid, add obeticholic acid
- Supportive treatment: cholestyramine for pruritus
- Liver transplantation

Primary Sclerosing Cholangitis

Definition: an autoimmune disorder characterised by intrahepatic and/or extrahepatic bile duct destruction and scarring

Buzzwords:
- **Risk factors:** male, 32–41 years of age, inflammatory bowel disease (IBD) (particularly ulcerative colitis (UC))
- **Presentation:** initially asymptomatic. Symptoms develop late and include abdominal pain, jaundice, pruritus, fatigue, fever and weight loss

Investigations:
- **Blood:** cholestatic picture (ALP or GGT>ALT or AST)
- **MRCP:** to confirm diagnosis. Biliary tree has a beaded appearance
- **Liver biopsy** (ONLY if an unclear diagnosis or if PSC/PBC-overlap syndrome is suspected): onion peel scarring

Differentials: gallstones, liver disease

Management:
- Ursodeoxycholic acid: improves liver biochemistry but there is no evidence that it improves outcomes
- Supportive treatment: cholestyramine for pruritus
- Screen for oesophageal varices
- Endoscopic balloon dilatation

LOWER GASTROINTESTINAL DISORDERS
Malnutrition

Definition: a state of nutritional imbalance, most commonly involving protein, micronutrient and energy intake. This condition includes overnutrition (obesity) and undernutrition. While commonly associated with children, undernutrition is also prevalent in elderly and hospitalised individuals. Overnutrition is associated with an increased risk of noncommunicable diseases. Other states of malnutrition may be related to micronutrients, which typically impacts pregnant females and children, who have higher micronutrient requirements/hormone production.

Buzzwords:
- **Risk factors:** disorders of absorption (e.g., coeliac disease, Crohn's disease); disordered eating (e.g., anorexia, bulimia); chronic infections (e.g., HIV); states of increased metabolic activity (e.g., excessive exercise, cancer), prematurity in babies
- **Presentation:** largely depends on the type of malnutrition present but often includes fatigue, cognitive impairment, stunted growth in children, wasting, oedema, increased susceptibility to infection, impaired wound healing
- **Complications:** refeeding syndrome – monitor fluid balance, glucose levels, phosphate, magnesium and potassium

Investigations:
- **Body mass index (BMI) assessment** (18.5–25 kg/m² = normal range). For babies and children, accurate growth-chart plotting

- **Malnutrition Universal Screening Tool** (MUST)
- Assess **percentage of weight loss** (if applicable)
- **Blood tests:** assess all micronutrients (e.g., vitamin B12, folate, iron, Ca, PO_4, Mg, albumin, vitamin D), thyroid function tests (TFTs), coeliac screen

Differentials: conditions with an increased metabolic demand (e.g., malignancy), conditions of malabsorption (e.g., coeliac disease), depression, dementia

Management:
- Treat any underlying conditions
- Dietician review and nutritional supplementation
- Monitor for refeeding syndrome

Coeliac Disease

Definition: small bowel inflammation triggered by gluten exposure in genetically predisposed individuals. Gluten is a protein found in wheat, barley and rye

Buzzwords:
- **Risk factors:** genetics (HLA-DQ2.5 shows a very strong association), gluten exposure
- **Presentation:**
  - **Malabsorption:** diarrhoea, steatorrhea, weight loss, failure to thrive
  - **Other symptoms:** anaemia, neuropathy, ataxia, depression, osteomalacia, osteoporosis, short stature, lymphoma, liver disease, dermatitis herpetiformis

Investigations:
- **Blood whilst on gluten-rich diet:** IgA-EMA, tissue transglutaminase (TTG) or IgG-DGP present
- **Stool sample** (to rule out other differentials): infective organism (present in gastroenteritis), faecal calprotectin (present in IBD along with other inflammatory processes within the bowel)
- **Duodenal biopsy** whilst on a gluten-rich diet: villous atrophy
- **Genetic testing** is only done if coeliac disease is suspected but the patient fails to respond to a gluten-free diet.
- **HLA-DQ2.5** is positive in ≥90%
- **HLA-DQ8** is positive in ~10%
  - If HLA-DR2.5/8 negative, you can rule out coeliac disease. A positive HLA test on its own is not enough to diagnose coeliac disease

Differentials: gastroenteritis, irritable bowel syndrome (IBS), IBD

Management: gluten-free diet

Crohn's Disease

Definition: a chronic, relapsing-remitting inflammatory disease of the GI tract. IBD is an umbrella term used to describe three main disorders: Crohn's disease, UC (see Table 10.7) and IBD unclassified (if a definitive diagnosis of Crohn's disease or UC cannot be made). Crohn's disease is thought to be caused by an environmental trigger in a genetically susceptible individual.

Buzzwords:
- **Risk factors:** smoking is a risk factor (as opposed to in UC for which smoking is protective), family history, infectious gastroenteritis, appendicectomy, drugs (e.g., NSAIDs, combined oral contraceptive pills)
- **Presentation:**
  - **GI manifestations:** generalised abdominal pain, vomiting, diarrhoea, tenesmus, faecal urgency, +/- mucus in stool, +/- blood in stool
  - **Extra-GI manifestations related to disease activity:** pauci-articular arthritis (≤four joints affected), erythema nodosum, aphthous mouth ulcers, episcleritis, metabolic bone disease, clubbing

TABLE 10.7	**Crohn's Disease vs Ulcerative Colitis**	
	Crohn's Disease	**Ulcerative Colitis**
Affected site(s) in GI tract	Anywhere from mouth to anus	Only colon and rectum
Lesions	• Skip lesions • Cobblestone appearance (see Fig 10.7) • Full thickness of intestinal wall affected	• Continuous lesions • Pseudopolyps • Only intestinal mucosa affected
Complications	Fistula Adhesions Abscess Malignancy anywhere in the GI tract	Toxic megacolon Perforation Obstruction Colorectal carcinoma

GI, Gastrointestinal.

- **Extra-GI manifestations not related to disease activity:** axial arthritis, polyarticular arthritis, pyoderma gangrenosum, psoriasis, uveitis, hepatobiliary conditions (e.g., PSC, pericholangitis, steatosis, autoimmune hepatitis, cirrhosis, gallstones)
- **In children:** weight loss, faltering growth or delayed puberty

Investigations:
- **Blood:** ↓ Hb, ↑ CRP, malabsorption (↓ ferritin/vitamin B12/folate/vitamin D/albumin)
- **Blood (to rule out other differentials):** IgA-EMA/ TTG/ IgG-DGP (present in coeliac disease)
- **Stool sample:** ↑ faecal calprotectin (>200 μg/g)
- **Stool sample (to rule out other differentials):** infective organism (may be present in gastroenteritis), increased risk of *Clostridium difficile*
- **Endoscopy + biopsy:** cobblestone appearance (see Fig 10.7), full thickness of intestinal wall affected
- **CT/MRI/barium studies:** to identify complications, such as fistulas, obstruction, abscesses
- **Colonoscopy:** to monitor for risk of malignancy

Differentials: UC, coeliac disease, infective gastroenteritis, IBS

Management:
Inducing remission:
1. **Monotherapy:**
   - **First line:** corticosteroids (PO prednisolone, PO methylprednisolone or IV hydrocortisone)
   - **Second line:** budesonide (particularly for mild–to-moderate terminal ileal disease)
   - **Third line:** aminosalicylates (e.g., mesalazine or sulfasalazine)
2. **Add-on therapy:** consider if there have been ≥2 inflammatory episodes in the last 12 months or the glucocorticoid dose cannot be tapered. Test thiopurine methyltransferase (TPMT) activity first
   - **If TPMT activity is normal:** offer glucocorticoid or budesonide + **normal-dose thiopurine drug** (e.g., azathioprine or mercaptopurine)
   - **If TPMT activity is reduced:** offer glucocorticoid or budesonide + **low-dose thiopurine drug** (e.g., azathioprine or mercaptopurine)
   - **If TPMT activity is deficient:** offer glucocorticoid or budesonide + **methotrexate**
3. **Biological agents** (e.g., infliximab or adalimumab) as monotherapy or combination therapy if previous steps fail

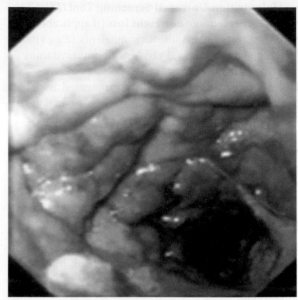

Fig 10.7 Cobblestone Appearance in Crohn's Disease (Lichtenstein, G. R. (2020). Inflammatory bowel disease (Fig. 132.1). In *Goldman-Cecil Medicine, 2-volume Set.* Elsevier. Copyright © 2020 Elsevier Inc. All rights reserved.)

Maintenance of remission:
- **First line:** thiopurine drug (e.g., azathioprine or mercaptopurine)
- **Second line:** methotrexate

Ulcerative Colitis

Definition: IBD affecting the rectum and colon to a variable extent (see Fig 10.8):
- **Ulcerative proctitis** (common in adults): inflammation of the rectum only
- **Left-sided colitis:** inflammation of the rectum, sigmoid colon and descending colon
- **Extensive pancolitis** (common in children): inflammation of the entire colon

Buzzwords:
- **Risk factors:** family history, drugs (e.g., NSAIDs), no appendectomy, not smoking
- **Presentation:**
  - **GI manifestations:** generalised abdominal pain, diarrhoea, tenesmus, faecal urgency, blood in stools
  - **Extra-GI manifestations related to disease activity:** same as Crohn's disease with the addition of venous thromboembolism

Proctitis   Left sided colitis   Extensive (Pan) colitis

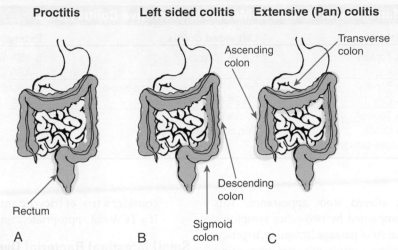

Fig 10.8 Ulcerative Colitis and the Extent of the Condition (A) Proctitis, (B) left-sided colitis and (C) extensive colitis. (Illustrated by Hollie Blaber)

- **Extra-GI manifestations not related to disease activity:** same as Crohn's disease except for psoriasis, which is not common in UC
- **In children:** same as Crohn's disease

Investigations:
- **Bloods:** ↓ Hb, ↑ CRP, malabsorption (low ferritin/vitamin B12/folate/vitamin D/albumin)
- **Blood (to rule out other differentials):** IgA-EMA/TTG/IgG-DGP (present in coeliac disease)
- **Stool sample:** raised faecal calprotectin (>200 µg/g)
- **Stool sample (to rule out other differentials):** infective organism (may be present in gastroenteritis), increased risk of *C. difficile*
- **Endoscopy + biopsy:** pseudopolyps, only mucosa is affected
- **CT/MRI/barium studies:** identifies complications, such as toxic megacolon, obstruction, perforation
- **Monitoring:** blood tests for assessing malnutrition, colonoscopy for risk of malignancy

Differentials: Crohn's disease, coeliac, infective gastroenteritis, IBS

Management:

Manage acute flare: determine severity using Truelove and Witt criteria
- **Mild-to-moderate flare:** corticosteroids and/or aminosalicylates (5-ASA) (e.g., sulfasalazine, mesalazine, Pentasa). Route and choice of drug depends on disease extent (see Table 10.8)
- **Moderate-to-severe flare (all extents of disease):** biologics and Janus-kinase inhibitors

- **Severe flare (all extents of disease):** admit to hospital
  - **First line:** IV corticosteroids for 72 h. If contraindicated, then IV ciclosporin or consider surgery
  - **Second line:** IV corticosteroids + IV ciclosporin. If ciclosporin is contraindicated, then infliximab or consider surgery

Maintenance of remission:
- 5-ASA after a mild-to-moderate flare
- Azathioprine or mercaptopurine oral after a severe episode or if two or more flare-ups have occurred in the last 12 months or if 5-ASA alone is not effective

Irritable Bowel Syndrome

Definition: chronic relapsing disorder characterised by changes in the bowel habits. Classified into four subtypes according to the Rome IV classification system:
- Diarrhoea predominant (IBS-D) – most common
- Constipation predominant (IBS-C)
- Mixed (IBS-M)
- Unclassified (IBS-U)

Buzzwords:
- **Risk factors:** unknown. Possible risk factors include genetics, infection, inflammation, diet, drugs, stress, anxiety, depression
- **Presentation:**
  - **Consider IBS** if at least **6 months** of **A**bdominal pain, **B**loating, **C**hange in bowel habits (**mnemonic 'ABC'**)
  - **Diagnose IBS** if abdominal pain is relieved by defaecation **OR** associated with altered stool

TABLE 10.8   Management of Mild-to-Moderate Ulcerative Colitis Flares

	Proctitis	Left-sided Colitis	Extensive Colitis
STEP 1	5-ASA Topical	5-ASA Topical	5-ASA Topical 5-ASA Oral High Dose
STEP 2	5-ASA Topical 5-ASA Oral	5-ASA Topical or Corticosteroid Topical 5-ASA Oral High Dose	Corticosteroid Topical 5-ASA Oral
STEP 3	5-ASA Topical 5-ASA Oral Corticosteroid Oral or Topical	5-ASA Oral Corticosteroids Oral	

5-ASA, Aminosalicylates.

frequency **OR** altered stool appearance. This should be accompanied by two other symptoms including altered stool passage (straining, urgency, tenesmus), bloating, symptoms worse after eating and mucus in stools.

Investigations:
- **Stool sample (to rule out other differentials):** faecal calprotectin (high in IBD), infective organism (may be present in gastroenteritis)
- **Blood (to rule out other differentials):** coeliac screen, thyroid function disease, inflammatory markers in IBD
- **Abdominal x-ray, USS, colonoscopy (to rule out other differentials):** diverticular disease, gallstones, pancreatitis, malignancy

Differentials:
- **Constipation:** hypothyroidism, drug induced (morphine), malignancy
- **Diarrhoea:** IBD, coeliac disease, infections, hyperthyroidism, drugs (e.g., laxatives, antibiotics), malignancy
- **Abdominal pain:** diverticular disease, gallstones, pancreatitis, peptic ulcer, anxiety

Management:
1. Identify and avoid triggers
2. Dietary changes: high-fibre diet for IBS-C, avoid a high-fibre diet in IBS-D, FODMAP dietary approach
3. Medication:
   - **IBS-D:** loperamide (antimotility drug), trial of gluten-free diet
   - **IBS-C:** laxatives. If unsuccessful, then consider a trial of additional laxatives, such as prucalopride or linaclotide (secretory drug)
   - **Abdominal pain:** antispasmodic drugs, such as mebeverine hydrochloride, alverine citrate or peppermint oil when required. If unsuccessful,

consider a trial of tricyclic antidepressants (TCA). If a TCA not appropriate, consider an SSRI.

Small Intestinal Bacterial Overgrowth

Definition: a condition closely associated with IBS, in which there is an increase in the bacteria of the bowel. This overgrowth alters the dynamics of the gut microbiota and damages the gut mucosa. The pathophysiology is complex but is thought to occur due to a breakdown of the built-in defence mechanisms that normally keep gut bacteria under control, including bile acid/gastric acid/pancreatic enzyme secretion, peristalsis, the intestinal immune system and the presence of valves to prevent retrograde spread.

Buzzwords:
- **Risk factors:** immunodeficiency, motility disorders, chronic pancreatitis, long-term PPI use, intestinal obstruction (leading to stagnation of contents), liver cirrhosis
- **Presentation:** bloating, diarrhoea, anaemia, weight loss, features of malabsorption or malnutrition

Investigations:
- **Blood:** ↓ Hb, vitamin deficiencies, hypocalcaemia
- **Hydrogen breath test:** an increase in exhaled hydrogen following ingestion of glucose or lactulose
- **OGD with jejunal aspirate for culture:** $\geq 10^5$ bacteria/mL

Differentials: IBS, coeliac disease, chronic pancreatitis

Management:
1. Treat any underlying conditions or precipitating factors if possible
2. Nutritional supports: dietary advice, supplementation, may require NG or NJ feeding
3. Antibiotics: avoid long-term, broad-spectrum therapy as this increases the risk of complications like *C. difficile* infection or antibiotic resistance

THE ONE-LINE ROUND-UP!

Here are some key words to help you remember each condition/concept.

Condition/Concept	One-line Description
Oral hairy leucoplakia	Painless, white patches, self-resolving
Aphthous ulcers	Painful, small, round ulcers
Oral candidiasis	Generalised white plaques, can be scraped off
Oral lichen planus	Lace-like, white inflammation of mucosa
GORD	Dyspepsia, ALARM, H. pylori
Barrett's oesophagus	Premalignant change to columnar epithelium
Peptic ulcers	H. pylori, gastric: worse with food, duodenal: better with food
Viral hepatitis	A&E: faeco-oral, B,C&D: blood borne. D only exists with B.
NAFLD	Fatty liver in the absence of alcohol excess
ALD	Fatty/cirrhosed liver with a history of alcohol excess
Cirrhosis	Portal hypertension, increased risk of HCC
Ascites	SAAG
SBP	Ascitic tap and IV antibiotics
Alpha-1-antitrypsin deficiency	Mutation of SERPINA-1, neutrophil elastase build-up, paracinar emphysema

Condition/Concept	One-line Description
Hereditary hemochromatosis	HFE mutation, iron overload, venesection
Wilson's disease	ATPB7 mutation, COPPER AAA
Autoimmune hepatitis	Type 1 (AN/ASMA), Type 2 (LKM-1/LC-1)
Primary biliary cholangitis	Intrahepatic duct destruction, AMA, female
Primary sclerosing cholangitis	Intra or extrahepatic duct destruction, associated with UC, beaded appearance on MRCP
Malnutrition	High refeeding risk
Coeliac disease	HLA DQ2 association, tissue transglutaminase, villous atrophy
Crohn's disease	Mouth to anus, transmural lesions, skip lesions, cobblestone appearance
UC	Colon and rectum, continuous lesions, Truelove and Witts criteria,
IBS	6 months of ABC
SIBO	Bacterial overgrowth, overlap with IBS

READING LIST: GASTROENTEROLOGY IN AN HOUR

Oral disorders
Oral Hairy Leucoplakia
Patient info. (2016). *Leukoplakia*. https://patient.info/doctor/leukoplakia-pro. [Accessed June 2020].

Aphthous Ulcers
NICE. (2017). *CKS: Aphthous ulcers*. https://cks.nice.org.uk/topics/aphthous-ulcer/ [Accessed June 2020].

Oral Candidiasis
NICE. (2017). *CKS: Candida – oral*. https://cks.nice.org.uk/topics/candida-oral/. [Accessed June 2020].

Oral Lichen Planus
British Association of Dermatologists. (2019). *Oral lichen planus*. https://www.bad.org.uk/shared/get-file.ashx-?id=111&itemtype=document [Accessed June 2020].

Upper Gastrointestinal Disorders
GORD
NICE. (2018). *CKS: Dyspepsia*. https://cks.nice.org.uk/topics/dyspepsia-unidentified-cause/ [Accessed June 2020].

BSG. (2020). *Physiology and function in patients with complex gastrointestinal reflux disease*. https://www.bsg.org.uk/web-education-articles-list/physiology-and-function-in-patients-with-complex-gastrointestinal-reflux-disease/ [Accessed November 2020].

Barrett's Oesophagus
NICE. (2018). *CKS: Dyspepsia*. https://cks.nice.org.uk/topics/dyspepsia-unidentified-cause/ [Accessed June 2020].

BSG. (2020). *Physiology and function in patients with complex gastrointestinal reflux disease*. https://www.bsg.org.uk/web-education-articles-list/physiology-and-function-in-patients-with-complex-gastrointestinal-reflux-disease/ [Accessed November 2020].

Patient info. (2017). *Barrett's oesophagus*. https://patient.info/doctor/barretts-oesophagus-pro [Accessed June 2020].

NICE Guidelines. (2019). *Gastro-oesophageal reflux disease and dyspepsia in adults: Investigation and management.* https://www.nice.org.uk/Guidance/CG184 [Accessed June 2020].

NICE Guidance. (2011). *Interventional procedures guidance [IPG407].* https://www.nice.org.uk/Guidance/IPG407 [Accessed June 2020].

Peptic Ulcers And *H. Pylori*

NICE. (2019). *CKS: dyspepsia – proven peptic ulcer.* https://cks.nice.org.uk/topics/dyspepsia-proven-peptic-ulcer/ [Accessed June 2020].

BNF. (2020). *Peptic ulcer disease.* https://bnf.nice.org.uk/treatment-summary/peptic-ulcer-disease.html [Accessed June 2020].

Hepatobiliary disorders

Jaundice

Patient info. (2015). *Jaundice.* https://patient.info/doctor/jaundice-pro [Accessed April 2021].

NICE. (2020). *CKS: Jaundice in adults.* https://cks.nice.org.uk/topics/jaundice-in-adults/ [Accessed April 2021].

Abnormal Liver Function Tests

Patient info. (2015). *Abnormal liver function tests.* https://patient.info/digestive-health/abnormal-liver-function-tests-leaflet [Accessed 2020].

BMJ Best Practice. (2020). *Assessment of liver dysfunction.* https://bestpractice.bmj.com/topics/en-gb/1122 [Accessed March 2021].

Lab Tests Online. https://labtestsonline.org.uk/tests/liver-blood-tests [Accessed March 2021].

Martin, P., & Friedman, L. (2018). Assessment of liver function and diagnostic studies. *Handbook of liver disease*, 1–17 Elsevier.

Hepatitis A, B, C, D, E

NICE. (2021). *CKS: Hepatitis A.* https://cks.nice.org.uk/topics/hepatitis-a/ [Accessed March 2021].

World Health Organization. (2020). *Hepatitis B.* https://www.who.int/news-room/fact-sheets/detail/hepatitis-b [Accessed November 2020].

NICE. (2020). *CKS: Hepatitis B.* https://cks.nice.org.uk/topics/hepatitis-b/ [Accessed November 2020].

World Health Organization. (2020). *Hepatitis C.* https://www.who.int/news-room/fact-sheets/detail/hepatitis-c [Accessed November 2020].

NICE. (2020). *CKS: Hepatitis C.* https://cks.nice.org.uk/topics/hepatitis-c/ [Accessed November 2020].

Booth, J. C. L., O'Grady, J., & Neuberger, J. (2001). Clinical guidelines on the management of hepatitis C. *Gut, 49*, I1–I21.

World Health Organisation. (2020). *Hepatitis D.* https://www.who.int/news-room/fact-sheets/detail/hepatitis-d [Accessed March 2021].

Patient info. (2014). *Viral hepatitis (particularly D and E).* https://patient.info/doctor/viral-hepatitis-particularly-d-and-e [Accessed March 2021].

Centers for Disease Control and Prevention. (2020). *Hepatitis D questions and answers for health professionals.* https://www.cdc.gov/hepatitis/hbv/hbvfaq.htm [Accessed March 2021].

Public Health England. (2014). *Hepatitis E: Symptoms, transmission, treatment and prevention.* https://www.gov.uk/government/publications/hepatitis-e-symptoms-transmission-prevention-treatment/hepatitis-e-symptoms-transmission-treatment-and-prevention [Accessed November 2020].

World Health Organization. (2020). *Hepatitis E.* https://www.who.int/news-room/fact-sheets/detail/hepatitis-e [Accessed November 2020].

Nonalcoholic Fatty Liver Disease

NICE. (2016). *CKS: Non-alcoholic fatty liver disease (NAFLD).* https://cks.nice.org.uk/topics/non-alcoholic-fatty-liver-disease-nafld/ [Accessed February 2021].

BMJ Best Practice. (2019). *Hepatic steatosis.* https://bestpractice.bmj.com/topics/en-gb/796 [Accessed February 2021].

British Society of Gastroenterology. (2020). *NAFLD – diagnosis, assessment and management.* https://www.bsg.org.uk/web-education-articles-list/nafld-diagnosis-assessment-and-management/ [Accessed February 2021].

Alcohol-related Liver Disease

BMJ Best Practice. (2019). *Alcoholic liver disease.* https://bestpractice.bmj.com/topics/en-gb/1116 [Accessed February 2021].

British Society of Gastroenterology. (2014). *BSL – BASL decompensated cirrhosis care bundle – first 24 hours.* https://www.bsg.org.uk/clinical-resource/bsg-basl-decompensated-cirrhosis-care-bundle-first-24-hours/ [Accessed February 2021].

Liver Cirrhosis

British Society of Gastroenterology. (2014). *BSL – BASL decompensated cirrhosis care bundle – first 24 hours.* https://www.bsg.org.uk/clinical-resource/bsg-basl-decompensated-cirrhosis-care-bundle-first-24-hours/ [Accessed February 2021].

NICE Guidelines. (2016). *NG50: Cirrhosis in over 16s: Assessment and management* https://www.nice.org.uk/guidance/ng50 [Accessed March 2021]..

Ascites

Medscape. (2018). *Serum-ascites albumin gradient (SAAG) interpretation.* https://emedicine.medscape.com/article/2172621-overview [Accessed June 2020].

BSG. (2006). *Guidelines on the management of ascites in cirrhosis.* https://www.bsg.org.uk/clinical-resource/guidelines-on-the-management-of-ascites-in-cirrhosis/ [Accessed July 2020].

Spontaneous Bacterial Peritonitis

BMJ Best Practice. (2020). *Spontaneous bacterial peritonitis.* https://bestpractice.bmj.com/topics/en-gb/793 [Accessed February 2021].

Aithal, G. P., Palaniyappan, N., China, L., et al. (2021). Guidelines on the management of ascites in cirrhosis. *Gut, 70,* 9–29.

Alpha-1-Antitrypsin Deficiency

National Center for Advancing Translational Sciences. (2020). *Alpha-1 antitrypsin deficiency.* https://ncats.nih.gov/adst/projects [Accessed November 2020].

BMJ Best Practice. (2020). *Alpha-1 antitrypsin deficiency.* https://bestpractice.bmj.com/topics/en-gb/1075 [Accessed November 2020].

Hereditary Haemochromatosis

British Liver Trust. *Haemochromatosis.* https://britishlivertrust.org.uk/information-and-support/living-with-a-liver-condition/liver-conditions/haemochromatosis/. [Accessed Nov 2020].

Haemochromatosis UK. http://www.haemochromatosis.org.uk. [Accessed Nov 2020].

Fitzsimons, E. J., Cullis, J. O., Thomas, D. W., Tsochatzis, E., & Griffiths, W. J. H. (2018). Diagnosis and therapy of genetic haemochromatosis (review and 2017 update). *Br J Haematol, 181,* 293–303.

Wilson's Disease

Genetics Home Reference. (2020). *Wilson's disease.* https://ghr.nlm.nih.gov/condition/wilson-disease#genes. [Accessed July 2020].

British Liver Trust. https://britishlivertrust.org.uk/information-and-support/living-with-a-liver-condition/liver-conditions/wilsons-disease/. [Accessed July 2020].

Autoimmune Hepatitis

British Society of Gastroenterology. (2011). *Guidelines for management of autoimmune hepatitis.* https://www.bsg.org.uk/clinical-resource/bsg-guidelines-for-the-management-of-autoimmune-hepatitis/ [Accessed July 2020].

Primary Biliary Cholangitis (PBC)

British Society of Gastroenterology. (2018). *UK-PBC primary biliary cholangitis treatment and management guidelines.* https://www.bsg.org.uk/clinical-resource/bsg-and-ukpbc-primary-biliary-cholangitis-treatment-and-management-guidelines/ [Accessed July 2020].

Primary Sclerosing Cholangitis (PSC)

British Society of Gastroenterology. (2019). *UK-PSC guidelines for the diagnosis and management of primary sclerosing cholangitis.* https://www.bsg.org.uk/clinical-resource/bsg-and-uk-psc-guidelines-for-the-diagnosis-and-management-of-primary-sclerosing-cholangitis/ [Accessed July 2020].

Lower Gastrointestinal Disorders
Malnutrition

World Health Organisation. (2020). *Malnutrition.* https://www.who.int/news-room/fact-sheets/detail/malnutrition [Accessed March 2021].

Patient info. (2016). *Malnutrition.* https://patient.info/doctor/malnutrition [Accessed March 2021].

Coeliac Disease

NICE CKS. (2020). *Coeliac disease.* https://cks.nice.org.uk/topics/coeliac-disease/ [Accessed July 2020].

Ludvigsson, J. F., Bai, J. C., Biagi, F., et al. (2014). Diagnosis and management of adult coeliac disease: guidelines from the British Society of Gastroenterology. *Gut, 63,* 1210–1228.

Crohn's Disease

NICE. (2020). *Crohn's disease.* https://cks.nice.org.uk/topics/crohns-disease/ [Accessed July 2020].

NICE Guidelines. (2019). *NG129: Crohn's disease* https://www.nice.org.uk/guidance/ng129 [Accessed July 2020].

Lamb, C. A., Kennedy, N. A., Raine, T., et al. (2019). British Society of Gastroenterology consensus guidelines on the management of inflammatory bowel disease in adults. *Gut, 68,* s1–s106.

BNF Treatment Summaries. (2019). *Crohn's disease* https://bnf.nice.org.uk/treatment-summary/crohns-disease.html [Accessed July 2020].

Ulcerative Colitis

NICE Guidelines. (2019). *NG130: Ulcerative colitis.* https://www.nice.org.uk/guidance/ng130 [Accessed July 2020].

NICE. (2020). *CKS: Ulcerative colitis.* https://cks.nice.org.uk/topics/ulcerative-colitis/ [Accessed July 2020].

Irritable Bowel Syndrome

NICE. (2020). *CKS: Irritable bowel syndrome.* https://cks.nice.org.uk/topics/irritable-bowel-syndrome/ [Accessed July 2020].

BNF Treatment Summaries. *Constipation.* https://bnf.nice.org.uk/treatment-summary/constipation.html [Accessed March 2021].

Small Intestinal Bacterial Overgrowth

Bures, J. (2010). Small intestinal bacterial overgrowth syndrome. *World Journal of Gastroenterology, 16,* 2978.

Patient info. (2016). *Blind loop syndrome.* https://patient.info/doctor/blind-loop-syndrome [Accessed February 2021].

11

Haematology in an Hour

Viola Mendonca, Julia Wolf and Rebecca Allam

OUTLINE

HAEMATOLOGY KEY PRINCIPLES

Coagulation cascade: the recruitment of proteins leading to fibrin formation and, subsequently, a stable blood clot (see Fig 11.1 and Table 11.1)

- Activated partial thromboplastin time (APTT): provides information about the **INTRINSIC** and common pathway
- Partial thromboplastin time (PTT): provides information about the **EXTRINSIC** and common pathway

Formation of a Primary Platelet Plug: Primary platelet plugs form at sites of vessel damage. This process is dependent on the plasma glycoprotein, von Willebrand factor (vWF), which circulates in globular form and forms multimers. Globular vWF binds to subendothelial collagen at sites of vessel damage. Then, due to the high shear forces present in blood vessels, vWF unravels, revealing its platelet-binding domain, which binds reversibly to GP1b on platelets and leads to platelet capture at sites of vessel damage (Fig 11.2A). The multimeric structure of vWF and, therefore, its platelet-tethering ability, is controlled by the metalloprotease, ADAMTS13. ADAMTS13 cleaves vWF into smaller multimers (Fig 11.2B).

Fibrinolysis: the breakdown of fibrin (an insoluble 3D polymer that forms the meshwork for clots). **D-dimer** is a fibrin degradation product that it is produced when a clot is degraded by fibrinolysis (Fig 11.3).

Platelet recruitment happens by:
- Thromboxane A_2: a product of arachidonic acid and cyclooxygenase 1
- Adenosine diphosphate: binds to receptors $P2Y_1$ and $P2Y_{12}$ on the surface of platelets

Leads to the activation of the platelet receptor, GpIIb/IIIa, which causes platelet aggregation

Haematopoiesis: a differentiation process that leads to the formation of different types of blood cells (Fig 11.4)

PANCYTOPAENIA

Definition: a reduction in all cell lines (i.e., red cells, white cells and platelets). Can have many causes, although can simplistically be subdivided into problems related to production in the bone marrow vs increased destruction peripherally (see Table 11.2).

Buzzwords:
- **Risk factors:** chemotherapy, radiotherapy, systemic lupus erythematosus (SLE)
- **Presentation:** fatigue, breathlessness, chest pain (anaemia), recurrent infections (neutropenia), bruising, bleeding, petechiae (see Figs 11.5–11.7)

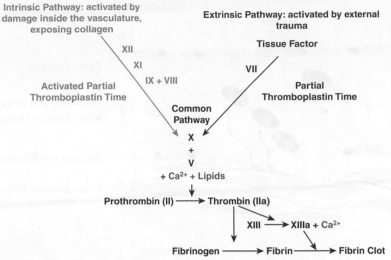

Fig 11.1 Coagulation cascade. (Illustrated by Viola Mendonca.)

TABLE 11.1   Activated Partial Thromboplastin Time (APTT) and Partial Thromboplastin Time (PTT)

APTT	PTT	Causes
Prolonged	Normal	Deficiency of intrinsic factors (XII, XI, IX, VIII), lupus anticoagulant (in vitro artefact) Von Willebrand disease, haemophilia A (factor VIII deficiency) and haemophilia B (factor XI deficiency)
Prolonged	Prolonged	Common pathway deficiency (X,V,II), multiple clotting factor deficiencies (e.g., V and VIII), disseminated intravascular coagulation, liver disease
Prolonged	Prolonged (PTT< APTT)	Patient might be on unfractionated heparin
Prolonged (APTT<PTT)	Prolonged	Patient might be on warfarin, vitamin K deficiency

ANAEMIA

Definition: low haemoglobin. See Table 11.3 for the different types of anaemia.

Investigations: a full blood count (FBC) (haemoglobin (Hb), mean corpuscular volume (MCV) and mean corpuscular haemoglobin concentration (MCHC)) is used to diagnose anaemia and to determine the type of anaemia.

- **Hb:** anaemia is diagnosed if Hb <130 g/L in males or <120 g/L in nonpregnant females
- **MCV:**
  - Low <80 fL (microcytic)
  - Normal 80-100 fL (normocytic)
  - High >100 fL (macrocytic)

- **MCHC:**
  - Low (hypochromic)
  - Normal (normochromic)
  - High (hyperchromic)

Iron-deficiency Anaemia

Definition: microcytic, hypochromic anaemia. Low iron levels in the body lead to decreased red blood cell production. Most common cause of microcytic anaemia globally

Buzzwords:
- **Risk factors:** pregnancy, menorrhagia, poor oral intake, vegetarian or vegan diet, malabsorption (e.g., coeliac disease), malignancy
- **Presentation:** dyspnoea, fatigue, chest pain, palpitations, cognitive dysfunction, restless leg syndrome, vertigo

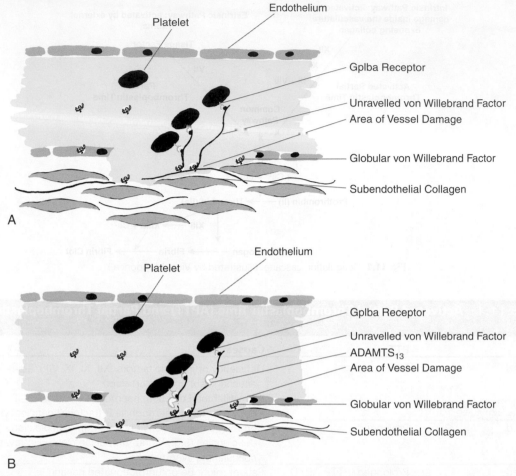

Fig 11.2 (A) Formation of a primary platelet plug and (B) control of a primary platelet plug. (Illustrated by Hollie Blaber.)

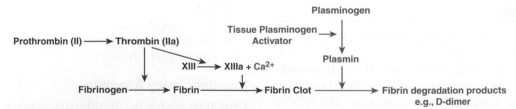

Fig 11.3 Fibrin clot formation (*red*) vs fibrinolysis (*blue*). (Illustrated by Viola Mendonca.)

Investigations:
- **Blood:** FBC (↓ Hb, ↓ MCV, ↓ MCHC)
- ***Serum ferritin:** low (<15 micrograms/L if no infection/inflammation present, <100 micrograms/L if infection/inflammation present)

- **Blood film:** microcytic hypochromic cells (Fig 11.8) with anisocytosis (different sizes) and pencil poikilocytosis (abnormal shape)

Differentials: anaemia of chronic disease, thalassaemia
Management: find and treat the underlying cause.

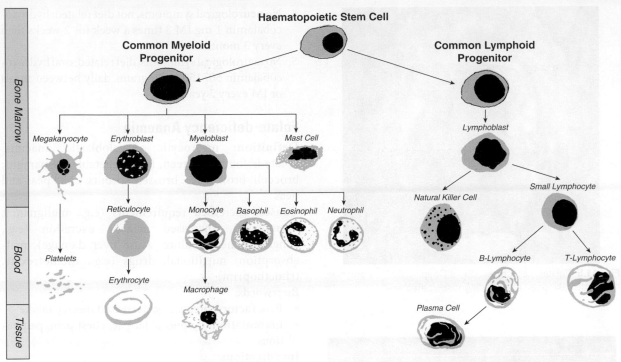

Fig 11.4 Haematopoiesis. (Illustrated by Hollie Blaber.)

Labels within figure: Haematopoietic Stem Cell; Common Myeloid Progenitor; Common Lymphoid Progenitor; Bone Marrow; Blood; Tissue; Megakaryocyte; Erythroblast; Myeloblast; Mast Cell; Lymphoblast; Reticulocyte; Monocyte; Basophil; Eosinophil; Neutrophil; Natural Killer Cell; Small Lymphocyte; Platelets; Erythrocyte; Macrophage; B-Lymphocyte; T-Lymphocyte; Plasma Cell

TABLE 11.2 Bone Marrow Problems vs Peripheral Destruction

Bone Marrow Problems	Peripheral Destruction
Severe folate/ vitamin B12 deficiency	Immune destruction (e.g., systemic lupus erythematosus)
Malignant infiltration (primary or metastatic)	Disseminated intravascular coagulation
Myelofibrosis	Sepsis
Aplastic anaemia (hypoplasia of bone marrow for many reasons, including genetic conditions)	Splenomegaly
Viruses (e.g., human immunodeficiency virus)	Microangiopathy
Drug-induced myelosuppression (e.g., chemotherapy)	Drugs

- Iron supplements: ferrous sulphate 200 mg tablets PO OD to be continued for 3 months after correction of the iron deficiency

Vitamin B12-Deficiency Anaemia

Definition: vitamin B12 is found in eggs, meat, salmon, cod, milk and dairy products. Vitamin B12 deficiency leads to a megaloblastic anaemia (red blood cells with immature nuclei). **Causes:** decreased intrinsic factor (e.g., pernicious anaemia), decreased absorption (e.g., terminal ileum defect), nutritional, drugs (e.g., colchicine, metformin, proton-pump inhibitors)

Buzzwords:
- **Risk factors:** vegan diet, gastric surgery, autoimmune disease
- **Presentation:** dyspnoea, fatigue, chest pain, palpitations, symmetrical neuropathy, psychiatric disturbances, indigestion, glossitis

Investigations:
- **Blood:** FBC (↓ Hb, ↑ MCV), vitamin B12 levels (<200 ng/L), anti-intrinsic factor antibodies (found in pernicious anaemia)
- **Blood film:** hypersegmented neutrophils (see Fig 11.9), oval macrocytes, megaloblasts

Differentials: folic acid–deficiency anaemia, myelodysplastic syndrome, alcoholic liver disease

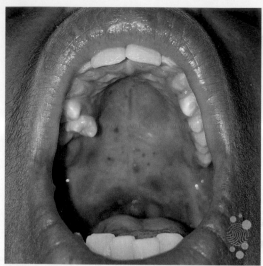

Fig 11.5 Palatal petechiae. (Skin Deep. (2022). Petechiae. https://dftbskindeep.com/all-diagnoses/petechiae/)

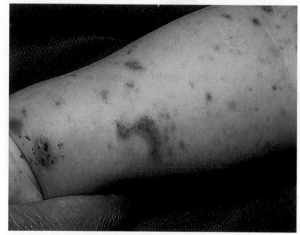

Fig 11.6 Petechiae in lighter skin. (Singh, S. B. (2011). Petechial rash (Case 55, Fig. 98.1). In *Pediatrics a Competency-Based Companion*. Elsevier. Copyright © 2011 Elsevier Inc. All rights reserved.)

Management:
1. Find underlying cause
2. Dietary advice
3. Neurological symptoms: hydroxocobalamin 1 mg intramuscularly on alternative days until no more improvement (minimum 3 weeks), then every 2 months

4. No neurological symptoms, not diet related: hydroxocobalamin 1 mg IM 3 times a week for 2 weeks then every 3 months
5. No neurological symptoms, diet related: oral hydroxocobalamin 50–150 micrograms daily between meals or IM every 2 years

Folate deficiency Anaemia

Definition: macrocytic megaloblastic anaemia. Folate is found in green, leafy vegetables; asparagus; broccoli; brown rice; brussels sprouts; chickpeas and peas

Causes: increased requirements (e.g., malignancy, haemolysis), increased urinary excretion (e.g., congestive heart failure, acute liver damage), malabsorption, nutritional, drugs (e.g., methotrexate, trimethoprim)

Buzzwords:
- **Risk factors:** pregnancy, decreased dietary intake
- **Presentation:** dyspnoea, fatigue, chest pain, palpitations

Investigations:
- **Blood:** FBC ($\downarrow$ Hb, $\uparrow$ MCV), folate levels (<3 micrograms/L)
- **Blood film:** hypersegmented neutrophils, oval macrocytes, megaloblasts

Differentials: vitamin B12-deficiency anaemia, myelodysplastic syndrome, alcohol-related liver disease

Management:
1. Find underlying cause (and rule out a vitamin B12 deficiency, since vitamin B12 replacement needs to be performed **before** folate replacement)
2. Dietary advice
3. Oral folic acid 5 mg for 4 months, for prophylaxis in pregnancy 400 mcg daily until week 12

Haemolytic Anaemia

Definition: increased rate of destruction of red blood cells. **Causes:**
- **Inherited:** red blood cell enzyme abnormalities (e.g., glucose-6-phosphate dehydrogenase (G6PD) deficiency), red blood cell membrane abnormalities, haemoglobin abnormalities (e.g., thalassaemia, sickle cell disease)
- **Acquired:** drugs, transfusion reaction, microangiopathic haemolytic anaemia (MAHA) (e.g., thrombotic thrombocytopenic purpura (TTP), haemolytic

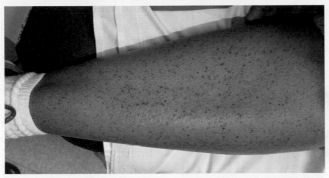

Fig 11.7 Petechiae in darker skin. (With permission from Flanagan, S. M., & Lombardi, D. (2018). Immune thrombocytopenic purpura (Fig. 2). *Visual Journal of Emergency Medicine*. Publisher: Elsevier. © 2017 Elsevier Inc. All rights reserved.)

TABLE 11.3 Microcytic, Normocytic and Macrocytic Anaemias

Microcytic (Mnemonic: TAILS)	Normocytic (Mnemonic: AAAH)	Macrocytic (Mnemonic: ABCDEF)
Thalassaemia	Anaemia of chronic disease	Alcohol/chronic liver disease
Anaemia of chronic disease	Acute blood loss	B12 deficiency
Iron deficiency	Aplastic anaemia	Compensatory reticulocytosis (can be
Lead poisoning	Haemolytic	seen in haemolysis)
Sideroblastic anaemia		Drugs (e.g., methotrexate, phenytoin)
		Endocrine (hypothyroidism)
		Folate deficiency

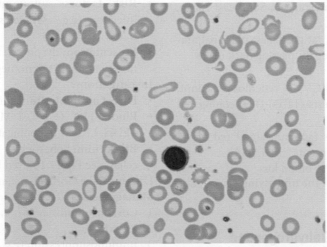

Fig 11.8 Blood Film Showing Hypochromic Cells in Iron-Deficiency Anaemia (With permission from Hayter, J., & Thomas, A. (2021). Investigation and management of anaemia (Fig. 1). *Medicine*. Elsevier. © 2021 Published by Elsevier Ltd.)

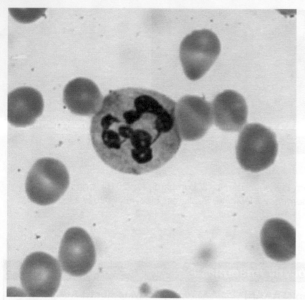

Fig 11.9 Hypersegmented neutrophil. (With permission from Ed Uthman, Houston, TX, USA, CC BY 2.0, via Wikimedia Commons. https://commons.wikimedia.org/wiki/File:Hyperlobated_Neutrophil_(8612790151).jpg.)

uraemic syndrome (HUS), disseminated intravascular coagulation (DIC))

Buzzwords:

- **Risk factors:** autoimmune disorders, malignancy, ethnic origin (e.g., Mediterranean, Southeast Asian, African)
- **Presentation:** dyspnoea, fatigue, chest pain, palpitations, jaundice, splenomegaly, passing dark urine

Investigations:

- **Blood:** FBC (↓ Hb, ↑ MCV), ↑ reticulocyte count, ↑ LDH, liver function tests (LFTs) (↑ unconjugated bilirubin), ↓ haptoglobin
- **Blood film:** spherocytes (sphere-shaped red blood cells), red blood cell fragments (in MAHA)

Differentials: anaemia due to blood loss

Management: find and treat the underlying cause. Folic acid supplementation

Glucose-6-phosphate Dehydrogenase Deficiency

Definition: G6PD is an enzyme that replenishes reduced glutathione, protecting red blood cells from oxidant stress. Without it, a cell is more susceptible to oxidant stress, which leads to intravascular haemolysis

Buzzwords:

- **Risk factors:** family history (X-linked), Greek, Cypriot, Arab, Italian, Afro-Caribbean, infections, fava beans, moth balls, drugs (e.g., dapsone, fluoroquinolones, nitrofurantoin, sulphonamides)
- **Presentation:** neonatal jaundice, acute haemolytic anaemia (in response to oxidative stress)

Investigations:

- **Blood:** FBC (↓ Hb, ↑ MCV), ↑ reticulocyte count, ↑ LDH, LFTs (↑ unconjugated bilirubin), ↓ haptoglobin
- **Blood film:** spherocytes (sphere-shaped red blood cells), red blood cell fragments
- **G6PD assay**
- **Blood film:** Heinz bodies (precipitated Hb), bite cells (where the spleen removes Heinz bodies)

Differentials: sickle cell disease, autoimmune haemolytic anaemia

Management:

1. Avoid oxidant stress
2. Blood transfusion for acute haemolysis

Autoimmune Haemolytic Anaemia

Definition: autoantibodies against the body's own red blood cells

Buzzwords:

- **Risk factors:** autoimmune disease, malignancy, infection (e.g., *Mycoplasma pneumoniae*, Epstein-Barr virus (EBV))
- **Presentation:** dyspnoea, fatigue, chest pain, palpitations, jaundice, splenomegaly, passing dark urine

Investigations:

- **Direct antiglobulin test** is positive
- **Blood:** FBC (↓ Hb, ↑ MCV), ↑ reticulocyte count, ↑ LDH, LFTs (↑ unconjugated bilirubin), ↑ haptoglobin
- **Blood film:** spherocytes ('sphere-shaped' red blood cells – see Fig 11.10), red blood cell fragments

Differentials: G6PD deficiency, sickle cell disease

Management:

1. Corticosteroid
2. Rituximab
3. Immunosuppression (e.g., azathioprine)
4. Splenectomy
5. Intravenous immunoglobulin (IVIG) for emergencies

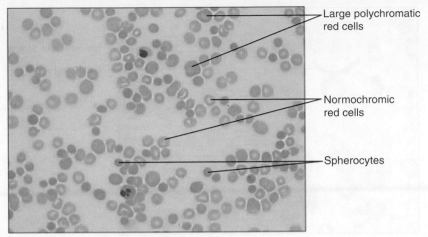

Large polychromatic red cells

Normochromic red cells

Spherocytes

Fig 11.10 Blood film showing spherocytes in autoimmune haemolytic anaemia. (With permission from Newland, A. C, MacCallum, P., & Davies, J. (2019). Haematology (Fig. 12.8). In *Medical sciences*. Elsevier. Copyright © 2019 Elsevier Ltd. All rights reserved.)

Sickle Cell Disease

Definition: mutation in the β chains of haemoglobin leading to the formation of Hb S, which has a low affinity for oxygen
- Carrier: sickle cell trait (often asymptomatic)
- Affected (homozygous): sickle cell disease

Buzzwords:
- **Risk factors:** Afro-Caribbean, also from the Middle East, India, Eastern Mediterranean and South and Central America
- **Presentation:** vaso-occlusive crisis (e.g., pain, priapism), acute chest crisis, stroke, haemolytic anaemia, aplastic crisis (profound anaemia), splenic sequestration, leg ulcers, incidental finding on screening

Investigations:
- **Blood:** FBC (Hb 60–90 g/L), ↑ LDH, ↑ reticulocytes, LFTs (↑ unconjugated bilirubin)
- **Blood film:** sickle cells, target cells, Pappenheimer bodies (granules of iron), Howell-Jolly bodies (DNA remnants) (See Fig 11.11)
- **Haemoglobin electrophoresis and high-performance liquid chromatography (HPLC):** Hb S
- **Sickle solubility test:** positive
- **Guthrie test** (newborn blood-spot test): positive
- **Chest x-ray (CXR) and arterial blood gas (ABG):** if suspicious for acute chest syndrome

Differentials: iron deficiency anaemia, anaemia of chronic disease, haemolytic anaemia

Management:
- **Prevention of sickle cell crisis**
  - **Avoid precipitants** (e.g. cold weather, dehydration, infection, hypoxia).
  - **Vaccination** against *peumococcus, haemophilus, meningococcus, influenza*
  - **Prophylactic oral penicillin** (patients are hyposplenic and need protection against encapsulated bacteria)
  - Exchange transfusions for some patients
- **Treating sickle cell pain:** Analgesia (WHO pain ladder), Hydroxycarbamide
- **Treating anaemia:** Folic acid, blood transfusions
- **Allogenic Stem Cell Transplantation** is the only cure.

Thalassaemia

Definition: a genetic disorder leading to an imbalance of haemoglobin chains (a deficiency of either α or β chains)
- The α chains are coded for by four alleles on Chromosome 16
  - If two are deleted = trait
  - If three are deleted = Hb H disease (Hb H is a tetramer of β chains)

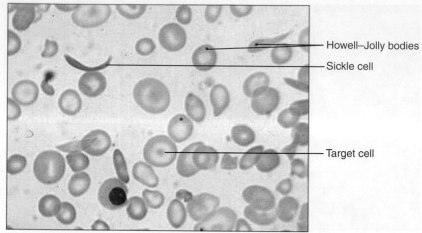

Fig 11.11 Blood film showing Howell-Jolly bodies, sickle cells and target cells in sickle cell anaemia. (With permission from Newland, A. C, MacCallum, P., & Davies, J. (2019). Haematology (Fig. 12.20). In *Medical sciences*. Elsevier. Copyright © 2019 Elsevier Ltd. All rights reserved.)

- If four are deleted = Hb Barts (hydrops fetalis, death in utero)
- The β chains are coded by two alleles on Chromosome 11
  - If one is deleted = trait
  - If two are deleted = Major/Cooley

Buzzwords:
- **Risk factors:** family history, ethnic origin (e.g. Mediterranean, Southeast Asian, African)
- **Presentation:**
  - **Major/Hb H disease** (often in childhood): failure to thrive, hepatosplenomegaly, bone expansion (classically, frontal bossing), jaundice, gallstones
  - **Trait:** usually asymptomatic or with mild anaemia, dyspnoea, fatigue, headache

Investigations:
- **Blood:** FBC (↓ Hb, ↓ MCV, ↓ MCHC, ↓ MCH (<25 Pg), ↑ RBC (due to reticulocytosis))
- **Blood film:** microcytic hypochromic cells with target cells, reticulocytosis
- **Haemoglobin electrophoresis** (can detect the presence of Hb chains)
  - α thalassaemia: Hb H
  - β thalassaemia: Hb Foetal (Hb F), Hb A2
- **HPLC** (quantifies the fraction of Hb chains)
  - α thalassaemia: Hb H
  - β thalassaemia: Hb F, Hb A2

Differentials: iron-deficiency anaemia, anaemia of chronic disease, haemolytic anaemia

Management:
1. Blood transfusions
2. Folic acid supplementation
3. Iron chelation

THROMBOCYTOPENIA

Immune Thrombocytopenic Purpura

Definition: a condition caused by immune destruction of platelets causing macrophages to prematurely remove them from the circulation, decreasing the platelet lifespan from 10 days to a few hours. Can be acute or chronic. Usually self-resolves in children but often requires treatment in adults. **Causes:** idiopathic (primary). In children, post-vaccination or after a viral infection (e.g., chickenpox or infectious mononucleosis). Mainly in adults, may be secondary to hepatitis C, HIV, *Helicobacter pylori* infection, chronic lymphocytic leukaemia (CLL), Hodgkin lymphoma, autoimmune haemolytic anaemia

Buzzwords:
- **Risk factors:** women of childbearing age, age <10 or >65 years
- **Presentation:** bruising, petechiae, epistaxis, oral blood blisters (wet petechiae), intracranial haemorrhage (very rare)

Investigations:
- **Blood:** FBC (↓ platelets)
- **Blood film:** low platelets, large platelets are frequently seen

Differentials: TTP, DIC

Management:
- In children, often resolves spontaneously
- Platelet transfusion for life-threatening bleeding or if emergency surgery is required
- High-dose corticosteroids and high-dose IVIG
- Thrombopoietin-receptor agonists in chronic cases (e.g., eltrombopag and romiplostim)
- Rituximab
- Mycophenolate mofetil (MMF)

Heparin-induced Thrombocytopenia

Definition: thrombocytopenia induced by heparin exposure (mainly to unfractionated heparin because it is made from pig intestine, which causes IgG immune–mediated destruction of platelets). Platelets can release procoagulant microparticles, causing thrombosis. The 4 Ts score has a good negative predictive value (See Table 11.4)
- Score 1–3 = low probability of heparin-induced thrombocytopenia (HIT)
- Score 4–5 = intermediate probability of HIT
- Score 6–8 = high probability of HIT

Buzzwords:
- **Risk factors:** unfractionated heparin (high risk), low molecular weight heparin (LMWH), females, middle to older age, history of trauma or orthopaedic surgery

- **Presentation:** new clots, skin necrosis, fall in platelets by greater than 30% between 5–10 days of heparin use

Investigations:
- **Blood:** FBC (at least a 30% decrease in platelets)
- **ELISA:** for IgG heparin-PF4

Differentials: TTP, drug-induced thrombocytopenic purpura

Management: stop heparin. Alternative anticoagulation with danaparoid sodium, fondaparinux, argatroban (warfarin should not be used until the platelet count normalises due to an increased thrombosis risk at initiation)

Disseminated Intravascular Coagulation

Definition: an excessive and inappropriate activation of the coagulation pathway, which leads to the consumption of platelets and coagulation factors.

Buzzwords:
- **Risk factors:** sepsis, acute promyelocytic leukaemia, obstetrical complications (e.g., amniotic fluid embolism, placental abruption, pre-eclampsia), trauma, malignancy
- **Presentation:** oozing blood from venepuncture sites and wounds. Bleeding from gastrointestinal/urogenital tract. Thrombus formation in the skin, brain, kidneys and distal circulation (gangrene of fingers and toes)

Investigations:
- **Blood:** FBC (↓ platelets), coagulation screen (prolonged APTT and PTT), D-dimer (raised), fibrinogen (<1)

TABLE 11.4	Scoring of the 4 T Categories for Heparin-induced Thrombocytopenia		
4 T Category	**2 Points**	**1 Point**	**0 Point**
Thrombocytopenia	Platelet count fall >50% and platelet nadir >20×10⁹/L	Platelet count fall 30%–50% or platelet nadir 10–19×10⁹/L	Platelet count fall <30% or platelet nadir <10×10⁹/L
Timing of platelet count fall	Clear onset 5–10 days, or platelet fall <1 day with prior heparin exposure in the last 30 days	Fall within 5–10 days, or after 10 days or fall <1 day with prior heparin exposure in 30–100 days	Platelet count fall <4 days without recent exposure
Thrombosis of other sequalae	New thrombosis (e.g., skin necrosis)	Progressive or recurrent thrombosis	None
Other causes of thrombocytopenia	None	Possible	Definite

- **Blood film:** schistocytes (red blood cell fragments) from microangiopathic haemolytic anaemia (fibrin deposits in microcirculation, which shreds red blood cells and causes thrombosis)

Differentials: severe liver failure, vitamin K deficiency, HIT

Management:

- Treat the underlying cause
- If bleeding: fresh frozen plasma (FFP), platelets, cryoprecipitate, fibrinogen concentrate, red blood cell transfusion
- Support: hypotension, hypoxia, acidosis

Haemolytic Uraemic Syndrome

Definition: a triad of microangiopathic haemolytic anaemia, acute kidney injury and thrombocytopenia. Often seen in children. Causes: *Shigella* and *Escherichia coli* 0157 infection.

Buzzwords:

- **Risk factors:** ingestion of contaminated food or water, local outbreaks
- **Presentation:** first diarrhoea then jaundice, fatigue, shortness of breath, headache, decreased urine output, petechiae

Investigations:

- **Blood:** FBC (↓ Hb, ↓ platelets), ↑ reticulocytes, LFTs (↑ bilirubin), ↑ LDH, U&E (↑ creatinine and ↑ urea)
- **Blood film:** schistocytes (red blood cell fragments)
- **Stool culture:** *Shigella*, *E. coli* 0157

Differentials: TTP, malignant hypertension, SLE

Management: IV fluids. Haemodialysis for renal failure

Thrombotic Thrombocytopenic Purpura

Definition: an autoimmune disease with antibody formation against ADAMTS13. ADAMTS13, which usually cleaves vWF, is reduced. Ultra-large multimers of vWF have a greater ability to bind to platelets (compared with the shorter form), therefore leading to thrombosis. Untreated mortality is >90%. **Causes:** idiopathic, autoimmune disease, sepsis, drugs (e.g., ciclosporin, clopidogrel)

Buzzwords:

- **Risk factors:** pregnancy, female, Black ethnicity
- **Presentation:** microangiopathic haemolytic anaemia (tiredness, shortness of breath), thrombocytopenia (purpura), fever, neurological dysfunction

(fluctuating cerebral dysfunction), renal failure (decreased urine output)

Investigations:

- **Blood:** FBC (↓ Hb, ↓ platelets), ↑ reticulocytes, LFTs (↑ unconjugated bilirubin), ↑ LDH, U&E (↑ creatinine and ↑ urea), coagulation screen (APTT and PTT normal – differentiates from DIC)
- **Blood film:** schistocytes (red blood cell fragments), thrombocytopenia

Differentials: HUS, DIC, malignant hypertension

Management:

1. This condition represents an emergency and treatment should be started within 4 h:
   a. Plasma exchange: removal of plasma and replacement with either FFP or cryosupernatant to remove the autoantibodies and replace ADAMTS13
   b. Steroids (methylprednisolone or prednisolone)
2. Rituximab
3. Caplacizumab (anti-vWF antibody): inhibits binding of platelets to the ultra-large multimers of vWF
4. LMWH + aspirin once platelet count >50×10⁹/L

INHERITED THROMBOPHILIA

Thrombophilia refers to a group of conditions that predispose patients to blood clots. Most blood clots have a multifactorial aetiology. Heritable causes are rare, and testing for thrombophilia in unselected patients with venous thromboembolic disease is not indicated.

Factor V Leiden

Definition: Factor V Leiden is caused by a mutation in the factor V gene, which causes resistance to activated protein C. The mutation exhibits incomplete penetrance, which means that most people with the mutation will not experience thromboses. It is the most common inherited thrombophilia.

Buzzwords:

- **Risk factors:** family history
- **Presentation:** venous thrombosis

Investigations

- **APTT:** shortened (or failure of prolongation when activated protein C is added to the plasma)
- **Activated protein C resistance:** positive
- **PCR for factor V Leiden:** positive

Differentials: antiphospholipid syndrome, protein C or S deficiencies, antithrombin III deficiency

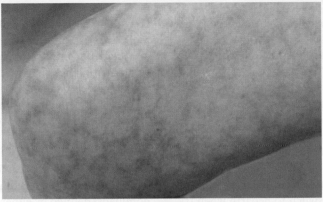

Fig 11.12 Livedo reticularis in lighter skin. (With permission from Barbhaiya, M., Salmon, J. E., & Erkan, D. (2021). Antiphospholipid syndrome (Fig. 87.2). In *Firestein & Kelley's textbook of rheumatology, 2-volume set.* Copyright © 2021 Elsevier Inc. All rights reserved.)

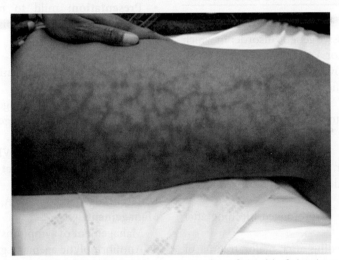

Fig 11.13 Livedo reticularis in darker skin. (With permission from Saks, M., & Isenberg, D. (2016). Livedo reticularis on the bilateral thighs (Fig. 1). *Visual Journal of Emergency Medicine.* Copyright © 2015 Elsevier Inc. All rights reserved.)

Management: anticoagulation if symptomatic (presents with venous thromboembolism (VTE)), homozygous (rare, but risk of VTE significantly higher) or with a strong family history of factor V Leiden and VTE

ACQUIRED THROMBOPHILIA

Antiphospholipid Syndrome

Definition: an acquired autoimmune disorder linked to venous or arterial thrombosis with or without obstetrical complications (e.g., recurrent miscarriages) with persistent antiphospholipid antibodies.

Buzzwords:

- **Risk factors:** female, around 30s, autoimmune diseases (e.g., SLE)
- **Presentation:** recurrent miscarriages, venous/arterial/small vessel thrombosis, unexplained thrombocytopenia, livedo reticularis (Figs 11.12, 11.13)

Investigations:

- **Antiphospholipid antibodies** (two occasions, 12 weeks apart):
  - Cardiolipin antibodies (IgG, IgM, and sometimes IgA)
  - Lupus anticoagulant assay

- Anti-β2 glycoprotein-1 (IgG, IgM)
- **Blood:** FBC (normal/↓ platelets), coagulation screen (APTT prolonged)

Differentials: factor V Leiden, SLE, other causes of thrombophilia (see factor V Leiden)

Management:

1. **Lifestyle:** avoid smoking, regular exercise, management of cardiovascular risk factors
2. **After first venous event:** lifelong warfarin (**INR 2–3**)
3. **After second venous event:** lifelong warfarin (**INR 3–4**)
4. In recurrent miscarriage: LMWH and aspirin
5. NB: women who are on warfarin (because of previous thrombosis) should switch to heparin when trying to conceive or at confirmation of conception

INHERITED COAGULATION DISORDERS

Haemophilia A and B

Definition: X-linked recessive genetic disorder in which there is a decrease in factor VIII (A) or factor IX (B). Mutations can arise de novo. The severity depends on the degree of the factor deficiency.

Buzzwords:

- **Risk factors:** family history, almost exclusively affecting males (X-linked)
- **Presentation**
  - **Severe:** age <1 year, spontaneous bleeding into joints and muscles, delayed and prolonged bleeding
  - **Moderate:** excessive or prolonged bleeding after minor trauma
  - **Mild:** excessive bleeding after major trauma or surgery (e.g., dental extraction)

Investigations:

- **Blood:** coagulation screen (APTT prolonged, PTT normal), FBC (normal platelets)
- **Plasma factor VIII and IX:**
  - severe: <0.01 international units (IU)/mL
  - moderate: 0.01 to 0.05 IU/mL
  - mild: >0.05 but <0.40 IU/mL

Differentials: Von Willebrand disease (vWD), deficiency of other coagulation factors, platelet dysfunction, nonaccidental injury

Management:

1. Antifibrinolytic agent (e.g., tranexamic acid)
2. Desmopressin (DDAVP)
3. Factor concentrate replacement (for treatment and primary prophylaxis in severe and moderate cases)

4. Emicizumab (for primary prophylaxis in severe patients and in those with inhibitors)
5. Due to risk of inhibitory antibodies forming against factor concentrates, bypass agents to overcome these autoantibodies may be necessary for acute presentations (e.g., factor VIII inhibitor–bypassing agent (FEIBA) contains prothrombin and factor Xa or recombinant FVIIa (Novoseven))

Von Willebrand Disease

Definition: vWF is a carrier protein for factor VIII. vWD is an inherited bleeding disorder (often autosomal dominant) defined by either a quantitative or qualitative defect in vWF.

Buzzwords:

- **Risk factors:** family history (but can be de novo)
- **Presentation:** mild to moderate mucocutaneous bleeding pattern (e.g., epistaxis, menorrhagia, post-tooth extraction)

Investigations:

- **vWF antigen:** <0.30 IU/mL with a bleeding history is diagnostic
- **APTT:** normal or prolonged if FVIII is low
- **Specialist tests to gauge function** – e.g., FVIII concentration (FVIII:C), VWF ristocetin cofactor activity (VWF:Rco), VWF-collagen binding assay, ristocetin-induced platelet agglutination (RIPA) and genetic analysis

Differentials: haemophilia A, platelet dysfunction

Management:

1. Management of symptoms
2. Antifibrinolytic agents (e.g., tranexamic acid)
3. DDAVP: stimulates release of the vWF stored in endothelial cells
4. vWF-containing concentrate

ACQUIRED COAGULATION DISORDERS

Vitamin K Deficiency

Definition: vitamin K is a fat-soluble vitamin required for formation of factors II, VII, IX, X, protein C and S. If a deficiency occurs in the first 12 weeks of infancy, it is known as haemorrhagic disease of the newborn

Buzzwords:

- **Risk factors:** malnutrition, malabsorption (e.g., coeliac disease, cystic fibrosis), liver disease, poor placental transfer, liver disease

- **Presentation:**
  - Neonate: intracranial haemorrhage, gastrointestinal bleeding, bleeding after circumcision
  - Older patient: easy bruising, mucocutaneous bleeds, postsurgical bleeds

Investigations:
- **Blood:** coagulation screen (PTT prolonged)

Differentials: DIC, nonaccidental injury

Management:
1. Prophylactic vitamin K at birth (IM)
2. Oral vitamin K supplementation

MALIGNANCY

Acute vs Chronic Leukaemia

Acute leukaemia: clonal disorders (originating from a single abnormal cell) that often progress rapidly and can affect patients of all ages. Haematopoietic cells halt during differentiation in the early stages of development in the bone marrow. These immature cells (known as **blast cells**) accumulate in the bone marrow. Leukaemia cells may infiltrate lymph nodes (leading to lymphadenopathy) or infiltrate the spleen/liver (causing hepatosplenomegaly). As blasts build up in the bone marrow, they will affect the production of other cell lines, such as red blood cells, platelets and white blood cells (see Table 11.5).

Chronic leukaemia: malignant process affecting mature haematopoietic cells

Acute Myeloid Leukaemia

Definition: a rapidly progressive, malignant process that causes a halt in the differentiation of myeloid progenitor cells. Acute myeloid leukaemia (AML) is the most common form of acute leukaemia in adults.

Buzzwords:
- **Risk factors:** previous chemotherapy/radiotherapy, previous myelodysplasia, Down syndrome
- **Presentation:** median onset at 65 years of age. unexplained fever, gum hypertrophy, skin infiltration

Investigations:
- **Blood:** FBC (↓ Hb, ↓ platelets, ↓ neutrophils, ↑ WCC (usually increased due to blasts but may be low))
- **Blood film:** myeloid blast cells (cytoplasm is filled with granules or Auer rods) (See Fig 11.14)
- **Bone marrow aspirate:** myeloid blast cells
- **Cytogenetics and immunophenotyping**

TABLE 11.5 Common Presenting Features Associated with the Interruption of Different Cell Lines

Cell Line Affected	Presentation
Red blood cells	↓ haemoglobin, pallor, fatigue, breathlessness
Platelets	↓ platelets, bruising, petechiae, bleeding
White cells	↓ immunity, persistent/recurrent/life-threatening infections

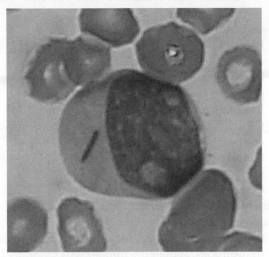

Fig 11.14 Blood film showing a myeloblast with an Auer rod. (With permission from Mourao, P., CC BY-SA 3.0, via Wikimedia Commons. *https://commons.wikimedia.org/wiki/File:Myeloblast_with_Auer_Rod_smear_2009-11-23_cropped.jpg*.)

Differentials: acute lymphoblastic leukaemia (ALL), myelodysplastic syndrome, myelofibrosis

Management:
1. Supportive treatment for bone marrow failure (transfusions, antibiotics, tumour lysis syndrome)
2. Combination chemotherapy (e.g., daunorubicin and cytarabine)
3. Allogenic stem cell transplant (in high-risk and fit patients)
4. Best supportive/palliative care (in patients not fit for treatment)

Prognosis: poor in the elderly: <10% of those at 70 years of age achieve long-term remission

Acute Lymphoblastic Leukaemia

Definition: a rapidly progressive malignant process that causes a halt in the differentiation of lymphoid progenitors. ALL can involve B or T cells. Most common childhood cancer (majority <6 years of age).

Buzzwords:

- **Risk factors:** most common in children, previous chemotherapy, Down syndrome
- **Presentation:** unexplained fever, bone pain, testicular enlargement
  - If CNS invasion: headaches, isolated cranial nerve palsies
  - **Tumour lysis syndrome** (see Palliative Care/Oncology in an Hour)

Investigations:

- **Blood:** FBC (↓ Hb, ↓ platelets, ↓ neutrophils, ↑ WCC (usually increased due to blasts but may be low))
- **Blood film:** blast cells (scanty cytoplasm without granules)
- **Bone marrow aspirate:** blast cells
- **CXR:** look for a mediastinal mass (indicative of T-cell disease)
- **Lumbar puncture:** for assessment of CNS involvement
- **Cytogenetics and immunophenotyping**

Differentials: AML, reactive lymphocytosis

Management:

1. **Supportive** treatment for bone marrow failure (transfusions, antibiotics, tumour lysis syndrome)
2. **Intensive chemotherapy regime** for 2 years (girls) or 3 years (boys) (induction of remission, consolidation, cranial prophylaxis, intensification and maintenance)

Prognosis: good in children – a cure can be expected in 90%. Poor in adults. T-cell ALL has a worse prognosis than B-cell ALL

Chronic Lymphocytic Leukaemia

Definition: a malignancy of mature B cells, which display impaired apoptosis and functioning. There is a risk of transformation to a high-grade lymphoma (**Richter's transformation**).

Buzzwords:

- **Risk factors:** increasing age, male, Caucasian
- **Presentation:** lymphadenopathy (cervical, axillary, inguinal – large, nontender, rubbery), hepatosplenomegaly, recurrent infections, immune-mediated complications (e.g., haemolysis, ITP)

Investigations:

- **Blood:** FBC (normocytic normochromic anaemia, ↑ WCC, ↓ platelets)
- **Blood film:** mature, small lymphocytes, **smudge/smear cells** (because lymphocytes are more fragile) (Fig 11.15)
- **Bone marrow aspirate:** infiltration of other bone marrow with lymphocytes
- **Cytogenetics and immunophenotyping**

Differentials: lymphoma

Management: indolent disease that often requires only active monitoring

1. **Supportive treatment against infections:** vaccination, low threshold for antibiotics
2. **Chemotherapy:** fludarabine, cyclophosphamide, rituximab (FCR) for fit patients requiring treatment
3. **If high risk (determined by cytogenetics):** Ibrutinib (a Bruton-kinase inhibitor), Idelalisib (phosphoinositide 3–kinase inhibitor), Venetoclax (BCL-2 inhibitor)

Prognostic scores: Rai or Binet classification systems (incorporate factors such as organ enlargement, haemoglobin, lymphocytosis, platelet count)

Chronic Myeloid Leukaemia

Definition: a malignant haematopoietic disorder caused by a reciprocal translocation between Chromosome 9 and Chromosome 22 [t(9,22)]. This leads to the formation of the *BCR-ABL* gene on Chromosome 22, known as the Philadelphia chromosome. The BCR-ABL protein is a tyrosine kinase enzyme that is permanently switched 'on', leading to increased proliferation and decreased apoptosis. It can develop into AML (**blast transformation**)

Buzzwords:

- **Risk factors:** increased age, radiation exposure (rare)
- **Presentation:** splenomegaly, B symptoms (fever, weight loss, night sweats), symptoms of anaemia or thrombocytopaenia.

Investigations:

- **Blood:** FBC (normocytic normochromic anaemia, ↑ WCC, ↑ basophils/eosinophils, ↑/↓ platelets)
- **Blood film/bone marrow aspirate:** hypercellular with granulocytes at different stages of proliferation
- **Cytogenetic analysis:** Philadelphia chromosome (*BCR-ABL* gene)

Differentials: AML

Management: tyrosine-kinase inhibitor (e.g., imatinib, nilotinib, dasatinib)

Prognostic scores: Sokal, Hasford, EUTOS, which factor in the patient's age, blasts on peripheral blood, platelet count, and spleen size

Myelodysplastic Syndromes

Definition: a clonal disorder of haematopoietic stem cells characterised by ineffective haematopoiesis and peripheral cytopenia (can affect all cell lines or just one).

Buzzwords:

- **Risk factors:** age, previous radiation, previous chemotherapy, inherited haematological disorder (e.g., Fanconi anaemia)
- **Presentation:** median onset at 70 years of age, fatigue, breathlessness (anaemia), recurrent infections (neutropenia), bruising, bleeding (thrombocytopenia)

Investigations:

- **Blood:** FBC (macrocytic anaemia, ↓ platelets, ↓ neutrophils), ↓ reticulocytes
- **Blood film:** macrocytic red blood cells, nucleated red blood cells, decreased platelets, myeloblasts may be seen; features of dysplasia
- **Bone marrow biopsy:** hypercellular
  - Erythroid dysplasia: ring sideroblasts (iron deposition in mitochondria of erythroblasts – Pappenheimer body).
  - Myeloid dysplasia: nucleus hyposegmentation
  - Megakaryocyte dysplasia: monolobulated nuclei

- **Cytogenetics:** linked to prognosis, often loss of chromosome 5 or 7

Differentials: vitamin B12/folate-deficiency anaemia, alcohol excess, aplastic anaemia, AML, viral infection

Management: calculate risk of transformation using the revised International Prognostic Scoring System for MDS (IPSS-R)

- Low-risk disease:
  - **Stimulating agents:** erythropoietin (EPO), romiplostim (stimulates platelets), granulocyte colony–stimulating factor
  - **Transfusion:** blood or platelet
  - **Antibiotics:** prophylactic
  - Lenalidomide
- High-risk disease:
  - **Intensive chemotherapy** with allogenic stem cell transplantation if fit
  - **Azacitidine** (DNA methyltransferase inhibitors) if not fit

Prognosis: often progresses to AML

Lymphoma

Definition: accumulation of malignant lymphocytes in the lymph nodes and lymphoid tissue (e.g., spleen).

B symptoms such as **unexplained fever, weight loss by more than 10% in 6 months and night sweats** may be present. If present, a B will follow the stage (e.g., Stage IB). If absent, an A will follow the stage (e.g., Stage IA)

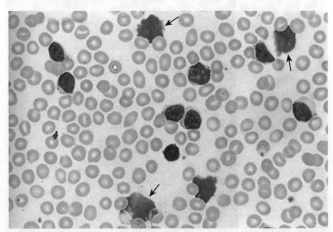

Fig 11.15 Blood film showing smear cells in chronic lymphocytic leukaemia. (With permission from Kumar, D. P. J., & Clark, M. L. (2021). Haematology and oncology (Fig. 6.15). In *Kumar & Clark's cases in clinical medicine.* Elsevier. Copyright © 2021 Elsevier Ltd. All rights reserved.)

Hodgkin Lymphoma

Definition: an accumulation of malignant B cell–lineage lymphocytes characterised by the presence of Reed-Sternberg cells. A Reed-Sternberg cell is a binucleate cell derived from a B cell (Fig 11.16).

Buzzwords:

- **Risk factors:** HIV, EBV, bimodal age distribution (20–30 and >70 years of age)
- **Presentation:** painless lymphadenopathy (commonly cervical), mediastinal involvement +/- splenomegaly, B symptoms, pruritus, alcohol-induced pain in lymph nodes, symptoms of cytopenias

Investigations:

- **Blood:** FBC (normocytic normochromic anaemia, ↑ basophils/eosinophils, ↑ neutrophils, in advanced disease there is ↓ lymphocytes), ↑ LDH
- **Blood film/bone marrow aspirate: Reed-Sternberg cell ('owl eyes' appearance)** with reactive inflammatory cells
- **Biopsy** (histology)
- **PET/CT:** staging (Table 11.6)

Differentials: non-Hodgkin lymphoma, infectious mononucleosis, lymphadenopathy from other malignancies

Management:

1. **Chemotherapy +/- radiotherapy:** e.g., ABVD (doxorubicin, bleomycin, vinblastine, dacarbazine)

2. **Supportive treatment:** e.g., transfusions, tumour lysis prophylaxis

Prognosis: good – approximately 80% can be cured. However, there is a risk of secondary cancers

Non-Hodgkin Lymphoma

Definition: all other lymphomas that *don't have* Reed-Sternberg cells present. These can be derived from B cells, T cells or natural killer cells.

Buzzwords:

- **Risk factors:** HIV, EBV, autoimmune conditions (e.g., Hashimoto's, coeliac disease, Sjögren's syndrome)
- **Presentation:** localised or generalised lymphadenopathy, hepatosplenomegaly, B symptoms, compressive symptoms from large lymph nodes

TABLE 11.6   Ann Arbor Staging System for Lymphoma

ANN ARBOR STAGING OF LYMPHOMAS	
Stage I	One lymph node area involved
Stage II	Two or more lymph node areas on the *same side of the diaphragm*
Stage III	Lymph nodes *above and below* the diaphragm
Stage IV	Diffuse or disseminated disease (e.g., bone marrow, liver)

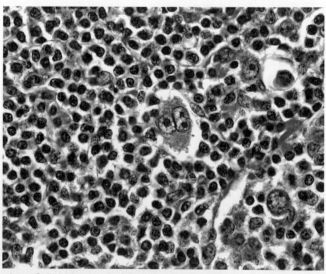

Fig 11.16 Reed-Sternberg Cell. (Uthman, E. CC BY-SA 2.0, via Wikimedia Commons. https://commons.wikimedia.org/wiki/File:Hodgkin_Disease,_ Reed-Sternberg_Cell.jpg.)

Investigations:

- **Blood:** FBC (can be normal; if bone marrow infiltration, may see normocytic normochromic anaemia, ↓ platelets, ↓ neutrophils), ↑ LDH
- **Blood film/lymph node biopsy:** lymphoma cells
- **HIV screening** (associated with a poorer prognosis in diffuse large B-cell lymphoma)
- **PET/CT:** staging

Differentials: Hodgkin lymphoma, reactive lymphadenopathy (e.g., infectious mononucleosis), CLL, ALL

Management: chemotherapy +/- monoclonal antibody therapy (e.g., R-CHOP); Ibrutinib (a Bruton-kinase inhibitor), Venetoclax (BCL-2 inhibitor) +/- rituximab

Monoclonal Gammopathy of Undetermined Significance (MGUS)

Definition: a malignant clonal haematopoietic disorder characterised by the production of a paraprotein in the absence of end-organ damage. A paraprotein is an abnormal monoclonal immunoglobulin produced by plasma cells. A plasma cell is a B cell that has been primed by an antigen-presenting cell in a lymphoid organ

Buzzwords:

- **Risk factors:** increasing age (>50 years)
- **Presentation:** incidental finding, no clinical symptoms

Investigations:

- **Serum immunoglobulin electrophoresis**: paraprotein <30 g/L, free kappa or lambda light chain ratio may be disrupted
- **Bone marrow aspirate** (if done): plasma cells comprise up to 10%

Differentials: multiple myeloma, amyloidosis, Waldenström macroglobulinaemia

Management: follow-up. Measure paraprotein levels and assess for symptoms every 6–12 months

Prognosis: 1% a year will go on to develop multiple myeloma

Multiple Myeloma

Definition: a malignant disease of plasma cells characterised by the presence of a paraprotein or light chains in the serum or urine and end-organ damage

Buzzwords:

- **Risk factors:** MGUS, age (rare under the age of 40 years), high-dose radiation, ethnicity (twice more common in Afro-Caribbeans than Caucasians)

- **Presentation: mnemonic CRAB**
  - **H**yper**C**alcaemia
  - **R**enal impairment (due to light chain deposition)/ Recurrent infections (deficient antibody production)
  - **A**naemia
  - **B**one disease (due to osteolysis → pathological fractures, back pain)

Investigations:

- **Blood:** FBC (normocytic normochromic anaemia, ↑ ESR), ↑ LDH, U&E (↑ urea, ↑ creatinine), bone profile (↑ adjusted calcium)
- **Serum free light chains:** elevated levels of kappa and lambda
- **Serum protein electrophoresis:** paraprotein present
- **Immunofixation:** to identify the specific type of paraprotein
- **Serum immunoglobulins:** decreased IgA, IgG, IgM – immunoparesis
- **Blood film:** Rouleaux formation (coin stacking of erythrocytes) (Fig 11.17)
- **Urine:** free light chains (**Bence Jones** proteins)
- **Bone marrow aspirate and trephine:** plasma cells >10%
- **Imaging:** MRI, CT, PET

Differentials: MGUS, amyloidosis, Waldenström macroglobulinaemia

Management:

- Supportive treatment
- Chemotherapy: bortezomib (proteosome inhibitor), thalidomide, dexamethasone (VTD) in fit patient; lenalidomide and dexamethasone in unfit
- Autologous stem cell transplantation for fit patients

Prognosis: median survival is 7–10 years.

Waldenström Macroglobulinaemia

Definition: a low-grade, clonal, B-cell disorder characterised by the production of monoclonal IgM paraproteins and bone marrow infiltration by lymphoplasmacytic cells

Buzzwords:

- **Risk factors:** IgM MGUS, family history, male, age >50 years
- **Presentation:** lymphadenopathy, hepatosplenomegaly, B symptoms, peripheral neuropathy, hyperviscosity syndrome (visual changes, headaches, shortness of breath), bleeding tendency (macroglobulin interferes

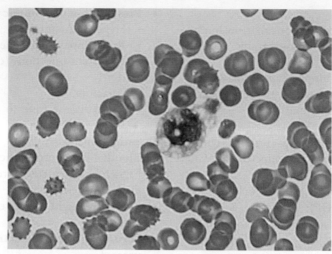

Fig 11.17 Blood film showing rouleaux formation. (With permission from John M. Bennett, MD.)

with platelet and coagulation factor function), cryoglobulinemia (may present with Raynaud's phenomenon)

Investigations:
- **Blood:** FBC (↓ Hb, ↓ WCC, ↓ neutrophils, ↓ platelets), ↑ LDH
- **Serum protein electrophoresis:** large amounts of IgM paraprotein
- **Cryoglobulins:** may be present
- **Blood film:** lymphoplasmacytoid cells
- **Bone marrow aspirate/lymph node biopsy:** lymphoplasmacytoid cells
- **Cytogenetic analysis:** *MYD88* mutation
- **PET/CT:** staging

Differentials: IgM MGUS, multiple myeloma, CLL

Management:
- If asymptomatic: active monitoring
- If symptomatic: combination chemotherapy with monoclonal antibody therapy (e.g., cyclophosphamide, fludarabine, bendamustine, bortezomib, rituximab)

MYELOPROLIFERATIVE DISORDERS/ NEOPLASMS

Clonal disorders caused by mutations in haematopoietic progenitor cells that lead to proliferation of one or more cell lines.

Polycythaemia Vera

Definition: a primary bone marrow disorder causing an increase in clonal red cell production. Can develop into myelofibrosis or AML

Buzzwords:
- **Risk factors:** family history, age >40 years
- **Presentation:** facial plethora, pruritus made worse by heat, hyperviscosity syndrome (headache, blurred vision), thrombosis, haemorrhage

Investigations:
- **Blood:** FBC (↑ Hb, ↑ haematocrit, ↑ WCC, ↑ platelets), ↓ EPO
- **Blood film:** packed with erythrocytes
- **Janus kinase 2 (*JAK2*) mutation:** present (95% have *JAK2* V617F)
- **Bone marrow trephine biopsy:** hypercellular
- **Cytogenetics:** prognostication – likelihood to transform to myelofibrosis or AML

Differentials: secondary polycythaemia, CML, essential thrombocythaemia

Management:
- Cardiovascular risk factor **management**
- Daily 75 mg aspirin for risk reduction for thrombosis
- Aim for haematocrit below 0.45
- Venesection
- Hydroxycarbamide (if at high risk of thrombosis)
- Ruxolitinib (JAK2 inhibitor)

Essential Thrombocythaemia

Definition: a primary bone marrow disorder causing an increase in clonal platelet production. Can develop into myelofibrosis or AML

Buzzwords:

- **Risk factors:** genetic mutations (e.g., *JAK2*, *CALR*, *MPL*), age >50 years
- **Presentation:** often an incidental finding, hyperviscosity syndrome (headache, blurred vision), thrombosis, erythromelalgia (burning pain, redness and warmth in extremities relieved by aspirin), haemorrhage (due to acquired vWD at a platelet count >1000 $\times 10^9$/L)

Investigations:

- **Blood:** FBC (↑ platelets, ↑ WCC, ↔/↑ Hb and haematocrit, ESR normal), CRP (normal)
- **Blood film:** increased number and size of platelets
- **Bone marrow biopsy:** increased megakaryocytes-enlarged, mature, hyperlobulated nuclei (staghorn nuclei)
- **Cytogenetics:** *JAK2*, *CALR*, *MPL* (for diagnosis), rule out CML

Differentials: myelodysplastic syndrome, CML, reactive thrombocytosis, iron-deficiency anaemia

Management:

1. Cardiovascular risk factor management
2. Daily 75 mg aspirin
3. Hydroxycarbamide (if at high risk of thrombosis)

Primary Myelofibrosis

Definition: primary bone marrow fibrosis due to clonal proliferation of a multipotent haematopoietic progenitor cell

Buzzwords:

- **Risk factors:** myeloproliferative disorder, radiation exposure, industrial solvents exposure, middle-aged and elderly
- **Presentation:** symptoms of cytopenias, hepatosplenomegaly (due to extramedullary haematopoiesis), portal hypertension and ascites, B symptoms

Investigations:

- **Blood:** FBC (↓ Hb, ↑ WCC, ↑ platelets (the latter two decrease in advanced disease)), ↑ LDH

- **Blood film:** leucoerythroblastic (granulocyte precursor cells and nucleated red blood cells) with 'tear drop' erythrocytes
- **USS abdomen:** for hepatosplenomegaly
- **Bone marrow trephine biopsy:** fibrotic marrow, increased megakaryocytes
- **Cytogenetics:** *JAK2*, *CALR*, *MPL*, rule out CML

Differentials: myeloproliferative disorders, myelodysplastic syndrome, CML

Management:

- **Symptom control:** anaemia (transfusions, EPO), thrombocytopaenia (transfusion), pruritis (antihistamines), splenomegaly (ruxolitinib)
- **Hydroxycarbamide:** for high counts
- **Allogeneic stem cell transplantation:** only curative option, only for very fit patients

Prognosis: 10%–20% transform to AML. Median survival is 3–5 years

HYPOSPLENISM

Definition: decreased function of the spleen. The spleen is involved in the removal of old and abnormal red cells and plays a role in immune function against encapsulated bacteria

Buzzwords:

- **Causes:** splenectomy, sickle cell disease, coeliac disease
- **Presentation:** sepsis from bacterial infections (e.g., *Haemophilus influenza* type B, *Neisseria meningitidis*, *Streptococcus pneumoniae*)

Investigations:

- **Blood:** FBC (↑ platelets, ↑ neutrophils), ↑ reticulocytes
- **Blood film:** acanthocytes (spiky red blood cells), target cells, Pappenheimer bodies, Howell-Jolly bodies (DNA remnants)

Management:

1. Counsel patients about their increased susceptibility to infection, especially meningitis, and the importance of vaccination
2. Prophylactic oral antibiotics (e.g., penicillin V) (lifelong)
3. Vaccination against *Pneumococcus*, *Haemophilus*, *Meningococcus*, *Influenza*

THE ONE-LINE ROUND-UP!

Here are some key words to help you remember each condition/concept.

Condition/Concept	One-line Description
Thalassaemia	Mediterranean, Southeast Asian, African with target cells
Iron-deficiency anaemia	Menorrhagia, vegan diet, serum ferritin <15 μg/L
Haemolytic anaemia	Decreased half-life of red blood cells, increased LDH, decreased haptoglobin
B12 deficiency	Found in eggs, meat, salmon, cod, milk
Folate deficiency	Found in asparagus, broccoli, brown rice, brussels sprouts, chickpeas
Sickle cell anaemia	Afro-Caribbeans, sticky red blood cells causing occlusions in the spleen, brain
ITP	Post-viral infection in children
HIT	>50% fall in platelet count, 5–10 days post-exposure to heparin
DIC	Excessive clot formation and fibrinolysis
HUS	Acute kidney injury
TTP	Large multimers of vWF binding to platelets and causing thrombosis in kidneys and brain
Factor V Leiden	Activated protein C resistance, family history of venous thrombosis
APLS	Recurrent miscarriages and thrombosis, females in 30s
Haemophilia	Increased bleeding in males of the family
VWD	Increased mucocutaneous bleeding (e.g., epistaxis, menorrhagia)
Vitamin K deficiency	Haemorrhagic disease of the newborn
AML	Halt in differentiation of myeloid cells accumulating in the bone marrow, adults

Condition/Concept	One-line Description
ALL	Halt in differentiation of lymphoid cells accumulating in the bone marrow, <6 years of age
CLL	Western world, elderly, lymphadenopathy, recurrent infection, smudge cells
CML	Philadelphia chromosome, splenomegaly, B symptoms, tyrosine-kinase inhibitors
MDS	Ineffective haematopoiesis leading to peripheral cytopenia, median onset at 70 years of age
HL	Lymphadenopathy, alcohol-induced pain, Reed-Sternberg cells
NHL	Lymphadenopathy, HIV, EBV, autoimmune conditions (e.g., Hashimoto's, coeliac, Sjögren's)
MGUS	Presence of paraprotein, no end-organ damage
MM	CRAB
Waldenström macroglobulinaemia	IgM paraprotein due to a clonal B-cell disorder, over 50 years of age, hyperviscosity syndrome, lymphadenopathy, peripheral neuropathy, bleeding tendency
PV	Increased red blood cells, hyperviscosity syndrome, JAK2 mutations
ET	Increased platelets, hyperviscosity syndrome, erythromelalgia
MF	Scarring of bone marrow, eventually causing cytopenias, middle-aged and elderly
Hyposplenism	Increased chance of infection (e.g., Pneumococcus, Haemophilus, Meningococcus)

READING LIST: HAEMATOLOGY IN AN HOUR

Haematology Key Principles

Hoffbrand, A. V., & Steensma, D. P. (2020). Chapter 24: Platelets, blood coagulation and haemostasis. In *Hoffbrand's essential haematology*. Wiley-Blackwell.

Pancytopaenia

Bain, B. J. (2020). Chapter 6: Miscellaneous anaemias, pancytopenia and the myelodysplastic syndromes. In *Haematology: A core curriculum*. World Scientific Publishing Europe Ltd.

Pancytopenia and the Myelodysplastic Syndromes

Hoffbrand, A. V., & Steensma, D. P. (2020). Chapter 22-Aplastic anaemia and bone marrow failure. In *Hoffbrand's essential haematology*. Wiley-Blackwell.

Thalassaemia

British Society of Haematology. (2010). Significant haemoglobinopathies: Guidelines for screening and diagnosis. *The British Journal of Haematology*, 149, 35–49.

BMJ Best Practice. (2019). *Alpha-thalassaemia*. https://bestpractice.bmj.com/topics/en-gb/250. [Accessed April 21].

Iron-deficiency Anaemia

NICE. (2018). *CKS: Anaemia – iron deficiency*. https://cks.nice.org.uk/topics/anaemia-iron-deficiency/. [Accessed April 2021].

Haemolytic Anaemia

Bain, B. J. (2020). Chapter 5: Haemoglobinopathies and haemolytic anaemias. In *Haematology: A core curriculum*. World Scientific Publishing Europe Ltd.

Hoffbrand, A. V., & Steensma, D. P. (2020). Chapter 6: Haemolytic anaemias. In *Hoffbrand's essential haematology*. Wiley-Blackwell.

Glucose-6-Phosphate Dehydrogenase Deficiency

Bain, B. J. (2020). Chapter 5: Haemoglobinopathies and haemolytic anaemias. In *Haematology: A core curriculum*. World Scientific Publishing Europe Ltd.

Hoffbrand, A. V., & Steensma, D. P. (2020). Chapter 6: Haemolytic anaemias. In *Hoffbrand's essential haematology*. Wiley-Blackwell.

Autoimmune Haemolytic Anaemia

Bain, B. J. (2020). Chapter 5: Haemoglobinopathies and haemolytic anaemias. In *Haematology: A core curriculum*. World Scientific Publishing Europe Ltd.

Hoffbrand, A. V., & Steensma, D. P. (2020). Chapter 6: Haemolytic anaemias. In *Hoffbrand's essential haematology*. Wiley-Blackwell.

BNF. *Treatment summary: Anaemias*. https://bnf.nice.org.uk/treatment-summary/anaemia-iron-deficiency.html. [Accessed April 2021]

B12-deficiency Anaemia

NICE. (2018). *CKS: Anaemia – B12 and folate deficiency*. https://cks.nice.org.uk/topics/anaemia-b12-folate-deficiency/. [Accessed April 2021].

British Society of Haematology. (2014). Guidelines for the diagnosis and treatment of cobalamin and folate disorders. *The British Journal of Haematology*, 166, 496–513.

Folate-deficiency Anaemia

NICE. (2018). *CKS: Anaemia – B12 and folate deficiency*. https://cks.nice.org.uk/topics/anaemia-b12-folate-deficiency/. [Accessed April 2021].

Sickle Cell Disease

Bain, B. J. (2020). Chapter 5: Haemoglobinopathies and haemolytic anaemias. In *Haematology: A core curriculum*. World Scientific Publishing Europe Ltd.

Hoffbrand, A. V., & Steensma, D. P. (2020). Chapter 7: Genetic disorders of haemoglobin. In *Hoffbrand's essential haematology*. Wiley-Blackwell.

NICE. (2016). *CKS: Sickle cell disease*. https://cks.nice.org.uk/topics/sickle-cell-disease/. [Accessed April 2021].

Immune Thrombocytopenic Purpura

Bain, B. J. (2020). Chapter 11: Platelets, coagulation and haemostasis. In *Haematology: A core curriculum*. World Scientific Publishing Europe Ltd.

Hoffbrand, A. V., & Steensma, D. P. (2020). Chapter 25: Bleeding disorders: Vascular and platelet abnormalities. In *Hoffbrand's essential haematology*. Wiley-Blackwell.

BMJ Best Practice. (2019). *Immune thrombocytopenia*. https://bestpractice.bmj.com/topics/en-gb/138. [Accessed April 2021].

Heparin-induced Thrombocytopenia

Bain, B. J. (2020). Chapter 12: Thrombosis and its management. In *Haematology: A core curriculum*. World Scientific Publishing Europe Ltd.

Hoffbrand, A. V., & Steensma, D. P. (2020). Chapter 28: Thrombosis 2: treatment. In *Hoffbrand's essential haematology*. Wiley-Blackwell.

Cuker, A., Gimotty, P., Crowther, M., & Warkentin, T. (2012). Predictive value of the 4Ts scoring system for heparin-induced thrombocytopenia: A systematic review and meta-analysis. *Blood*, 120, 4160–4167.

BNF. *Drugs: Enoxaparin sodium*. https://bnf.nice.org.uk/drug/enoxaparin-sodium.html. [Accessed April 2021]

Disseminated Intravascular Coagulation

Bain, B. J. (2020). Chapter 11: Platelets, coagulation and haemostasis. In *Haematology: A core curriculum*. World Scientific Publishing Europe Ltd.

Hoffbrand, A. V., & Steensma, D. P. (2020). Chapter 26: Coagulation disorders. In *Hoffbrand's essential haematology*. Wiley-Blackwell.

Haemolytic Uraemic Syndrome

Bain, B. J. (2020). Chapter 5: Haemoglobinopathies and haemolytic anaemias. In *Haematology: A core curriculum*. World Scientific Publishing Europe Ltd.

Hoffbrand, A. V., & Steensma, D. P. (2020). Chapter 25: Bleeding disorders: vascular and platelet abnormalities. In *Hoffbrand's essential haematology*. Wiley-Blackwell.

Thrombotic Thrombocytopenia Purpura

Bain, B. J. (2020). Chapter 11: Platelets, coagulation and haemostasis. In *Haematology: A core curriculum*. World Scientific Publishing Europe Ltd.

Hoffbrand, A. V., & Steensma, D. P. (2020). Chapter 25: Bleeding disorders: Vascular and platelet abnormalities. In *Hoffbrand's essential haematology*. Wiley-Blackwell.

BMJ Best Practice. (2019). *Thrombotic thrombocytopenic purpura*. https://bestpractice.bmj.com/topics/en-gb/715#:~:text=An%20urgent%20haematological%20consultation%20is,an%20adjunctive%20therapy%20in%20adults. [Accessed April 2021].

Factor V Leiden

BMJ Best Practice. (2019). *Hypercoagulable state*. https://bestpractice.bmj.com/topics/en-gb/889#:~:text=Hypercoagulable%20state%20(also%20known%20as,contribute%20to%20the%20hypercoagulable%20state. [Accessed April 2021].

Antiphospholipid Syndrome

British Society of Haematology. (2012). Guidelines on the investigation and management of antiphospholipid syndrome. *The British Journal of Haematology*, *157*, 47–58.

Hoffbrand, A. V., & Steensma, D. P. (2020). Chapter 27: Thrombosis 1: Pathogenesis and diagnosis. In *Hoffbrand's essential haematology*. Wiley-Blackwell.

Clunie, G., Wilkinson, N., Nikiphorou, E., & Jadon, D. (2018). *Oxford handbook of rheumatology* (4th ed.). Oxford University Press.

Patient info. (2015). *Antiphospholipid syndrome*. https://patient.info/doctor/antiphospholipid-syndrome-pro. [Accessed 24 August 2020].

Haemophilia A and B

NICE. (2016). *CKS: Bruising*. https://cks.nice.org.uk/topics/bruising/ [Accessed April 2021].

BMJ Best Practice. (2019). *Haemophilia*. https://bestpractice.bmj.com/topics/en-gb/468. [Accessed April 2021].

Von Willebrand Disease

NICE. (2016). *CKS: Bruising*. https://cks.nice.org.uk/topics/bruising/. [Accessed April 2021].

BMJ Best Practice. (2018). *Von Willebrand disease*. https://bestpractice.bmj.com/topics/en-gb/365. [Accessed April 2021].

Vitamin K Deficiency

NICE. (2016). *CKS: Bruising*. https://cks.nice.org.uk/topics/bruising/. [Accessed April 2021].

Lab tests online. (2017). *Vitamin K deficiency*. https://labtestsonline.org.uk/conditions/vitamin-k-deficiency. [Accessed April 2021].

Acute Myeloid Leukaemia

Bain, B. J. (2020). Chapter 8: Leukaemias and lymphomas. In *Haematology: A core curriculum*. World Scientific Publishing Europe Ltd.

Hoffbrand, A. V., & Steensma, D. P. (2020). Chapter 13: Acute myeloid leukaemia. In *Hoffbrand's essential haematology*. Wiley-Blackwell.

NICE. (2020). *CKS: Haematological cancers-recognition and referral*. https://cks.nice.org.uk/topics/haematological-cancers-recognition-referral/. [Accessed April 2021].

Acute Lymphoblastic Leukaemia

Bain, B. J. (2020). Chapter 8: Leukaemias and lymphomas. In *Haematology: A core curriculum*. World Scientific Publishing Europe Ltd.

Hoffbrand, A. V., & Steensma, D. P. (2020). Chapter 17: Acute lymphoblastic leukaemia. In *Hoffbrand's essential haematology*. Wiley-Blackwell.

NICE. (2020). *CKS: Haematological cancers-recognition and referral*. https://cks.nice.org.uk/topics/haematological-cancers-recognition-referral/. [Accessed April 2021].

Chronic Lymphocytic Leukaemia

Bain, B. J. (2020). Chapter 8: Leukaemias and lymphomas. In *Haematology: A core curriculum*. World Scientific Publishing Europe Ltd.

Hoffbrand, A. V., & Steensma, D. P. (2020). Chapter 18: The chronic lymphocytic leukaemias. In *Hoffbrand's essential haematology*. Wiley-Blackwell.

Chronic Myeloid Leukaemia

Bain, B. J. (2020). Chapter 8: Leukaemias and lymphomas. In *Haematology: A core curriculum*. World Scientific Publishing Europe Ltd.

Hoffbrand, A. V., & Steensma, D. P. (2020). Chapter 14: Chronic myeloid leukaemia. In *Hoffbrand's essential haematology*. Wiley-Blackwell.

NICE. (2020). *CKS: Polycythaemia/erythrocytosis*. https://cks.nice.org.uk/topics/polycythaemia-erythrocytosis/. [Accessed April 2021].

BMJ Best Practice. (2018). *Chronic myelogenous leukaemia*. https://bestpractice.bmj.com/topics/en-gb/276. [Accessed April 2021].

Myelodysplastic Syndromes

Bain, B. J. (2020). Chapter 6: Miscellaneous anaemias, pancytopenia and the myelodysplastic syndromes. In *Haematology: A core curriculum*. World Scientific Publishing Europe Ltd.

Hoffbrand, A. V., & Steensma, D. P. (2020). Chapter 16: Myelodysplastic syndromes. In *Hoffbrand's essential haematology*. Wiley-Blackwell.

Hodgkin Lymphoma

Bain, B. J. (2020). Chapter 8: Leukaemias and lymphomas. In *Haematology: A core curriculum*. World Scientific Publishing Europe Ltd.

Hoffbrand, A. V., & Steensma, D. P. (2020). Chapter 19: Hodgkin lymphoma. In *Hoffbrand's essential haematology*. Wiley-Blackwell.

Non-Hodgkin Lymphoma

Bain, B. J. (2020). Chapter 8: Leukaemias and lymphomas. In *Haematology: A core curriculum*. World Scientific Publishing Europe Ltd.

Hoffbrand, A. V., & Steensma, D. P. (2020). Chapter 20: Non-Hodgkin lymphomas. In *Hoffbrand's essential haematology*. Wiley-Blackwell.

Monoclonal Gammopathy of Undetermined Significance

Bain, B. J. (2020). Chapter 10: Multiple myeloma. In *Haematology: A core curriculum*. World Scientific Publishing Europe Ltd.

Hoffbrand, A. V., & Steensma, D. P. (2020). Chapter 21: Multiple myeloma and related plasma cell neoplasms. In *Hoffbrand's essential haematology*. Wiley-Blackwell.

Multiple Myeloma

Bain, B. J. (2020). Chapter 10: Multiple myeloma. In *Haematology: A core curriculum*. World Scientific Publishing Europe Ltd.

Hoffbrand, A. V., & Steensma, D. P. (2020). Chapter 21: Multiple myeloma and related plasma cell neoplasms. In *Hoffbrand's essential haematology*. Wiley-Blackwell.

MacMillan. (2018). *Cancer information and support: Myeloma*. https://www.macmillan.org.uk/cancer-information-and-support/myeloma. [Accessed 2021].

NICE Pathways. (2021). *Myeloma overview*. https://www.nice.org.uk/search?om=[%7B%22gst%22:[%22Published%22]%7D]&ps=15&q=myeloma&sp=on. [Accessed on April 2021].

Waldenström Macroglobulinaemia

Hoffbrand, A. V., & Steensma, D. P. (2020). Chapter 20: Non-Hodgkin lymphomas. In *Hoffbrand's essential haematology*. Wiley-Blackwell.

BMJ Best Practice. (2020). *Waldenström's macroglobulinaemia*. https://bestpractice.bmj.com/topics/en-gb/897#:~:text=Waldenstr%C3%B6m's%20macroglobulinaemia%20(WM)%20is%20an,paraprotein%20on%20a%20blood%20test. [Accessed April 2021].

Polycythaemia Vera

Bain, B. J. (2020). Chapter 9: Polycythaemia, thrombocytosis and the myeloproliferative neoplasms. In *Haematology: A core curriculum*. World Scientific Publishing Europe Ltd.

Hoffbrand, A. V., & Steensma, D. P. (2020). Chapter 15: Myeloproliferative neoplasms. In *Hoffbrand's essential haematology*. Wiley-Blackwell.

NICE. (2020). *CKS: Polycythaemia/erythrocytosis*. https://cks.nice.org.uk/topics/polycythaemia-erythrocytosis/. [Accessed April 2021].

BMJ Best Practice. (2018). *Polycythaemia vera*. https://bestpractice.bmj.com/topics/en-gb/178. [Accessed April 2021].

Essential Thrombocythaemia

Bain, B. J. (2020). Chapter 9: Polycythaemia, thrombocytosis and the myeloproliferative neoplasms. In *Haematology: A core curriculum*. World Scientific Publishing Europe Ltd.

Hoffbrand, A. V., & Steensma, D. P. (2020). Chapter 15: Myeloproliferative neoplasms. In *Hoffbrand's essential haematology*. Wiley-Blackwell.

Macmillan. (2019). *Cancer information and support: Blood cancer: Essential thrombocythaemia*. https://www.macmillan.org.uk/cancer-information-and-support/blood-cancer/essential-thrombocythaemia-et. [Accessed April 2021].

British Society of Haematology. (2010). Guideline for investigation and management of adults and children presenting with a thrombocytosis. *The British Journal of Haematology*, *149*, 352–375.

Primary Myelofibrosis

Bain, B. J. (2020). Chapter 9: Polycythaemia, thrombocytosis and the myeloproliferative neoplasms. In *Haematology: A core curriculum*. World Scientific Publishing Europe Ltd.

Hoffbrand, A. V., & Steensma, D. P. (2020). Chapter 15: Myeloproliferative neoplasms. In *Hoffbrand's essential haematology*. Wiley-Blackwell.

BMJ Best Practice. (2018). *Myelofibrosis*. https://bestpractice.bmj.com/topics/en-gb/1132. [Accessed April 2021].

Hyposplenism

Bain, B. J. (2020). Chapter 5: Haemoglobinopathies and haemolytic anaemias. In *Haematology: A core curriculum*. World Scientific Publishing Europe Ltd.

Hoffbrand, A. V., & Steensma, D. P. (2020). Chapter 10: The spleen. In *Hoffbrand's essential haematology*. Wiley-Blackwell.

12

Infectious Diseases in an Hour

*Yvonne Chang, Jeffrey Wu, Gregory Oxenham,
Berenice Aguirrezabala Armbruster, Hannah Punter
and Georgina Beckley*

INTRODUCTION

Antibacterial Classification

Antibacterials can be classified by their spectrum, activity and/or mode of action.

Spectrum:
- **Broad spectrum:** target both Gram-positive **and** Gram-negative bacteria
- **Narrow spectrum:** target only **one** type, either Gram-positive **or** Gram-negative bacteria

Gram Stain:

Gram-negative stains **pink** and Gram-positive stains **purple**. See Fig 12.1 to see the difference between the cell wall structures of Gram-positive and Gram-negative bacterias.

Activity:
- **Bactericidal** (irreversible): kills bacteria
- **Bacteriostatic** (reversible): slows down the growth of bacteria

Mode of action:
- **Cell wall synthesis inhibitors:**
  - Glycopeptides: vancomycin, teicoplanin
  - Beta lactams: Peni**cillin**s (e.g., Benzylpeni**cillin**, Fluclox**acillin**, Amoxi**cillin**), Cephalosporins (e.g., Cephalexin, Cefuroxime, Ceftazidime), Carbap**enem**s (e.g., Imip**enem**, Ertap**enem**, Merop**enem**)
- **Nucleic acid synthesis inhibitors:**
  - Folate synthesis inhibitors: Sulphonamides (e.g., Sulfamethoxazole), Trimethoprim
  - DNA gyrase inhibitors: Fluoroquinolones (e.g., Ciprofloxacin, Ofloxacin, Levofloxacin)
  - DNA strand inhibitors: Nitroimidazoles (e.g., Metronidazole)
  - RNA polymerase inhibitors: Rifamycins (e.g., Rifampicin)
- **Protein synthesis inhibitors:**
  - Chloramphenicol
  - Macrolides: clarithromycin, erythromycin, azithromycin
  - Lincosamides: clindamycin
  - Tetra**cyclines**: Tetra**cycline**, Doxy**cycline**
  - Aminoglycosides: gentamycin, streptomycin

Monitoring levels of antimicrobials

Peak (post-dose) level measured 1 h after administration and trough (pre-dose) levels are measured immediately before administration of the next dose

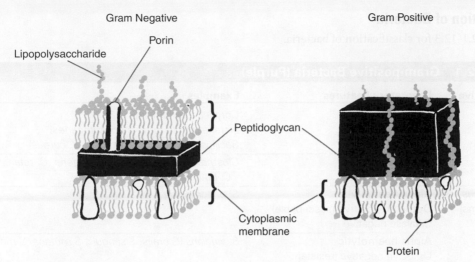

Fig 12.1 Structure of the cell wall in gram-negative vs gram-positive bacteria. (Illustrated by Hollie Blaber.)

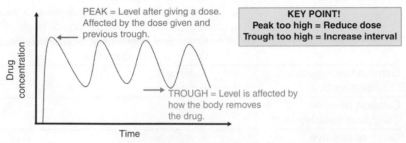

Fig 12.2 Peak and trough levels.

(see Fig 12.2). Antibiotics that require monitoring include:

- **Aminoglycosides:** gentamicin, tobramycin, amikacin
- **Glycopeptides:** vancomycin, teicoplanin

Serum samples should be sent after the 3rd or 4th dose. Subsequent levels should be checked twice weekly if renal function is stable or more frequently if renal function changes, since aminoglycosides are nephrotoxic.

Each antibiotic has its own peak and trough target levels.

Gentamicin levels:

- Gentamicin serum levels are taken 1 h before the third dose ('trough' concentration) and after the third dose ('peak' concentration).

- **Post-dose (peak) concentration:** reflects how much gentamicin has accumulated in the blood
- **Pre-dose (trough) concentration:** reflects how well the body is getting rid of gentamicin
- If the **pre-dose ('trough') concentration** is too high, the interval between doses must be increased to allow the body more time to get rid of the gentamicin (e.g., TDS to BD)
- If the **post-dose ('peak') concentration** is too high, the dose must be decreased

Vancomycin levels:

- Initial dosing should be based on body weight
- Subsequent dosing should be based on serum vancomycin concentration
- For drug monitoring, apply the same principles as with gentamicin

Classification of Bacteria

See Tables 12.1-12.3 for classification of bacteria.

TABLE 12.1	Gram-positive Bacteria (Purple)	
Gram Positive	**Laboratory Features**	**Examples**
Bacilli	Aerobic	*Corynebacterium* spp.
		Listeria spp. (e.g., *L. monocytogenes*)
		Bacillus spp. (e.g., *B. anthracis, B. cereus*)
	Anaerobic	*Clostridium* spp. (e.g., *C. perfringens, C. tetani, C. difficile, C. botulinum*)
Streptococcus (cocci chains)	Alpha haemolytic Optochin positive (susceptible) Catalase negative	*S. pneumoniae*
	Alpha haemolytic Optochin negative (resistant) Catalase negative	*S. viridians* (*S.oralis, S.sanguis, S.mutans, S.mitis*)
	Beta haemolytic Catalase negative	Group A: *S. pyogenes* Group B: *S. agalactiae* Group C: *S. esqui, S. esquisimilus, S. zooepiodemicus* Group D: *Enterococcus* spp., *S. bovis* Group F: *S. anguinosus, S. constellatus, S. intermedius* Group G: *S. dysgalactiae*
	Gamma haemolytic Catalase negative	*E. faecalis* *E. faecium*
Staphylococcus (cocci clusters)	Catalase positive Coagulase positive	*S. aureus*
	Catalase positive Coagulase negative	*S. epidermidis* *S. saprophyticus* *S. haemolyticus*

Classification of Viruses

See Table 12.4-12.6 for virus classification.

Notifiable Diseases

Some common diseases notifiable under the 2010 Health Protection (Notification) Regulations:

- Acute infectious hepatitis
- Acute poliomyelitis
- Anthrax
- Botulism
- Cholera
- SARS-CoV-2 (COVID-19)
- Diphtheria
- Enteric fever (typhoid or paratyphoid fever)
- Food poisoning
- Haemolytic uraemic syndrome (HUS)
- Infectious bloody diarrhoea
- Invasive group A streptococcal disease
- Legionnaires' disease
- Malaria
- Measles
- Meningococcal septicaemia
- Mumps
- Plague
- Rabies
- Rubella
- Severe acute respiratory syndrome (SARS)
- Scarlet fever
- Smallpox
- Tuberculosis
- Viral haemorrhagic fever (VHF)
- Whooping cough
- Yellow fever

TABLE 12.2 Gram-negative Bacteria (Pink)

Gram Negative	Laboratory Features	Examples
Coccoba-cilli	Parvo bacteria	*Hemophilus influenzae* *Bordetella pertussis* *Moraxella catarrhalis* *Brucella* spp.
Bacilli	Simple growth requirements: Aerobic Lactose fermenters	*Klebsiella pneumoniae* *Escherichia coli* *Enterobacter cloacae*
	Simple growth requirements: Aerobic Lactose nonfermenters Oxidase positive	*Pseudomonas aeruginosa* *Vibrio* spp.
	Simple growth requirements: Aerobic Lactose nonfermenters Oxidase negative	*Proteus mirabilis* *Shigella dysenteriae* *Salmonella* spp.
	Fastidious growth requirements	*Legionella pneumophilia* *Campylobacter* spp. *Helicobacter* spp. *Bartonella* spp.
Diplococci	Oxidase positive	*N. meningitidis* *N. gonorrhoea*

TABLE 12.3 Non-gram–staining Bacteria

Features	Examples
Obligate intracellular	*Chlamydia* spp. *Rickettsia* spp.
Acid-fast bacilli	*Mycobacteria* spp.
Spirochaetes	*Treponema* spp. *Borrelia* spp. *Leptospira* spp.
No cell wall	*Mycoplasma* spp.

TABLE 12.4 DNA Viruses

DNA Viruses	Laboratory Features	Examples
Adenoviridae	Capsid: nonenveloped (naked) Structure: icosahedral Nucleic acid type: double stranded	Common cold viruses
Herpesviridae	Capsid: enveloped Structure: icosahedral Nucleic acid type: double stranded	Herpes simplex virus Varicella zoster virus Cytomegalovirus Epstein-Barr virus
Poxviridae	Capsid: complex coats Structure: complex Nucleic acid type: double stranded	Smallpox virus Myxoma virus
Papovaviridae	Capsid: nonenveloped (naked) Structure: icosahedral Nucleic acid type: double stranded, circular	Human papillomavirus
Parvoviridae	Capsid: nonenveloped (naked) Structure: icosahedral Nucleic acid type: single stranded	Parvovirus B19

CNS INFECTIONS

Bacterial Meningitis

Definition: inflammation of the meninges caused by bacteria, predominantly *Streptococcus pneumoniae*, *Neisseria meningitidis* (meningococcus) and *Haemophilus influenzae* (all three are notifiable diseases)

For viral meningitis and encephalitis, see Neurololgy in an Hour

Buzzwords:

- **Risk factors:** crowded living conditions, exposure/close contact with an infected person, cranial anatomical defects, sickle cell disease
- **Presentation:** headache, neck stiffness, fever, altered mental status, vomiting, photophobia, seizures, rash (meningococcal meningitis/septicaemia – nonblanching purpura), papilledema, Kernig's sign (lower back pain on extension of knee while hip is flexed at 90°)
- **Complications:** shock, seizures, ↑ intracranial pressure, disseminated intravascular coagulation (DIC),

TABLE 12.5 RNA Viruses

RNA Viruses	Laboratory Features	Examples
Reoviridae	Capsid: nonenveloped (naked) Structure: icosahedral Nucleic acid type: double stranded	Rotavirus
Herpesviridae	Capsid: nonenveloped (naked) Structure: icosahedral Nucleic acid type: single stranded	Hepatitis B virus
Picornaviridae	Capsid: nonenveloped (naked) Structure: icosahedral Nucleic acid type: single stranded	Hepatitis A virus Enterovirus Rhinovirus Poliovirus Coxsackie virus
Flaviviridae	Capsid: enveloped Structure: icosahedral Nucleic acid type: single stranded	Dengue virus Hepatitis C virus Yellow fever virus Zika virus
Coronaviridae	Capsid: enveloped Structure: helical Nucleic acid type: single stranded	Severe acute respiratory syndrome coronavirus 2 (SARS-Cov-2) Middle East Respiratory virus (MERS)
Filoviridae	Capsid: enveloped Structure: helical Nucleic acid type: single stranded (-)	Ebola virus
Orthomyxoviridae	Capsid: enveloped Structure: helical Nucleic acid type: single stranded (-)	Influenza viruses A, B and C
Paramyxoviridae	Capsid: enveloped Structure: helical Nucleic acid type: single stranded (-)	Measles virus Mumps virus Respiratory syncytial virus
Rhabdoviridae	Capsid: enveloped Structure: helical Nucleic acid type: single stranded (-)	Rabies virus
Matonaviridae	Capsid: enveloped Structure: icosahedral Nucleic acid type: single stranded (+)	Rubella virus

TABLE 12.6 Reverse-transcribing Viruses that Encode a Reverse Transcriptase

Reverse-transcribing Viruses	Laboratory Features	Examples
Retroviridae	Capsid: enveloped Structure: complex Nucleic acid type: single stranded RNA (+)	Human immunodeficiency virus
Hepadnaviridae	Capsid: enveloped Structure: icosahedral Nucleic acid type: double stranded DNA	Hepatitis B virus

Waterhouse-Friderichsen syndrome (in meningococcal infection)

Investigations:
- **Blood cultures** ideally within 1 h of symptom onset and before antibiotic treatment
- **VBG:** acidosis, ↑ lactate (septic shock)
- **Full blood count (FBC):** ↑ WCC, ↓ RBC, ↓ platelets, ↑ CRP
- **Blood glucose:** ↑/↓ glucose
- **U&Es:** ↓ K, ↓ Ca, ↓ Mg
- **Coagulation screen:** ↑ prothrombin time, ↑ D-dimer, ↓ fibrinogen
- **Lumbar puncture** (within 1 h of symptom onset): cerebrospinal fluid (CSF) (↑ protein, ↑ lactate, ↓ glucose, ↑ neutrophils)

Differentials: encephalitis, viral meningitis, tuberculous meningitis, fungal meningitis

Management: IV antibacterials, corticosteroids, supportive (fluids, oxygen)
- *S. pneumoniae*: ceftriaxone/cefotaxime/benzylpenicillin/chloramphenicol/vancomycin
- *N. meningitidis*: ceftriaxone/cefotaxime/cefepime (benzylpenicillin on first suspicion)
- *H. influenzae*: ceftriaxone or cefotaxime

GASTROINTESTINAL INFECTIONS

See Table 12.7 for a summary of organisms causing dysentery or watery diarrhoea.

Bloody Diarrhoea
Campylobacter Enteritis
Definition: intestinal infection caused by *Campylobacter jejuni*

TABLE 12.7 Diarrhoea Presentations and Associated Organisms

Bloody Diarrhoea (Dysentery)	Watery Diarrhoea
Campylobacter jejuni E. coli O157:H7 Other Shiga toxin–producing E. coli Salmonella spp. Shigella spp.	Bacillus cereus Listeria monocytogenes Enterotoxigenic E. coli (ETEC – traveller's diarrhoea) Clostridium perfringens Clostridium difficile Giardia lamblia

Buzzwords:

- **Risk factors:** exposure to poultry/farm animals, eating undercooked chicken, recent foreign travel, human immunodeficiency virus (HIV) infection, immunocompromise, proton-pump inhibitor (PPI) use
- **Presentation:** self-limiting bloody diarrhoea (5–7 days), abdominal pain
- **Complications:** reactive arthritis, Guillain-Barre syndrome (GBS), bacteraemia
  - *Campylobacter* is the most implicated gastrointestinal (GI) infection in GBS

Investigations:

- **Stool microscopy, culture and sensitivity (MC&S):** RBCs and neutrophils in stool
- **FBC:** normal or neutrophilia

Differentials: *Salmonella* gastroenteritis, *Shigella* gastroenteritis, *E. coli* gastroenteritis, cholera, viral gastroenteritides

Management:

- Rehydration: oral rehydration solutions, IV fluids for nausea and vomiting
- Antibacterials: azithromycin, for severe infections and the immunocompromised (high fever, bacteraemia, grossly bloody diarrhoea, symptoms >1 week)

E. coli O157:H7 and Other Shiga Toxin–producing *E. coli* Infections

Definition: *E. coli* O157:H7 is a strain of Shiga toxin–producing *E. coli* that is known to cause a bloody diarrhoeal illness.

Buzzwords:

- **Risk factors:** contaminated water, undercooked meat (ground beef), travel, poor hygiene, contact with infected person, age <5 or >60 years

- **Presentation:** incubation is 3–4 days, bloody diarrhoea, abdominal pain, fever, oliguria
- **Complications:** dehydration, haemolytic uraemic syndrome (HUS), acute kidney injury (AKI)

Investigations:

- **Stool MC&S**
- **Blood:** FBC (↑ WCC; ↓ platelets in HUS); U&Es (AKI, ↓ K); ↑ CRP
- **Imaging:** abdominal X-ray (AXR) to rule out toxic megacolon

Differentials: intussusception, amoebiasis, viral gastroenteritis, noninfectious food poisoning (e.g., mushrooms/toxins), ischaemic colitis

Management:

- Oral/IV rehydration
- Management of HUS

Salmonella Gastroenteritis

Definition: non-typhoidal gastroenteritis that is self-limited. Most commonly caused by *Salmonella enteritidis*. Incubation is 6–72 h.

Buzzwords:

- **Risk factors:** poultry, raw milk, undercooked eggs, age <12 months or >50 years, low gastric acidity, diabetes
- **Presentation:** bloody diarrhoea, nausea/vomiting, fever, myalgia, abdominal pain
- **Complications:** dehydration, reactive arthritis, bacteraemia

Investigations:

- **Stool MC&S**
- **Blood culture**

Differentials: shigellosis, *Campylobacter* infection, yersiniosis, cholera

Management:

- Oral/IV rehydration, reduced osmolarity oral rehydration solution
- Antibacterials: ciprofloxacin, azithromycin, ceftriaxone for severe infections lasting >5 days, immunocompromised or bacteraemia

Shigellosis

Definition: most important pathogen is *Shigella dysenteriae* (cause of HUS, Shiga-toxin producing), others can cause a self-limited diarrhoeal illness

Buzzwords:

- **Risk factors:** contaminated water or food, age <5 or >50 years, travel to endemic areas

- **Presentation:** diarrhoea, abdominal cramps/pain, fever, tenesmus, oliguria
- **Complications:** dehydration, reactive arthritis, HUS, AKI

Investigations:
- **Stool MC&S**
- **Blood:** U&Es (↑ urea, AKI→ HUS); FBC (↑ WCC, ↓ platelets→ HUS)
- **Imaging:** AXR to rule out toxic megacolon

Differentials: viral gastroenteritis, parasitic diarrhoea, amoebiasis

Management:
- Oral/IV rehydration
- Management of HUS
- **Antibacterials** are indicated: ciprofloxacin, azithromycin

Watery Diarrhoea
Bacillus cereus

Definition: cause of food poisoning due to its toxin. Common sources include leftover rice and sauces kept at room temperature for a long period of time, typically at take-aways. Incubation period is 1-16 h.

Buzzwords:
- **Risk factors:** food not cooked to sufficiently high temperatures or stored incorrectly
- **Presentation:** self-limiting, watery diarrhoea and/or vomiting, cramping abdominal pain
- **Complications:** dehydration

Investigations:
- **Stool MC&S**

Differentials: other causes of food poisoning

Management:
- Oral rehydration

Listeriosis

Definition: Foodborne infection caused by *Listeria monocytogenes*. Responsible for local outbreaks related to contaminated food.

Buzzwords:
- **Risk factors:** raw, undercooked or processed meats; soft cheeses; unpasteurised milk; pregnancy; older adults; neonates
- **Presentation:** headache, fever, diarrhoea, abdominal pain, flu-like symptoms in pregnancy, altered mental status (CNS involvement)
- **Complications:** in pregnancy – septic abortion, stillbirth; listerial meningitis, listerial endocarditis

Investigations:
- **Blood:** FBC (↑ WCC, ↓ platelets); blood culture (bacteraemia)
- **Urine BHCG:** – to rule out pregnancy (causes severe disease)
- **Imaging:** brain MRI or CT – if suspicion of CNS infection
- **Lumbar puncture:** if symptoms or signs of meningitis

Differentials: other bacterial gastroenteritides or meningitides, brain abscesses, viral gastroenteritides

Management:
- Oral/IV rehydration
- **Antibacterials (In Severe Disease):** Amoxicillin or Trimethoprim/Sulfamethoxazole (if penicillin allergy) for 3 to 5 days. Ampicillin is first-line treatment, with gentamicin used for systemic or CNS involvement for up to 21 days. Benzylpenicillin – strongly indicated

Traveller's Diarrhoea (TD)

Definition: three or more unformed stools in 24 h accompanied by fever, nausea, vomiting, cramps or tenesmus during a trip abroad. Most common causes are enterotoxigenic *E. coli* and enteroaggregative *E. coli*.

Buzzwords:
- **Risk factors:** contaminated food or water, travel to high-risk areas (Latin America, South and Southeast Asia), decreased stomach acidity
- **Presentation:** self-limiting diarrhoea (3–5 days), see 'Definition'
- **Complications:** post-traveller's diarrhoea lactose intolerance and/or irritable bowel syndrome (IBS), pseudomembranous colitis

Investigations:
- **Stool MC&S** (not always necessary)
- **Stool ova and parasite exam:** to rule out giardiasis
- ***C. difficile* stool toxin:** to rule out *C. difficile*

Differentials: food poisoning, pseudomembranous colitis, malabsorption, coeliac disease

Management:
- Oral rehydration
- **Antibacterials (in severe disease):** azithromycin, rifaximin, fluoroquinolones

Clostridium perfringens

Definition: can cause food poisoning. Caused by the endotoxins produced in anaerobic conditions from the spores of *C. perfringens*. Incubation period is 8–18 h.

Buzzwords:
- **Risk factors:** undercooked food (meat products)
- **Presentation:** abdominal pain, diarrhoea, vomiting
- **Complications:** dehydration

Investigations:
- **Stool MC&S**
- **PCR:** to identify the enterotoxin (not routinely done)

Differentials: other causes of food poisoning, IBS, malabsorption

Management:
- Oral/IV hydration

Clostridium difficile

Definition: an infection of the colon caused by *C. difficile,* characterised by colonic inflammation and pseudomembrane formation.

Buzzwords:
- **Risk factors:** *broad-spectrum* antimicrobial use (e.g., penicillins, clindamycin, cephalosporins), advancing age, low stomach acidity (PPI use), hospital stays, nursing homes
- **Presentation:** diarrhoea, abdominal pain and tenderness, fever
- **Complications:** toxic megacolon, ileus, perforation, peritonitis, shock

Investigations:
- **Stool MC&S** for other gastrointestinal pathogens
- **Stool *C. difficile* toxin panel**
- **Blood:** FBC (leucocytosis); U&Es; ↑ CRP; VBG (↑ lactate)
- **Imaging:** AXR to rule out toxic megacolon

Differentials: ischaemic colitis, bacterial or viral gastroenteritis, inflammatory bowel disease (IBD)

Management:
- Stop the offending antibiotic(s). Admit and isolate in a side room
- Oral/IV rehydration
- Antibiotics: oral vancomycin/fidaxomicin or metronidazole, IV metronidazole/rectal vancomycin in patients with ileus

Giardiasis

Definition: an enteric infection caused by *Giardia lamblia*, a eukaryotic, flagellated, binucleated protozoa

Buzzwords:
- **Risk factors:** contaminated water/food, endemic areas

- **Presentation:** watery diarrhoea, frequent belching (sulphuric smell), bloating
- **Complications:** dehydration, weight loss, malabsorption, post-*Giardia* lactose intolerance

Investigations:
- **Immunocard STAT!:** completed in 10–12 min – lateral flow immunoassay for detection of *Giardia* in stools
- **Stool MC&S:** presence of cysts and trophozoites
- **Stool antigen detection:** ELISA and direct fluorescence antibody – positive for cell wall

Differentials: *Cryptosporidium parvum* infection, Rotavirus gastroenteritis, *C. difficile* diarrhoea, microscopic colitis, coeliac disease, IBD

Management:
- Oral/IV rehydration
- Antibiotics: metronidazole/tinidazole

Clostridium botulinum

Definition: causes the clinical syndrome of botulism, an acute flaccid paralytic illness resulting from ingestion of a neurotoxin produced by *C. botulinum*. Notifiable disease

Buzzwords:
- **Risk factors:** home-canned vegetables, fruits, meat and fish products, fermented food, ingestion of honey or soil in infants, intravenous drug use (IVDU)
- **Presentation:** blurred vision and diplopia, ptosis, dysarthria, dysphagia, symmetrical descending flaccid paralysis, loss of deep tendon reflexes, respiratory dysfunction (diaphragmatic and accessory muscle weakness), urinary retention, constipation, hypotonia and feeding difficulties in infants, **no sensory deficits**
- **Complications:** death from respiratory muscle paralysis, chronic muscle weakness, chronic dyspnoea, permanent diplopia

Investigations:
- **Detection of the toxin** in serum, gastric secretions, stool and food samples

Differentials: Miller-Fisher syndrome, GBS, myasthenia gravis

Management:
- Supportive: intubation for respiratory paralysis
- Urgent antitoxin administration

Viral Gastroenteritis

Definition: enteric infection caused by viruses (e.g., *Norovirus* and *Rotavirus*)

Buzzwords:

- **Risk factors:** contaminated food/water, close contact with infected people, poor hygiene, winter months
- **Presentation:** watery diarrhoea, nausea, fever, abdominal pain. Projectile vomiting with *Norovirus* infection
- **Complications:** severe dehydration, electrolyte imbalance, AKI

Investigations:

- **Stool MC&S:** rule out bacterial causes; microscopy for ova and parasites
- **Stool or vomitus for viral PCR**

Differentials: bacterial gastroenteritides, protozoal infection, helminthic infection

Management:

- Oral/IV rehydration

Whipple's Disease

Definition: a chronic multisystem disease caused by the Gram-positive bacteria, *Tropheryma whipplei*

Buzzwords:

- **Risk factors:** age >50 years, male, Caucasian
- **Presentation:** diarrhoea, weight loss, arthralgia, abdominal pain, lymphadenopathy, steatorrhea, neurological involvement
- **Complications:** severe CNS infection, arthritis

Investigations:

- ***Upper GI endoscopy with duodenal biopsies:** histology (foamy Periodic acid-Schiff (PAS)-positive macrophages)
- **Blood:** FBC (anaemia); liver function tests (LFTs) (low albumin); CRP/ESR (elevated)

Differentials: seronegative rheumatoid arthritis; sarcoidosis; coeliac disease; tropical sprue; Crohn's disease with reactive arthritis

Management:

- IV ceftriaxone for 14 days, then oral trimethoprim/sulfamethoxazole for 1 year

Typhoid Fever

Definition: an enteric infection transmitted via the faecal-oral route and caused by *Salmonella enterica*, serotype *S. typhi*.

Buzzwords:

- **Risk factors:** overcrowded living conditions in endemic areas; poor sanitation; contaminated food/water

- **Presentation: high fever** increasing in a stepwise pattern, dull frontal headache, abdominal pain, **constipation**, hepatosplenomegaly, relative bradycardia, rose spots
- **Complications:** hepatitis, bowel perforation, GI bleed, chronic biliary carriage

Investigations:

- ***Blood culture:** isolate organism
- **Blood:** FBC (leucopoenia, thrombocytopaenia); LFTs (raised transaminases)
- **Stool MC&S**
- **Typhidot-M:** ELISA kit that detects IgM and IgG against the outer membrane protein of *S. typhi*

Differentials: malaria, dengue, typhus, leptospirosis

Management:

- Antibiotics: fluoroquinolones, azithromycin and ceftriaxone, chloramphenicol, ampicillin

RESPIRATORY INFECTIONS

Tuberculosis

Definition: a disease caused by *Mycobacterium tuberculosis* (most common organism), which predominantly affects the lungs but can also cause disease at extrapulmonary sites

- **Active TB:** evidence of symptomatic/progressive disease in the lungs/other organs
- **Latent TB:** persistent immune reaction to mycobacterial antigens without clinically active disease. May progress to active disease if immunosuppression/intercurrent illness.

Buzzwords:

- **Risk factors:** contact with someone with active TB, socioeconomic deprivation, high-prevalence area
- **Risk factors for developing active TB:** immunosuppression, comorbidity (e.g., HIV, diabetes mellitus (DM), malnutrition), IVDU, alcohol dependence
- **Presentation:**
  - **General symptoms:** weight loss, fever, night sweats, anorexia
  - **Pulmonary symptoms:** persistent productive cough, dyspnoea, haemoptysis
  - **Extrapulmonary symptoms:** lymphadenopathy (typically painless/rubbery, bone/joint pains), spinal TB (known as Pott's disease), abdominal/pelvic pain +/- obstruction, sterile pyuria (renal TB), meningism, skin lesions (e.g., erythema nodosum, lupus vulgaris, scrofuloderma (see Fig 12.3))

- **Children:** may present with delayed growth, poor weight gain, fatigue
- **Post-TB complications:** bronchiectasis, COPD, aspergilloma in the TB cavity

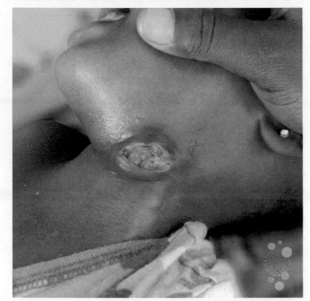

Fig 12.3 Scrofuloderma: an ulcerated abscess secondary to a tuberculosis infection in the skin. (Skin Deep. (2022). Scrofuloderma. https://dftbskindeep.com/all-diagnoses/scrofuloderma/.)

Investigations:
- **Sputum for acid-fast bacilli (AFB) + MC/S:** to confirm the diagnosis and guide antibiotic treatment
- **Urine for AFB:** if renal involvement
- **CSF for AFB and mycobacterial culture:** if CNS involvement
- **Mycobacterial blood cultures:** if systemic involvement
- **CXR:** cavitation, effusion, lymphadenopathy, infiltrates (mainly in the upper lobes). Latent TB may show upper lobe changes.
- **Focused radiological biopsy/LP:** for extrapulmonary (e.g., spinal CT + biopsy for suspected Pott's. See Fig 12.4)
- **Interferon gamma release assay (e.g., QuantiFERON):** test for *latent TB*
- **Mantoux test:** test for *latent TB (less reliable)*
- **HIV:** common coinfection
- **HbA1c:** DM is a common risk factor
- **FBC, U&Es, LFTs:** at baseline, for monitoring of treatment side effects

Differentials: lung cancer, pneumonia, aspergillosis, lymphoma, sarcoidosis, granulomatosis with polyangiitis

Management:
1. Specialist TB team and admission to hospital if unwell

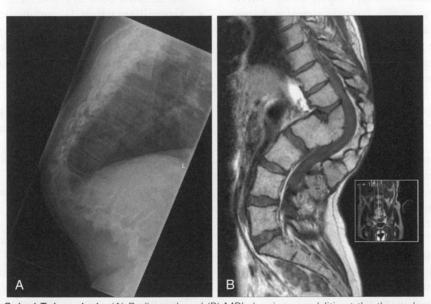

Fig 12.4 Spinal Tuberculosis. (A) Radiograph and (B) MRI showing spondylitis at the thoracolumbar junction. (With permission from de Nijs, R. N. J. (2011) Spinal tuberculosis (Fig. 1). The Lancet, Elsevier. Copyright © 2011 Elsevier Ltd. All rights reserved.)

2. Contact tracing/screening
3. Notify public health england (PHE) – **notifiable disease**
4. Enhanced care (e.g., observed treatment) required for underserved groups at risk of poor adherence, including homeless, history of drug misuse, multidrug-resistant TB (MDRTB), incarcerated
5. If active TB:
   a. Two months of **R**ifampicin, **I**soniazid **P**yrazinamide and **E**thambutol (monitor visual fields) **(RIPE)**
   b. Followed by 4 months of rifampicin and isoniazid
6. If MDRTB: 18–24 months of treatment with at least six drugs
7. If evidence of central nervous system involvement: longer course required with dexamethasone
8. **If latent TB:** everyone under the age of 65 years with latent TB should be treated with 3 months of isoniazid (with pyridoxine) and rifampicin *or* 6 months of isoniazid (with pyridoxine)

Aspergillosis

Definition: a collection of diseases caused by spores from the *Aspergillus* spp. of fungi, primarily affecting the respiratory tract but also causing nail, skin and upper respiratory tract infections. The main *pulmonary* presentations are as follows:

- **Allergic bronchopulmonary aspergillosis (ABPA):** hypersensitivity reaction, happens almost exclusively in people with asthma/cystic fibrosis (CF)
- **Aspergilloma:** presence of a fungal ball (mycetoma) in a pre-existing lung cavity
- **Invasive aspergillosis (IA):** disseminated fungal infection in immunocompromised. Often starts in the lungs but spreads to other organs

Buzzwords:
- **Risk factors:**
  - **ABPA:** asthma, CF, bronchiectasis
  - **Aspergilloma:** cavitating lung disease (e.g., TB, lung abscess, sarcoidosis)
  - **IA:** immunosuppression (e.g., AIDS, chemotherapy, organ transplant, critical care patient)
- **Presentation:**
  - **ABPA:** recurrent/worsening asthma exacerbations, deteriorating CF, cough +/- sputum
  - **Aspergilloma:** asymptomatic, massive haemoptysis, round opacity in cavity
  - **IA:** cough/fever/dyspnoea, haemoptysis, multiorgan failure, hypoxia, thrombosis

Investigations:
- **Blood:** ↑ eosinophils, ↑ serum IgE
- **Spirometry:** obstructive in ABPA
- **Sputum cultures:** *Aspergillus*
- **Blood for fungal markers, β-D-glucan and galactomannan:** raised in invasive/systemic infection
- **CXR:**
  - **ABPA:** upper lobe consolidation
  - **Aspergilloma:** opacity in cavity
- **High-resolution CT:**
  - **ABPA:** bronchiectasis
  - **Aspergilloma:** mycetoma
  - **IA:** consolidation, halo, collapse
- **Bronchioalveolar lavage (BAL):** detect *Aspergillus* in IA
- **Biopsy:** required for IA diagnosis
- **AFB sputum:** especially if there is a cavity on CXR, assess for TB

Differentials:
- **ABPA:** community-acquired pneumonia, asthma, interstitial lung disease
- **Aspergilloma:** lung abscess, lung cancer, TB, other fungal infections
- **IA:** sepsis of other origin, other fungal

Management:
- **ABPA:** prednisolone for acute attacks, may need maintenance dose. Itraconazole.
- **Aspergilloma:** treat if symptomatic, surgical excision of solitary lesions. Limited success with antifungals
- **IA:** treat if suspected before confirmation. Voriconazole is first-line agent. High risk of requiring critical care

Influenza

Definition: an acute respiratory illness caused by influenza viruses that is spread via respiratory droplets. Incubation period is 2–7 days.

Influenza A is more frequent and more virulent, causing outbreaks, epidemics and pandemics with severe clinical illness. Influenza B causes a less severe clinical illness.

Buzzwords:
- **Risk factors:** winter months (December to March in the United Kingdom), age <6 months and >65 years, chronic cardiovascular/respiratory conditions, chronic kidney disease, diabetes, obesity, pregnancy
- **Presentation:** coryza, rhinorrhoea, cough, fever, chills, headache, myalgia, sore throat, conjunctival injection

- **Complications:** acute bronchitis, bacterial/viral pneumonia, otitis media

Investigations:

- Clinical diagnosis
- **PCR** of nasopharyngeal swab, nasal aspirate or sputum
- **CXR:** should be normal, rules out consolidation

Differentials: COVID-19, bacterial pneumonia, respiratory syncytial virus (RSV) infection, parainfluenza

Management:

- Oral/IV hydration, rest, stay off work/school (at least 1 week)
- Simple analgesia
- Oseltamivir or zanamivir for patients at high risk of developing serious complications

Infectious Mononucleosis

Definition: an infection caused by the Epstein-Barr virus (EBV), also known as glandular fever, transmitted via saliva ('kissing' disease). Incubation period is 4–7 weeks.

Buzzwords:

- **Risk factors:** sharing food and drinks, kissing, sexual contact, blood transfusion
- **Presentation:** triad of fever, pharyngitis, lymphadenopathy
- **Complications:** antibiotic-induced rash (usually ampicillin, but not an allergy), upper airway obstruction, splenomegaly risking splenic rupture, haemolytic anaemia, jaundice, chronic fatigue

Investigations:

- **Blood:** FBC (lymphocytosis with atypical lymphocytes), LFTs (increased ALT)
- **Monospot test:** to detect heterophile antibodies
- **EBV:** specific antibodies
- **US abdomen:** possibly splenomegaly

Differentials: group A streptococcal pharyngitis, acute HIV infection, rubella, Adenovirus infection, CMV infection

Management:

- Supportive treatment
- Refrain from strenuous physical activities and contact sports (risk of splenic rupture) for up to 8 weeks

SKIN AND SOFT TISSUE INFECTIONS

Gas Gangrene

Definition: a deep bacterial infection of the soft tissue and muscles caused by *Clostridium* spp. (90% by *Clostridium perfringens*), producing myonecrosis and gas in tissues. Mostly associated with deep penetrating trauma but can occur spontaneously.

Buzzwords:

- **Risk factors:** recent trauma (including weeks earlier), immunocompromise, farm and animal work
- **Presentation:** general systemic symptoms, tissue crepitus on palpation, necrotic sores, localised inflammation
- **Complications:** death, septic shock, amputation

Investigations:

- Clinical diagnosis
- **X-ray/CT/USS:** gas in tissue (see Fig 12.5)
- **Wound swab with MC&S:** Gram-positive anaerobic bacilli identified on culture

Differentials: cellulitis, necrotising fasciitis

Management:

- Antibiotics: penicillin or clindamycin, plus metronidazole
- Urgent surgical debridement

Folliculitis

Definition: inflammation of the hair follicles. This condition can be caused by a bacterial infection (commonly *S. aureus*), viral/fungal infection, occlusion or irritation

Buzzwords:

- **Risk factors:** DM; immunocompromise; thick, curly hair; shaving against the direction of hair growth; humidity; tight clothing; hot tubs (*Pseudomonas* spp.)
- **Presentation:** tender, red lesions in a follicular pattern, pustules may also be present
- **Complications:** scarring, progression to a furuncle/carbuncle/abscess

Investigations:

- Clinical diagnosis
- **Skin swab:** for microscopy and culture

Differentials: acne vulgaris, impetigo, insect bites, milia, miliaria

Management:

- Conservative management: keep affected area clean and dry, avoid risk factors
- Systemic antibiotics for severe/complicated infection

Head Lice (*Pediculosis capitis*)

Definition: an infestation with the head louse, *Pediculus humanus capitis*

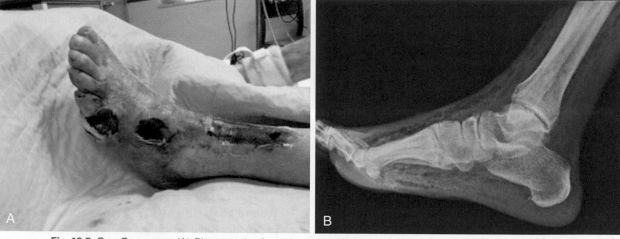

Fig 12.5 Gas Gangrene. (A) Photograph of gas gangrene. This patient required an emergency above-knee amputation. (B) Gas in the soft tissues on a lateral radiograph of the foot (With permission from Reiner, M. M, Khoury, W. E., Canales, M. B., Chmielewski, R. A., Patel, K., Razzante, M. C., et al. (2017). Procalcitonin as a biomarker for predicting amputation level in lower extremity infections. *The Journal of Foot and Ankle Surgery.* Elsevier. © 2017 by the American College of Foot and Ankle Surgeons. All rights reserved.)

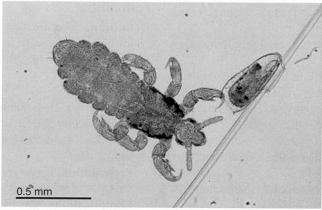

Fig 12.6 A head louse (*Pediculus humanus capitis*). (With permission from Bauer, I. (2019). Itchy critters: Preparing volunteer travelers for head lice infestation (Fig. 1). *Travel Medicine and Infectious Disease.* Elsevier © 2019 Elsevier Ltd. All rights reserved.)

Buzzwords:
- **Risk factors:** long hair, close contact with children, shared bedding, brushes and headwear
- **Presentation:** persistent scalp itch, visible nits (eggs) and lice (see Fig 12.6) in a severe infestation
- **Complications:** impetigo, anxiety and mental distress

Investigations:
- **Clinical diagnosis:** live lice required to confirm an active infestation

Differentials: eczema, seborrheic scales may resemble nits (can be distinguished by being easily brushed off while nits are firmly adherent)

Management:
- Topical insecticide: silicone or ester-based topicals. Malathion shampoo was used in the past but is associated with resistance. Treat the whole household simultaneously and wash clothes and bedding
- Wet combing to remove nits, dry-detection combing to monitor for recurrence

VECTOR-BORNE INFECTIONS

Malaria

Definition: an infection of the red blood cells caused by the protozoa, *Plasmodium* spp., transmitted through the bite of an infected female *Anopheles* mosquito and potentially by blood transfusions and organ transplantation.

Five known species: *Plasmodium falciparum* (**life threatening**), *Plasmodium vivax*, *Plasmodium ovale*, *Plasmodium malariae*, *Plasmodium knowlesi*

   P. vivax and *P. ovale* have a dormant liver stage and can relapse.

Buzzwords:

- **Risk factors:** mosquito bites, travel to endemic areas, lack of chemoprophylaxis, absence of physical barriers to mosquitoes (e.g., bed nets)
- **Presentation: cyclical fever.** Paroxysms of chills, high fever, sweats. Headache, myalgia, arthralgia, diarrhoea, abdominal pain, nausea, vomiting, hepatosplenomegaly, seizures (in cerebral malaria), hypotension, confusion
- **Complications:** cerebral malaria (associated with *P. falciparum*), jaundice, pulmonary oedema, hypoglycaemia, severe haemolytic anaemia, AKI (blackwater fever in *P. falciparum* malaria due to haemoglobinuria), metabolic acidosis

Investigations:

- **Blood film: thick** (parasite detection) and **thin** (parasite identification and parasitaemia level quantification) **smears** with Giemsa stain. Parasitaemia level >2% – high → severe disease (see Fig 12.7)
- **Rapid diagnostic tests** (malarial dipstick tests): OptiMAL-IT, Paracheck-Pf
- **Blood:** FBC (thrombocytopaenia, haemolytic anaemia), U&Es (prerenal AKI, haemoglobinuria, myoglobinuria), LFTs (↑ bilirubin)
- **Urine analysis:** RBC++ (could be due to myoglobinuria), proteinuria

Differentials: dengue fever, Zika virus, Chikungunya, yellow fever, typhoid, leptospirosis

Management:

- Antimalarials:
  - Artemisinin derivatives: artemisinin, artemether-lumefantrine, artesunate
  - Quinoline derivatives: quinine, chloroquine, mefloquine
  - Antifolates: pyrimethamine, sulphonamides

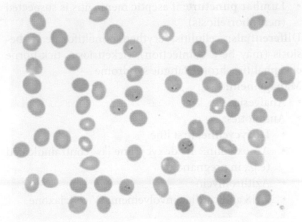

Fig 12.7 Malaria. Parasites are seen as dark rings inside the red blood cells. (With permission from Gutman, J., & Arguin, P. M. (2018). *Plasmodium* species (malaria) (Fig. 271.2). In *Principles and practice of pediatric infectious diseases.* Elsevier. Copyright © 2018 Elsevier Inc. All rights reserved.)

- Ribosomal inhibitors: doxycycline, tetracycline, clindamycin
- Supportive therapy for AKI, pulmonary oedema

Lyme Disease

Definition: an infection caused by the spirochaete, *Borrelia burgdorferi*, and spread by the vector, the *Ixodes* tick

Buzzwords:

- **Risk factors:** tick bites, travel to endemic areas (e.g., New Forest and Salisbury Plain in the United Kingdom; central European and Scandinavian countries; Northeast, mid-Atlantic, and upper Midwest regions of the United States), outdoor activities in endemic areas
- **Presentation:** erythema chronicum migrans (bull's eye rash), Bell's palsy, arthralgia, myalgia, fatigue, fever, headache
- **Complications:** peripheral neuropathy, cranial neuropathy, aseptic meningitis, heart block, perimyocarditis, arthritis and joint effusions

Investigations:

- **Clinical diagnosis:** in the presence of erythema chronicum migrans and risk factors
- **Blood:** serology – enzyme immunoassay (EIA) for confirmation but only positive after 4 weeks of symptoms, Western blot for Lyme-specific IgM and IgG

- **Lumbar puncture:** if aseptic meningitis is suspected (neuroborreliosis)

Differentials: cellulitis, erythema multiforme, babesiosis (may be a coinfection), rickettsiosis, tick-borne encephalitis, chronic fatigue syndrome

Management:
- Analgesia
- Antibiotics.
  - **Doxycycline:** first line
  - Amoxicillin: if doxycycline is contraindicated (e.g., in pregnancy)
  - Azithromycin
  - CNS and cardiac involvement: IV ceftriaxone

THE ONE-LINE ROUND-UP!

Here are some key words to help you remember each condition/concept.

Condition/Concept	One-line Description
Drug monitoring	Peak too high: reduce dose; trough too high: space out doses
Bacterial meningitis	S. pneumoniae, N. meningitidis, H. influenzae
Campylobacter	Undercooked chicken, most common GI infection associated with GBS
E. coli O157	Bloody diarrhoea, ground beef, HUS
Salmonella gastro	Animal source, 6–72-h incubation period
Shigellosis	Returning traveller, risk of HUS
B. cereus	Leftover rice
Listeria	Soft cheese, risk in pregnancy
Traveller's diarrhoea	Self-limited, usually E. coli
C. perfringens	Food poisoning and gas gangrene
C. difficile	Pseudomembranous colitis
Giardiasis	Diarrhoea/malabsorption in a returning traveller
Botulism	Descending paralysis, home-canned food, honey in infants
Viral gastro	Sick contacts, dehydration
Whipple's	Chronic diarrhoea, PAS macrophages, arthritis
Typhoid	Constipation, fever, relative bradycardia, rose spots
TB	AFB, RIPE

Condition/Concept	One-line Description
Aspergillosis	ABPA – asthmatics, Aspergilloma in TB cavity
Influenza	Respiratory droplets, winter months, myalgia
Infectious mono	Amoxicillin causes rash, splenomegaly
Gas gangrene	C. perfringens, gas on imaging
Folliculitis	Follows follicular pattern
Head lice	Wet combing, itchy-headed school child
Malaria	Falciparum most deadly
Lyme disease	Tick + neuropathy + bull's eye

READING LIST: INFECTIOUS DISEASES IN AN HOUR

Notifiable Diseases

Gov.uk. (2021). *Notifiable diseases and causative organisms.* https://www.gov.uk/guidance/notifiable-diseases-and-causative-organisms-how-to-report#list-of-notifiable-diseases – [Accessed Jan 2021].

Bacterial Meningitis

BMJ Best Practice. (2021). *Bacterial meningitis.* https://best-practice.bmj.com/topics/en-gb/3000104 Accessed Jan 2021.

BMJ Best Practice. (2021). *Meningococcal disease.* https://best-practice.bmj.com/topics/en-gb/3000175 [Accessed Jan 2021].

***Campylobacter* Enteritis**

BMJ Best Practice. (2021). *Campylobacter infection.* https://best-practice.bmj.com/topics/en-gb/1175 [Accessed Feb 2021].

***E. coli* O157:H7 And Other Shiga-toxin Producing *E. coli* Infections**

Health Protection Scotland. (2018). *Escherichia coli O157 (STEC).* https://www.hps.scot.nhs.uk/web-resources-container/guidance-for-the-public-health-management-of-escherichia-coli-o157-and-other-shiga-toxin-producing-stec-infections/ [Accessed Feb 2021].

Patient info. (2014). *Escherichia coli O157.* https://patient.info/doctor/escherichia-coli-o157 [Accessed Feb 2021].

Health Protection Scotland. (2018). *Guidance for the public health management of Escherichia coli O157 and other Shiga toxin-producing (STEC) infections.* https://hps-pubsrepo.blob.core.windows.net/hps-website/nss/2032/documents/1_SHPN-Guidance-Ecoli-shiga-STEC.pdf [Accessed Mar 2021].

Salmonella Gastroenteritis

BMJ Best Practice. (2021). *Salmonellosis*. https://bestpractice.bmj.com/topics/en-gb/817 [Accessed Dec 2021].

Patient info. (2016). *Salmonella gastroenteritis*. https://patient.info/doctor/salmonella-gastroenteritis [Accessed Dec 2021].

Shigellosis

BMJ Best Practice. (2021). *Shigella infection*. https://bestpractice.bmj.com/topics/en-gb/1174 Accessed Feb 2021.

Centers for Disease Control and Prevention. (2019). *Shigellosis. CDC Yellow Book 2020*. Oxford University Press.

Bacillus cereus

BMJ Best Practice. (2021). *Food poisoning*. https://bestpractice.bmj.com/topics/en-gb/203 [Accessed Jan 2021].

Listeriosis

BMJ Best Practice. (2021). *Listeriosis*. https://bestpractice.bmj.com/topics/en-gb/914 [Accessed Jan 2021].

Shane, A., Mody, R., Crump, J., et al. (2017). 2017 Infectious Diseases Society of America clinical practice guidelines for the diagnosis and management of infectious diarrhea. *Clin Infect Dis, 65*, e45–e80.

Traveller's Diarrhoea (TD)

BMJ Best Practice. (2021). *Traveller's diarrhoea*. https://bestpractice.bmj.com/topics/en-gb/601 [Accessed Feb 2021].

Centers for Disease Control and Prevention. (2019). *Traveller's diarrhea. CDC Yellow Book 2020*. Oxford University Press.

Clostridium perfringens

GP notebook. (2020). *Clostridium perfringens (food poisoning)*. https://gpnotebook.com/en-gb/simplepage.cfm?ID=986710020 [Accessed Mar 2021].

Clostridium difficile

Public Health England. (2013). *Updated guidance on the management and treatment of Clostridium difficile infection*. https://assets.publishing.service.gov.uk/government/uploads/system/uploads/attachment_data/file/321891/Clostridium_difficile_management_and_treatment.pdf [Accessed Mar 2021].

BMJ Best Practice. (2021). *Clostridium difficile-associated disease*. https://bestpractice.bmj.com/topics/en-gb/230 [Accessed Jan 2021].

Giardiasis

BMJ Best Practice. (2021). *Giardiasis*. https://bestpractice.bmj.com/topics/en-gb/353 [Accessed Dec 2020].

Centers for Disease Control and Prevention. (2019). *Giardiasis. CDC Yellow Book 2020*. Oxford University Press.

Clostridium botulinum

Public Health England. (2018). *Botulism: clinical and public health management*. https://www.gov.uk/government/publications/botulism-clinical-and-public-health-management/botulism-clinical-and-public-health-management [Accessed Dec 2020].

BMJ Best Practice. (2021). *Botulism*. https://bestpractice.bmj.com/topics/en-gb/810 [Accessed Dec 2020].

Viral Gastroenteritis

BMJ Best Practice. (2020). *Viral gastroenteritis in adults*. https://bestpractice.bmj.com/topics/en-gb/3000126 [Accessed Jan 2021].

Shane, A., Mody, R., Crump, J., et al. (2017). 2017 Infectious Diseases Society of America clinical practice guidelines for the diagnosis and management of infectious diarrhea. *Clin Infect Dis, 65*, e45–e80.

Whipple's Disease

BMJ Best Practice. (2020). *Whipple's disease*. https://bestpractice.bmj.com/topics/en-gb/467 [Accessed Jan 2021].

UpToDate. (2020). *Whipple's disease*. https://www.uptodate.com/contents/whipples-disease?search=whipples%20disease&source=search_result&selectedTitle=1~75&usage_type=default&display_rank=1#H19 [Accessed December 2021].

Typhoid Fever

BMJ Best Practice. (2020). *Typhoid infection*. https://bestpractice.bmj.com/topics/en-gb/221 [Accessed Jan 2021].

Centers for Disease Control and Prevention. (2019). Typhoid and paratyphoid fever. In *CDC Yellow Book 2020*. Oxford University Press.

Tuberculosis

NICE. (2019). *CKS: Tuberculosis*. https://cks.nice.org.uk/topics/tuberculosis/ [Accessed Dec 2020].

NICE. (2019). *NG33: Tuberculosis*. https://www.nice.org.uk/guidance/ng33 [Accessed Dec 2020].

Aspergillosis

Akuthota, P. (2020). *Clinical manifestations and diagnosis of allergic bronchopulmonary aspergillosis*. UpToDate. https://www.uptodate.com/contents/clinical-manifestations-and-diagnosis-of-allergic-bronchopulmonary-aspergillosis?search=allergic%20bronchopulmonary%20aspergillosis&source=search_result&selectedTitle=1~50&usage_type=default&display_rank=1 [Accessed August 2020].

Henderson, R. (2016). *Aspergillosis. Patient info*. https://patient.info/doctor/aspergillosis [Accessed August 2020].

Wilkinson, I., Raine, T., Wiles, K., Goodhart, A., Hall, C., & O'Neill, H. (2017). Fungi and the lung. In *Oxford handbook of clinical medicine* (10th ed.), (p. 177).

Influenza

BMJ Best Practice. (2021). *Influenza infection*. https://bestpractice.bmj.com/topics/en-gb/6 [Accessed Jan 2021].

NICE. (2020). *CKS: Influenza – seasonal*. https://cks.nice.org.uk/topics/influenza-seasonal/ [Accessed Jan 2021].

Infectious Mononucleosis

BMJ Best Practice. (2021). *Infectious mononucleosis*. https://bestpractice.bmj.com/topics/en-gb/123 [Accessed Dec 2020].

NICE. *CKS: Glandular fever (infectious mononucleosis)*. https://cks.nice.org.uk/topics/glandular-fever-infectious-mononucleosis/ [Accessed Dec 2020].

Patient info. (2021). *Glandular fever*. https://patient.info/ears-nose-throat-mouth/sore-throat-2/glandular-fever-infectious-mononucleosis [Accessed Dec 2020].

Gas Gangrene

BMJ Best Practice. (2020). *Gangrene*. https://bestpractice.bmj.com/topics/en-gb/1015 [Accessed Dec 2020].

Buboltz, J., & Murphy-Lavoie, H. (2021). *Gas gangrene. Stat Pearls*. StatPearls Publishing. https://www.ncbi.nlm.nih.gov/books/NBK560552/ [Accessed Dec 2020].

Folliculitis

DermNet, N. Z. (2014). *Folliculitis*. https://dermnetnz.org/topics/folliculitis [Accessed Dec 2020].

GP Notebook. (2018). *Folliculitis: differential diagnosis*. https://gpnotebook.com/en-gb/simplepage.cfm?ID=1664417821&linkID=15611. [Accessed Dec 2020].

Head Lice *(Pediculosis capitis)*

NICE. CKS: Head lice. https://cks.nice.org.uk/topics/head-lice/ [Accessed Dec 2020]

Malaria

BMJ Best Practice. (2020). *Malaria infection*. https://bestpractice.bmj.com/topics/en-gb/3000122 [Accessed Feb 2021].

NICE. CKS: Malaria. https://cks.nice.org.uk/topics/malaria/ [Accessed Feb 2021]

Centers for Disease Control and Prevention. (2019). Malaria. In *CDC yellow book 2020*. Oxford University Press.

Lyme Disease

BMJ Best Practice. (2020). *Lyme disease*. https://bestpractice.bmj.com/topics/en-gb/224 [Accessed Mar 2021].

NICE. (2018). *NG95: Lyme disease*. https://www.nice.org.uk/guidance/ng95 [Accessed Mar 2021].

Török, E., Moran, E., & Cooke, F. (2017). *Oxford handbook of infectious diseases and microbiology* (2nd ed.). Oxford University Press, 338–340.

Centers for Disease Control and Prevention. (2019). Lyme disease. In *CDC yellow book 2020*. Oxford University Press.

13

Neurology in an Hour

Dominic Mahoney, Dillon Vyas, Osamuyimen Omoragbon, Hannah Punter, Mark Lam, Berenice Aguirrezabala Armbruster, Gregory Oxenham, and Matthew Smith

OUTLINE

NEUROANATOMY

Where is the Lesion?

Neurological diagnoses rely heavily on the history and clinical examination. Imaging and laboratory tests often only help to confirm or refine a diagnosis. Before determining which condition may have caused a patient's problem, try to determine where the abnormality is located in the nervous system (see Table 13.1 and 13.2).

HEADACHE

Definition:

- **Primary headache**: majority of headaches. No underlying sinister or structural pathologies. Migraines are one example that cause significant morbidity.
- **Secondary headache**: occurs secondary to an underlying pathology. Treated by addressing the cause, often serious

Buzzwords:

- **Risk factors**: see individual conditions

- **Presentation:** see individual conditions and Fig 13.1
  - **Red-flag features** *(indications for neuroimaging)*: sudden onset, severe (thunderclap), focal neurologic deficit, fever, photophobia, neck stiffness, seizure, reduced consciousness, cognitive impairment, vomiting, papilloedema, visual disturbances, dizziness, prolonged and progressive in nature, high-pressure features (i.e., worse with lying down)

Investigations: guided by presentation. All patients presenting with headache should have:

- **Fundoscopy:** may show papilloedema, which is indicative of a raised intracranial pressure (ICP)
- **Neurological exam:** may identify a focal neurological deficit

Further investigations and management strategies are detailed in individual sections.

Migraine

Definition: a primary headache disorder (cause unknown) characterised by mild to severe headaches that may be associated with auras and other characteristic features (see Presentation)

TABLE 13.1   Localising Neurological Lesions

Location of the Lesion	Possible Consequences of Damage
CENTRAL NERVOUS SYSTEM	
Cerebral cortex	Weakness (UMN), sensory impairment, visual impairment, cognitive or memory disturbances, character changes (depending on the area affected)
Pons and medulla	Cranial nerve impairment potentially causing ophthalmoplegia, bulbar dysfunction (speech and swallowing problems), facial weakness, etc. Limb weakness and sensory changes caused by damage to the descending neural tracts Disorders of arousal
Cerebellum	Ataxia, nystagmus, dysarthria
Spinal cord	UMN below lesion, LMN at the roots exiting at the level of the lesion Acute flaccid paralysis in spinal shock (see Neurosurgery in an Hour)
PERIPHERAL NERVOUS SYSTEM	
Autonomic nervous system	Bladder and bowel disturbances, orthostatic hypotension, excess or lack of sweating, pupillary abnormalities
Spinal nerve root and conus medullaris	Weakness, loss of sensation, neuropathic pain, bladder and bowel disturbances (if cauda equina)
Motor nerve	Weakness, muscle wasting (if chronic)
Sensory nerve	Loss/impairment of sensation, neuropathic pain
MUSCLE AND NEUROMUSCULAR JUNCTION	
Neuromuscular junction	Weakness (fatigable), ptosis, complex ophthalmoplegia
Muscle	Weakness, wasting (if chronic)

LMN, Lower motor neuron; UMN, upper motor neuron.

- **Episodic:** highly variable, one per year to several times per week
- **Chronic:** migraine attacks on 15 or more days per month for 3 months or longer. Features of a migraine headache must be present on at least 8 days per month

TABLE 13.2   Upper vs Lower Motor Neuron Lesions

	Upper Motor Neuron Lesion	Lower Motor Neuron Lesion
Inspection	Normal/spastic posture	Fasciculations, muscle wasting
Tone	Increased (spasticity)	Normal/decreased (flaccid paralysis)
Power	Decreased	Decreased
Reflexes	Increased	Decreased or absent

Buzzwords:
- **Risk factors:** female, family history, high caffeine intake, obesity
- **Presentation:**
  - Headache: unilateral, pulsating, moderate/severe, aggravated by movement/exertion
  - Additional features: nausea +/- vomiting, photophobia, phonophobia, aura (e.g., visual disturbances, paresthesias, transient motor symptoms)
  - Triggers: mnemonic **CHOCOLATE** – **cho**colate, **c**heese, **h**ormones, **c**affeine, alco**h**ol, **a**nxiety, **t**ravel, **e**xercise + sleep disturbance

Investigations:
- **Headache diary:** preceding features, severity, duration and medication trials should be recorded. The Migraine Disability Assessment is used to assess disability in migraine sufferers.
- **CT/MRI (only if the patient presents with red-flag features):** normal, higher risk of non-specific white matter lesions for age on MRI

Differentials: see Table 13.3

Management:
1. Avoid precipitants and disruptions to the daily routine. Sleep hygiene and good hydration.
2. Simple analgesia: paracetamol, nonsteroidal anti-inflammatory drugs (NSAIDs). Opioids are usually unhelpful, and it is vital that simple analgesia is used only to treat episodic migraines or flares of chronic migraine (<10 days per month) because there is a high risk of paradoxical medication-overuse headaches if used >15 days/month
3. Triptans (for episodic migraines)
4. Prokinetic antiemetics (e.g., metoclopramide): improves oral medication absorption whilst alleviating nausea

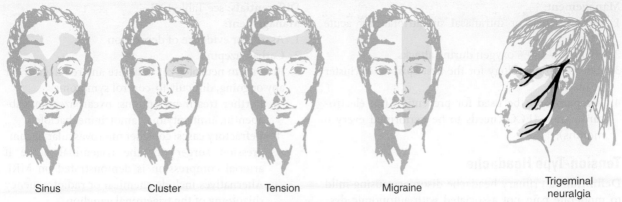

| Sinus | Cluster | Tension | Migraine | Trigeminal neuralgia |

Fig 13.1 Classical Distributions of Pain (*yellow*) with Different Types of Headaches. (Illustrated by Hollie Blaber.)

5. Preventative medications (e.g., propranolol, topiramate, amitriptyline and nonpharmacological adjuncts) can be offered if there is a significant impact on the quality of life, and acute analgesia has not been effective. Botulinum toxin injections and anti-CGRP monoclonal antibodies are available for refractory migraines (i.e., a failure of three preventative medications and headaches on >15 days per month).

NB: combined oral contraceptive pills are contraindicated in patients with migraine with aura.

Medication-overuse headaches are treated by withdrawal of simple analgesia, with codeine being a particular offender.

Cluster Headache

Definition: a primary headache disorder characterised by clusters of multiple attacks. May be classified as:
- Episodic cluster headache: bouts last >1 week and are separated by >4 weeks
- Chronic cluster headache: bouts either last all year or are separated by <1 month of remission

Part of a collection of primary headache disorders known as 'trigeminal autonomic cephalgias', which also include paroxysmal hemicrania and short-lasting, unilateral, neuralgiform headache attacks with conjunctival injection and tearing (SUNCT)

Buzzwords:
- **Risk factors:** male (M:F incidence is approximately 5:1), 3rd and 4th decades of life
- **Presentation:**
  - **Headache:** recurrent, very severe, unilateral pain lasting 15–180 min with multiple attacks per day/

TABLE 13.3	Differentials for Headache
Primary Headache	**Secondary Headache**
• Migraine • Tension-type headache • Cluster headaches	• Subarachnoid haemorrhage • Giant cell arteritis • Cerebral venous sinus thrombosis • Idiopathic intracranial hypertension • Space-occupying lesion (e.g., malignancy) • Meningitis/encephalitis • Carotid/vertebral artery dissection • Preeclampsia • Medication-overuse headache • Sinus headache

week, forming a 'cluster' of headaches that settles for weeks/months but then returns. Pain around the orbital area +/− temporal area with a seasonal rhythmicity to the clusters
- **Additional features:** Horner's syndrome, conjunctival injection, nasal congestion. In contrast to migraine (with which patients desire to stay still), patients with cluster headaches will tend to clutch the area of pain and pace around.

Investigations:
- **MRI:** usually normal, rarely a hypothalamic hamartoma

Differentials: see Table 13.3

Management:
1. Intramuscular or intranasal sumatriptan for acute attacks
2. High-flow 100% oxygen during attacks
3. Referral to neurology for the first episode of cluster headaches
4. Verapamil can be used for prevention (an electrocardiogram (ECG) needs to be performed every 6 months).

Tension-Type Headache

Definition: a primary headache disorder causing mild to moderate pain not associated with autonomic dysfunction

Buzzwords:
- **Risk factors:** stress, disturbed sleep
- **Presentation:**
  - Headache: lasts 30 min–7 days; bilateral, nonpulsatile, mild-to-moderate pain; pericranial tenderness
  - Additional features: no nausea/vomiting

Investigations: clinical diagnosis (look out for red-flag features that suggest that the headache is not a tension-type headache (TTH))

Differentials: see Table 13.3

Management:
- Simple analgesia: paracetamol, NSAIDs. If used regularly, the patient is at risk of developing a medication-overuse headache
- Sleep hygiene, adequate hydration
- Acupuncture
- Amitriptyline

Trigeminal Neuralgia

Definition: severe pain in the distribution of a sensory branch of the trigeminal nerve (typically the maxillary branch), sometimes resulting from vascular compression of the nerve root

Buzzwords:
- **Risk factors:** multiple sclerosis (MS), female
- **Presentation:** episodic, unilateral, neuropathic pain in the distribution of the trigeminal nerve. Can be triggered by chewing, touching the face or even wind
  - **Red flags** (suggestive of a sinister underlying cause): age of onset <40 years, family history of MS, deafness, optic neuritis, oral or skin lesions

Investigations:
- **MRI** (if persistent): evidence of compression of the trigeminal nerve by the superior cerebellar artery (50%)

Differentials: see Table 13.3
Management:
1. Assess for evidence of depression
2. Carbamazepine
3. Referral to neurology if there are any red flags or for any ongoing, difficult-to-control symptoms
   a. Further treatment options: oxcarbazepine, gabapentin, amitriptyline, lamotrigine, baclofen
   b. Refractory cases: consider microvascular decompression surgery of the trigeminal nerve if arterial compression is demonstrated on MRI. Alternatives include chemical or radiofrequency rhizotomy of the trigeminal ganglion

NB: trigeminal neuralgia can occasionally be a symptom of MS, either during a first episode or subsequent relapse.

EPILEPSY AND SEIZURES

- **Seizures and epilepsy** are two separate concepts that are inextricably linked. Seizures are a symptom caused by abnormal electrical activity in the brain. Seizures can be an isolated phenomenon caused by factors acutely affecting brain function (e.g., an acute head injury, drug use), but, often, no cause is ever identified.
- Epilepsy simply means an ongoing tendency to have seizures. This condition can be linked to a clearly observable brain lesion (e.g., a brain tumour, scarring from an old brain injury), can be part of a defined collection of symptoms known as an epilepsy syndrome (in which a genetic cause has been discovered or is suspected) or can develop without any clear cause.
- In general, **2%–5%** of the population will experience a seizure at some point in their lives. Of these, 40% will go on to have further seizures, usually indicating that they have epilepsy.
- **Single isolated seizures are not usually treated with drugs** unless there is an ongoing risk of further occurrences (see Epilepsy section).

Seizure

Definition: neurological dysfunction caused by a transient period of abnormal synchronised neuronal discharges. Seizures are classified by:
1. **Seizure origin:** focal or generalised?
2. **Level of awareness:** is awareness preserved? (Extremely rare during generalised seizures)
3. **Ictal phenomena:** what is the patient's behaviour during the seizure?

TABLE 13.4	**Presentations of Seizures**	
Seizure Type	**Presentation**	**First-line Antiepileptic Drugs (see Epilepsy Section)**
Generalised: discharge from both hemispheres, usually with a loss of consciousness and NO aura		
Absence	<60 sec of unresponsiveness, staring into space, may lead to falling behind in school	Valproate
Tonic-clonic	Fall to the ground then rhythmical contractions	Levetiracetam Valproate Lamotrigine
Myoclonic	Brief, jerking movements of limbs (consciousness usually retained)	Valproate Levetiracetam
Tonic	Stiff, increased tone	Valproate Levetiracetam
Atonic	Floppy, falling to the floor	Valproate Levetiracetam
Focal: seizure starts in a specific location and is often associated with an aura. May remain conscious or may become generalised, leading to a tonic-clonic seizure		
Frontal	Motor phenomenon	Lamotrigine Carbamazepine Levetiracetam Valproate
Temporal	Auditory, sensory or cognitive aura (e.g., 'déjà vu')	
Occipital	Visual aura	
Parietal	Contralateral altered sensation	

Buzzwords:

- **Risk factors:**
  - **Generalised:** epilepsy, head trauma, family history of epilepsy, alcohol withdrawal, hypoglycaemia, electrolyte disturbances
  - **Focal**: epilepsy, tumour, focal brain injury, stroke, intracranial infection
- **Presentation**: see Table 13.4

For acute investigations and management strategies for different types of seizures, including status epilepticus, see Emergency Medicine in an Hour.

Epilepsy

Definition: a neurological disorder involving recurrent seizures. This condition is defined as:

- Two or more unprovoked epileptic fits
- One unprovoked seizure with an increased risk of further seizures
- An epilepsy syndrome characterised by a specific pattern of seizures

Buzzwords:

- **Risk factors:** premature birth, febrile seizure, hippocampal sclerosis, genetic conditions associated with epilepsy (e.g., tuberous sclerosis or neurofibromatosis), brain developmental malformations, family

history, previous head trauma, previous intracranial infection, brain tumour, cerebrovascular disease, neurodegenerative disorder

- **Presentations:** epilepsy can be categorised into specific epilepsy syndromes, some of which may be caused by specific genetic mutations. However, many patients with epilepsy are not found to have a specific cause or epilepsy syndrome. In these cases, epilepsy is categorised by the type of seizure (see Table 13.4).
- **Examples of epilepsy syndromes:**
  - **Idiopathic generalised epilepsy**: sudden-onset, tonic-clonic seizures. A clear cause is not identified in this common epilepsy type. Although it is suspected to have a genetic basis, few associated genes have been identified.
  - **Temporal lobe epilepsy**: déjà vu, epigastric rising with or without impaired awareness. May generalise. Frequently associated with hippocampal sclerosis
  - **Juvenile myoclonic epilepsy**: tonic-clonic, absence and early-morning myoclonic seizures. Photosensitive. 10% of epilepsy cases, onset typically in adolescence
  - **Infantile spasms**: 3–12 months of age; violent spasms of the head, trunk and limbs; developmental regression. May or may not be associated

with a structural brain disorder or genetic mutation. Typically displays an electroencephalogram (EEG) pattern of 'hypsarrhythmia'

- **Childhood absence seizures**: 4–12 years of age, unresponsive for 30 sec. Individuals frequently grow out of this condition and do not have epilepsy in adulthood

Investigations:

- **Electrocardiogram (ECG):** to rule out a cardiac cause
- **EEG**: interictal EEG. If normal, does NOT rule out epilepsy
- **MRI:** to look for focal causes
- **PET/SPECT:** to identify hypometabolic changes in complex cases
- **Metabolic profiling or genetic testing** (if developmental arrest or regression)

Differentials: nonepileptic attack disorder, syncope, cardiac arrhythmia

Management:

1. Antiepileptic drugs (AEDs) (see Seizure Types for general recommendations):
    a. Monotherapy if possible (see Table 13.5 for common side effects)
    b. Rescue medication (buccal midazolam) if prolonged seizures
    c. The decision to start a medication is generally made after the occurrence of two seizures. This decision is made in consultation with the patient, and the ideal drug is the one that is best suited to the patient and the type of epilepsy
2. Epilepsy surgery: usually only performed for focal seizures for which a triggering lesion can be identified
3. Ketogenic diet
4. Vagal nerve stimulation

In the United Kingdom, patients must be instructed to inform the Driver and Vehicle Licensing Agency (DVLA) and will likely have their driving licences revoked for a period of time (typically for *6 months after an unprovoked seizure* or *12 months from the last seizure in patients with epilepsy*)

STROKE

Stroke

Definition:

- **Stroke:** a clinical syndrome of cerebrovascular origin characterised by the rapid onset of a focal or global

TABLE 13.5 Common Side Effects of Antiepileptic Drugs

Medication	Side Effects
Valproate[a]	TERATOGENIC, weight gain, hair loss, liver function impairment
Carbamazepine	Rash, hyponatraemia, P450 inducer, may worsen absence or myoclonic epilepsy
Lamotrigine	Rash, insomnia, ataxia, may worsen absence or myoclonic epilepsy
Ethosuximide	Nausea and vomiting
Levetiracetam	Irritability and mood disturbance

[a]Valproate is contraindicated in women of child-bearing age

neurological deficit with symptoms lasting longer than 24 h. Strokes can be subdivided into:

- **Ischaemic:** a vessel occlusion or stenosis with symptoms that are highly dependent on the area of brain ischaemia (see Fig 13.2)
- **Haemorrhagic:** a vessel rupture with symptoms affected by the pressure created by the haemorrhage
- **Transient ischaemic attack (TIA):** a neurological deficit caused by cerebral hypoperfusion with a resolution of symptoms within 24 h

Buzzwords:

- **Risk factors (mnemonic ASCOD):**
    - **A**therosclerosis (the internal carotid artery is commonly affected): hypercholesterolaemia, diabetes mellitus (DM), smoking, hypertension (HTN), >55 years of age
    - **S**mall vessel disease (for lacunar infarcts): HTN, smoking, DM
    - **C**ardioembolic: atrial fibrillation (AF), valvular heart disease, previous myocardial infarction (MI), endocarditis, patent foramen ovale
    - **O**ther: systemic lupus erythematosus (SLE), antiphospholipid syndrome, disseminated intravascular coagulation, sickle cell disease
    - **D**issection
- **Presentation: Bamford/Oxford Stroke Classification System**
    - **Total Anterior Circulation Stroke (TACS):** patient demonstrates all three of the following findings:
        1. unilateral weakness or sensory loss of the face, arm and leg

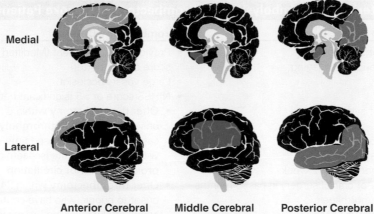

Fig 13.2 Stroke Territories. (Illustrated by Hollie Blaber.)

2. homonymous hemianopia
3. higher cerebral dysfunction (e.g., dysphasia, visuospatial loss)

- **Partial Anterior Circulation Stroke (PACS):** two of the three mentioned above
- **Posterior Circulation Stroke (POCS):** one of the following:
  - cranial nerve palsy
  - contralateral motor or sensory deficit
  - bilateral motor/sensory loss
  - cerebellar dysfunction (mnemonic **DANISH** = **D**ysdiadochokinesis, **A**taxia, **N**ystagmus, **I**ntention tremor, **S**lurred speech, **H**ypotonia/ heel-shin test positive)
  - isolated homonymous hemianopia
- **Lacunar stroke (LACS):** affects the basal ganglia and internal capsule, presenting as one of the following:
  - pure motor deficit
  - pure sensory deficit
  - ataxic hemiparesis

Even though a stroke represents an UMN lesion, patients can initially present with LMN signs such as flaccid paralysis or hyporeflexia and then subsequently develop UMN signs over time (e.g., spastic paralysis) (see Table 13.1).

Differentials: space-occupying lesion, hypoglycaemia, migraine, seizure, Bell's palsy, vasculitis, encephalitis

Investigations and Management: see section on Ischaemic and Haemorrhagic Stroke

Ischaemic Stroke

The management of ischaemic stroke can be divided into distinct phases:

1. **Reperfusion:** restoring blood supply to brain. This phase is time dependent and is usually triggered by the ambulance crew prior to arrival at the hospital
   a. **CT head/angiogram:** to determine the extent of the established infarct and to rule out a cerebral bleed or stroke mimic (note: often the CT scan is normal in the early phases, even with extensive strokes)
   b. **Establish and quantify the neurological deficit:** the standardised National Institutes of Health Stroke Scale (NIHSS) score is used
   c. **Establish the time of onset and circumstances:** this step is vital and includes determining whether the patient is on anticoagulation and performing a focused medical history
   d. **Blood sugar:** hypoglycaemia is an easy-to-miss stroke mimic
   e. **Consideration for thrombolysis**
      i. Thrombolysis is an option if there is a clear history of stroke and the onset is within 4.5 hours (this excludes wake-up strokes)
      ii. Several exclusions apply (see Table 13.6)
      iii. The blood pressure (BP) must be below 185 mm Hg systolic. Can attempt to lower with IV labetalol
      iv. The stroke needs to be severe enough to justify the risk. An NIHSS score of 5 or more is acceptable; however, a disabling isolated deficit scoring less can be considered

TABLE 13.6 **Criteria for Thrombolysis and Thrombectomy in Stroke Patients**

Thrombolysis Criteria	Thrombectomy Criteria

• <4.5 h since onset of symptoms
• Haemorrhage ruled out with imaging
• >18 years of age
Exclusion criteria
  • Seizure at onset of symptoms
  • INR >1.7
  • NIHSS score of <5 or >25
  • BP >180 mm Hg systolic
  • Recent major surgery within 2 weeks
  • Stroke, head injury or cranial surgery in past 3 months
  • Previous brain haemorrhage
  • On DOAC or therapeutic LMWH
	• Previously independent (Modified Rankin Scale (mRS) score of 2 or better)
	• Large vessel occlusion
	• NIHSS score of >5 (significant neurological deficit)
	• Offer **thrombectomy** within 6 hours of symptoms onset together with **thrombolysis** (if not contraindicated and within licensed time window) for people with confirmed acute ischaemic stroke involving the **proximal anterior circulation**
	• Offer **thrombectomy** within 24 hours of symptoms onset to people who have confirmed acute ischaemic stroke involving the **proximal anterior/posterior circulation and** there is **potential to salvage brain tissue** (low ASPECT score on CT imaging)

DOAC, Direct oral anticoagulant; LMWH, low-molecular-weight heparin; mRS, Modified Rankin Scale; NIHSS, National Institutes of Health Stroke Scale.

v. The outcome is improved the quicker the patient is assessed and treated – 'time is brain'

vi. Risk of intracranial haemorrhage

f. **Consideration for thrombectomy**: the intraarterial removal of a clot by interventional radiology

  i. Considered if CT angiogram (CTA) shows occlusion of a large, proximal artery

  ii. An option for those who are not eligible for thrombolysis

  iii. Can be considered up to 24 h after onset, although the outcome is less favourable further from onset

2. **Early management**

a. **Aspirin:** aspirin 300 mg is given as soon as possible if thrombolysis or thrombectomy are not performed, otherwise it is given 24 h later

b. **Assessment of swallowing:** patients with large strokes will have impaired swallowing, placing them at risk of choking and aspiration. NG tube placement

c. **Prevention of deep vein thrombosis (DVT):** patients are likely to be immobile for some time, increasing their risk of developing a DVT. Pneumatic calf compression devices are preferred in the first 2 weeks because enoxaparin increases the risk of haemorrhagic transformation

d. **Acute BP:** should not be lowered acutely, as the BP helps to maintain the cerebral perfusion pressure

e. **Management of blood sugar:** improved outcomes are seen with acute control of blood sugar

3. **Assessment: establish the cause of the stroke**

a. **Bloods:** FBC, U&Es, LFTs, clotting, cholesterol, HbA1c, plasma viscosity

b. **ECG:** 50% of strokes are caused by AF. Comorbid MI is also seen

c. **Carotid doppler assessment:** to assess for carotid stenosis

d. **Echocardiogram:** to look for a cardiac thrombus as a source of emboli

e. **Ambulatory cardiac monitoring:** paroxysmal AF may not be seen on ECGs performed in the hospital

f. **MR angiogram (MRA):** overlap with carotid doppler, can also assess the posterior circulation

4. **Prevention**

a. Continue aspirin 300 mg for 2 weeks, then lifelong clopidogrel 75 mg

b. If found to have AF, start anticoagulation rather than clopidogrel at 2 weeks (there is a risk of haemorrhagic transformation if started too early)

c. Aim for a long-term BP of <135/85 mm Hg

d. Statin

e. Long-term blood sugar control if high

f. Carotid endarterectomy (if >50% carotid stenosis on the symptomatic side)

5. **Rehabilitation: optimise recovery, ideally initiated as soon as safe**

a. Physiotherapy

b. Occupational therapy

c. Speech therapy

6. Patients must not drive for 1 month following a TIA or stroke and must prove that they are safe to drive after this timeframe

Haemorrhagic Stroke

Occur less frequently than ischaemic strokes

1. **Early management**

   a. CT scan demonstrates a haemorrhagic stroke

   b. NIHSS score to quantify the neurological deficit

   c. Reverse anticoagulation: liaise with haematology, stop antiplatelets

   d. BP control: the outcome is improved if the BP is lowered to below 140 mm Hg systolic

      i Treat aggressively with IV labetalol or a GTN infusion within the first 6 h of onset

   e. If hydrocephalus or oedema is causing a mass effect, consider referral to neurosurgery

      i. This tends to be a life-saving intervention rather than improving the level of disability. Consider the patient's premorbid functional status

   f. Prevention of DVT: pneumatic compression stockings

2. **Assessment and prevention**

   a. CT angiogram/MRI: to look for an underlying tumour or vascular malformation

      i. This often needs to be repeated after 3 months due to the obscuring effect of blood

   b. BP control

3. **Rehabilitation**

   a. Therapies as per ischaemic stroke

Transient Ischaemic Attack

Definition: stroke symptoms with complete resolution within 24 h. Represents an important warning sign of an impending stroke.

1. TIA risk stratification scores (e.g., ABCD2) are not recommended to guide management. Instead, all patients should be referred to a TIA clinic within 24 h for consideration of further investigations

2. Aspirin 300 mg

3. If the bleeding risk is not excessive, patients are usually started on daily aspirin 75 mg and clopidogrel 75 mg for 1 month, stepping down to lifelong clopidogrel alone

4. Investigations as per ischaemic stroke

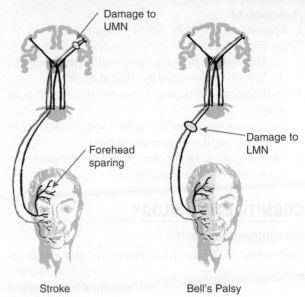

Fig 13.3 Stroke vs Bell's Palsy. *LMN,* Lower motor neuron; *UMN,* upper motor neuron. (Illustrated by Hollie Blaber.)

5. Secondary prevention (see Ischaemic Stroke)

   NB: driving regulations in the United Kingdom require a 1-month period of driving cessation for stroke and TIA unless there is a disqualifying neurological deficit

BELL'S PALSY

Definition: an acute, unilateral facial nerve weakness or paralysis of rapid onset and with unknown cause. This condition may be caused by inflammation and oedema of CNVII, causing compression and damage.

Buzzwords:

- **Risk factors:** herpes simplex virus (HSV), varicella-zoster virus (VZV), DM, immunocompromise, obesity, HTN, respiratory conditions, pregnancy

- **Presentation:** facial weakness (non-forehead sparing see Fig 13.3), ear and postauricular pain, failure of eye closure (*Bell's sign*), taste changes, dry eye, dry mouth, hyperacusis

Investigations:

- Diagnosis of exclusion (i.e., no other deficit identified besides a LMN facial palsy)

- No routine investigations required unless other differentials are suspected (e.g., stroke, malignancy, Lyme disease, cholesteatoma, sarcoidosis, MS)

Differentials: cerebrovascular event, Ramsay-Hunt syndrome, Lyme disease, otitis media, cholesteatoma, parotid gland tumour

Management:
1. Reassurance: recovery in 3 to 4 months
2. Eye protection
   a. Lubrication: hypromellose, sodium hyaluronate
   b. Tape for keeping the eye shut at night
3. Prednisolone (if patient presents within <72 h of symptom onset)
   a. Various regimens. 60 mg for 1 week then taper to 10 mg per day to stop is common
4. Examination of the ear canal: if herpetic vesicles, aciclovir (Ramsey-Hunt syndrome)

COGNITIVE NEUROLOGY

Meningoencephalitis

Definition: an acute inflammation of the meninges and brain tissue leading to neurological dysfunction. Causes confusion with or without focal neurological deficits

Encephalitis
- **Viral:** HSV 1 & 2, VZV, cytomegalovirus (CMV), Epstein-Barr virus (EBV), human herpesvirus 6 (HHV6), enterovirus, Japanese encephalitis, West Nile virus
- **Autoimmune:** anti-NMDA, anti-LGI1, antineuronal (paraneoplastic)–associated antibody syndromes

Meningoencephalitis
- **Bacterial:** *Neisseria meningitidis*, *Streptococcus pneumoniae*, *Listeria*, tuberculosis (TB), rickettsia, Lyme disease (see Infectious Diseases in an Hour)
- **Protozoan:** *Toxoplasma*
- **Fungal:** cryptococcal
- **Treponemal:** syphilis (chronic)

Buzzwords:
- **Risk factors:** immunosuppression, young or elderly, pregnancy, recent travel. Autoimmune type may be associated with an occult cancer
- **Presentation:** fever, headache, confusion, progressive drowsiness and coma, seizures, focal neurological deficit, neck stiffness

Investigations:
- **Bloods:** elevated inflammatory markers with bacterial causes, paired glucose for lumbar puncture (LP)
- **Blood culture:** to detect bacteraemia and culture the pathogen
- **CT head/MRI:** CT head is often normal but may occasionally show hydrocephalus or cerebral oedema if severe

- **LP:** cell count, protein, glucose, opening pressure, culture, viral PCR (initial brain imaging is obligatory)
  - Polymorphic picture: bacterial
  - Lymphocytic picture: viral, autoimmune, TB, less common types of bacteria
  - Glucose: should be >two-thirds of the serum value. Low in bacterial infections and very low in TB
  - Protein: elevated with infections, markedly increased with bacterial and TB infections
  - Raised opening pressure in bacterial, fungal and TB infections. Therapeutic drainage may improve symptoms
- **Consider antibody testing for autoimmune encephalitis** (dependent on MRI findings and lack of an infective agent)
- **Consider CT of the body for autoimmune encephalitis** (50% are associated with occult malignancies)

Management:
- **IV antibiotics:** ceftriaxone, amoxicillin if elderly, young, pregnant or immunosuppressed
- **IV aciclovir:** for HSV encephalitis
- **Dexamethasone for suspected bacterial meningitis**
- **Adjust treatment as indicated by investigations and cultures**
  - Negative culture/cell count: consider stopping antibiotics/dexamethasone. Treat bacterial causes as per local microbiology guidelines if confirmed (for at least 1 week)
  - Negative HSV PCR: consider stopping aciclovir. If positive, treat for 14 days and then repeat the LP to ensure negativity (21 days if immunosuppressed)
- If the infection screen is negative and there is a concern for autoimmune encephalitis: consider treatment with pulsed steroids and plasma exchange
  - Antibody testing will usually take weeks to return and confirm the diagnosis
- If concerned about TB, start quadruple therapy (rifampicin, isoniazid, pyrazinamide, ethambutol) with dexamethasone

Delirium

Definition: an acute reversible state of confusion, tending to affect the elderly and triggered by a non-neurological stressor. There are many causes of delirium, which can be remembered using the mnemonic:

- PINCHME: Pain, Infection, Nutrition, Constipation, Hydration, Medication, Environment

See Anaesthetics and Critical Care in an Hour for disordered consciousness

Buzzwords:
- **Risk factors**: >65 years of age, cognitive impairment, surgery, comorbidities, polypharmacy, visual or hearing impairments
- **Presentation**: inattention, impaired cognition, visual/auditory hallucinations, altered psychomotor activity
  - Hyperactive delirium: restlessness, agitation, wandering
  - Hypoactive delirium: drowsy, quiet, withdrawn, reduced oral intake

Investigations:
- **Scoring systems:**
  - Confusion Assessment Method (CAM)
    - Acute onset and fluctuating course *AND*
    - Inattention *AND EITHER*
    - Disorganized thinking *OR*
    - Altered level of consciousness
  - **4AT:** Alertness, AMT4 (age, date of birth, place, current year), Attention (months of the year backwards), Acute change or fluctuating course. A score of 4 or above indicates possible delirium +/- cognitive impairment. A score of 1-3 indicates possible cognitive impairment. A score of 0 indicates delirium or severe cognitive impairment unlikely (but delirium is still possible if acute change or fluctuating course is questionable).
- **Confusion screen:**
  - Capillary blood glucose (CBG)
  - Bloods (baseline blood tests (FBC, U&E, LFTs, CRP, clotting), TSH, vitamin B12, folate, bone profile): may show an infection or deranged values
  - CT/MRI head: may show acute intracranial pathology (e.g., subdural haematoma)
  - Other investigations are guided by the differentials (e.g., a chest x-ray (CXR) for suspected pneumonia)
  - Depression screen

Differentials: dementia, cerebrovascular event, sepsis, electrolyte imbalances, renal failure, encephalitis

Management:
- Treat underlying cause
- Conservative: same place, same staff, pictures from home, twiddlemuff

- Drug therapy: should be avoided if possible. Only indicated if patients are at risk to themselves or others

Dementia

Definition: a progressive decline in cognitive function significantly impacting activities of daily living (ADLs). This condition may affect both cognitive domains and social behaviours. There are four main types of dementia:
- Alzheimer's disease
- Vascular dementia
- Dementia with Lewy bodies
- Frontotemporal lobe dementia

This section will cover the general workup of anyone presenting with cognitive decline.

Buzzwords: see specific section

Investigations: it is important to rule out any reversible causes of cognitive decline, to determine a baseline and to monitor the patient's response to therapy
- **Cognitive testing** (e.g., the Mini-Mental State Exam, Montreal Cognitive Assessment, Addenbrooke's Cognitive Examination-Revised): to characterise the specific domains affected and to monitor changes in cognitive function
- **Bloods**: to rule out acute causes of confusion or organic causes (see Delirium)
- **CT**: to assess for differentials, may show age-related/involutional changes. See relevant sections for results expected for specific conditions
- **MRI**: more sensitive. Can characterise the specific type of dementia. See relevant sections for results expected for specific conditions

Differentials: delirium, depression, normal pressure hydrocephalus, vitamin B12 deficiency, Wernicke-Korsakoff's syndrome, Creutzfeldt-Jakob disease

Management: all patients should receive the management steps described below. See individual conditions for additional disease-specific management strategies
- If sudden onset, rule out reversible causes and treat accordingly
- Referral to a memory assessment clinic (referral to neurology for younger, rapid-onset cases)
- In the United Kingdom, patients must inform the DVLA
- Monitor for evidence of behavioural and psychological symptoms of dementia
- If patients become acutely agitated, nonpharmacological treatments should be used first. If these fail and patients are a danger to themselves or others,

TABLE 13.7 Side Effects: Acetylcholinesterase Inhibitors and Glutamate-receptor Antagonists

Drug Class	Side Effects
Acetylcholinesterase inhibitors	Increased risk of falls (dizziness, drowsiness, syncope), urinary incontinence, weight loss, headache, gastrointestinal disturbances
Glutamate-receptor antagonist	Increased risk of falls (impaired balance, dizziness, drowsiness), constipation, hypertension, hypersensitivity

very low–dose haloperidol (do NOT use in patients with Parkinson's disease (PD) nor in dementia with Lewy bodies) or lorazepam can be used

- End-of-life care in dementia should be discussed and carefully planned while the patient still has capacity.

Alzheimer's Disease

Definition: a neurodegenerative disorder caused by deposits of amyloid-beta plaques (extracellularly) and tau neurofibrillary tangles (intracellularly) in the brain, causing neuronal dysfunction and eventual cerebral atrophy. Most cases are sporadic, although a small number of cases have a genetic cause.

Buzzwords:

- **Risk factors:** advancing age (strongest risk factor), learning difficulties, stroke, depression, heavy alcohol consumption, low educational attainment, low social engagement/support, genetic predisposition
  - **Early-onset (< 65 years of age):** Is associated with mutations in the genes encoding **Presenilin 1 protein** (*PSEN1* gene in Chromosome 1), **Presenilin 2 protein** (*PSEN2* gene in Chromosome 2), and **Amyloid precursor protein** (*APP* gene in Chromosome 21)
  - **Late-onset (> 65 years of age):** *APOE* gene encodes **Apolipoprotein E protein**. There are different alleles in humans. Carrying the *APOE e4* **allele** increases the risk of late-onset Alzheimer's Disease. Carrying the *APOE e2 allele* is protective.
- **Presentation:** mnemonic: '4 A's'
  - Amnesia (short-term memory dysfunction, long-term memory is relatively spared)

- Apraxia (inability to perform and plan motor tasks)
- Aphasia (inability to comprehend and formulate words)
- Agnosia (inability to recognise things using one (or more) senses)

Investigations:

- **CT/MRI:** diffuse cerebral atrophy (there is a predilection for the temporal lobes early in the disease course), enlargement of the cortical sulci and increased size of the ventricles

Management:

- **Mild-to-moderate disease:** monotherapy with acetylcholinesterase (AChE) inhibitors (e.g., donepezil, galantamine, rivastigmine). See table 13.7 for side effects
- **Moderate-to-severe disease:** monotherapy with a glutamate-receptor antagonist (memantine). See table 13.7 for side effects
- **AChE intolerant/contraindicated:** monotherapy with memantine
- **Already taking AChE but effect is suboptimal:** consider adding memantine

Vascular Dementia

Definition: cognitive impairment caused by a gradual cerebrovascular compromise

Buzzwords:

- **Risk factors:** Mnemonic ASCOD (see Stroke Risk Factors)
- **Presentation:** stepwise deterioration, gait disturbance ('marche à petits pas' = short-stepping gait), apathy, disinhibition, problem-solving difficulties

Investigations:

- **CT:** evidence of small-vessel disease, diffuse hypodensities
- **MRI** (more sensitive): small-vessel disease, microhaemorrhages

Management:

- Cardiovascular risk factor management
- Only consider AChE inhibitors (donepezil, galantamine, rivastigmine) if patients have comorbid Alzheimer's disease, dementia with Lewy bodies or PD

Dementia With Lewy Bodies

Definition: dementia occurring as a result of **alpha-synuclein** cytoplasmic inclusions (a.k.a., Lewy bodies) within nerve cells, impacting their functioning and resulting in cognitive impairment. Key definitions are:

- **Lewy body dementia:** cognitive decline before or within the first year of developing parkinsonism
- **PD dementia:** dementia that develops after at least 1 year of having features of PD

Buzzwords:

- **Risk factors:** increasing age, male, family history
- **Presentation:** visual hallucinations (often of small people and animals (a.k.a., Lilliputian hallucinations)), REM sleep behaviour disorder, parkinsonism (bradykinesia, rigidity, tremor, postural instability), fluctuations in cognition and alertness

Investigations:

- **DaTscan:** reduced uptake of dopamine in the basal ganglia

Management:

- Mild, moderate or severe: donepezil or rivastigmine
- If donepezil or rivastigmine intolerant/contraindicated: consider galantamine
- If AChE inhibitors contraindicated: consider memantine
- Other things to consider:
  - Levodopa/carbidopa may be used if patient has concomitant motor features of PD
  - Clonazepam or melatonin may be used if patient has REM sleep behaviour disorder
  - DO NOT use dopamine receptor antagonists such as haloperidol or metoclopramide

Frontotemporal Dementia

Definition: a neurodegenerative disease of the frontal and temporal lobes occurring as a result of intraneuronal deposits. There are several types of frontotemporal dementia (FTD) causing similar symptom profiles. Most common:

- **FTD-tau:** intraneuronal and glial inclusions of tau (a microtubule protein) associated with mutations in the gene *MAPT*
- **FTD-ubiquitin (Pick bodies):** deposits of the TDP-43 protein associated with mutations in *PGRN* genes

Buzzwords:

- **Risk factors:** family history, increasing age
- **Presentation:** early changes in personality, behaviour and language

- **Behavioural variant** (focal atrophy of the frontal lobes): apathy, disinhibition, obsessive-compulsive disorder (OCD), craving sweet foods
- **Progressive nonfluent aphasia:** loss of speech fluency and grammar
- **Semantic variant/fluent aphasia** (atrophy of the dominant temporal lobe): receptive aphasia, inability to name objects, preserved speech

Investigations:

- **MRI:** cerebral atrophy, predominantly affecting the frontal and temporal lobes
- **Genetic testing:** if a clear family history is apparent. Also, increasingly being used for sporadic cases (where de novo mutations are seen)

Management:

- Social support and educating patients/families/carers
- Benzodiazepines can be used for acute restlessness
- Selective serotonin reuptake inhibitors (SSRIs) can be used for compulsions, and mirtazapine can be used for sleep disturbances

Normal Pressure Hydrocephalus

Definition: a form of communicating hydrocephalus without a raised ICP, causing gradual cognitive and mobility symptoms

Buzzwords:

- **Risk factors:** >40 years of age, vascular disease
- **Presentation:** remember the following triad:
  - **Whacky:** behavioural changes with cognitive impairment
  - **Wobbly:** gait disturbances; broad-based, shuffling gait
  - **Wet:** urinary incontinence, urgency, frequency, nocturia

Investigations:

- **CT and MRI:** dilated ventricles, crowded vertex, widened sylvian fissures
- **CSF drainage:** large-volume removal of cerebrospinal fluid (CSF) as a therapeutic test of the potential response to surgery (rapid, temporary improvement in symptoms)

Differentials: dementia, obstructive hydrocephalus, enlarged ventricles secondary to cerebral atrophy

Management:

- If appropriate for surgery: ventriculoperitoneal shunt
- If not a candidate for surgery: Vascular risk factor management

MOVEMENT DISORDERS

Parkinsonism

Definition: an umbrella term used to describe the clinical syndrome of bradykinesia, tremor, rigidity and/or postural instability

Causes of parkinsonism:

• Idiopathic PD
• Parkinson-plus syndromes (parkinsonism + other features): progressive supranuclear palsy (PSP), multisystem atrophy (MSA), corticobulbar degeneration, Lewy body dementia (see Table 13.8)
• Drug-induced parkinsonism: antipsychotics, antiemetics, lithium, methyldopa

Idiopathic Parkinson's Disease

Definition: a movement disorder associated with a loss of dopaminergic neurons in the substantia nigra, eventually becoming a diffuse whole-brain condition. Deposits of alpha-synuclein (Lewy bodies) are present within neurons

Buzzwords:

• **Risk factors:** most commonly sporadic, but hereditary cases can occur with younger presentations
• **Presentation:**
  • **Motor symptoms:** bradykinesia, tremor (resting, pill rolling), cog-wheel rigidity (with tremor), lead-pipe rigidity (without tremor), postural instability

• **Non-motor symptoms:** autonomic dysfunction (urinary frequency, postural hypotension, hypersalivation), REM sleep behaviour disorder, depression

Investigations:

• **DaTscan:** reduced uptake of dopamine in the basal ganglia

Differentials: Parkinson-plus syndromes, drug-induced parkinsonism (antipsychotics, antimuscarinics), vascular parkinsonism, Wilson's disease, neurosyphilis, benign essential tremor

Management:

NB: Parkinson's medications are *critical medications* and MUST be given at the correct time. This is particularly important for hospital inpatients

1. Medications for motor symptoms (combinations can be used):
   • Levodopa: Madopar/Sinemet (see Table 13.9 for side effects)
   • Dopamine-receptor agonists: pramipexole, ropinirole, rotigotine (see Table 13.9 for side effects)
   • Monoamine oxidase-B inhibitors: rasagiline or selegiline hydrochloride
   • COMT inhibitors: entacapone
   • Amantadine can help with dyskinesias associated with levodopa treatment

TABLE 13.8 Parkinson-plus Syndromes

Parkinson-plus Syndrome	Buzzwords
Progressive supranuclear palsy	Recurrent falls, slurred speech, swallowing difficulties, vertical gaze impairment, poor response to levodopa
Multisystem atrophy	Cerebellar signs, autonomic dysfunction (erectile dysfunction, incontinence, postural hypotension), poor response to levodopa
Corticobulbar degeneration	Asymmetric apraxia, alien limb syndrome, aphasia, poor response to levodopa
Lewy body dementia	Cognitive decline within 12 months of Parkinson's disease diagnosis, hallucinations

TABLE 13.9 Side Effects: Levodopa and Dopamine-Receptor Agonists

Medication	Side Effect
Levodopa	Somnolence, nausea, peak-dose dyskinesia. *On-off effect* is seen, in which symptoms of Parkinson's disease return towards the end of the dose; however, this side effect is a consequence of disease progression. NB: do not stop levodopa abruptly as this can increase the risk of akinesia and neuroleptic malignant syndrome
Dopamine-receptor agonists (e.g., pramipexole, ropinirole, rotigotine)	Impulse-control disorder, visual hallucinations and daytime sleepiness. Avoid dopamine agonists in patients at high risk of impulse-control disorder

2. Deep brain stimulation may be used to treat problematic motor fluctuations by reducing the required levodopa dose
3. In individuals in whom surgery is not appropriate, duodopa (levodopa delivered continuously by a jejunal tube) or apomorphine infusions can be considered
4. Do not give haloperidol, chlorpromazine or metoclopramide to patients with PD

Benign Essential Tremor

Definition: a rhythmic, involuntary, oscillatory movement of the body, particularly the upper limbs. It is the most common movement disorder and is typically present only during movement.

Buzzwords:

- **Risk factors:** highly heritable between generations, although no gene has yet been identified
- **Presentation:** bilateral, symmetrical tremor, often seen in the hands but can also be seen in the head and neck overlapping with cervical dystonia. Tremor occurs with movement, particularly marked during actions with outstretched arms and affecting handwriting. Should be absent at rest, with no gait disturbances. Alcohol can improve the symptoms.

Investigations:

- **DaTscan** (if atypical features, raises concern for PD)

Differentials: PD, hyperthyroidism, drug induced (e.g., lithium, methylphenidate)

Management: if the tremor has no effect on ADLs, management is conservative. Otherwise:

1. Propranolol or primidone
2. Second-line options include gabapentin, benzodiazepine, levetiracetam, topiramate, deep brain stimulation

Huntington's Disease

Definition: an *autosomal dominant* condition characterised by more than 36 CAG repeats in the Huntington's gene (*HTT*) on Chromosome 4. These mutations lead to the formation of an abnormal Huntingtin protein. Huntington's disease is associated with **genetic anticipation** (i.e., an increase in the number of trinucleotides repeats over successive generations leads to an increase in disease severity and earlier onset).

Buzzwords:

- **Risk factors:** family history
- **Presentation:** increased irritability and depression, dementia, impaired cognitive executive function, chorea (starts with fidgety movements progressing to choreiform movements)

Investigation:

- Genetic testing: >36 CAG repeats

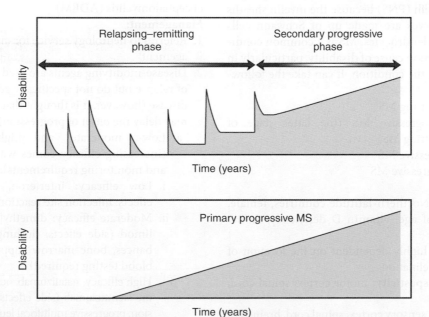

Fig 13.4 Clinical Patterns of Multiple Sclerosis *(MS).* (With permission from Jarman, P. (2017). Neurological disease. In *Kumar and Clark's clinical medicine.* Elsevier. Copyright © 2017 Elsevier Ltd. All rights reserved.)

- CT/MRI: loss of the caudate nucleus, later cerebral atrophy

Differentials: tardive dyskinesia, Wilson's disease, benign hereditary chorea, structural lesion affecting the basal ganglia

Management:

- Currently no cure
- Management involves symptoms control:
  - **Chorea:** dopamine antagonists, VMAT inhibitors (e.g., tetrabenazine), clonazepam
  - **Psychosis:** antipsychotics (e.g., haloperidol, quetiapine, clozapine)
  - **Depression:** SSRIs

MOTOR AND SENSORY DISORDERS

Central Nervous System

Multiple Sclerosis

Definition: an autoimmune inflammatory disease resulting in demyelination at multiple sites in the central nervous system (CNS). In its most common form, relapsing-remitting MS, acute episodes of inflammatory demyelination are seen, causing 'relapses' that often recover. Eventually, axonal loss is seen, at which point symptoms become progressive.

Remember: there is no involvement of the peripheral nervous system (PNS) because the myelin sheaths of peripheral nerves are made up of Schwann cells rather than oligodendrocytes. MS is a common condition and is a common cause of disability, particularly in the later stages of the condition. It can take the following forms (see Fig 13.4):

- Relapsing-remitting MS
- Secondary progressive MS (the latter stage of relapsing-remitting MS)
- Primary progressive MS
- Relapsing progressive MS

Buzzwords:

- **Risk factors:** Northern-latitude countries, female, 20–40 years of age, vitamin D deficiency, family history
- **Presentation:** highly dependent on the location of the focal demyelination
  - **Weakness, spasticity:** motor cortex, spinal cord, brainstem
  - **Numbness:** sensory cortex, spinal cord, brainstem
  - **Ataxia:** brainstem/cerebellum
  - **Bladder dysfunction:** spinal cord

- **Optic neuritis** (reduced visual acuity, painful eye movements, loss of colour vision): optic nerve
- **Intranuclear ophthalmoplegia** (damage to the medial longitudinal fasciculus (MLF), resulting in an inability to adduct the affected eye and nystagmus in the contralateral eye causing diplopia): brainstem
- **Uhthoff's phenomenon:** heat worsens symptoms
- **Lhermitte's sign:** a sudden electric-shock pain running down the spine when flexing the neck

Investigations:

- **MRI:** T2 hyperintensities in the periventricular, juxtacortical (between the grey and white matter), infratentorial and spinal regions (see Radiology in an Hour)
- **CSF:** oligoclonal bands in the CSF but not the serum
- **Revised McDonald's criteria for relapsing MS are met if:** more likely diagnoses have been excluded and there is demonstrated dissemination in *time and space*
  - Time: 2× clinical relapses or new brain lesions on sequential scans (oligoclonal bands count as an additional 'relapse')
  - Space: relapses relate to different brain areas or lesions are in different areas on scans

Differentials: sarcoidosis, SLE, human immunodeficiency virus (HIV), progressive multifocal leukoencephalopathy, antiphospholipid syndrome, neuromyelitis optica (NMO)-spectrum disorder, acute disseminated encephalomyelitis (ADEM)

Management:

1. Referral to neurology service for diagnosis and management
2. Disease-modifying agents are used to reduce the risk of relapse but do not specifically address progressive disease (however, it is thought that reducing relapses may delay the onset of progression)
   a. Low-, moderate- and high-efficacy agents (increasing efficacy comes with increasing risk and monitoring requirements):
      i. Low efficacy: interferon, glatiramer (side effects: injection site reactions and fever)
      ii. Moderate efficacy: dimethyl fumarate, fingolimod (side effects: flushing, cardiac disturbances, bone marrow suppression – regular blood testing required)
      iii. High efficacy: natalizumab, ocrelizumab, cladribine alemtuzumab (side effects: immunosuppression, progressive multifocal leukoencephalopathy, new autoimmune disease, bone marrow suppression – regular blood testing required)

b. Typically, disease-modifying treatments are started after two relapses occur within 2 years

3. Ocrelizumab has recently been licenced for primary progressive MS

4. Symptomatic management of complications, including spasticity, fatigue, neuropathic pain, mood, bladder and bowel symptoms

   a. Baclofen/physiotherapy for spasticity, antidepressants, intermittent self-catheterisation, colonic irrigation systems

5. Acute relapse: methylprednisolone can be used, but it only improves the time to resolution and does not change the final outcome. Typically only used if relapses are disabling

Neuromyelitis Optica

Definition: an antibody-mediated autoimmune disease of the CNS characterized by optic neuritis and myelitis
Buzzwords:

- **Risk factors**: family history of autoimmune disorders, existing autoimmune condition
- **Presentation**: uni/bilateral eye pain and vision loss (optic neuritis – without recovery), weakness, sensory loss, bladder dysfunction due to rapid-onset and severe spinal cord inflammation – 'longitudinally extensive transverse myelitis'. Severe nausea and hiccoughing (area postrema syndrome – spinal inflammation can extend to the lower brainstem)

Investigations:

- **Antibodies:** anti-aquaporin 4 positive, less commonly anti-MOG positive
- **MRI brain/spinal cord:** optic nerve inflammation, brain lesions are unusual, lesions extending >3 vertebrae (longitudinally extensive transverse myelitis)
- **Lumbar puncture:** raised WCC and protein (in some cases), absent oligoclonal bands
- **Visual-evoked potentials:** positive response time

Differentials: spinal cord infarct, MS, vasculitis, ADEM, SLE, paraneoplastic disorders, sarcoidosis
Management:

- Rescue therapy: high-dose methylprednisolone +/- plasmapheresis +/- IV immunoglobulin (IVIG)
- Maintenance therapy: long-term prednisolone, immune modulators (e.g., azathioprine, methotrexate, rituximab)
- Bladder and bowel care, DVT prophylaxis (if severe spinal disorder)

- Some cases can be rapid and have effects on ventilation, particularly if there is cervical spine involvement
- Rehabilitation
- Management of residual symptoms
  - Baclofen: spasticity
  - Intermittent self-catheterisation

Prognosis: relapsing condition without a progressive element. Relapses are severe, and recovery can be limited, unlike with MS. Long-term immunosuppression prevents relapses, which must be addressed urgently when they present

Subacute Combined Degeneration of the Cord

Definition: a myelopathy resulting from a vitamin B12 (cobalamin) deficiency, specifically affecting the dorsal columns of the spinal cord. This condition can present concurrently or without a B12 peripheral neuropathy.
Buzzwords:

- **Risk factors:** nutritional deficiency, vegan diet, pernicious anaemia, resection of terminal ileum/short bowel syndrome. A 'functional B12 deficiency' is commonly seen in people who extensively overuse recreational nitrous oxide. In these cases, B12 levels can be normal but the reaction is blocked
- **Presentation:** distal paresthesias and numbness, sensory ataxia causing gait disturbances, reduced vibration and proprioception sensation

Investigations:

- **Bloods:** low vitamin B12 level (can be normal in nitrous oxide use in which homocysteine and methylmalonic acid levels are elevated instead). Megaloblastic anaemia is often NOT seen in people with a neurological B12 deficiency
- **Parietal cell antibodies:** if concern for pernicious anaemia
- **MRI:** T2/FLAIR hyperintensity in the dorsal columns – typically seen in the thoracic cord first and then progresses rostrally and/or caudally

Differentials: neurosyphilis, MS, copper deficiency, peripheral neuropathy (sensory ataxia)
Management:

1 Vitamin B12 supplementation (high-dose regimen)
2 Folate supplementation may aid in reversal of associated haematological disorders if present. However, vitamin B12 must be replaced first to avoid an exacerbation of neurological symptoms.
3 Cessation of nitrous oxide use if relevant

Peripheral Nervous System
Guillain-Barré Syndrome (GBS)

Definition: an acute inflammatory polyneuropathy (usually) resulting in a symmetrical, ascending muscle weakness. Guillain-Barré syndrome (GBS) is among the most common causes of acute neuromuscular weakness.

Buzzwords:

- **Risk factors:** occurs sporadically, half of cases are preceded by a gastrointestinal or upper respiratory infection (e.g., *Campylobacter jejuni*, influenza, CMV, EBV)
- **Presentation:** progressive, ascending sensorimotor deficit and autonomic dysfunction (cardiac arrythmias, blood pressure lability)
  - Symptoms reach their worst point (nadir) by week 4 – if longer, consider an alternative diagnosis (e.g., chronic inflammatory demyelinating polyneuropathy (CIDP))
  - Symptoms can affect motor or sensory nerves in isolation
  - Variants exist such as Miller-Fisher syndrome, specifically causing ophthalmoplegia and ataxia

Investigations:

- **ABG:** may show type 2 respiratory failure (an indication that ventilation is required) if severe
- **Lung function testing:** forced vital capacity (FVC). If the FVC <1.5 L, ventilation in the ITU may be required
- **Bloods:** inflammatory markers are normal. Rule out thyrotoxicosis (Basedow's paraplegia), Lyme disease serology, HIV, syphilis
  - Cases can be associated with positive antiganglioside antibodies
- **Lumbar puncture:** ↑/↔ protein, ↔ WCC; raised protein without WCC = 'albuminocytological dissociation'
- **Nerve conduction studies:** demyelination is consistent with GBS

Differentials: Lyme disease, heavy metal poisoning, acute intermittent porphyria, Basedow's paraplegia

Management:

1. IVIG or plasma exchange is associated with a reduced time on ventilation and a faster recovery. Used if rapidly progressive and/or affecting motor function
2. Monitoring of respiratory function, supportive ventilation if required
3. Nutritional support (NG tube)
4. DVT prophylaxis
5. Rehabilitation – recovery can last months or more

A related condition called chronic inflammatory demyelinating polyneuropathy (CIDP) can have a similar presentation, with a symmetrical, length-dependent peripheral nerve demyelination. CIDP features:

- Characterised by multiple relapses and a more chronic picture; however, it can have similar symptoms
- Management principles are similar (not as acute)
- Many patients require long-term immunosuppression for prevention of relapses
- It is considered to be a different condition than GBS despite their similarities (autoimmune vs parainfectious)

Charcot-Marie-Tooth Disease

Definition: a genetic condition affecting motor and sensory nerves. There are multiple subtypes of this disease that vary in their presentations and genetics.

Buzzwords:

- **Risk factors:** family history
- **Presentation:** often the 1st and 2nd decades of life but variable onset; atrophy and weakness of the distal musculature ('champagne-bottle legs'); a high-stepping gait due to foot-drop; areflexia; orthopaedic deformities (e.g., pes cavus)

Investigations:

- Nerve conduction studies/electromyography: axonal neuropathy

Differentials: diabetic neuropathy, myopathy, chronic inflammatory polyneuropathy

Management:

- Orthopaedic deformities may be managed with physiotherapy, splinting and, possibly, corrective surgery
- No disease-modifying treatments are currently available. Severity is highly variable, but life expectancy is generally unaffected

Diabetic Neuropathy

Definition: a complication of DM leading to a symmetrical and distal polyneuropathy of the motor, sensory and autonomic fibres.

Buzzwords:

- **Risk factors:** poor diabetic control, increased duration of DM, smoking, HTN, coronary heart disease
- **Presentation:**
  - **Sensory neuropathy:** tingling and numbness (typically in a stocking-glove distribution, see Fig 13.5), neuropathic pain (most common)

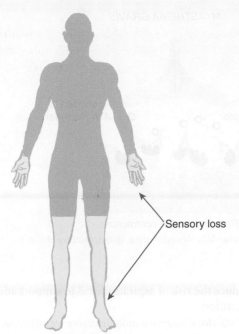

Fig 13.5 Glove and Stocking Distribution of Sensory Loss. (Illustrated by Hollie Blaber.)

- **Motor neuropathy:** weakness, muscle wasting
- **Autonomic neuropathy:** slow stomach emptying (gastroparesis), urinary incontinence, excessive sweating, impotence (also caused by microvascular disease)

Investigations:
- **Nerve conduction studies:** symmetrical, length-dependent axonal neuropathy
- Often a **clinical diagnosis** in the context of DM (see Endocrinology in an Hour)

Differentials: hypothyroidism, vitamin B12 deficiency, paraneoplastic neuropathy, chronic inflammatory polyneuropathy

Management:
- Optimise diabetic control
- **Neuropathic pain:** duloxetine (first line) (see Chronic Pain in Palliative Care and Oncology in an Hour)
- Ensure the patient receives diabetic foot care because of high risk of developing ulcers/infections

Sciatica

Definition: also known as lumbar radiculopathy. Radiculopathy describes the clinical features associated with the dysfunction of a specific nerve root. Sciatica occurs when the lumbosacral nerve roots (L4-S1) forming the sciatic nerve become inflamed or compressed. Causes include intervertebral disc herniation, spondylolisthesis and spinal stenosis.

Buzzwords:
- **Risk factors:** age, heavy manual labour, obesity, psychosocial stress, osteoporosis
- **Presentation:** no history of significant trauma, pain radiating down the leg to below the knee into the foot and toes (sciatic nerve distribution), neurogenic claudication (leg and buttock pain on walking), can be unilateral or bilateral, relieved by sitting and flexion, positive straight-leg raise (provokes similar pain)

Investigations:
- Usually a clinical diagnosis (make sure you exclude red flag symptoms/signs)
- Imaging is indicated if associated with intractable symptoms or weakness. MRI may show a compressed spinal nerve/disc prolapse (see Neurosurgery in an Hour).

Differentials: metastatic spinal disease, cauda equina, spondylarthritis, vertebral collapse

Management:
- Education about the chronic nature of back pain
- Physical activity +/- cognitive behavioural therapy (CBT)
- Benzodiazepines, gabapentin and steroids are not recommended
- Low-dose NSAIDs (for a short time) with paracetamol
- **Interventions (if nonsurgical treatment has failed):** consider referral for nerve root injections/spinal-decompression surgery

Motor Neuron Disease

Definition: Motor neuron disease (MND) refers to a family of neurodegenerative conditions characterised by a progressive loss of motor nerves. There are four subtypes:
- **Amyotrophic lateral sclerosis (ALS):** most common form of MND, affecting the CNS and peripheral motor nerves (mixed UMN/LMN signs)
- **Progressive bulbar palsy:** only affects the bulbar nerves
- **Progressive muscular atrophy:** only affects LMNs
- **Primary lateral sclerosis:** pure CNS loss of motor nerves

Buzzwords:
- **Risk factors:** familial, geographical cluster distribution (e.g., increased cases in the Western Pacific); lymphoproliferative disease, >40 years of age, male

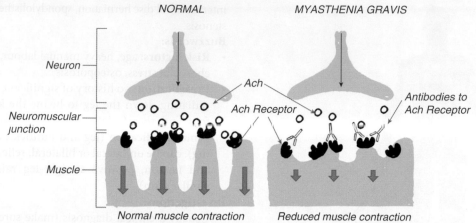

NORMAL   *MYASTHENIA GRAVIS*

Fig 13.6 The Neuromuscular Junction in Myasthenia Gravis. *ACh,* Acetylcholine. (Illustrated by Hollie Blaber.)

- **Presentation:** weakness (frequently distal-to-proximal progression), UMN signs (e.g., hyperreflexia, spasticity), LMN signs (e.g., flaccidity, fasciculations), sialorrhea, neck drop
  - 15% of patients with MND will develop frontal dementia, significant cross-over in the pathologies of FTD and MND
  - Never involves autonomic (bladder, bowel) or sensory nerve dysfunction

Investigations:
- **Bloods:** lab tests often normal
- **Neurophysiological testing:** evidence of denervation of multiple body segments on nerve conduction studies and electromyogram (EMG)
- **MRI:** to exclude alternative diagnoses, particularly cervical stenosis

Differentials: multifocal motor neuropathy, myasthenia gravis (MG), syringomyelia/syringobulbia, Kennedy's disease, late-onset spinal muscular atrophy

Management:
1. Multidisciplinary approach: include the patient and family members to establish wishes for future care
2. Riluzole: delays ventilator dependence and prolongs the life expectancy by months only; little effect on functional improvement
3. Symptomatic relief: antimuscarinics for sialorrhea, splints may aid function (e.g., thumb splint facilitating opposition in an affected hand), mobility assistance
4. Feeding support: insertion of a gastrostomy feeding tube (PEG or RIG) at the appropriate time point to reduce the risk of aspiration and to support adequate nutrition
5. Ventilatory support: non-invasive ventilation, often starting overnight, with an aim of improving the quality of life and life expectancy
6. End-of-life care when appropriate, recognising the patient's wishes – mean life expectancy with ALS is 2 years

NEUROMUSCULAR JUNCTION DISORDERS

Myasthenia Gravis

Definition: an autoimmune condition characterised by the development of antibodies to post-synaptic nicotinic acetylcholine receptors in the neuromuscular junction ('**blocking auto-antibodies**').

Buzzwords:
- **Risk factors:** other autoimmune diseases, peak in females between 20 and 30 years of age, peak in males at 50+ years of age, can be a paraneoplastic disorder with associated cancer
- **Presentation:**
  - **Fatigable muscle weakness:** worse with repetitive movement and towards the end of the day. Weakness tends to be proximal, affecting the ability to stand/walk, or it affects the bulbar muscles, impairing speech/swallowing
  - **Ocular symptoms:** ptosis (worse in the evenings), diplopia (complex ophthalmoplegia on examination)

- **Myasthenic crisis:** acute respiratory failure potentially requiring mechanical ventilation (breathlessness, complete dysphagia)
- 50% of MG cases only ever affect the ocular muscles, causing diplopia and ptosis. 'Generalised' MG (affecting the bulbar or body muscles) usually progresses from an ocular onset

Investigations:
- **Antibodies:** anti-AChR antibodies (90%), anti-MUSK antibodies (5%)
- **Nerve-conduction studies/electromyography:** decreased response to repetitive stimulation in nerve conduction studies, increased jitter on single-fibre EMG
- **CT thorax:** 10%–15% patients will have an associated thymic mass
  - A small percentage are malignant.

Differentials: Lambert-Eaton myasthenic syndrome (LAMS)

Management:
1. Anticholinesterases (e.g., pyridostigmine): inhibit the breakdown of acetylcholine (ACh) in the synapse to increase the intra-synaptic concentration of ACh. Often adequate to control purely ocular MG
2. Oral corticosteroids are effective for achieving remission – generalised MG
3. Immunosuppressants (e.g., azathioprine, methotrexate and mycophenolate) are used as steroid-sparing agents in the long term if there is a recurrence of symptoms after weaning of steroids
4. Thymectomy in selected younger patients (can be curative) and for a malignant thymic mass
5. Treatment of myasthenic crisis:
   a. Monitoring of respiratory function (FVC) and mechanical ventilation if required (FVC <1.5 L is concerning)
   b. Plasma exchange or IVIG
6. Nutritional support: NG tube
7. Care needs to be taken when prescribing medications, as many can idiosyncratically worsen symptoms. Common examples: ciprofloxacin/gentamicin/beta blockers

Lambert-Eaton Myasthenic Syndrome

Definition: an autoimmune condition resulting in the production of antibodies sensitive to pre-synaptic voltage-gated calcium channels (VGCC)

Buzzwords:
- **Risk factors:** >50% cases are associated with cancer; female
- **Presentation:** proximal weakness; hypo-/areflexia; weakness **improves** with activity; dry mouth

Investigations:
- **Antibodies:** antibodies against VGCCs
- **Nerve-conduction studies:** short bursts of exercise or high-frequency stimulation increase the amplitude of the detected signal
- **CT thorax, abdomen and pelvis (CT TAP):** advised, as there is a strong association with malignancies (especially small cell lung cancer)

Differentials: MG, myopathy, CIDP

Management:
1. Treatment of underlying cancer if identified
2. Anticholinesterases (e.g., pyridostigmine) may confer some symptomatic relief
3. Aminopyridines (e.g., 3,4-diaminopyridine) prolong the time during which VGCCs remain open, indirectly increasing the amount of acetylcholine in the neuromuscular junction
4. Immunotherapy: plasma exchange, IVIG and steroids

MUSCLE DISORDERS

Myositis Including Dermatomyositis

Definition: an autoimmune-mediated inflammation of the muscles

Buzzwords:
- **Risk factors:** underlying cancer (can be paraneoplastic), interstitial lung disease (seen together with anti-synthetase syndrome), a recently started medication (e.g., statins), post-viral infection
- **Presentation:**
  - Weakness and muscle pain: proximal (difficulty standing, stairs)
  - Diminished or absent reflexes: usually not chronic enough to cause wasting
  - Rash in dermatomyositis: heliotrope (eyes), Gottron's papules (finger joints) (see Rheumatology in an Hour)
  - Rhabdomyolysis, renal failure and myoglobinuria in severe cases (necrotising myositis)

Investigations:
- **Bloods:** markedly raised creatine kinase (CK), signs of renal impairment if severe

- **Antibody testing:** ANA positive, anti-Jo, anti-synthetase antibodies (e.g. PL7), anti-HMGCoA antibodies (necrotising myositis)
- **EMG:** myopathic picture
- **MRI muscles:** inflammation visualised – can also help locate a target for biopsy
- **Muscle biopsy:** inflammatory infiltration, muscle degeneration
- **CT TAP:** may show an underlying cancer

Differentials: MG, genetic myopathy, fibromyalgia
Management: dependent on the extent and cause

- If underlying cancer is discovered: treatment of cancer
- Cessation of precipitating drugs
- Immunosuppression: corticosteroids, IVIG, cyclophosphamide
- Renal support (dialysis) if needed whilst recovering

Inclusion body myositis is an acquired inflammatory cause of muscle weakness affecting people over 50 years of age. Features include:

- Insidious onset
- Affects the flexor muscles disproportionately
- No benefit with immunosuppression
- The cause is not known

Myotonic Dystrophy

Definition: an autosomal-dominant condition caused by mutations in the *DMPK* gene (DM1) or *CNBP* gene (DM2), causing progressive muscular weakness
Buzzwords:

- **Risk factors:** family history
- **Presentation:** distal weakness (hands/feet), facial and neck weakness (including ptosis), respiratory weakness, learning disabilities, frontal balding, cataracts, cardiac dysfunction, myotonia (delay in muscle relaxation after contraction)

Investigations:

- **Bloods:** mildly raised CK
- **Genetic testing:** abnormality in *DMPK* or *CBNP*

Differentials: muscular dystrophies
Management: mostly supportive, may include:

- Orthotics and mobility aids
- Yearly ECG due to a risk of cardiac conduction abnormalities – pacemaker may be needed
- Ventilatory support
- Mexiletine may improve symptoms

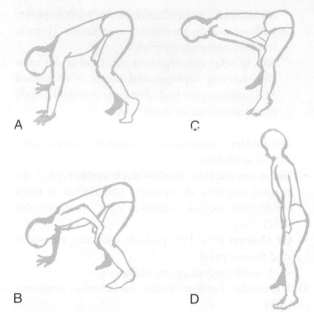

Fig 13.7 Demonstration of How a Patient with Duchenne's Muscular Dystrophy Can Get Off the Floor. The patient must roll onto their front and use their arms to push up their legs to standing. (Illustrated by Hollie Blaber.)

Duchenne's Muscular Dystrophy

Definition: an X-linked recessive disorder characterised by a mutation in the gene encoding the dystrophin protein. It is a progressive disease with no cure currently. Becker's muscular dystrophy is a similar X-linked condition affecting the dystrophin gene but has a much more variable course and is often less severe
Buzzwords:

- **Risk factors:** family history, male (X-linked disorder)
- **Presentation:** difficulty walking in childhood, progressive muscle wasting (see Fig 13.7), proximal weakness and toe walking, Gower's manoeuvre, calf pseudohypertrophy, often wheelchair-bound by adolescence, associated with a cardiomyopathy that may result in arrhythmias

Investigations:

- **Blood:** ⇈ CK
- **Genetic testing:** abnormality in the dystrophin gene

Differentials: Becker's muscular dystrophy, spinomuscular atrophy, other hereditary myopathies
Management: supportive, may include:

- Corticosteroids: appear to slow disease progression

- Splints and physiotherapy
- Corrective spinal surgery considered in cases of severe spinal deformity
- Ventilatory support later in the disease process

Many other hereditary myopathies exist:

- These vary in their pattern of muscle involvement, age of onset and severity (most being less severe than Duchenne's)
- Early symptoms can involve inappropriate muscle pain with trivial exercise, difficulty partaking in exercise with a later second-wind phenomena and some may have flares of symptoms associated with myoglobinuria
- Muscle biopsy and genetic testing is required to make the diagnosis

CEREBELLAR ATAXIA

Definition: a dysfunction of the cerebellum causing symptoms of impaired coordination. This condition can be caused by a structural lesion (e.g., stroke/brain tumour) or acquired causes (e.g., infection, inflammation or toxins), or degenerative as part of a genetic mutation later

Buzzwords:

- **Risk factors:** family history (genetic), malignancy (paraneoplastic, posterior fossa metastasis), chronic alcohol abuse, long-term medication use (e.g., phenytoin, barbiturates), coeliac disease, VZV infection
- **Presentation:**
  - Incoordination (gait, fine movement or both), dysarthria
  - Nystagmus, intention tremor, past pointing
  - Onset depends on the cause; genetic causes commonly have an adult and even elderly onset
- **Investigations:**
  - **Consider MRI brain:** may show cerebellar lesion (infarct, tumour, inflammatory), cerebellar volume loss in chronic ataxia
  - **Bloods:** baseline bloods (FBC, U&E, LFTs, CRP, Clotting), TFTs, Vitamin B12. Other bloods to be requested based on likely cause
  - **Genetic testing panel:** suspected genetic ataxia

Management

- Treat underlying cause
- Supportive care: speech and language therapy, physiotherapy, mobility aids

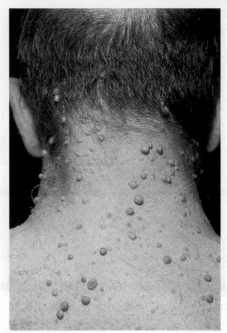

Fig 13.8 Neurofibromatosis. (With permission from Chapman, S. (2018). Cutaneous manifestations of internal disease. In *Skin disease*. Elsevier. Copyright © 2018 Elsevier Inc. All rights reserved.)

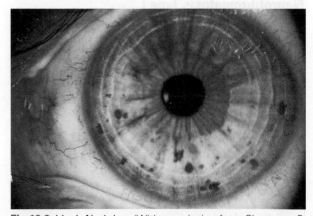

Fig 13.9 Lisch Nodules. (With permission from Chapman, S. (2018). Cutaneous manifestations of internal disease. In *Skin disease*. Elsevier. Copyright © 2018 Elsevier Inc. All rights reserved.)

PHAKOMATOSES

Neurocutaneous conditions causing abnormalities of the skin as well as the nervous system, many involving cellular overgrowth

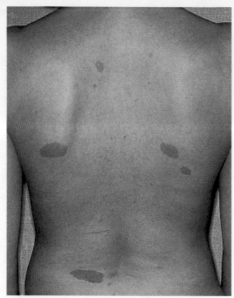

Fig 13.10 Café-au-lait Spots. (With permission from Chapman, S. (2018). Cutaneous manifestations of internal disease. In *Skin disease*. Elsevier. Copyright © 2018 Elsevier Inc. All rights reserved.)

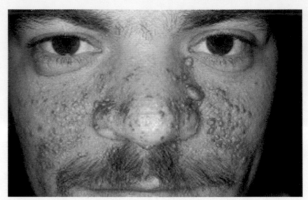

Fig 13.11 Adenoma Sebaceum. (With permission from Chapman, S. (2018). Cutaneous manifestations of internal disease. In *Skin disease*. Elsevier. Copyright © 2018 Elsevier Inc. All rights reserved.)

Neurofibromatosis Type I

Definition: an autosomal-dominant genetic condition characterised by a predisposition to develop pigmented skin lesions, neurofibromas and glial tumours as a result of a mutation in the **NF1 gene** located on Chromosome 17.

Buzzwords:
- **Risk factors:** family history
- **Presentation:** Mnemonic **6, 2, 2, BOA**
  - **≥6** café au lait spots (see Fig 13.10)
  - **≥2** neurofibromas (see Fig. 13.8)
  - **≥2** Lisch nodules (hamartomas of the iris) (see Fig 13.9)
  - Bony dysplasia
  - Optic pathway glioma
  - Axillary or groin freckling

Investigations:
- **MRI brain or spine** if new focal symptoms: may demonstrate tumour growth, such as a plexiform neuroma
- **Ophthalmological assessment:** screening for an optic nerve glioma (annually between the ages of 2 and 7 years)

Differentials:
- **Neurofibromatosis:** Neurofibromatosis Type II
- **Café-au-lait patches:** hereditary non-polyposis cancer of the colon

Management: there is currently no cure. Treatment involves regular monitoring, physiotherapy, psychological support, pain management and surgery.
- **Surgery** – such as neurofibromatosis excision, optic nerve glioma excision, bony deformity correction surgery

Neurofibromatosis Type II

Definition: an autosomal-dominant genetic condition characterised by an increased propensity to develop meningiomas, schwannomas and ependymomas of the spinal cord as a result of a mutation in the **NF2 gene** on Chromosome 22.

Buzzwords:
- **Risk factors:** family history
- **Presentation:**
  - **Vestibular schwannomas:** tinnitus, hearing impairment and vertigo (may be bilateral)
  - **Meningiomas and gliomas:** focal neurological deficits
  - **Spinal cord ependymomas:** pain, weakness and sensory disturbances

Investigations:
- MRI brain or spine: tumours as above may be seen
- Audiology: to monitor hearing loss precipitated by CN VIII tumours

Differentials: isolated meningioma or acoustic neuroma

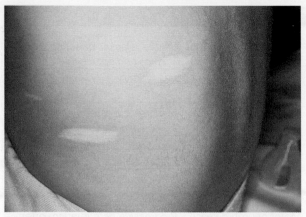

Fig 13.12 Hypomelanotic Macules. (With permission from Chapman, S. (2018). Cutaneous manifestations of internal disease. In *Skin disease.* Elsevier. Copyright © 2018 Elsevier Inc. All rights reserved.)

Management: due to the high propensity for recurrence, the quality of life and preservation of function should be the aims of treatment rather than remission.

Tuberous Sclerosis

Definition: a genetic condition resulting from mutations in the *TSC1* gene on Chromosome 9 (which codes for the hamartin protein) and/or the *TSC2* gene on Chromosome 16 (which codes for the tuberin protein). Mutations in these genes lead to the formation of benign tumours (hamartomas) at multiple sites in the body.

Buzzwords:
- **Risk factors:** family history
- **Presentation:** triad of seizures, learning disabilities and adenoma sebaceum (see Fig. 13.11). Lesions may include subependymal nodules, angiomyolipomata, retinal hamartomas and shagreen patches. Hypomelanotic macules may be seen (see Fig 13.12)

Investigations:
- **MRI brain:** should be considered in patients presenting with seizures; may demonstrate tubers in the cortex of the brain or subependymal nodules/giant cell astrocytomas, all of which are associated with tuberous sclerosis (TS)

Differentials: multiple endocrine neoplasia (MEN) 1, epilepsy

Management:
- Epilepsy: anti-epileptic drugs, surgery may be considered if refractory to medication

- Surgery may also be considered for the removal of tumours causing a local mass effect

CHRONIC FATIGUE SYNDROME/MYALGIC ENCEPHALOMYELITIS

Definition: There is no universally accepted definition of chronic fatigue syndrome/myalgic encephalomyelitis, and both terms are used interchangeably. A disabling condition characterised by new-onset fatigue exacerbated by minimal activity levels with additional symptoms of unknown aetiology

Buzzwords:
- **Risk factors:** female, lower educational attainment, lower socioeconomic status, high body mass index, low levels of physical activity, viral infections, inflammatory/immune/endocrine dysfunction
- **Presentation:** new or specific onset of symptoms, post-exertional malaise or fatigue (>4 months) unexplained by alternative diagnoses, insomnia, cognitive dysfunction, pain not relieved by rest

Investigations:
- Diagnosis of exclusion
- Investigations guided by differentials

Differentials: anaemia, malignancy, depression, hyper/hypothyroidism, chronic kidney disease, DM, coeliac disease, HIV, myopathy, demyelinating disease

Management:
Lifestyle advice and symptom control:
- Insomnia: sleep hygiene
- Fatigue: low level of physical activity (graded exercise therapy), limit rest periods to 30 min or less
- Relaxation techniques
- Well-balanced diet
- Pain: if chronic and associated with insomnia, consider a low-dose tricyclic antidepressant (e.g., amitriptyline)

INSOMNIA

Definition: a sleep disorder that results in impaired functioning

Buzzwords:
- **Risk factors:** stress, psychiatric disorders, chronic medical disorders, substance misuse, environmental changes, female
- **Presentation:** difficulty initiating/maintaining sleep, early awakening, non-restorative sleep, impaired daytime functioning, daytime stimulant use to remain alert

Investigations: sleep diary

THE ONE-LINE ROUND-UP!

Here are some key words to help you remember each condition/concept.

Condition	One-line Description
Migraine	Triggers = CHOCOLATE
Cluster headache	Unilateral orbital pain
Tension headache	Bilateral pain
Trigeminal neuralgia	Unilateral pain in the distribution of the trigeminal nerve
Seizure	Abnormal synchronised neuronal discharge
Epilepsy	Disorder of recurrent seizures
Ischaemic stroke	TACS, PACS, POCS, LACS – Time is brain
Haemorrhagic stroke	Acute blood pressure control
TIA	Resolution within 24 h
Bell's palsy	Not forehead sparing
Meningoencephalitis	Fever, headache, confusion
Delirium	PINCHME
Alzheimer's	Apraxia, aphasia, agnosia
Vascular dementia	Stepwise deterioration
Lewy body dementia	Cognitive decline within 1 year of PD
Frontotemporal dementia	Personality and behavioural changes
Normal pressure hydrocephalus	Whacky, wobbly, wet
Idiopathic Parkinson's disease	Bradykinesia, tremor, rigidity, postural instability
Benign essential tremor	Bilateral tremor on action only
Huntington's disease	Autosomal dominant, choreiform movement
Multiple sclerosis	Disseminated in time and space

Neuromyelitis optica	Severe relapses affecting the spine and optic nerve
Subacute combined degeneration	Vitamin B12 deficiency
Guillain-Barré	Symmetrical ascending weakness and numbness
Charcot-Marie-Tooth	Sensory and motor, distal to proximal
Diabetic neuropathy	Glove and stocking
Sciatica	Pain radiates below knee
Motor neuron disease	Progressive deterioration, often mixed UMN and LMN signs
Myasthenia gravis	Fatiguability, ptosis, bulbar
LEMS	Weakness improves with activity
Myositis/dermatomyositis	Find trigger (drug/cancer). Heliotrope/Gottron's in dermatomyositis
Myotonic dystrophy	Distal weakness, frontal balding
Duchenne muscular dystrophy	X-linked, gross motor delay
Cerebellar ataxia	Uncoordinated, nystagmus, past pointing
NF Type I	Neurofibromas, Lisch nodules, glioma, café au lait
NF Type II	Vestibular schwannoma, meningioma, spinal cord ependymoma
Tuberous sclerosis	Hamartomas, seizures and learning difficulties
Chronic fatigue syndrome	Post-exertional malaise
Insomnia	Find trigger, sleep diary

Differentials: poor sleep hygiene, depression, obstructive sleep apnoea, restless legs syndrome, narcolepsy

Management:
- Sleep hygiene education: e.g. regular bedtime, cool room
- CBT for insomnia
- Short-term zopiclone: no more than 2 weeks, caution in elderly
- Melatonin if >55 years of age

Prognosis: acute insomnia resolves within weeks once the trigger is identified. Chronic insomnia can last for years

READING LIST: NEUROLOGY IN AN HOUR

Headache

NICE. (2019). *CKS: Headache.* [https://cks.nice.org.uk/topics/headache-assessment/- Accessed March 2022].

Classification Committee of The International Headache Society. (2013). *International classification of headache disorders.* http://ichd-3.org.

Migraine

Clark, C., Howard, R., Rossor, M., & Shorvon, S. (2016). In *Neurology: A queen square textbook.* Wiley-Blackwell.

Jones, H. R., Srinivasan, J., Allam, G. J., & Baker, R. A. (2012). In *Netter's neurology.* Elsevier.

NICE. (2020). *CKS: Migraines.* [https://cks.nice.org.uk/topics/migraine/- Accessed March 2022].

Cluster Headache

Manji, H., Connolly, S., Kitchen, N., Lambert, C., & Mehta, A. (2014). In *Oxford handbook of neurology.* Oxford University Press.

Clark, C., Howard, R., Rossor, M., & Shorvon, S. (2016). In *Neurology: A queen square textbook.* Wiley-Blackwell.

NICE. (2017). *CKS: Cluster headaches.* [https://cks.nice.org.uk/topics/headache-cluster/- Accessed March 2022].

Tension Headache

Olesen, J. (2018). Headache classification Committee of the International Headache Society (IHS): The international classification of headache disorders, abstracts. *Cephalalgia, 38*, 1–211.

NICE. (2017). *CKS: Tension–type headaches.* [https://cks.nice.org.uk/topics/headache-tension-type/- Accessed March 2022].

Trigeminal Neuralgia

NICE. (2018). *CKS: Trigeminal neuralgia.* [https://cks.nice.org.uk/topics/trigeminal-neuralgia/. Accessed March 2022].

Seizure

Leone, M., Bottacchi, E., Beghi, E., et al. (2002). Risk factors for a first generalized tonic-clonic seizure in adults. *Neurology Science, 23*, 99–106.

Fisher, R., Cross, J., French, J., et al. (2017). Operational classification of seizure types by the International League Against Epilepsy: position paper of the ILAE Commission for classification and Terminology. *Epilepsia, 58*, 522–530.

Epilepsy

NICE. (2020). *NICE Pathways, diagnosing and classifying epilepsy.* https://pathways.nice.org.uk/pathways/epilepsy- Accessed March 2022.

NICE. (2021). *CKS: Epilepsy.* [https://cks.nice.org.uk/topics/epilepsy/- Accessed March 2022].

ILAE. (2020). *Diagnostic manual.* [http://epilepsydiagnosis.org].

BNF. (2021). *Side effects: Valproate, carbamazepine, lamotrigine, ethosuximide.* https://bnf.nice.org.uk/- Accessed 2021.

Stroke

Amarenco, P., Bogousslavsky, J., Caplan, L. R., et al. (2013). The ASCOD phenotyping of ischemic stroke (Updated ASCO Phenotyping). *Cerebrovascular Disorders, 36*, 1–5.

Bamford, J., Sandercock, P., Dennis, M., et al. (1988). A prospective study of acute cerebrovascular disease in the community: The Oxfordshire Community Stroke Project 1981-86. 1. Methodology, demography and incident cases of first-ever stroke. *Journal of Neurology Neurosurgery Psychiatry, 51*, 1373–1380.

Nor, A. M., Davis, J., Sen, B., et al. (2005). The Recognition of Stroke in the Emergency Room (ROSIER) scale: Development and validation of a stroke recognition instrument. *Lancet Neurology, 4*, 727–734.

NICE Guidelines. (2019). *NG128, stroke and transient ischaemic attack in over 16s: Diagnosis and initial management.* [https://www.nice.org.uk/guidance/ng128- Accessed March 2022].

Ortiz, G. A., & L. Sacco, R. (2014). *National Institutes of Health Stroke Scale (NIHSS). Wiley StatsRef: Statistics reference online.* https://onlinelibrary.wiley.com/doi/full/10.1002/9781118445112.stat06823.

Bell's Palsy

NICE. (2019). *CKS: Bell's palsy.* [https://cks.nice.org.uk/topics/bells-palsy/- Accessed March 2022].

Meningo-encephalitis

NICE. (2015). *CG102: Meningitis (bacterial) and meningococcal septicaemia in under 16s: Recognition, diagnosis and management.* [https://www.nice.org.uk/guidance/cg102- Accessed March 2022].

Patient info. (2015). *Encephalitis.* [https://patient.info/doctor/encephalitis-pro- Accessed March 2022].

BMJ Best Practice. (2021). 2015). *Encephalitis.* https://bestpractice.bmj.com/topics/en-gb/436- Accessed March 2022].

BMJ Best Practice. (2021). *Viral meningitis.* [https://bestpractice.bmj.com/topics/en-gb/3000242- Accessed March 2022].

Delirium

NICE Guidelines. (2019). *CG103: Delirium: Prevention, diagnosis and management.* [https://www.nice.org.uk/guidance/cg103- Accessed March 2022].

SIGN. (2019). *Guideline 157: Risk reduction and management of delirium.* [https://www.bgs.org.uk/resources/sign-157-risk-reduction-and-management-of-delirium#:~:text=This%20guideline%20provides%20recommendations%20based,most%20common%20of%20medical%20emergencies- Accessed March 2022].

Dementia

NICE. (2020). *CKS: Dementia.* [https://cks.nice.org.uk/topics/dementia/- Accessed March 2022].

Alzheimer's Disease

Weller, J., & Budson, A. (2018). Current understanding of Alzheimer's disease diagnosis and treatment. *F1000Research, 7*(F1000 Faculty Rev), 1161.

Bondi, M. W., Edmonds, E. C., & Salmon, D. P. (2017) Alzheimer's disease: Past, present, and future. *Journal International Neuropsychology Society, 23*, 818.

BNF. (2021). *Side effects: AChE inhibitors and memantine.* [https://bnf.nice.org.uk/- Accessed 2021].

BMJ Visual Summary. (2018). *Pharmacological management for people with dementia.* https://www.bmj.com/content/bmj/suppl/2018/06/27/bmj.k2438.DC1/Dementia_v19_web.pdf.

NICE. (2020). *CKS: Dementia.* [https://cks.nice.org.uk/topics/dementia/- Accessed March 2022].

EMedicine. (2018). *Alzheimer disease imaging.* https://emedicine.medscape.com/article/336281-overview#:~:text=The%20initial%20criteria%20for%20CT,increased%20size%20of%20the%20ventricles.

Vascular Dementia

Lee, A. Y. (2011). Vascular dementia. *Chonnam Medical Journal, 47*, 66.

Johns, P. (2014). *Clinical neuroscience E-book.* Elsevier Health Sciences.

BMJ Visual Summary. (2018). *Pharmacological management for people with dementia.* https://www.bmj.com/content/bmj/suppl/2018/06/27/bmj.k2438.DC1/Dementia_v19_web.pdf.

NICE. (2020). *CKS: Dementia.* [https://cks.nice.org.uk/topics/dementia/- Accessed March 2022].

Dementia With Lewy Bodies

Johns, P. (2014). *Clinical neuroscience E-book.* Elsevier Health Sciences.

BMJ Visual Summary. (2018). *Pharmacological management for people with dementia.* https://www.bmj.com/content/bmj/suppl/2018/06/27/bmj.k2438.DC1/Dementia_v19_web.pdf.

NICE. (2020). *CKS: Dementia.* [https://cks.nice.org.uk/topics/dementia/- Accessed March 2022].

Fronto-Temporal Dementia (FTD)

Young, J. J., Lavakumar, M., Tampi, D., Balachandran, S., & Tampi, R. R. (2018). Frontotemporal dementia: Latest evidence and clinical implications. *Therapy Advances Psychopharmacology, 8*, 33–48.

Warren, J. D., Rohrer, J. D., & Rossor, M. N. (2013). Frontotemporal dementia. *BMJ, 347.*

Normal Pressure Hydrocephalus

Greenberg, M. S. (2020). In *Handbook of neurosurgery.* Thieme.

Parkinsonism

NICE. (2018). *CKS: Parkinson's disease.* [https://cks.nice.org.uk/topics/parkinsons-disease/- Accessed June 2021].

Idiopathic Parkinson's Disease

Kalia, L. V., & Lang, A. E. (2015). Parkinson's disease. *Lancet, 386*, 896–912.

BNF. (2021). *Parkinson's disease.* [https://bnf.nice.org.uk/- Accessed 2021].

Benign Essential Tremor

Smaga, S. (2003). Tremor. *American Family Physician, 68*, 1545–1552.

GP Notebook. (2018). *Benign essential tremor.* https://gpnotebook.com/simplepage.cfm?id=1986723889.

Ninds.nih.gov. (2021). *Tremor Fact Sheet | National Institute of Neurological Disorders and Stroke.* https://www.ninds.nih.gov/Disorders/Patient-Caregiver-Education/Fact-Sheets/Tremor-Fact-Sheet. [Accessed 19 February 2021].

Huntington's Disease

Huntington's Disease Association. (2021). *Huntington's disease.* https://www.hda.org.uk/huntingtons-disease/what-is-huntingtons-disease. [Accessed 6 March 2021].

Patient info. (2016). *Huntington's disease. About Huntington's disease (HD).* https://patient.info/doctor/huntingtons-disease-pro. [Accessed 6 March 2021].

Chial, H. (2008). Huntington's disease: The discovery of the Huntingtin gene. *Nature Education, 1*, 71.

Multiple Sclerosis (MS)

Thompson, A. J., Banwell, B. L., Barkhof, F., et al. (2017). Diagnosis of multiple sclerosis: 2017 revisions of the McDonald criteria. *Lancet Neurology, 17*, 162–173.

Reich, D. S., Lucchinetti, C. F., & Calabresi, P. A. (2018). Multiple sclerosis. *New England Journal of Medicine, 378*, 169–180. https://doi.org/10.1056/NEJMra1401483

NICE. (2020). *CKS: Multiple sclerosis.* [https://cks.nice.org.uk/topics/multiple-sclerosis/- Accessed March 2022].

Neuromyelitis Optica

Rarediseases.org. (2018). *Neuromyelitis optica spectrum disorder.* [https://rarediseases.org/rare-diseases/neuromyelitis-optica/#:~:text=Neuromyelitis%20optica%20spectrum%20disorder%20(NMOSD,the%20spinal%20cord%20(myelitis).- Accessed March 2022].

NMOUK. (2021). *Neuromyelitis optica.* http://www.nmouk.nhs.uk/healthcare-professionals/management-of-nmo.

National Institute of Neurological Disorders and Stroke. (2021). *Neuromyelitis optica.* https://www.ninds.nih.

gov/Disorders/All-Disorders/Neuromyelitis-optica-Information-Page.

Subacute Combined Degeneration of the Cord
Manji, H., Connolly, S., Kitchen, N., Lambert, C., & Mehta, A. (2014). In *Oxford handbook of neurology*. Oxford University Press.
Jankovic, J., Mazziotta, J. C., Pomeroy, S. L., & Daroff, R. B. (2015). In *Bradley's neurology in clinical practice*. Elsevier.

Guillain-Barré Syndrome (GBS)
Clark, C., Howard, R., Rossor, M., & Shorvon, S. (2016). In *Neurology: A queen Square Textbook*. Wiley-Blackwell.
FP Notebook. (2021). *Guillain-Barre syndrome*. https://fp-notebook.com/Neuro/Demyelinating/GlnBrSyndrm.htm.

Charcot-Marie-Tooth Disease
Jones, H. R., Srinivasan, J., Allam, G. J., & Baker, R. A. (2012). In *Netter's neurology*. Elsevier.
Clark, C., Howard, R., Rossor, M., & Shorvon, S. (2016). In *Neurology: A queen square textbook*. Wiley-Blackwell.

Diabetic Neuropathy
NICE. (2019). *NG19: Diabetic foot problems: Prevention and management*. [https://www.nice.org.uk/guidance/ng19- Accessed March 2022].
Diabetes UK. (2021). *Peripheral neuropathy*. https://www.diabetes.org.uk/guide-to-diabetes/complications/nerves_neuropathy.
Patient info. (2020). *Diabetic neuropathy*. [https://patient.info/diabetes/diabetes-mellitus-leaflet/diabetic-neuropathy#:~:text=Motor%20neuropathy&text=Diabetic%20neuropathy%20may%20also%20cause,of%20blood%20glucose%20levels%20improves.- Accessed March 2022].

Sciatica
NICE. (2020). *NG59: Low back pain and sciatica in over 16s: Assessment and management*. [https://www.nice.org.uk/guidance/ng59- Accessed March 2022].
Bernstein, I., & Carville, S. (2017). Low back pain and sciatica: Summary of NICE guidance. *BMJ, 356*, 6748.

Motor Neuron Disease (MND)
Clark, C., Howard, R., Rossor, M., & Shorvon, S. (2016). In *Neurology: A queen square textbook*. Wiley-Blackwell.
Jones, H. R., Srinivasan, J., Allam, G. J., & Baker, R. A. (2012). In *Netter's neurology*. Elsevier.
NICE. (2019). *NG42: Motor neurone disease: Assessment and management*. [https://www.nice.org.uk/guidance/ng42- Accessed March 2022].

Myasthenia Gravis
Jones, H. R., Srinivasan, J., Allam, G. J., & Baker, R. A. (2012). In *Netter's neurology*. Elsevier.

Clark, C., Howard, R., Rossor, M., & Shorvon, S. (2016). In *Neurology: A queen square textbook*. Wiley-Blackwell.
Sussman, J., Farrugia, M., Maddison, P., Hill, M., Leite, M., & Hilton-Jones, D. (2018). The Association of British Neurologists' myasthenia gravis guidelines. *Annual New York Academy Science, 1412*, 166–169.

Lambert-Eaton Myasthenic Syndrome
Jones, H. R., Srinivasan, J., Allam, G. J., & Baker, R. A. (2012). In *Netter's neurology*. Elsevier.
Clark, C., Howard, R., Rossor, M., & Shorvon, S. (2016). In *Neurology: A queen square textbook*. Wiley-Blackwell.
NHS UK. (2019). *Conditions: Lambert-Eaton myasthenic syndrome*. [https://www.nhs.uk/conditions/lambert-eaton-myasthenic-syndrome/#:~:text=Lambert%2DEaton%20myasthenic%20syndrome%20(LEMS,a%20range%20of%20other%20symptoms.- Accessed March 2022].

Myositis Including Dermatomyositis
Schmidt, J. (2018). Current classification and management of inflammatory myopathies. *Journal of Neuromuscular Disorders, 5*, 109–129.

Myotonic Dystrophy
Turner, C., & Hilton-Jones, D. (2010). The myotonic dystrophies: Diagnosis and management. *Journal of Neurology Neurosurgery Psychiatry, 81*, 358–367.
Muscular Dystrophy UK. (Myotonic dystrophy. http://musculardystrophyuk.org.

Duchenne's Muscular Dystrophy
Jones, H. R., Srinivasan, J., Allam, G. J., & Baker, R. A. (2012). In *Netter's neurology*. Elsevier.
Manji, H., Connolly, S., Kitchen, N., Lambert, C., & Mehta, A. (2014). In *Oxford handbook of neurology*. Oxford University Press.
Clark, C., Howard, R., Rossor, M., & Shorvon, S. (2016). In *Neurology: A queen square textbook*. Wiley-Blackwell.

Cerebellar Ataxia
Bird, T. D. (2019). Hereditary ataxia overview. In M. P. Adam, H. H. Ardinger, R. A. Pagon, et al. (Eds.), *GeneReviews*. https://www.ncbi.nlm.nih.gov/books/NBK1138/.

Neurofibromatosis Type I
Batchelor, T. T., Nishikawa, R., Tarbell, N. J., & Weller, M. (2017). *Oxford textbook of neuro-oncology*. Oxford University Press.
Ferner, R. E., Huson, S. M., Thomas, N., et al. (2007). Guidelines for the diagnosis and management of individuals with neurofibromatosis 1. *Journal of Medical Genetics, 44*, 81–88.
Patient info. (2014). *Neurofibromatosis*. [https://patient.info/doctor/neurofibromatosis-pro- Accessed March 2022].

Neurofibromatosis Type II

Batchelor, T. T., Nishikawa, R., Tarbell, N. J., & Weller, M. (2017). *Oxford textbook of neuro-oncology.* Oxford University Press.

Tuberous Sclerosis

Batchelor, T. T., Nishikawa, R., Tarbell, N. J., & Weller, M. (2017). *Oxford textbook of neuro-oncology.* Oxford University Press.

Chronic Fatigue Syndrome (CFS)/Myalgic Encephalomyelitis (ME)

NICE. (2020). *CKS: Tiredness/fatigue in adults.* [https://cks.nice.org.uk/topics/tiredness-fatigue-in-adults/- Accessed March 2022].

NICE. (2007). *CG53: Chronic fatigue syndrome/myalgic encephalomyelitis (or encephalopathy): Diagnosis and management.* [https://www.nice.org.uk/guidance/cg53- Accessed June 2021].

Insomnia

BMJ Best Practice. (2019). *Insomnia.* [https://bestpractice.bmj.com/topics/en-gb/227- Accessed March 2022].

NICE. (2020). *CKS: Insomnia.* [https://cks.nice.org.uk/topics/insomnia/- Accessed March 2022].

14

Neurosurgery in an Hour

Dominic Mahoney, Dillon Vyas, Berenice Aguirrezabala Armbruster and Matthew Boissaud-Cooke

NEUROANATOMY

Brain

For brain anatomy and function see Table 14.1 and Fig 14.1.

Meninges

Definition: the connective tissue surrounding the brain and spinal cord that provides protection (Fig 14.2). The meninges consist of:

- **Dura mater:** outer layer of meninges composed of thick connective tissue. Attached to the sutures
- **Arachnoid mater:** a thinner membrane contiguous with the dura mater with trabecular projections traversing the subarachnoid space through which the cerebrospinal fluid (CSF) flows. Arachnoid granulations allow the CSF to pass from the subarachnoid spine into the dural sinus
- **Pia mater:** the finest and innermost membrane of the meninges. It is intimately associated with the cortex and runs into all sulci.

Spinal Cord

- The spinal cord begins at the level of the foramen magnum.
- In adults, the spinal cord terminates as the conus medullaris at approximately the L1/L2 vertebral level. The spinal cord terminates at lower vertebral levels in infants.
- The cauda equina continues below the level of the conus medullaris into the lumbar cistern within the thecal sac.
- The meninges descend from the foramen magnum and terminate at the S2 vertebral level.
- Spinal cord histology:
  - **Ventral horn:** contains cell bodies of the lower motor neurons (LMNs). Axons exit ventrally to enter the ventral rootlets and roots before entering the spinal nerve proper.
  - **Dorsal horn:** contains cell bodies of second-order neurons that project cranially. The cell bodies of the primary sensory neurons reside in the dorsal root ganglion. The dorsal horn receives the axons of these neurons, which enter the dorsal horn via the dorsal rootlets/roots.
  - **Lateral horn:** contains the efferent motor neurons of the sympathetic nervous system from the T1–L2 spinal level.
  - **Ascending tracts:** there are numerous ascending sensory tracts that convey a range of sensory modalities to the cerebellum and cerebrum.
  - **Descending tracts:** pyramidal and extrapyramidal motor tracts descend through the spinal cord, with their axons terminating at the appropriate level to control the LMNs.
- Figs 14.3 and 14.4 show cross-sections through the spinal cord.

TABLE 14.1   Brain Anatomy

Part of Brain	Function
Hemispheres (Fig. 14.1)	
Frontal lobe	Primary motor area, premotor cortex, supplementary motor area (motor control) Broca's area (dominant hemisphere, expressive dysphasia) Frontal eye fields (saccadic eye movements) Prefrontal cortex (personality, motivation)
Parietal lobe	Primary somatosensory area (sensation), optic radiation (visual fields)
Temporal lobe	Hippocampus (memory), amygdala (emotion, autonomic nervous system), transverse temporal gyrus (primary auditory cortex), optic radiation (visual fields)
Occipital lobe	Primary and secondary visual cortex (vision)
Brainstem	
Midbrain	• **Houses nuclei for the following cranial nerves:** Oculomotor nerve (parasympathetics), trochlear nerve. • **Other nuclei:** substantia nigra, red nucleus. • **Motor tracts:** corticospinal tracts passing through the crus cerebri (cerebral peduncle).
Pons	• **Houses nuclei for the following cranial nerves:** Trigeminal nerve, abducens nerve, facial nerve (parasympathetics), vestibulocochlear nerve (CNVIII nuclei overlaps with the medulla) • **Other nuclei:** pneumotaxic (upper pons, inhibits respiration) and apneustic (lower pons, stimulates respiration) centres; pontine • **Motor tracts:** corticospinal tracts pass through the pons basis
Medulla	• **Houses nuclei for the following cranial nerves:** Glossopharyngeal nerve (parasympathetics), vagus nerve (parasympathetics), accessory nerve, hypoglossal nerve • **Other nuclei:** inferior olive, area postrema (nausea and vomiting), respiratory control nuclei • **Motor tracts:** corticospinal tracts pass through the medullary pyramids
Other	
Cerebellum The 'little brain'	Role in coordination of motor functions, balance and speech production
Diencephalon	**Thalamus:** large subcortical grey matter nucleus composed of multiple nuclei. Acts as a relay centre for most inputs and outputs to and from the cerebral cortex **Hypothalamus:** located anteroinferiorly to the thalamus. Vital role in coordinating homeostasis and control of the endocrine system. Connected to the pituitary gland **Pineal gland:** small gland that releases melatonin and plays a role in the sleep-wake cycle
Hippocampus	Grey matter structure found in the medial temporal lobe, with a role in spatial memory
Basal ganglia	Structures: caudate nucleus, putamen, globus pallidus interna/externa Role in extrapyramidal motor function

- Table 14.2 and Figs 14.5 and 14.6 show the ascending and descending tract pathways.

Peripheral Nerves

- Ventral root(let)s and dorsal root(let)s join to form a peripheral nerve proper, which passes through the intervertebral foramen.
- The peripheral nerve proper divides into a ventral ramus and dorsal ramus.

- There are 31 pairs of paired peripheral nerves (8 cervical, 12 thoracic, 5 lumbar, 5 sacral and 1 coccygeal). There are only seven cervical vertebrae; therefore, there is a mismatch between the number of vertebrae and peripheral nerves. The exiting of spinal nerves relative to their respective vertebra is as follows:
  - C1–C7 peripheral nerves exit **ABOVE** their respective pedicles (i.e., C5 nerve root exits at the C4/5 vertebral level)

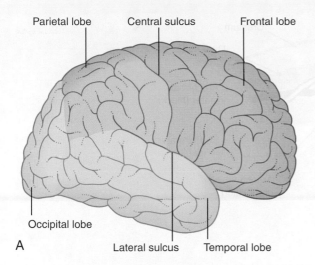

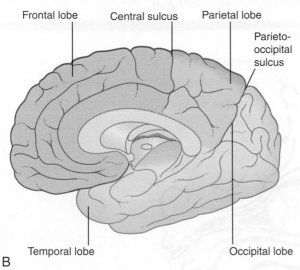

Fig. 14.1 Brain Hemispheres. (A) Lateral surface and (B) medial surface. (With permission from Mtui, E. (2016). *Fitzgerald's clinical neuroanatomy* (Fig. 2.1, 7th ed.). Philadelphia: Elsevier.)

- C8 peripheral nerve exits between C7 and the T1 pedicle (C7/T1 vertebral level)
- T1 and below peripheral nerves exit **BELOW** their respective pedicles (i.e., L4 nerve root exits at the L4/5 vertebral level)

Assessment of Spinal Cord Injury

There are numerous types of spinal cord injuries (SCIs). The extent and type of SCI can be classified using the International Standards for Neurological Classification of SCIs, which was devised by the American Spinal Injury Association. This systematic review of all dermatomes and myotomes permits an identification of the level of neurological injury (see Fig. 14.7 and Table 14.3).

Cranial Nerves (see Table 14.4)

Arterial Blood Supply to the Brain (see Fig. 14.8)

NEUROPHYSIOLOGY

Intracranial Pressure

- **Monro-Kellie doctrine:** the skull is a vault with a fixed volume, and the brain, arterial and venous blood and CSF are incompressible. Therefore, an increase in the volume of one of these elements will result in an increased intracranial pressure (ICP).
- **CSF production:** produced by the choroid plexus in the lateral, 3rd and 4th ventricles. Approximately 500 mL of CSF is produced per day. The total CSF volume in an adult (ventricular system and subarachnoid space) is approximately 150 mL at any one point.
- **Hydrocephalus:** excess CSF caused by an obstruction to CSF drainage or increased CSF production.
- **Cerebral oedema:** accumulation of water in the brain parenchyma. Types include:
  - Vasogenic oedema, cytotoxic oedema, interstitial oedema
- **Herniation syndromes** (in the context of a raised ICP):
  - Subfalcine herniation
  - Uncal herniation
  - Tonsillar herniation

BRAIN INJURY AND INTRACRANIAL HAEMORRHAGE

Traumatic Brain Injury

Definition: the application of an external force to the head resulting in a disruption of normal brain functioning. Traumatic brain injuries (TBIs) can be classified using the Glasgow Coma Scale (GCS) into mild (GCS score 13–15), moderate (GCS score 9–12) or severe (GCS score 3–8).

Buzzwords:

- **Risk factors:** blunt injury (most common aetiology; e.g., fall, assault, motor vehicle accident) vs a penetrating injury (e.g., gunshot wound, stabbing)
- **Presentation:** headache, nausea, vomiting, amnesia, seizures, CSF otorrhoea/rhinorrhoea (base of skull

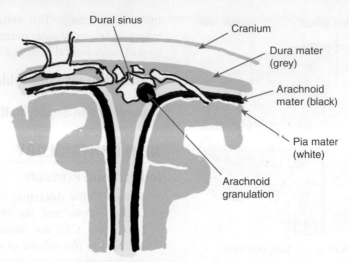

Fig. 14.2 The Meninges. (Illustrated by Hollie Blaber.)

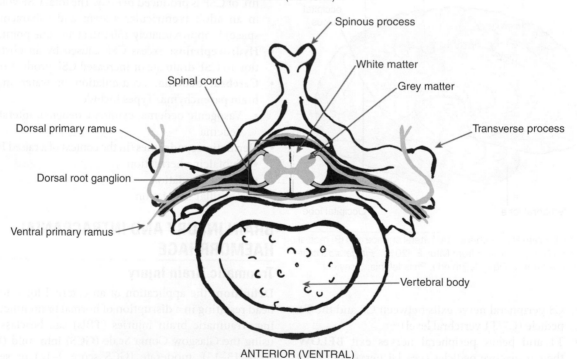

Fig. 14.3 Cross-section: Vertebra and Spinal Cord. (Illustrated by Hollie Blaber.)

fracture), focal neurological deficit, reduced level of consciousness, associated injuries

Investigations:

- **CT head:** may show scalp haematoma, skull fractures, pneumocephalus, extra-axial blood (e.g., extradural,

subdural, subarachnoid), intra-axial blood (e.g., contusions, intracerebral/intraventricular haemorrhage), cerebral swelling (e.g., sulcal effacement, loss of basal cisterns), herniation syndromes (e.g., subfalcine, uncal, tonsillar)

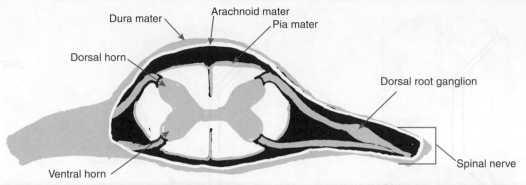

Fig. 14.4 Cross-section: Spinal Cord. (Illustrated by Hollie Blaber.)

TABLE 14.2	**Ascending and Descending Tract Pathways**			
Tract	Function	Level of Decussation	Injury to Cortex	Injury to Spinal Cord
Afferent: Sensory Nerves from the Periphery to the CNS				
Spinothalamic	Pain and temperature	Level of entry in the spinal cord	Contralateral loss of sensation	Contralateral loss of sensation
Dorsal column	Fine touch, vibration and conscious pro-prioception	In the brain stem	Contralateral loss of sensation (except in brainstem injuries!)	Ipsilateral loss of sensation
Efferent: Motor Nerves from the CNS to the Periphery				
Corticospinal tract	Conscious motor control	90% at medulla (other 10% decussate at the level of innervation)	Contralateral loss of power	Ipsilateral loss of power

- **CT angiogram:** may show vascular injury (e.g., arterial dissection, dural venous sinus injury)
- **Trauma CT:** depends on the extent of the trauma. To identify any associated injuries
- **MRI head:** not used acutely for TBIs. Useful for diffuse axonal injury

Management:
- Manage according to Advanced Trauma Life Support (ATLS)/local/national guidelines. The aim of treatment is to prevent secondary injury.
- Treatment depends on the severity of the head injury and any associated injuries.
- Nonoperative interventions:
  - Neurological observation
  - Antiepileptic drugs (AEDs): seizure prophylaxis for 7 days (seek advice from neurosurgery)
  - Medical management of a raised ICP: tiered approach to interventions (e.g., head of bed elevation, straight neck, avoid hypoxia/hypotension, treat seizures, osmotherapy (e.g., mannitol, hypertonic saline), sedation and paralysis, hyperventilate to hypocarbia, phenobarbitone (burst suppression))
- Operative interventions:
  - ICP monitoring
  - Removal of a mass lesion: extradural haematoma, acute subdural haematoma, intracerebral haemorrhage
  - Treatment of medically refractory ICP: CSF diversion (external ventricular drainage), decompressive craniectomy
- Neurorehabilitation

Aneurysmal Subarachnoid Haemorrhage

Definition: a bleed in the subarachnoid space (See Fig. 14.9). The most frequent cause of a subarachnoid haemorrhage (SAH) is trauma, but they may also occur spontaneously from aneurysmal rupture.

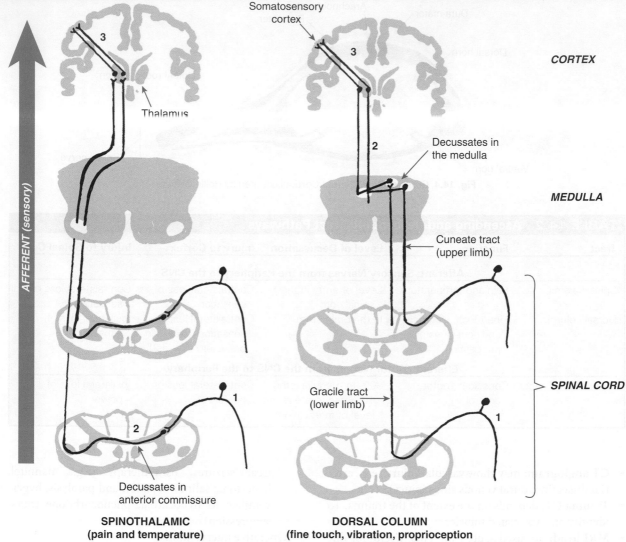

Fig. 14.5 Spinothalamic Pathway vs Dorsal Column Pathway. (Illustrated by Hollie Blaber.)

Buzzwords:

- **Risk factors for aneurysm development:** hypertension (HTN), smoking, female, family history, connective tissue disease (e.g., Ehlers-Danlos disease, polycystic kidney disease), trauma, infection, drug abuse
- **Risk factors for aneurysmal rupture:** HTN, smoking, age, site/size of aneurysm, previous SAH
- **Presentation:** sudden-onset thunderclap headache, nausea, vomiting, focal neurological deficits, meningism (photophobia, nuchal rigidity), seizures, loss of consciousness/collapse, low GCS

Investigations:

- **CT head:** hyperdensity in the sulci/cisterns +/- intracerebral haemorrhage +/- intraventricular haemorrhage +/- hydrocephalus (see Radiology in an Hour)
- **CT angiogram (CTA):** identification of an aneurysm or other vascular lesion
- **Lumbar puncture (LP)** (if negative CT at 12 h after symptom onset): xanthochromia (positive in nearly 100% of SAH patients within this timeframe)
- ***Catheter angiogram/digital subtraction angiography*:** the gold-standard imaging technique for intracranial aneurysms

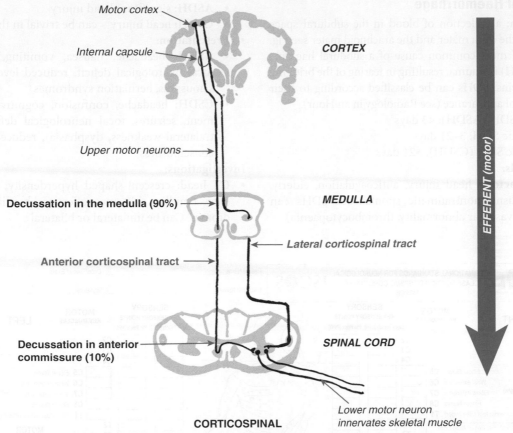

Motor cortex

Internal capsule

CORTEX

Upper motor neurons

EFFERENT (motor)

Decussation in the medulla (90%) → **MEDULLA**

→ *Lateral corticospinal tract*

Anterior corticospinal tract →

SPINAL CORD

Decussation in anterior commissure (10%)

Lower motor neuron innervates skeletal muscle

CORTICOSPINAL

Fig. 14.6 Anatomy of the Corticospinal Tract. (Illustrated by Hollie Blaber.)

- **MR imaging/angiogram:** can be used for the diagnosis and monitoring of aneurysms
- **Bloods:** daily electrolyte monitoring to identify electrolyte abnormalities. Hyponatraemia from syndrome of inappropriate ADH secretion (SIADH) or cerebral salt wasting (CSW) can occur
- **Electrocardiogram (ECG):** SAH is frequently associated with electrocardiographic abnormalities, most commonly U waves and deeply inverted T waves

Differentials for a thunderclap headache: pituitary apoplexy, cerebral venous sinus thrombosis, arterial dissection, primary thunderclap headache, reversible cerebral reversible constriction, ischaemic/haemorrhagic stroke

Management:
- Resuscitation as required
- Referral to neurosurgery to guide further management (multiple grading systems can be used: World Federation of Neurosurgical Societies grade, Fisher grade)

- Securing the aneurysm
  - Endovascular methods: coiling, flow diversion
  - Surgical methods: clipping, bypass method
- Prevention, identification and treatment of complications
  - Rebleeding: secure the aneurysm
  - Hydrocephalus: CSF diversion (e.g., external ventricular device, permanent shunt)
  - Delayed cerebral ischaemia: nimodipine, trial of HTN
  - Electrolyte abnormalities (e.g., SIADH, CSW): salt/fluid replacement
  - Venous thromboembolism: thromboembolic-deterrent stockings, calf pumps, low-molecular-weight heparin
  - Seizures: anti-epileptic drugs (there is controversy regarding the administration of prophylactic anti-epileptic drugs to prevent seizures)
- Symptom control: analgesia, antiemetics and laxatives

Subdural Haemorrhage

Definition: a collection of blood in the subdural space (between the dura mater and the arachnoid mater see Fig. 14.9). The most common cause of a subdural haemorrhage (SDH) is trauma, resulting in tearing of the bridging cortical veins. SDHs can be classified according to their radiological appearance (see Radiology in an Hour).

- Acute SDH (ASDH): <3 days
- Subacute SDH: 3–21 days
- Chronic SDH (CSDH): >21 days

Buzzwords:

- **Risk factors:** head injury, anticoagulation, elderly, alcoholism, nontraumatic spontaneous SDHs can occur (vascular abnormality, thrombocytopaenia)
- **ASDH:** significant head injury
- **CSDH:** head injury – can be trivial in the elderly
- **Presentation:**
  - **ASDH:** headache, nausea, vomiting, seizures, focal neurological deficit, reduced level of consciousness, herniation syndromes
  - **CSDH:** headache, confusion, cognitive impairment, seizures, focal neurological deficit (contralateral weakness, dysphasia), reduced level of consciousness

Investigations:

- **CT head:** crescent-shaped hyperdensity; may also show a midline shift, mass effect and herniation syndromes. Can be unilateral or bilateral

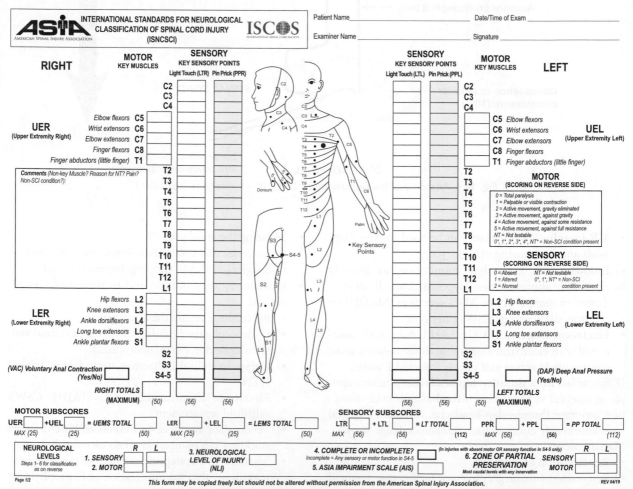

Fig. 14.7 American Spinal Injury Association Score (A) and (B). (With permission from American Spinal Injury Association. International Standards for Neurological Classification of Spinal Cord Injury (revised 2019). Richmond, VA.)

Muscle Function Grading

0 = Total paralysis

1 = Palpable or visible contraction

2 = Active movement, full range of motion (ROM) with gravity eliminated

3 = Active movement, full ROM against gravity

4 = Active movement, full ROM against gravity and moderate resistance in a muscle specific position

5 = (Normal) active movement, full ROM against gravity and full resistance in a functional muscle position expected from an otherwise unimpaired person

NT = Not testable (i.e. due to immobilization, severe pain such that the patient cannot be graded, amputation of limb, or contracture of > 50% of the normal ROM)

0*, 1*, 2*, 3*, 4*, NT* = Non-SCI condition present [a]

Sensory Grading

0 = Absent   1 = Altered, either decreased/impaired sensation or hypersensitivity

2 = Normal   NT = Not testable

0*, 1*, NT* = Non-SCI condition present [a]

[a] Note: Abnormal motor and sensory scores should be tagged with a '*' to indicate an impairment due to a non-SCI condition. The non-SCI condition should be explained in the comments box together with information about how the score is rated for classification purposes (at least normal / not normal for classification).

When to Test Non-Key Muscles:

In a patient with an apparent AIS B classification, non-key muscle functions more than 3 levels below the motor level on each side should be tested to most accurately classify the injury (differentiate between AIS B and C).

Movement	Root level
Shoulder: Flexion, extension, adbuction, adduction, internal and external rotation **Elbow:** Supination	C5
Elbow: Pronation **Wrist:** Flexion	C6
Finger: Flexion at proximal joint, extension **Thumb:** Flexion, extension and abduction in plane of thumb	C7
Finger: Flexion at MCP joint **Thumb:** Opposition, adduction and abduction perpendicular to palm	C8
Finger: Abduction of the index finger	T1
Hip: Adduction	L2
Hip: External rotation	L3
Hip: Extension, abduction, internal rotation **Knee:** Flexion **Ankle:** Inversion and eversion **Toe:** MP and IP extension	L4
Hallux and Toe: DIP and PIP flexion and abduction	L5
Hallux: Adduction	S1

ASIA Impairment Scale (AIS)

A = Complete. No sensory or motor function is preserved in the sacral segments S4-5.

B = Sensory Incomplete. Sensory but not motor function is preserved below the neurological level and includes the sacral segments S4-5 (light touch or pin prick at S4-5 or deep anal pressure) AND no motor function is preserved more than three levels below the motor level on either side of the body.

C = Motor Incomplete. Motor function is preserved at the most caudal sacral segments for voluntary anal contraction (VAC) OR the patient meets the criteria for sensory incomplete status (sensory function preserved at the most caudal sacral segments S4-5 by LT, PP or DAP), and has some sparing of motor function more than three levels below the ipsilateral motor level on either side of the body. (This includes key or non-key muscle functions to determine motor incomplete status.) For AIS C – less than half of key muscle functions below the single NLI have a muscle grade ≥ 3.

D = Motor Incomplete. Motor incomplete status as defined above, with at least half (half or more) of key muscle functions below the single NLI having a muscle grade ≥ 3.

E = Normal. If sensation and motor function as tested with the ISNCSCI are graded as normal in all segments, and the patient had prior deficits, then the AIS grade is E. Someone without an initial SCI does not receive an AIS grade.

Using ND: To document the sensory, motor and NLI levels, the ASIA Impairment Scale grade, and/or the zone of partial preservation (ZPP) when they are unable to be determined based on the examination results.

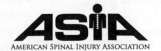

AMERICAN SPINAL INJURY ASSOCIATION

INTERNATIONAL STANDARDS FOR NEUROLOGICAL CLASSIFICATION OF SPINAL CORD INJURY

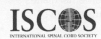

INTERNATIONAL SPINAL CORD SOCIETY

Page 2/2

Fig. 14.7, cont'd

Steps in Classification

The following order is recommended for determining the classification of individuals with SCI.

1. Determine sensory levels for right and left sides.
The sensory level is the most caudal, intact dermatome for both pin prick and light touch sensation.

2. Determine motor levels for right and left sides.
Defined by the lowest key muscle function that has a grade of at least 3 (on supine testing), providing the key muscle functions represented by segments above that level are judged to be intact (graded as a 5).
Note: in regions where there is no myotome to test, the motor level is presumed to be the same as the sensory level, if testable motor function above that level is also normal.

3. Determine the neurological level of injury (NLI).
This refers to the most caudal segment of the cord with intact sensation and antigravity (3 or more) muscle function strength, provided that there is normal (intact) sensory and motor function rostrally respectively.
The NLI is the most cephalad of the sensory and motor levels determined in steps 1 and 2.

4. Determine whether the injury is Complete or Incomplete.
(i.e. absence or presence of sacral sparing)
If voluntary anal contraction = No AND all S4-5 sensory scores = 0 AND deep anal pressure = No, then injury is Complete.
Otherwise, injury is Incomplete.

5. Determine ASIA Impairment Scale (AIS) Grade.
  Is injury <u>Complete</u>? If YES, AIS=A

  NO ↓

  Is injury <u>Motor Complete</u>? If YES, AIS=B

  NO ↓   (No=voluntary anal contraction OR motor function more than three levels below the <u>motor level</u> on a given side, if the patient has sensory incomplete classification)

  Are <u>at least half (half or more) of the key muscles below the neurological level of injury</u> graded 3 or better?

  NO ↓   YES ↓

  AIS=C   AIS=D

If sensation and motor function is normal in all segments, AIS=E
Note: AIS E is used in follow-up testing when an individual with a documented SCI has recovered normal function. If at initial testing no deficits are found, the individual is neurologically intact and the ASIA Impairment Scale does not apply.

6. Determine the zone of partial preservation (ZPP).
The ZPP is used only in injuries with absent motor (no VAC) OR sensory function (no DAP, no LT and no PP sensation) in the lowest sacral segments S4-5, and refers to those dermatomes and myotomes caudal to the sensory and motor levels that remain partially innervated. With sacral sparing of sensory function, the sensory ZPP is not applicable and therefore "NA" is recorded in the block of the worksheet. Accordingly, if VAC is present, the motor ZPP is not applicable and is noted as "NA".

TABLE 14.3   Peripheral Nerve Motor and Sensory Testing

Upper Limb Peripheral Nerve	Motor Testing	Sensory Testing
Musculocutaneous	Elbow flexion	Lateral aspect of forearm
Axillary	Shoulder abduction	Regimental badge area
Median	Thumb abduction	Pad of index finger
Ulnar	Finger abduction	Ulnar aspect of little finger
Radial	Wrist extension	Dorsal aspect of web space
Lower Limb Peripheral Nerve	*Motor Testing*	*Sensory Testing*
Femoral	Knee extension	Anterior thigh
Tibial	Ankle plantar flexion	Plantar aspect of foot
Superficial peroneal	Ankle eversion	Dorsum of foot
Deep peroneal	Ankle dorsiflexion	First web space of foot

Adapted with permission from White, T.O., Mackenzie, S.P., Gray, A.J., & Mcrae, R. (2016). *McRae's orthopaedic trauma and emergency fracture management.* Elsevier.

TABLE 14.4   Cranial Nerves

Cranial Nerve	Function	Common (And Not So Common) Pathologies
CN I – Olfactory	Olfaction (i.e., the detection of scent)	• Kallmann syndrome • Olfactory groove meningioma
CN II – Optic	Vision	Optic nerve: optic neuritis, ischaemic optic neuropathy, optic nerve glioma Optic chiasm: compression from a pituitary adenoma or craniopharyngioma Optic tract: stroke, tumour
CN III – Oculomotor	Innervation of the **levator palpebrae superioris** and **extraocular muscles** (except superior oblique and lateral rectus, mnemonic SO4 LR6) **Parasympathetic** control of the iris (miosis, constriction)	3rd nerve palsy – partial vs complete • Ptosis, 'down and out' pupil, dilated pupil Aetiology: • 'Medical 3rd nerve': diabetes, vasculitis. Spares outer pupillary fibres • 'Surgical 3rd nerve': PComA aneurysm, tumour, uncal herniation, trauma (raised ICP). Compresses outer pupillary fibres
CN IV – Trochlear	Innervation of the **superior oblique**	• Very fine nerve – can be damaged in trauma
CN V – Trigeminal	Sensation of the face and anterior 2/3 of the tongue Innervation of the muscles of mastication	• Trigeminal neuralgia
CN VI – Abducens	Innervation of the **lateral rectus**	• Prone to stretching in cases of raised ICP due to its long intracranial course (false localising sign)

CN VII – Facial	Innervation of the **muscles of facial expression**
	Parasympathetic control of the lacrimal, submandibular and submental glands
	Taste afferents from **anterior 2/3** of tongue
		• Facial nerve palsies (LMN vs UMN)
		  • Ramsay-Hunt syndrome
		  • Bell's palsy
		  • Vestibular schwannoma
		  • Stroke
		• Hemifacial spasm

CN VIII – Vestibulocochlear	Afferent conduction of hearing and balance from the cochlea and vestibular apparatus	• Cerebellopontine angle lesions (e.g., vestibular schwannoma, meningioma)
CN IX – Glossopharyngeal	**Sensation** from **posterior 1/3** of tongue and pharynx **Taste** from **posterior 1/3** of tongue Afferent signals from carotid bodies (chemoreceptor) and carotid sinuses (baroreceptor reflex) **Parasympathetic** control of parotid gland Innervation of stylopharyngeus	• Glossopharyngeal neuralgia • CN IX (like X and XI) is prone to injury from pathologies arising in/around the jugular foramen (e.g., glomus jugulare tumours, meningiomas, venous thrombosis)
CN X – Vagus	**General visceral afferents** from thoracic and abdominal organs (including aortic bodies) **Parasympathetic** control of the thoracic and abdominal viscera (up to distal 2/3 of transverse colon) Innervation of the pharyngeal and laryngeal musculature (including palatoglossus)	• Jugular foramen pathology (see CN IX)

TABLE 14.4   Cranial Nerves—cont'd

Cranial Nerve	Function	Common (And Not So Common) Pathologies
CN XI – Accessory	Innervation of the trapezius and sterno-cleidomastoid	• Prone to injury as it runs through the posterior triangle of the neck
CN XII – Hypoglossal	Innervation of all but one of the tongue muscles (palatoglossus)	• Due to imbalance in the strength of the genio-glossus, the protruded tongue will tend to deviate towards the weak side

ICP, Intracranial pressure; LMN, lower motor neuron; PComA, posterior communicating artery; UMN, upper motor neuron.

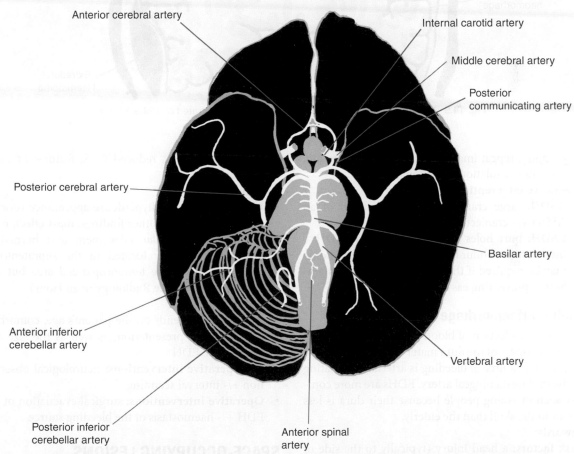

Fig. 14.8 Inferior Surface of the Brain with Cerebral Vasculature Depicting the Circle of Willis. (Illustrated by Hollie Blaber.)

- **ASDH:** hyperdense (bright) appearance, often associated with underlying brain parenchymal injuries
- **CSDH:** hypodense (dark) appearance

Differentials:
- **ASDH:** any traumatic intracranial lesion, ischaemic stroke

- **CSDH:** delirium, dementia, tumour, stroke

Management:

Depends on the patient's age, comorbidities and clinical presentation, as well as the size and location of the SDH.
- **Nonoperative interventions:** neurological observation, consider seizure prophylaxis if an acute

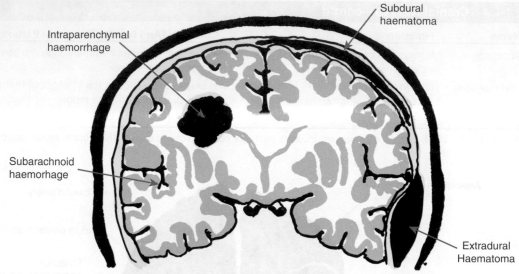

Fig. 14.9 Anatomy of an Intracranial Haemorrhage. (Illustrated by Hollie Blaber.)

head injury, repeat imaging if there is deterioration, reverse anticoagulation/coagulopathy

- **Operative interventions:**
  - **ASDH:** large craniotomy for evacuation of an ASDH +/- craniectomy
  - **CSDH:** burr holes for evacuation of a CSDH + insertion of subdural drain. A small craniotomy may be required if the CSDH has multiple membranes preventing easy drainage

Extradural Haemorrhage

Definition: a collection of blood between the skull and the external aspect of the dura mater (See Fig. 14.9). The most common source of bleeding is arterial, originating from the middle meningeal artery. EDHs are more commonly seen in young people because their dura is less adherent to the skull than the elderly.

Buzzwords:

- **Risk factors:** a head injury (typically to the side of the head) causing a fracture of the pterion (thin area of skull), which causes damage to the middle meningeal artery
- **Presentation:** headache, nausea, vomiting, seizure, reduced consciousness, focal neurological deficit (uncal herniation – contralateral hemiparesis, CN III palsy). Classical presentation: transient loss of consciousness followed by regaining consciousness for a period of time ('lucid interval') before subsequent

deterioration (e.g., reduced GCS, features of uncal herniation)

Investigations:

- **CT head:** biconvex hyperdense appearance (doesn't cross suture lines). Other findings: mass effect, midline shift, ventricular effacement and herniation syndromes. Usually located in the supratentorial compartment of the temporoparietal area but can occur elsewhere (see Radiology in an Hour)

Differentials: SDH

Management: depends on the patient's age, comorbidities and clinical presentation, as well as the size and location of the EDH

- **Nonoperative interventions:** neurological observation +/- interval scanning
- **Operative interventions:** surgical evacuation of the EDH +/- haemostasis of the bleeding source

SPACE-OCCUPYING LESIONS

Cerebral Abscess

Definition: a life-threatening condition. A collection of pus surrounded by a capsule within the brain parenchyma, preceded by cerebritis (inflammation of the brain). Rupturing of an abscess into the ventricle has a mortality rate of >80%. Cerebral abscesses arise from three routes:

- Direct inoculation (trauma, post-neurosurgery)

- Contiguous spread (sinusitis, otitis media, mastoiditis)
- Haematogenous spread from a distant source (e.g., dental infections, infective endocarditis, lung abscess)

Buzzwords:

- **Risk factors:** immunocompromise, chronic local infections (e.g., sinusitis, mastoiditis, otitis media), pulmonary conditions (e.g., lung abscess, pulmonary arteriovenous malformation (AVM)/arteriovenous fistula), congenital heart disease, chronic kidney disease, liver disease, cancer
- **Presentation:** features of a raised ICP (e.g., headache, nausea, vomiting, reduced consciousness), seizures, focal neurological deficit, features of infection (e.g., fever, sepsis, source of infection)

Investigations:

- **Bloods:** ↑/↔ WCC, ↑/↔ CRP, U&Es, LFTs
- **Cultures:** includes blood cultures, urine cultures and direct cultures from the cerebral abscess, although frequently negative. The most common isolated organisms include *Streptococcus* spp.
- **CT head:** ring-enhancing lesion with contrast (hyperdense rim with a central hypodense core) with peri-lesional low density (oedema) +/- ependymal enhancement (ventriculitis)
- **MRI head:** ring-enhancing lesion with gadolinium; restricted diffusion on diffusion-weighted imaging (DWI)
- **Identify primary source:** orthopantomogram (OPG), ECG, pulmonary imaging, CD4 count/HIV testing

Differentials: brain tumour, stroke, demyelination

Management:

1. Urgent neurosurgical referral
2. Operative intervention: obtaining a sample of brain pus is key to guiding antimicrobial therapy and reducing the ICP
   a. Needle aspiration of pus
   b. Excision of abscess
3. Nonoperative interventions
   a. Antimicrobial therapy: empirical vs targeted therapy with microbiology guidance; prolonged duration of 4–8 weeks
   b. Anti-epileptic drugs: treat seizures. Abscesses are strongly associated with seizures
   c. Identification of the primary source
4. Follow-up imaging/clinical evaluation/inflammatory markers to identify if the abscess is reaccumulating

Brain Tumours

Definition: a broad spectrum of tumours that can originate from any constituent of the CNS (brain parenchyma and meninges) or are secondary tumours deposited in the brain but originating from a primary cancer located elsewhere.

- **Primary brain tumours:** tumours are graded based on the presence/absence of certain histological features (e.g., **cellular atypia, mitotic activity, vascular proliferation, necrosis**). However, the use of molecular markers is becoming increasingly more frequent. Lower grade tumours are at risk of malignant transformation to a higher grade.
  - **Grade 1:** 0/4 histological features. Examples: pilocytic astrocytoma, choroid plexus papilloma, craniopharyngioma
  - **Grade 2:** 1/4 histological features. Examples: diffuse astrocytoma, central neurocytoma
  - **Grade 3:** 2/4 histological features. Examples: anaplastic astrocytoma, choroid plexus carcinoma
  - **Grade 4:** 3–4/4 histological features. Examples: glioblastoma, medulloblastoma
- **Secondary brain tumours:** the most common sources of cerebral metastases include lung cancers, breast cancers, renal cell carcinomas, melanomas and colorectal cancers.
- **Haematological tumours:** lymphomas can arise directly from within the brain without any systemic involvement (a primary CNS lymphoma) or can arise elsewhere and spread to the CNS (a secondary CNS lymphoma).

Buzzwords:

- **Risk factors:** genetic conditions/family history (e.g., neurofibromatosis type (NFT) 1/2, von Hippel Lindau syndrome, tuberous sclerosis, Li-Fraumeni syndrome), exposure to ionising radiation, age, overweight
- **Presentation:** incidental finding, headache (may/may not be due to a raised ICP), features of a raised ICP (e.g., headache – worse in the morning, with coughing/straining; nausea; vomiting; blurred vision; papilloedema), seizures, focal neurological deficit, endocrine dysfunction (pituitary tumours)

Investigations:

- **CT head (+/- contrast):** first-line investigation in an urgent setting. CT thorax, abdomen, pelvis (TAP) to identify a suspected primary cancer source

- **MRI scan:** to provide more detailed structural information about the tumour (multiple MR sequences used, including T1, T2, post-contrast, DWI, FLAIR)
- **Advanced MRI techniques:** functional MRI (location of the tumour in relation to eloquent areas), MR spectroscopy (chemical composition of the tumour)
- **Biopsy:** histopathology for morphology, molecular markers
- **Tumour markers (CSF, blood):** various pineal gland tumours can produce alpha-fetoprotein and/or human chorionic gonadotrophin

Differentials: cerebral abscess, ischaemic stroke, demyelination

Management: depends on the **patient's characteristics** (e.g., age, performance status, comorbidities, preferences) and the **tumour's characteristics** (e.g., size, location, type, extracranial disease, number of lesions, surgically accessible). A multidisciplinary team will discuss each case and determine management options, which may include:

- Observation: serial imaging
- Operative intervention: biopsy, surgical resection
- Chemotherapy: temozolomide, PCV (procarbazine, lomustine, vincristine)
- Radiotherapy: stereotactic radiosurgery (SRS) (single high-dose treatment), stereotactic radiotherapy (multiple lower-dose treatments but with the same total dose as SRS)
- Adjuncts
  - Steroids: reduce peritumoural oedema. Provide symptomatic relief and neurological improvement
  - Anti-epileptic drugs: treat seizures related to tumours

DISORDERS OF THE SPINE AND SPINAL CORD

Jefferson Fracture

Definition: a multifocal fracture of the C1 ring (think of how a polo mint usually breaks in at least two places around its circumference) (see Fig 14.10). Typically a stable injury if the transverse ligament is intact.

Buzzwords:

- **Risk factors:** axial loading (think of diving into a shallow pool)
- **Presentation:** most often neurologically intact (note the wide cross-sectional area of the vertebral canal at this level), neck pain, other traumatic cervical fractures/vertebral artery injuries

Investigations:

- **CT:** to assess the fracture pattern, stability and associated fractures; to indirectly assess the integrity of the transverse ligament (atlantodental interval)
- **MRI:** to directly assess the integrity of the transverse ligament; also indicated if there is a neurological deficit in order to identify spinal cord injuries
- **Radiographs:** the lateral masses of C1 are seen overhanging those of C2 bilaterally (rule of Spence = if total overhang of lateral masses >7 mm, it is an indirect indication that the integrity of the transverse ligament is compromised)

Differentials: congenital anomalies may appear radiologically similar

Management: all trauma patients should be assessed systematically according to the latest ATLS guidelines

1. Nonoperative intervention: external cervical immobilisation (hard collar, halo vest) if the transverse ligament is intact
2. Operative intervention: if the transverse ligament is not intact (an operative intervention is not always indicated though)

Odontoid Fracture

Definition: fracture of the odontoid peg of C2 caused by either a hyperextension or hyperflexion injury. Three fracture types according to the Anderson and D'Alonzo classification system:

- Type I = through the tip of the odontoid
- Type II = through the base of the odontoid neck
- Type III = through the body of C2

Buzzwords:

- **Risk factors:** high-energy trauma in a younger patient (e.g., road traffic collision, skiing accident, etc.); lower energy trauma in an elderly patient (e.g., simple fall)
- **Presentation:** most cases are neurologically intact (note the wide cross-sectional area of the vertebral canal at this level). Clinical features include neck pain, occipital neuralgia, altered scalp sensation, rarely a significant neurological deficit (e.g., tetraplegia)

Investigations:

- **Radiographs** (AP, lateral, open-mouth odontoid view of the cervical spine): to characterise the fracture
- **CT:** to assess the fracture pattern, stability and associated fractures
- **MRI:** indicated if there is a neurological deficit to identify spinal cord injuries

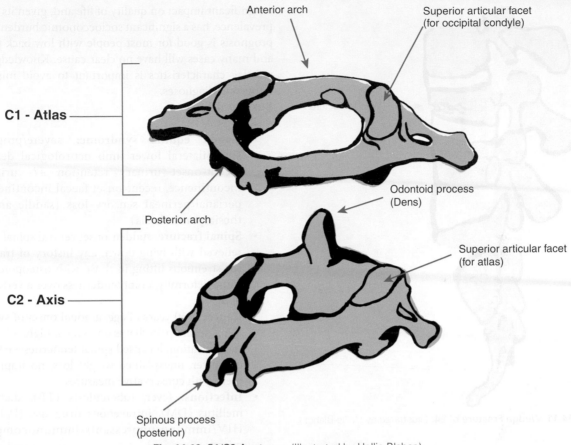

Fig. 14.10 C1/C2 Anatomy. (Illustrated by Hollie Blaber.)

Differentials: congenital defects and anatomical variants may give rise to the appearance of a fractured dens (i.e., os odontoideum)

Management: all trauma patients should be assessed systematically according to the latest ATLS guidelines. Management may be operative or nonoperative depending on the type of fracture, risk of nonunion and individual patient characteristics

- Type I: rare but a significant risk of instability; may require a halo vest or hard collar immobilisation
- Type II: depending on the patient and fracture characteristics some may heal with immobilisation alone; in other cases, an operative intervention is indicated
- Type III: often heals with immobilisation alone

Wedge Fracture

Definition: a compression fracture typically of the anterior vertebral column (see Fig 14.11). Wedge/compression fractures are not conventionally considered unstable and are not usually associated with any neurological impairment.

Buzzwords:
- **Risk factors:** osteoporosis, malignancy, trauma
- **Presentation:** pain at the site of fracture, focal spine tenderness, no neurological impairment

Investigations
- **X-ray:** reduced height of the vertebral body anteriorly with associated kyphosis
- **CT:** superior visualisation of fracture morphology compared with plain films
- **MRI:** bony injury may be visible on certain sequences (e.g., STIR). Neurological structures and posterior ligaments can also be visualised using MRI.

Differentials: spinal malignancy (e.g., metastasis, myeloma), discitis, spondylolysis

Management: all trauma patients should be assessed systematically according to the latest ATLS guidelines. Usually managed nonoperatively

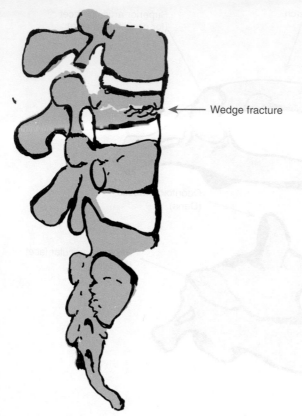

Wedge fracture ⟵

Fig. 14.11 Wedge Fracture of L4. (Illustrated by Hollie Blaber.)

1. **Nonoperative intervention:** analgesia, physical therapy (PT), treat underlying condition (e.g., osteoporosis – bisphosphonates, vitamin D and calcium replacement), serial imaging to assess for progressive deformity if clinically indicated
2. **Operative intervention:**
   a. Vertebroplasty/kyphoplasty: may provide faster pain relief and mitigate the risk of progressive deformity if an open surgical intervention is not indicated
   b. Open surgical decompression and stabilisation: significant loss of height, multiple fractures at consecutive levels, neurological deficits, disrupted posterior elements, progressive loss of height all may indicate instability and necessitate fusion

Low Back Pain

Definition: low back pain is a common symptom with a broad differential diagnosis. Low back pain can have

a significant impact on quality of life and, given its high prevalence, has a significant socioeconomic burden. The prognosis is good for most people with low back pain, and many cases will have no clear cause. Knowledge of red-flag characteristics is important to avoid missing important diagnoses.

Buzzwords:
- RED FLAGS:
  - **Cauda equina syndrome:** severe/progressive bilateral lower limb neurological deficit, recent-onset urinary retention +/- urinary incontinence, recent-onset faecal incontinence, perianal/perineal sensory loss (saddle anaesthesia/paraesthesia)
  - **Spinal fracture:** sudden-onset central spinal pain relieved with lying down, any history of trauma (or strenuous lifting in those with osteoporosis), spine deformity, point tenderness over a vertebral body
  - **Cancer:** >50 years of age, gradual onset of symptoms, severe pain that is ongoing at night +/- thoracic location, localised spinal tenderness, PMHx of cancer, unexplained weight loss, no improvement with conservative measures
  - **Infections:** fever, tuberculosis (TB), diabetes mellitus (DM), intravenous drug use (IVDU), HIV/immunosuppressants/immunocompromised
- **Presentation:** back pain, sciatica, radiculopathy, myelopathy, red flags

Investigations:
- **Radiographs:** limited use for low back pain
- **MRI:** utility for identifying spine pathology and compression of neural structures
- **Bloods:** raised inflammatory markers may indicate a spinal infection

Differentials: think red flags. Don't forget retroperitoneal, visceral and musculoskeletal conditions (e.g., abdominal aortic aneurysm, pancreatitis, renal colic, duodenal ulcer, hip osteoarthritis (OA))

Management:
- Nonspecific low back pain +/- radicular pain or neurogenic claudication: reassurance, lifestyle adjustments, physiotherapy, analgesia. If symptoms persist, then consider further investigation and/or spinal referral
- Red flag(s) present: emergent/urgent referral to Emergency Department/secondary care/tertiary care

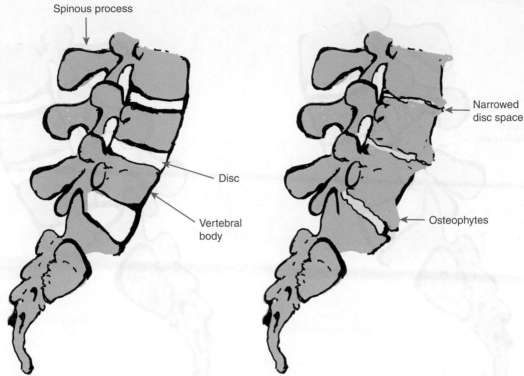

Fig. 14.12 Lumbar Spine, Normal (*left*) and with Spondylosis (*right*). (Illustrated by Hollie Blaber.)

for further assessment and investigation based on the suspected diagnosis

Spondylosis

Definition: Spondylosis is a nonspecific term referring to OA of the spinal column, most commonly affecting the cervical and lumbar spines. This condition may be caused by a combination of the following:

- Bony changes (e.g., osteophytes, bony spurs, spondylolisthesis). See Fig.14.12
- Soft-tissue changes (e.g., prolapsed intervertebral discs, ligamentum flavum hypertrophy, facet joint hypertrophy/cysts)

Buzzwords:

- **Risk factors:** abnormal loading (e.g., obesity, pregnancy, occupation, sports), smoking, osteoporosis, age
- **Presentation:** back/neck pain, radicular symptoms (e.g., brachialgia, sciatica), neurological deficits (e.g., myotome weakness, dermatomal sensory changes), neurogenic claudication (spinal stenosis)

Investigations:

- **Radiographs:** nonspecific degenerative findings (e.g., osteophytes, narrow disc space), scoliosis, spondylolisthesis
- **MRI:** degenerative findings (e.g., osteophytes, ligamentum flavum/facet joint hypertrophy, prolapsed disc), spinal stenosis, nerve root/spinal cord compression. MRI also provides useful information about compression of neural structures

Differentials: spinal metastasis, spondyloarthropathy, discitis, osteoporotic compression fractures

Management:

- **Nonoperative:** analgesia, physiotherapy, weight loss
- **Operative:** depends on the underlying diagnosis and patient characteristics. Surgical interventions include:
  - **Laminectomy:** removal of the lamina and ligamentum flavum to decompress the nerve roots, cauda equina or spinal cord
  - **Discectomy:** removal of a prolapsed intervertebral disc to decompress the nerve roots, cauda equina or spinal cord

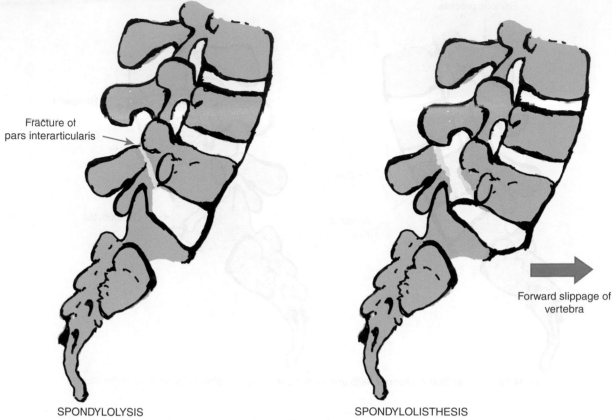

Fracture of pars interarticularis

Forward slippage of vertebra

SPONDYLOLYSIS   SPONDYLOLISTHESIS

Fig. 14.13 Spondylolysis and Spondylolisthesis. (Illustrated by Hollie Blaber.)

- **Foraminotomy:** decompressing a peripheral nerve as it passes through the intervertebral foramen
- **Interbody fusion:** removal of an intervertebral disc + replacement with artificial cage +/- insertion of instrumentation with the aim of fusing adjacent vertebrae

Spondylolisthesis and Spondylolysis

Definition:
- **Spondylolisthesis:** forward slippage of the vertebra above relative to the vertebra below, most commonly affecting the L5/S1 vertebral level (see Fig 14.13). Six different types based on their aetiology (Wiltse classification):
  - **Type 1:** congenital/dysplastic
  - **Type 2:** isthmic (spondylolysis)
  - **Type 3:** degenerative
  - **Type 4:** traumatic
  - **Type 5:** pathological
  - **Type 6:** iatrogenic

- **Spondylolysis** (isthmic spondylolisthesis): defect in the pars interarticularis (fracture) (see Fig. 14.13)

Buzzwords:
- **Risk factors:** depends on the aetiology (e.g., stress fracture from activity, bone disease, iatrogenic)
- **Presentation:** asymptomatic, back pain, radiculopathy, neurogenic claudication (unilateral/bilateral leg and buttock pain with walking, relieved by leaning forward), rarely cauda equina syndrome

Investigations:
- **Radiographs:** AP/lateral/oblique views to determine the extent and level of the spondylolisthesis pars defect; flexion/extension views to assess for instability
- **MRI:** to identify compression of neural structures

Differentials: prolapsed intervertebral disc, spondyloarthropathy, spinal metastasis, spinal fracture, vascular claudication

Management:
- **Nonoperative:** analgesia, physiotherapy

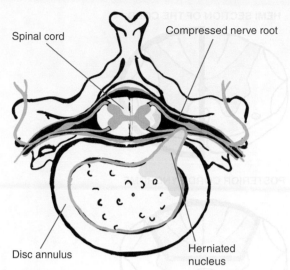

Spinal cord

Compressed nerve root

Disc annulus

Herniated nucleus

Fig. 14.14 Lumbar Disc Herniation. (Illustrated by Hollie Blaber.)

- **Operative intervention** may be required if there is evidence of radiculopathy, neurogenic claudication or myelopathy. Surgical techniques include decompression, instrumented fusion, interbody fusion

Prolapsed Intervertebral Disc

Definition: the intervertebral disc is composed of an inner **nucleus pulposus** and an outer **annulus fibrosus**. The nucleus pulposus becomes dehydrated with age and degeneration. The nucleus pulposus can herniate centrally through the annulus fibrosus to compress the thecal sac +/- cauda equina or (most commonly) posterolaterally to compress the nerve roots (see Fig. 14.14).

Buzzwords:
- **Risk factors:** workload, smoking, age, obesity
- **Presentation:**
  - **Lumbar disc prolapse:** low back pain, radicular pain (sciatica)/radiculopathy (Table 14.5), cauda equina syndrome. Radiculopathy describes the

clinical features associated with the dysfunction of a specific nerve root (e.g. myotomal weakness, dermatomal sensory changes, altered reflexes). Sciatica (a.k.a. lumbar radiculopathy) occurs when the lumbosacral nerve roots (L4-S1) forming the sciatic nerve become inflammed or compressed.
- **Cervical disc prolapse:** neck pain, radicular pain/radiculopathy, myelopathy

Investigations:
- **MRI:** to identify the level, extent and location of the disc prolapse +/- compression of neural structures

Differentials: spinal stenosis, spinal metastasis, spinal fracture

Management:
- **Nonoperative:** majority are treated conservatively with analgesia, lifestyle modifications and physiotherapy/exercise
- **Operative:** (micro)discectomy +/- laminectomy +/- nerve root decompression
  - **Indications:** persistent radicular pain despite adequate nonoperative treatments; progressive neurological deficit (foot drop)/cauda equina syndrome/severe pain despite adequate analgesia = urgent/emergent surgery

Cauda Equina Syndrome

Definition: a constellation of signs and symptoms arising from compression of the lumbar and sacral nerve roots that constitute the cauda equina. This condition is a surgical emergency because there is a risk of progression to irreversible paraplegia, incontinence and sexual dysfunction without prompt treatment. Compression can occur as a result of a space-occupying lesion compressing the nerve roots, most commonly a prolapsed intervertebral disc. Other causes include trauma (retropulsed fragment), spinal epidural abscess, spinal epidural haematoma, tumours or ischaemia/inflammation.

Buzzwords:
- **Risk factors:** osteoporosis, aging, cancer, infection

TABLE 14.5	**Physical Examination Findings in L4, L5 and S1 Radiculopathies**		
	Sensory Deficit	**Motor Weakness**	**Reduced Reflex**
L4 radiculopathy	Medial malleolus	Knee extension	Knee jerk
L5 radiculopathy	Dorsal foot (1st/2nd webspace)	Ankle dorsiflexion/1st toe extension; foot drop	Medial hamstring jerk
S1 radiculopathy	Lateral foot/malleolus	Ankle plantar flexion	Ankle jerk

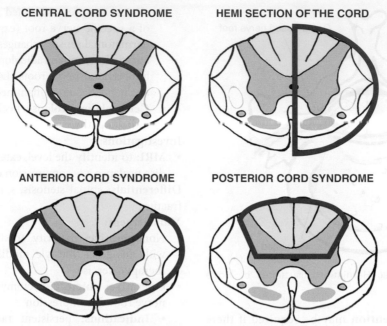

Fig. 14.15 Cord Syndromes. (Illustrated by Hollie Blaber.)

- **Presentation:** lower back pain +/- sciatica, lower limb weakness, sphincter disturbances (e.g., urinary retention, urinary and/or faecal incontinence, reduced anal tone), saddle anaesthesia (loss of sensation in the perineum, genitals, buttocks and around the anus)

Investigations:

- **Emergency MRI:** visualisation of the precise level at which the compression is occurring and the cause

Differentials: spinal metastasis, ankylosing spondylitis, discitis, osteoporotic compression fractures, sciatica, spondylosis

Management:

1. **Emergency referral** to neurosurgery/spine surgery services for consideration of an operative intervention
2. **Operative intervention:** laminectomy and discectomy (in cases of disc herniation). Relieves the compression by removing the culpable mass

Spinal Cord Injury

Definition:

- **SCI:** damage to the spinal cord resulting in temporary/permanent motor, sensory and/or autonomic dysfunction of the spinal cord
- **Complete SCI:** complete absence of motor and sensory function below the level of the SCI
- **Incomplete SCI:** varying levels of retained motor and/or sensory function below the level of the SCI.

There are various patterns of incomplete SCI lesions, including anterior cord syndrome, posterior cord syndrome, central cord syndrome and Brown-Sèquard syndrome. (see Fig. 14.15)

- **Spinal shock:** a transient loss of all spinal function below the level of a spinal cord reflex (areflexic flaccid paralysis) that returns gradually over time
- **Neurogenic shock:** associated with a cervical and high-thoracic SCI. Hypotension and bradyarrhythmias due to an interruption in sympathetic outflow
- **Autonomic dysreflexia:** abnormal and excessive sympathetic activity in response to stimuli after a SCI (T6 and above). Usually results in HTN, headaches and sweating above the level of the injury

Management:

- Treat the underlying aetiology
- Initial/early Nonoperative interventions: to prevent complications
  - Immobilisation: e.g. external cervical immobilisation
  - Cardiovascular and respiratory support: to prevent hypotension and hypoxia
  - DVT/PE prophylaxis
  - Peptic ulcer prevention: proton-pump inhibitor
  - Avoid/identify/treat autonomic dysreflexia
  - Avoid/treat hypothermia
  - Skin and pressure ulcer care

- Neurogenic bowel and bladder management: catheterisation, rectal stimulation, laxatives
- Avoid/treat spasticity
- Rehabilitation: inpatient specialised SCI rehabilitation, community rehabilitation
- Operative interventions (controversial)
  - Traction/reduction of fracture dislocations
  - Surgical decompression +/- stabilisation

Complete Spinal Cord Transection

Definition: a severe spinal injury in which the entire cord is transversely sectioned, associated with a significant level of trauma and resulting in a devastating impact on an individual's life. All descending and ascending white matter tracts are damaged at the level of injury, as well as segmental damage to the ventral and dorsal horns at the level of the injury

Buzzwords:

- **Causes:** significant level of trauma
- **Presentation:**
  - Loss of all sensory modalities at/below the level of the lesion
  - Paralysis (depends on the level of the injury): LMN signs at the level of the injury; UMN signs below the level of the injury. UMN signs seen below the lesion, while LMN signs may be seen at the level of ventral horn involvement
  - Associated traumatic injuries
  - Higher spinal level of injury associated with neurogenic shock/respiratory difficulties

Investigations:

- **CT:** a complete transection is most likely to present in the context of a major trauma. CT imaging will provide valuable information about the structural integrity of the spine.
- **MRI:** to assess the integrity/damage/level of spinal cord; assess other soft tissue injuries and prevertebral swelling

Differentials: incomplete spinal cord lesion; compressive pathology (e.g., tumour, haematoma), noncompressive pathology (e.g., transverse myelitis)

Management:

1. Assess according to the ATLS protocol
2. See section on management of SCIs
3. Surgical decompression +/- stabilisation

Central Cord Syndrome

Definition: the most common form of an incomplete SCI. Damage to the central part of the spinal cord, most likely affecting the cervical spinal cord and secondary to a hyperextension injury

Buzzwords:

- **Causes:** traumatic: hyperextension neck injury in an elderly patient with preexisting cervical spinal stenosis; nontraumatic: intramedullary spinal cord tumours, syringomyelia
- **Presentation:** depends on the level – assuming cervical central cord syndrome:
  - Pain and temperature sensory loss in the upper limbs (medial spinothalamic fibres affected first) in a cape-like distribution
  - Weakness (upper limb >>> lower limb; upper limb corticospinal fibres are located more medially than lower limb fibres; LMN weakness at the level of the lesion and UMN weakness below the level of the lesion)
  - Other: bowel and bladder disturbances

Investigations:

- **Radiographs:** lateral, AP, odontoid films to identify bony injuries and preexisting degenerative changes
- **CT:** to identify fractures and preexisting degenerative changes
- **MRI:** to identify spinal cord pathologies (e.g., haematoma, syrinx, contusion, oedema) or compression

Differentials: other forms of incomplete SCI

Management: See section on management of SCIs

Anterior Cord Syndrome

Definition: a form of incomplete SCI that affects the anterior two-thirds of the spinal cord (anterior spinal artery distribution). Affects the corticospinal tracts (weakness), spinothalamic tract (loss of pain/temperature sensation) and grey matter (ventral/lateral horn), with preservation of the dorsal columns

Buzzwords:

- **Causes:** ischaemia (anterior spinal artery infarction, abdominal aortic surgery), anterior compression (prolapsed disc, anterior bone fragment, tumour, epidural collection)
- **Presentation:** motor weakness (depends on the spinal level), dissociated sensory loss (loss of pain and temperature sensation but preservation of vibration and proprioception caused by damage to the spinothalamic tract but preservation of the dorsal column medial lemniscus pathway)

Investigations:

- **MRI:** to identify abnormalities within the spinal cord in the distribution of the anterior spinal artery;

identify compressive causes of anterior cord syndrome

Differentials: other causes of incomplete SCI, demyelination, Guillain-Barré syndrome

Management:
1. Treat the underlying aetiology
2. See section on management of SCIs
3. Surgical intervention in cases of compression or instability

Posterior Cord Syndrome

Definition: a rare form of incomplete SCI resulting in damage to the dorsal columns of the spinal cord. Very broad aetiology

Buzzwords:
- **Causes:** demyelination, metabolic (e.g., vitamin B12 deficiency, copper deficiency), infection (e.g., HIV, syphilis), compression (e.g., degenerative, epidural collection, tumour)
- **Presentation:** loss of proprioception and vibration sense below the level of the lesion; preservation of temperature and pain sensation and motor function. Lhermitte's sign (sudden electric-like pains originating in the neck and radiating down the spine)

Investigations:
- **Bloods:** possible megaloblastic anaemia with a vitamin B12 deficiency, HIV/syphilis serology
- **MRI:** T2/FLAIR hyperintensity in the dorsal columns of spinal cord, posterior spinal lesion

Differentials: broad differential diagnosis (see risk factors); other forms of incomplete SCI injury

Management:
Dependent on the underlying aetiology
- **Infection:** antibiotics
- **Metabolic deficiency:** supplementation
- **Demyelination:** steroids and immunomodulators
- **Compressive pathology:** surgical decompression

Brown-Séquard Syndrome

Definition: a clinical syndrome that occurs secondary to hemi-sectioning of the spinal cord, most commonly by a penetrating injury

Buzzwords:
- **Causes:** traumatic causes (usually a penetrating injury – e.g., stabbing, gunshot wound); nontraumatic causes (compressive pathology – e.g., epidural collection, tumour, AVM, disc herniation; noncompressive pathology – e.g., radiation, demyelination, inflammation, tumour)

- **Presentation:** clinical features are related to the side of the spinal cord that is affected
  - Ipsilateral pyramidal weakness below the level of the lesion (damage to the descending lateral corticospinal tract)
  - Ipsilateral loss of proprioception and vibration sense (damage to the ascending dorsal-column medial lemniscus; a pathway that has not yet decussated)
  - Contralateral loss of pain and temperature sensation below the level of lesion (damage to the ascending spinothalamic tract, decussation has already occurred at the level of neuron entry into the spinal cord)
  - Ipsilateral motor (LMN weakness) and sensory findings (all modalities) at the level of the lesion (damage to the ventral and dorsal horns at the lesion site)

Investigations:
- **MRI:** to assess the spinal cord and ligamentous injuries; findings dependent on the underlying aetiology
- **CT:** to assess for bony injuries, spinal instability, findings dependent on the underlying aetiology

Differentials: broad differential diagnosis (see causes); other forms of incomplete SCI

Management:
- Dependent on the underlying aetiology
- Treat trauma according to ATLS principles
- See section on management of SCIs

Syringomyelia

Definitions: This section focuses specifically on syringomyelia; however, a range of terms are encountered when reading about this topic:
- Syringomyelia: a cystic dilation within the substance of the spinal cord
- Syringobulbia: an extension of syringomyelia into the brainstem
- Hydromyelia: an abnormal dilation of the central canal of the spinal cord
- Syrinx: a general term used for an abnormal cystic dilation within the spinal cord

Buzzwords:
- **Risk factors:** congenital (Chiari I malformation – most common cause), acquired (post-traumatic, post-infectious, spinal cord tumour)
- **Presentation:** clinical features depend on the size and site of the syrinx. For a cervical syrinx:
  - Sensory loss ('cape-like' distribution = arms and back)

- Dissociated sensory loss (loss of temperature and pain sensation but preserved touch and joint position sense)
- UL >>> LL weakness (LMN pattern of weakness in the arms)
- See central cord syndrome

Investigations:
- **MRI:** most valuable study for identifying syringomyelia; with and without contrast. Also aids in identifying the underlying aetiology
- **CT scan/CT myelogram:** hypodense area may be visible within the cord. Similar appearance to CSF. Myelography may demonstrate effacement of the subarachnoid space where the syrinx causes an outward displacement of the spinal cord

Differentials: spinal intramedullary tumours, spinal intramedullary cysts, arachnoid cysts

Management:
1. Conservative management: incidental asymptomatic cases (without neoplasia) may be followed with serial MRIs
2. Surgical intervention: surgery can be considered in symptomatic cases. The aim is to improve CSF flow dynamics. Options include:
   a. Correcting the underlying aetiology: perform a decompression of the spinal cord
   b. CSF diversion: shunts (syrinx-subarachnoid space shunt)

THE ONE-LINE ROUND-UP!

Here are some key words to help you remember each condition/concept.

Condition/Concept	One-line Description
Raised ICP	Headache, papilloedema, Cushing's triad: bradycardia, hypertension, irregular breathing
Traumatic brain injury	Severity guided by the GCS, check for a base of skull fracture
Subarachnoid haemorrhage	Thunderclap headache, delayed xanthochromia
Subdural haemorrhage	Crescent on CT, middle meningeal artery
Extradural haemorrhage	Biconvex hyperdensity, elderly head injury
Cerebral abscess	Ring-enhancing lesion
Benign primary brain tumours	Meningioma, pituitary adenoma and craniopharyngioma
Malignant primary brain tumours	Glioblastoma, medulloblastoma
Secondary brain tumours	Lung, breast, colorectal, melanoma, renal
Jefferson fracture	Multifocal # of C1 (atlas)
Odontoid fractures	Anderson and D'Alonzo classification
Wedge fracture	Osteoporosis, normal neurology
Low back pain	Red flags = imaging
Spondylosis	Degenerative changes to the spine
Spondylolysis	Fracture of the pars interarticularis
Spondyloarthropathy	Inflammatory arthropathies affecting the axial skeleton
Spondylolisthesis	Slippage of one vertebra relative to another vertebra
Prolapsed disc	Radiculopathies
Cauda equina syndrome	Lower limb weakness, sphincter disturbance, saddle anaesthesia
Neurogenic shock	Hypotension and bradycardia after spinal injury
Spinal shock	Hyporeflexia below level of injury immediately after trauma
Central cord syndrome	Impaired sensation in a 'cape like' distribution
Complete transection of the spinal cord	UMN signs below level of transection
Anterior cord syndrome	Bilateral impaired pain and temperature sensation below the lesion
Posterior cord syndrome	Bilateral impaired fine touch, vibration and proprioception below the lesion
Hemi-section (Brown-Sequard)	Ipsilateral loss of fine touch, contralateral loss of pain and temperature sensation below the lesion
Syringomyelia	Chiari malformation

READING LIST: NEUROSURGERY IN AN HOUR

Neuroanatomy And Neurophysiology

Binder, D. K., Sonne, D. C., & Fischbein, N. J. (2010). *Cranial nerves: Anatomy, pathology and imaging*. Thieme.

Kirshblum, S. C., Burns, S. P., Biering-Sorensen, F., et al. (2011). International standards for neurological classification of spinal cord injury (revised 2011). *J Spinal Cord Med, 34*, 535–546. https://doi.org/10.1179/20457721 1X13207446293695.

White, T. O., Mackenzie, S. P., Gray, A. J., & Mcrae, R. (2016). *McRae's orthopaedic trauma and emergency fracture management*. Elsevier.

Traumatic Brain Injury

NICE. (2019). *CG 176: Head injury: Assessment and early management*. www.nice.org.uk/guidance/cg176. [Accessed March 2022].

Brain Trauma Foundation. (2016). *Guidelines for the management of severe traumatic brain injury* (4th ed.). http://braintrauma.org/guidelines/guidelines-for-the-management-of-severe-tbi-4th-ed#.

Aneurysmal Subarachnoid Haemorrhage (SAH)

Greenberg, M. S. (2020a). *Handbook of neurosurgery* (9th ed.). Thieme.

Liebenberg, W. A., & Johnson, R. D. (2018). *Neurosurgery for surgical trainees* (3rd ed.). Hippocrates Books.

Chatterjee, S. (2010). ECG changes in subarachnoid haemorrhage: A synopsis. *Netherlands Heart Journal, 19*, 31–34.

Subdural Haemorrhage

Osborn, A. G., Hedlund, G. L., & Salzman, K. L. (2018a). *Osborn's brain* (2nd ed.). Elsevier.

Extradural Haemorrhage (EDH)

Osborn, A. G., Hedlund, G. L., & Salzman, K. L. (2018b). *Osborn's brain* (2nd ed.). Elsevier.

Cerebral Abscess

Greenberg, M. S. (2020). *Handbook of neurosurgery* (9th ed.). Thieme.

Brain Tumours

Greenberg, M. S. (2020). *Handbook of neurosurgery* (9th ed.). Thieme.

Stupp, R., Mason, W. P., Van Den Bent, M. J., et al. (2005). Radiotherapy plus concomitant and adjuvant temozolomide for glioblastoma. *NEJM, 352*, 987–996.

Jefferson Fracture

Greenberg, M. S. (2020). *Handbook of neurosurgery* (9th ed.). Thieme.

Odontoid Fracture

Greenberg, M. S. (2020). *Handbook of neurosurgery* (9th ed.). Thieme.

Wedge Fracture

Greenberg, M. S. (2020). *Handbook of neurosurgery* (9th ed.). Thieme.

Low Back Pain

NICE. (2020). *CKS: Low back pain without radiculopathy*. www.cks.nice.org.uk/topics/back-pain-low-without-radiculopathy. [Accessed March 2022].

Spondylosis

Smith, C. P. (2012). *Essential revision notes for intercollegiate MRCS: Book 1*. PasTest Ltd.

Orthobullets. (n.d.). Cervical spondylosis – spine. https://www.orthobullets.com/spine/2029/cervical-spondylosis. [Accessed 1 March 2021].

Spondylolisthesis And Spondylolysis

Smith, C. P. (2012). *Essential revision notes for intercollegiate MRCS: Book 1*. PasTest Ltd.

Orthobullets. (n.d.). Degenerative spondylolisthesis – spine. https://www.orthobullets.com/spine/2039/degenerative-spondylolisthesis.

Prolapsed Intervertebral Disc

Orthobullets. (n.d.). Lumbar disc herniation – spine. https://www.orthobullets.com/spine/2035/lumbar-disc-herniation.

Cauda Equina Syndrome

Greenberg, M. S. (2020). *Handbook of neurosurgery* (9th ed.). Thieme.

British Association of Spinal Surgeons. (2016). *Standards of care for suspected and confirmed compressive cauda equina*. https://www.sbns.org.uk/index.php/download_file/view/994/87/.

Complete Spinal Cord Transection

Haines, D. E. (2003). *Neuroanatomy: An atlas of structures, sections and systems* (6th ed.). Lippincott Williams & Wilkins.

Greenberg, M. S. (2020). *Handbook of neurosurgery* (9th ed.). Thieme.

Central Cord Syndrome

Greenberg, M. S. (2020). *Handbook of neurosurgery* (9th ed.). Thieme.

Anterior Cord Syndrome

Haines, D. E. (2003). *Neuroanatomy: An atlas of structures, sections and systems* (6th ed.). Lippincott Williams & Wilkins.

Greenberg, M. S. (2020). *Handbook of neurosurgery* (9th ed.). Thieme.

Posterior Cord Syndrome

Manji, H., Connolly, S., Kitchen, N., Lambert, C., & Mehta, A. (2014). *Oxford handbook of neurology* (2nd ed.). Oxford University Press.

Jankovic, J., Mazziotta, J. C., Pomeroy, S. L., & Daroff, R. B. (2015). *Bradley's neurology in clinical practice* (7th ed.). Elsevier.

Brown-Sequard Syndrome

Haines, D. E. (2003). *Neuroanatomy: An atlas of structures, sections and systems* (6th ed.). Lippincott Williams & Wilkins.

Syringomyelia

Greenberg, M. S. (2020). *Handbook of neurosurgery* (9th ed.). Thieme.

15

Obstetrics and Gynaecology and Sexual Health in an Hour

Hannah Punter, Sanchita Sen, Patrick Horner and Ellie Crook

ANATOMY

See Fig 15.1 for a recap on your anatomy

THE MENSTRUAL CYCLE

Key Concepts

- The menstrual cycle lasts between 21–35 days, with an average of 4–5 days of bleeding each month.
- The cycle is under hormonal control (see Fig 15.2).
  - **Menstruation** (days 1–4): falling progesterone levels result in endometrial shedding
  - **Follicular phase** (days 1–13): pulses of gonadotrophin-releasing hormone (GnRH) stimulate luteinising hormone (LH) and follicle-stimulating hormone (FSH), causing follicular growth. Follicles produce oestrogen, suppressing FSH. Rising oestrogen levels cause an LH surge
  - **Ovulation** (day 14): ovum is released from the follicle following the LH surge
  - **Luteal phase** (days 14–28): the corpus luteum produces oestradiol and progesterone, supporting endometrial thickening. If the egg is not fertilised, the progesterone level then falls

- **Common disorders:**
  - **Amenorrhoea:** cessation of or failure to establish menstruation
  - **Menorrhagia:** heavy monthly bleeding impacting the quality of life
  - **Dysmenorrhoea:** painful menstruation
  - **Intermenstrual bleeding (IMB):** bleeding between the menstrual cycle
  - **Postmenopausal bleeding (PMB):** vaginal bleeding after menopause

OBSTETRICS

PREGNANCY OVERVIEW

Key Dates

See Fig 15.3 for the key dates during pregnancy.

SCREENING

- **Screening blood tests** (at the booking visit, see Fig 15.3)
  - Hepatitis B, human immunodeficiency virus (HIV), syphilis, sickle cell disease, thalassaemia, anaemia, blood group

ANATOMY

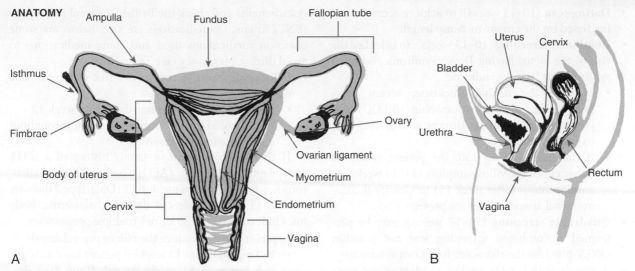

Fig 15.1 (A, B) **Overview of Anatomy for Obstetrics and Gynaecology.** (Illustrated by Hollie Blaber.)

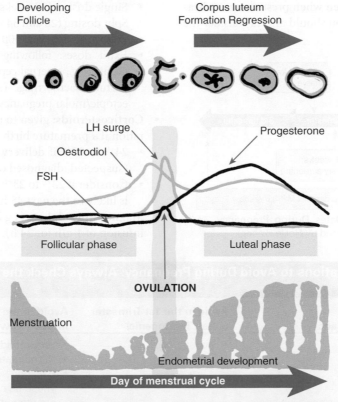

Fig 15.2 Illustration of the Menstrual Cycle. (Illustrated by Hollie Blaber.)

- **Dating scan** (10–13 weeks): to achieve accurate dating based on the crown-to-rump length
- **Combined screening** (10–13 weeks): to calculate the risk of the foetus having Down syndrome, Edwards syndrome or Patau's syndrome
  - Measure the nuchal thickness, serum beta-human chorionic gonadotrophin (β-hCG) and pregnancy associated plasma protein-A (PAPP-A) to generate a risk score
  - If the risk is >1 in 150, the patient is offered either chorionic villus sampling (11–14 weeks) or amniocentesis (after week 15) to identify if chromosomal abnormalities are present.
- **Quadruple screening** (14–17 weeks): may be performed if combined screening was not possible. ONLY provides the risk score for Down syndrome
- **Anomaly scan** (18–21 weeks): to identify any gross structural abnormalities

Prescribing in Pregnancy

Care should always be taken when prescribing medications during pregnancy. You should always consider the

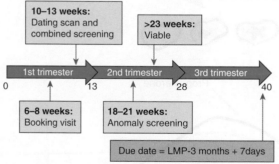

Fig 15.3 Timeline of Key Dates During Pregnancy. *LMP,* Last menstrual period. (Illustrated by Hollie Blaber.)

risks/benefits and check the British National Formulary (BNF) to ensure medications are safe. Below are some common medications used and some medications to avoid during pregnancy (see Table 15.1):

- **Folic acid:** given to reduce the risk of neural tube defects (NTDs)
  - Low risk: 400 micrograms daily until week 12
  - High risk: 5 mg daily until week 12 (or throughout if sickle cell or thalassemia)

  High risk if: personal or family history of a NTD, antiepileptic medications (AEDs), coeliac disease, malabsorption, type 1 diabetes mellitus (T1DM), type 2 diabetes mellitus (T2DM), sickle cell disease, thalassemia, body mass index (BMI) of >30 kg/m², multiple pregnancies
- **Aspirin:** given to reduce the risk of pre-eclampsia
  - 150 mg OD from 12 weeks if patient has one high-risk factor or >1 moderate-risk factor (see Pre-eclampsia section)
- **Anti D:** given if the mother is rhesus (Rh) negative to prevent haemolytic disease of the newborn
  - Single dosing (28 weeks): 1500 IU
  - Split dosing (28 and 34 weeks): 500 IU at each visit
  - Following delivery: 500 IU
  - Extra doses: following any potential sensitising events (e.g., external cephalic version (ECV), antepartum haemorrhage (APH), abdominal trauma, ectopic/molar pregnancy, termination, miscarriage)
- **Corticosteroids:** given to promote foetal lung maturation if a premature birth is likely
  - 24^{+0} to 33^{+6} if delivery is likely in the next 48 h (suspected, diagnosed or planned)
  - Consider if 23^{+0} to 23^{+6} OR 34^{+0} to 35^{+6} if delivery is likely in the next 48 h
- **Magnesium sulphate** (4 g IV bolus over 15 min, then infusion of 1 g/h for 24 h): given for neuroprotection

TABLE 15.1	**Medications to Avoid During Pregnancy: Always Check the British National Formulary!**	
Avoid Throughout Pregnancy	**Avoid in the 1st Trimester (Often Teratogenic)**	**Avoid in the 3rd Trimester (Often Impair Growth)**
• Methotrexate • Radioactive iodine • Lithium • Sodium valproate • Angiotensin-converting enzyme inhibitors • Isotretinoin • Mebendazole	• Trimethoprim	• Nonsteroidal antiinflammatory drugs • Nitrofurantoin • Dapsone These do not necessarily impair growth but are contraindicated for various reasons

- 24^{+0} to 29^{+6} if delivery is likely in the next 24 h (established preterm labour or planned)
- Consider if 23^{+0} to 23^{+6} OR 30^{+0} to 33^{+6} if delivery is likely in the next 24 h
- **Venous thromboembolism (VTE) prophylaxis:** pregnancy increases the risk of VTE.
  - Risk should be assessed at the booking appointment, during any hospital admissions and in the postpartum period.
  - Low-molecular-weight heparin (LMWH) may be required throughout pregnancy, from 28 weeks gestation or in the postpartum period depending on the individual's risk.
  - Risk factors include a previous VTE, thrombophilias, medical comorbidities, obesity, >35 years of age, parity ≥3, smoking, varicose veins, pre-eclampsia, immobility, family history, multiple pregnancy, lower segment caesarean section (LSCS), any operations in the puerperal period

PHYSIOLOGICAL CHANGES IN PREGNANCY

See Fig 15.4

ANTENATAL CONDITIONS

Intrauterine Growth Restriction

Definition: a slowing or ceasing of in utero foetal growth
- Symmetrical (normal proportions)
  - Uteroplacental insufficiency
  - Pre-eclampsia
  - Renal/cardiac disease
  - Multiple pregnancy
- Asymmetric (head size is preserved)
  - Idiopathic
  - Chromosomal abnormalities
  - TORCH (*Toxoplasma gondii*, other, *Rubella*, cytomegalovirus (CMV), herpes simplex virus (HSV), HIV)
  - Maternal smoking or substance abuse
  - Nutritional deficiencies

Buzzwords:
- **Risk factors:** >40 years of age, previous pregnancy with intrauterine growth restriction (IUGR), previous stillbirth, low PAPP-A, low maternal weight, vigorous exercise
- **Presentation:** small for gestational age (<10th centile for weight), dropping off the growth chart

Investigations:
- **Symphysial fundal height:** measuring less than the number of weeks pregnant − 2 cm (e.g., measuring less than 26cm at 28 weeks pregnant)
- **Ultrasound scan (USS) measuring the abdominal circumference and estimated foetal weight:** reduced
- **Umbilical artery doppler** (repeated twice weekly): to ensure ongoing good flow to the foetus

Differentials: small parents, ethnicity

Management:
1. Regular surveillance with an USS scan
2. Delivery by 37 weeks or from 34 weeks if growth becomes static

Gestational Diabetes Mellitus

Definition: glucose intolerance beginning during pregnancy

Buzzwords:
- **Risk factors:** previous pregnancy with gestational diabetes mellitus (GDM), previous macrosomia, BMI >30 kg/m², first-degree relative with DM, minority ethnic origin
- **Presentation:** asymptomatic, polyuria, polydipsia, large for gestational age (LGA)

Investigations:
- **Glucose tolerance test** (GTT) at 24–28 weeks
  - Fast from midnight
  - Fasting capillary glucose
  - Give 75 g fast-release glucose
  - Repeat capillary glucose after 2 h
  - GDM if Fasting glucose **>5.6 mmol/L** or glucose **>7.8mmol/L** after GTT (5678 rule)
- **USS every 4 weeks** from 28–36 weeks: to monitor growth and guide delivery planning

Differentials: LGA (obesity, polyhydramnios, fibroids, multiple pregnancies, tall), T2DM

Management:
1. Lifestyle advice
2. Metformin if target sugar levels are not reached in 1–2 weeks
3. Insulin (offer immediately if fasting glucose is >7 mmol/L)
4. Induction of labour at 37–39 weeks

Obstetric Cholestasis

Definition: an obstetrical condition resulting in pruritis without a rash and abnormal liver function. Increases the risk of premature birth

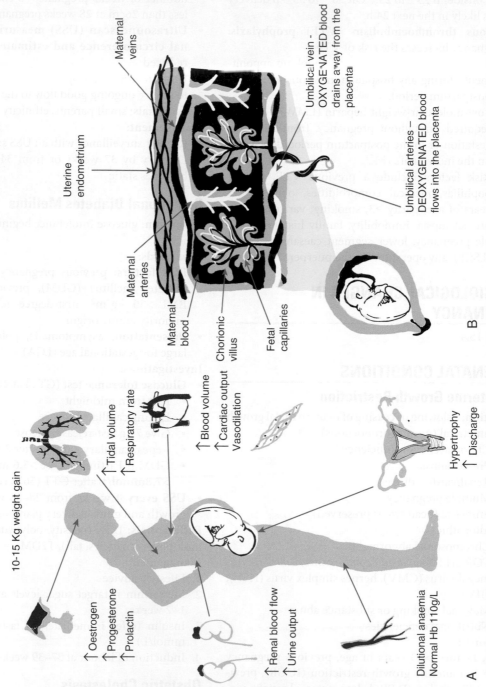

Fig 15.4 Physiological Changes in Pregnancy. (A) Maternal changes in pregnancy and (B) placental anatomy. (Illustrated by Hollie Blaber.)

Maternal veins

Uterine endometrium

Maternal arteries

Maternal blood

Chorionic villus

Fetal capillaries

Umbilical vein – OXYGENATED blood drains away from the placenta

Umbilical arteries – DEOXYGENATED blood flows into the placenta

B

↑ Tidal volume
↑ Respiratory rate

↑ Blood volume
↑ Cardiac output
Vasodilation

Hypertrophy
↑ Discharge

10-15 Kg weight gain

↑ Oestrogen
↑ Progesterone
↑ Prolactin

↑ Renal blood flow
↑ Urine output

Dilutional anaemia
Normal Hb 110g/L

A

Buzzwords:
- **Risk factors:** personal or family history of obstetric cholestasis (OC), multiple pregnancies, hepatitis C, gallstones
- **Presentation:** third trimester, **NO rash**, excoriation, itching of the hands and soles at night, pale stool, dark urine, jaundice

Investigations:
- **Blood:** ↑ alanine aminotransferase (ALT), ↑ alkaline phosphatase (ALP), ↑ bile acids

Differentials: cholecystitis, HELLP syndrome, acute hepatitis

Management:
1. Emollients and antihistamines
2. Ursodeoxycholic acid
3. Monitor liver function tests (LFTs) weekly

Gestational Hypertension

Definition: sustained hypertension (HTN) (>140/90 mmHg) after 20 weeks gestation in a previously normotensive patient. Resolves by 12 weeks postpartum

Buzzwords:
- **Risk factors:** nulliparity, multiple pregnancy, obesity, T1DM, migraines, Black or Hispanic
- **Presentation:** asymptomatic, screening

Investigations:
- **BP:** ×2 elevated readings (>140/90 mmHg) after 20 weeks gestation
- **Urine dip:** NO proteinuria
- **Bloods:** monitoring of the full blood count (FBC), LFTs, U&Es (weekly)

Differentials: pre-eclampsia, essential HTN

Management:
1. Labetalol PO aiming for a BP of 135/85 mm Hg
2. Nifedipine if asthmatic or other contraindications
3. If >160/110 mmHg, admit to hospital
4. Monitor the BP, blood tests and foetal wellbeing weekly

Pre-eclampsia

Definition: HTN with proteinuria as a result of impaired trophoblastic invasion. There is a spectrum of this disease:
- Pre-eclampsia: as above
- Eclampsia: pre-eclampsia with seizures
- HELLP syndrome: evidence of <u>H</u>aemolysis, <u>E</u>levated <u>L</u>iver enzymes and a <u>L</u>ow <u>P</u>latelet count

Buzzwords:
- **Risk factors:** see Table 15.2

TABLE 15.2 Risk Factors for Pre-eclampsia

High Risk	Moderate Risk
• Previous hypertensive disease in pregnancy	• Nulliparity
• Chronic kidney disease	• >40 years of age
• Autoimmune diseases	• >10 years pregnancy interval
• Type 1 diabetes mellitus/type 2 diabetes mellitus	• Body mass index >35 kg/m^2
• Chronic hypertension	• Family history of pre-eclampsia
	• Multiple pregnancies

TABLE 15.3 Types of Antepartum Haemorrhage

Term	Quantity of blood
Spotting	Streaks of blood in the underwear
Minor haemorrhage	<50 mL
Major haemorrhage	50–1000 mL
Massive haemorrhage	>1000 mL + shock

- **Presentation:** severe headache; swelling of the hands, face and feet; visual disturbances; right upper quadrant (RUQ) pain; vomiting; small for gestational age; reduced foetal movements, seizures

Investigations:
- **BP:** >140/90 mmHg
- **Urinalysis:** >30 mg/mmol of protein
- **Bloods:** ↑ LFTs, thrombocytopaenia
- **USS:** reduced foetal growth is common
- **Cardiotocography (CTG):** evidence of foetal distress prompts early delivery
- **Umbilical artery Doppler:** impaired end diastolic flow is a concerning sign suggesting delivery will be required soon

Differentials: essential HTN, gestational HTN, epilepsy

Management:

Pre-eclampsia:
1. Aspirin 150 mg OD from 12 weeks if one high-risk factor or >1 moderate-risk factor (see Table 15.2)
2. Admit to the hospital if there is any clinical concern or the BP >160/110 mmHg
3. Labetalol PO (nifedipine if contraindicated) for BP
4. Corticosteroids and IV magnesium given as per preterm birth guidelines – see Prescribing section earlier.
5. Aim to deliver within 24–48 h of 37 weeks gestation

Eclampsia:
1. ABCDE, move to the left lateral position, O$_2$ and IV access
2. 4 g IV MgSO$_4$ over 5 min
3. 1 g/hr MgSO$_4$ for 24-h maintenance
4. Labetalol to **gradually** lower the BP
5. Emergency LSCS

Antepartum Haemorrhage (APH)

Definition: bleeding from the genital tract after 24 weeks gestation (see Table 15.3)
Investigations:
- **Maternal observations:** tachycardia, hypotension and increased capillary refill time are concerning features
- **CTG/foetal heart auscultation:** possible foetal distress
Differentials:
- **Vaginal:** vaginitis, vaginal trauma
- **Cervix:** mucus show, ectropion

- **Uterus:** placenta previa, placental abruption, vasa previa

Placenta Previa

Definition: placenta covers the cervical os or is <2 cm away (see Fig 15.5)
Buzzwords:
- **Risk factors:** previous termination, placenta previa or LSCS; multiple pregnancy; increased maternal age; smoking; previous adherent placenta requiring manual removal
- **Presentation:** identified at the 20-week scan, APH
Investigations:
- **Anomaly USS at 20 weeks:** evidence of the placenta being close to or covering the cervical os
- **Transvaginal USS (TVUSS) at 32 weeks:** for monitoring, findings as above
- **Blood:** group and save and FBC

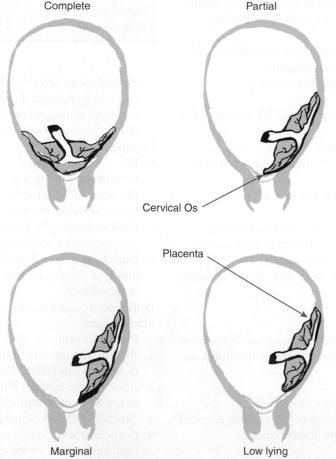

Fig 15.5 Different Types of Placenta Previa. (Illustrated by Hollie Blaber.)

Differentials: as per APH

Management:
- Asymptomatic:
  - Steroids at 34–36 weeks
  - LSCS at 36–37 weeks
- Recurrent bleeds
  - Steroids before 34 weeks
  - LSCS if at 34–36 weeks

Vasa Previa

Definition: foetal vessels run through the placental membranes unprotected, therefore increasing the risk of rupture and haemorrhage during pregnancy

Buzzwords:
- **Risk factors**: placenta previa
- **Presentation**: APH

Investigations:
- **TVUSS with colour Doppler imaging at the anomaly scan:** identifies evidence of foetal vessels in the placental membranes

Management:
1. **If ruptured:** emergency caesarean and neonatal resus
2. **Unruptured:** LSCS scheduled before natural labour

Placental Abruption

Definition: a partial or incomplete separation of the placenta from the uterine wall during pregnancy (see Fig 15.6)

Buzzwords:
- **Risk factors:** previous abruption, pre-eclampsia, foetal growth restriction, abdominal trauma, polyhydramnios, maternal thrombophilia
- **Presentation:** APH, woody uterus, abdominal pain, reduced foetal movements

Investigations:
- Clinical diagnosis
- **Blood:** including FBC, clotting, four units cross-matched, Kleihauer-Betke test (to quantify foeto-maternal haemorrhaging) if the mother is Rh D negative
- **CTG:** evidence of foetal distress
- **USS:** cannot rule out a placental abruption. Detects foetal heart pulsations and guides the timing and mode of delivery

Differentials: as per APH

Management:
1. ABCDE, immediate delivery if there is foetal or maternal compromise
2. Admit to hospital until bleeding has stopped
3. If between 24 and 34^{+6} weeks and likely to deliver, offer a single course of steroids
4. Active management of the third stage of labour is advised

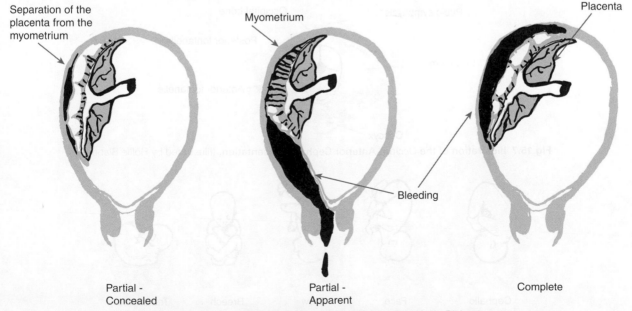

Separation of the placenta from the myometrium

Myometrium

Placenta

Bleeding

Partial - Concealed

Partial - Apparent

Complete

Fig 15.6 Types of Placental Abruption. (Illustrated by Hollie Blaber.)

LABOUR

Normal Labour

Definition: characterised by the onset of regular contractions and rupturing of membranes. Normally occurs spontaneously at 37–42 weeks

Monitoring/investigations:

- **Vaginal examination:** to establish cervix dilation and foetal presentation (see Figs 15.7 and 15.8)
- **Foetal heart auscultation**
- **4-hourly maternal observations**
- **Partogram:** monitors the progression of labour, foetal heart rate, liquor and foetal presentation
- **CTG:** tracing of the foetal heart rate and maternal contractions. Interpret by remembering **DR C BRAVADO** (see Table 15.4)
- **Foetal blood sampling (FBS)** (if evidence of foetal distress. NB: do not perform if HIV positive): a sample of blood is taken from the foetal scalp to identify foetal hypoxia
  - **pH ≥7.25 OR lactate ≤4.1 mmol/L = NORMAL.** Repeat if the foetal heart rate abnormality persists
  - **pH 7.21–7.24 OR lactate 4.2–4.8 mmol/L = BORDERLINE.** Repeat FBS within 30 min or consider delivery
  - **pH ≤7.2 OR lactate ≥4.9 = ABNORMAL.** Immediate delivery indicated

Presentation and foetal lie:

The foetus should be in the occiput anterior (OA) cephalic presentation (see Fig 15.7). Other presentations are shown in Fig 15.8 and may be associated with a prolonged labour.

Stages of labour: see Table 15.5

If poor progress is being made in stages 1 or 2 of labour, consider the **3 Ps**:

- **POWER:** effective uterine contractions? Maternal exhaustion?
- **PASSENGER:** presentation? Lie? Foetal abnormalities?
- **PASSAGE:** the bony pelvis, cervical dilatation

Induction of Labour

Definition: artificially starting the process or increasing the speed of labour

Buzzwords:

- **Indications:** post-dates (>42 weeks), premature rupture of membranes (PROM), preterm premature rupture of membranes (PPROM), DM, multiple pregnancy, IUGR, pre-eclampsia, maternal complications
- **Risks:** prolonged labour, increased rate of instrumental delivery, hyperstimulation, uterine rupture

Investigations:

- Confirm gestation from the **dating scan** performed at 12 weeks

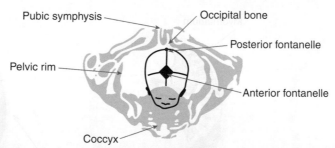

Pubic symphysis — Occipital bone

Posterior fontanelle

Pelvic rim —

Anterior fontanelle

Coccyx —

Fig 15.7 Illustration of the Occiput Anterior Cephalic Presentation. (Illustrated by Hollie Blaber.)

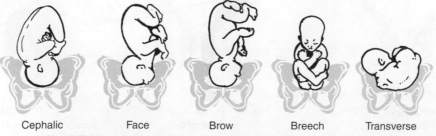

Cephalic　　Face　　Brow　　Breech　　Transverse

Fig 15.8 Illustration of Malpresentations. (Illustrated by Hollie Blaber.)

TABLE 15.4   Interpreting Cardiotocography (CTG) using Dr C BrAVADO

Feature	Definition	Reassuring	Concerning
Define risk	Why are you doing CTG? What risk factors does the patient have for foetal distress?		
Contractions	Strength and timing of maternal contractions		
Baseline rate	Average foetal heart rate	110–160 bpm	>160 bpm = foetal hypoxia, chorioamnionitis, anaemia **<100 bpm for >3 min** = cord compression, cord prolapse, epidural, rapid foetal descent
Variability	Variation from one beat to the next	5–25 bpm	Reduced variability (<5 bpm for >50 min) Increased variability (>25 bpm for >25 min)
Accelerations	Abrupt **increase** from baseline by >15 bpm for >15 sec	Generally reassuring	Alongside contractions
Decelerations (decel)	Abrupt **decrease** from baseline by >15 bpm for >15 sec	Early decel Variable decel associated with an acceleration	Late deceleration Prolonged decel (>3 min): perform foetal blood sampling or delivery Sinusoidal – very worrying feature. May suggest severe foetal hypoxia or anaemia
Overall impression	Is the CTG reassuring or concerning? Do you need to escalate? What further investigations are required?		

TABLE 15.5   Stages of Labour with Approximate Timings

Stage of Labour			Nulliparous	Multiparous
Stage 1 – initiation to full dilation of the cervix. At this stage, the amniotic membranes usually rupture	Latent phase	0–4-cm dilation		
	Active phase	4–10-cm dilation	1 cm/h	2 cm/h
Stage 2 – full dilation to delivery of the foetus	Passive phase	Full dilation till the head reaches the pelvic floor		
	Active phase	Active pushing	40 min (max 2 h)	20 min (max 1 h)
Stage 3 – delivery of foetus to delivery of placenta	Uterus contracts to compress blood vessels of the placenta and the placenta shears from the uterine wall		~15 mins Active management recommended Oxytocin or syntometrine given once shoulders have been delivered to decrease the risk of postpartum haemorrhage	

- **Palpate the foetal lie and presentation:** low lying, well engaged, cephalic
- **CTG**
- **Vaginal examination:** Bishop's score (see Table 15.6)

Management:
1. Membrane sweep offered at 40 and 41 weeks
2. If Bishop's score <8 (see Table 15.6), offer vaginal prostaglandins (pessary or gel)
3. Cook balloon
4. Amniotomy (head must be engaged)
5. Syntocinon

Fetal Distress

Definition: evidence of foetal distress suggested by CTG or FBS

Buzzwords:
- **Risk factors:** induction, prolonged labour
- **Presentation:** meconium-stained liquor, foetal tachycardia, foetal bradycardia, decelerations, loss of variability

Investigations:
- **CTG:** see above
- **FBS:** see above

Management:
1. Left lateral position
2. Maternal IV fluids and O_2
3. Delivery method guided by investigations

Breech

Definition: an inappropriate presentation of the foetus into the canal with the feet first

Buzzwords:
- **Risk factors:** polyhydramnios, foetal abnormalities, multiple pregnancy, uterine abnormalities

- **Presentation:** detected at scan or via abdominal palpation, prolonged labour

Investigations:
- **USS:** to confirm the foetal position
- **CTG:** to monitor for foetal distress

Management:
1. Watch and wait
2. ECV: an attempt to manually turn the baby. Can be performed from 36 weeks (primiparous) or 37 weeks (multiparous)
- USS before and after ECV
- Anti-D required if mother is Rh negative
3. Discuss risks of a vaginal vs LSCS birth – higher perinatal mortality rate with vaginal birth

Operative/Instrumental Deliveries

See Table 15.7 for a summary of operative and instrumental deliveries

Preterm Labour

Definition: regular painful contractions with cervical changes before 37 weeks

Buzzwords:
- **Risk factors:** previous preterm labour (PTL), cervical surgery, multiple pregnancy, uterine abnormalities, urinary tract infection (UTI), sexually transmitted infection (STI), low BMI, smoking, pre-eclampsia
- **Presentation:** regular contractions, abdominal pain, mucus plug

TABLE 15.6 Bishop's Scoring of Cervical Favourability

	BISHOP'S SCORE			
	0	1	2	3
Cervix dilation (cm)	<1	1–2	2–4	>4
Length of cervix (cm)	>4	2–4	1–2	<1
Station (cm from spines)	-3	-2	-1	0 or below
Consistency	Firm	Average	Soft	
Position	Posterior	Central	Anterior	

TABLE 15.7 Overview of Operative and Instrumental Deliveries

	Description	Indication	Benefits and Risks
Episiotomy	Incision made in the perineum (see Fig. 15.9)	Perineum tearing or likely to tear	Benefits: to reduce severity of a tear Risks: infection
Ventouse	Cap applied to foetal occiput and low-level suction applied. Paired cord blood samples should be analysed	To assist with maternal power. Requirements: full dilation, below spine, empty bladder, adequate analgesia	Benefit: assist with power, avoid LSCS Risk: failure, cephalohaematoma or foetal scalp swelling
Forceps	Instrument that assists with delivery Paired cord blood samples should be analysed	Failure to progress *Maximum three pulls* Requires a pudendal nerve block	Benefit: avoid LSCS Risk: failure, increased risk of tear, facial bruising, skull fracture
Caesarean	Incision (Pfannenstiel) and removal of foetus through the abdomen	Type 1: emergency – within 30 min Type 2: urgent – within 75 min Type 3: scheduled early delivery Type 4: elective	Benefit: rapid delivery Risk: haemorrhage, wound infection, VTE, complications in future pregnancies. Increased risk to baby

LSCS, Lower segment caesarean section; VTE, venous thromboembolism.

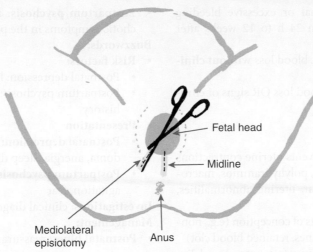

Fig 15.9 Mediolateral Episiotomy at 45 to 60 Degrees From the Midline. (Illustrated by Hollie Blaber.)

Investigations:
- **USS of cervical length**: <15 mm suggestive of PTL
- **Vaginal swab**: Actim Partus (after 22 weeks pregnancy), quantitative foetal fibronectin (from 30 weeks gestation) >50 ng/mL

Differentials: UTI, cervical discharge, placental abruption, symphysis pubis dysfunction, appendicitis

Management:
Prevention: cervical cerclage in the second trimester or vaginal progesterone
1. 2 × 12 mg IM of betamethasone 24 h apart if <36 weeks
2. 4 g IV magnesium sulphate over 15 min and 1g/h until birth or for 24 h
3. Consider tocolysis to allow for completion of steroids

Premature Rupture of Membranes

Definition: a rupture of the amniotic membrane before the onset of labour. If this occurs before 37 weeks, it is termed a preterm premature rupture of membranes (PPROM). After 37 weeks, it is called a premature rupture of membranes (PROM)

Buzzwords:
- **Risk factors**: UTI, STI
- **Presentation**: vaginal discharge, mucus show, no contractions

Investigations:
- **Aseptic speculum examination**: pooling of amniotic fluid
- **Insulin-like growth factor binding protein-1 test or placental alpha-microglobulin-1** (if no pooling): positive
- **CTG**: no evidence of foetal distress is reassuring

Management:
1. Admit for 48–72 h
2. Erythromycin PO QDS for 10 days
3. Consider giving steroids (if <37 weeks) and discuss most appropriate mode of delivery with senior

Cord Prolapse

Definition: a protrusion of the umbilical cord through the cervix past the presenting part of the foetus. **This is an emergency**.

Buzzwords:
- **Risk factors:** unstable lie, amniotomy, polyhydramnios
- **Presentation:** palpable cord, foetal distress

Investigations: clinical diagnosis, immediate management required

Management:
1. Manually elevate the presenting part of the foetus or fill the bladder
2. Left lateral position with head-down or knee-to-chest position
3. LSCS

POSTPARTUM

Postpartum Haemorrhage

Definition:
- **Primary postpartum haemorrhage (PPH)**: >500 mL blood loss from the birth canal within 24 h of delivery

- **Secondary PPH**: abnormal or excessive bleeding from the birth canal from 24 h to 12 weeks after delivery
- **Minor PPH**: 500–1000 mL blood loss **without clinical shock**
- **Major PPH**: >1000 mL blood loss OR signs of **clinical shock**

Buzzwords:
- **Risk factors**: the 4 Ts
  - **Tone**: anything that prevents uterine contractions (e.g., multiple gestation, polyhydramnios, macrosomia, prolonged labour, uterine abnormalities, uterine infection)
  - **Tissue**: retained products of conception (e.g., nonintact placental membranes, retained blood clot)
  - **Trauma**: genital tract injury (e.g., operative delivery, malposition)
  - **Thrombin**: any clotting abnormalities (e.g., preexisting coagulopathy, HELLP syndrome, disseminated intravascular coagulation (DIC), history of PPH)
- **Presentation**: bleeding +/-shock

Investigations: should not delay management
- Regular observations and electrocardiogram (ECG) monitoring
- **Blood**: FBC, coagulation profile, cross match
- Weigh all swabs to estimate the blood loss

Management:
1. Call for help: activate the major haemorrhage protocol. **Blood products should be given as soon as available** with fluid resuscitation until blood is available
2. ABCDE
3. Rub uterine fundus to stimulate contraction
4. Catheterise
5. Uterotonics (e.g., oxytocin, ergometrine and carboprost)
6. Tranexamic acid may be considered
7. Surgical management (e.g., intrauterine balloon tamponade, brace sutures, uterine devascularisation, hysterectomy)

Postpartum Mental Health

Definition:
- **Postnatal blues**: a low mood or mood lability in the first 3–10 days postpartum
- **Postnatal depression**: gradual onset of persistent low mood, anhedonia and anergia over 2 weeks after birth

- **Postpartum psychosis**: rapid development of psychotic symptoms in the postnatal period

Buzzwords:
- **Risk factors:**
  - Postnatal depression: history of depression
  - Postpartum psychosis: bipolar, family or personal history
- **Presentation**
  - **Postnatal depression:** persistent low mood, anhedonia, anergia, sleep disturbances
  - **Postpartum psychosis:** hallucinations, delusions, agitation, fear

Investigations: clinical diagnosis

Management:
- **Postnatal blues:** reassurance and support

THE ONE-LINE ROUND-UP!

Here are some key words to help you remember each condition/concept.

Condition/Concept	One-line Description
IUGR	Symmetric vs asymmetric
GDM	5678 rule
OC	Itching with no rash
Gestational HTN	Hypertension without proteinuria
Pre-eclampsia	Hypertension with proteinuria
Eclampsia	Seizures
HELLP syndrome	**H**aemolysis, **E**levated **L**iver enzymes, **L**ow **P**latelet count
Placenta praevia	Placenta <2 cm from os
Vasa praevia	Vessels in the placental membranes
Placental abruption	Woody uterus
CTG	Dr C BRAVADO
Induction of labour	Bishop's score
Foetal distress	CTG or FBS
Breech	Feet first
PTL	<37 weeks
PROM	Amniotic membrane rupture before labour
Cord prolapse	EMERGENCY
PPH	Tone, tissue, trauma, thrombin
Postnatal blues	3–10 days postpartum
Postnatal depression	Low mood, anhedonia, anergia
Postnatal psychosis	Hallucinations, delusions

- **Postnatal depression:** see management of depression (see Psychiatry in an Hour)
- **Postpartum psychosis:** urgent referral to a specialist psychiatrist

GYNAECOLOGY

CONTRACEPTION

This section will cover reversible contraception methods. Other forms of contraception, such as fertility awareness methods and male or female sterilisation, may also be used in practice.

Four distinct mechanisms of action:
- Suppress ovulation
- Thicken mucus
- Increase hostility of the endometrium
- Decrease tubal motility

Barrier method

Description: condoms or diaphragms used during sexual intercourse
Primary mode of action (MOA): prevents semen from reaching the ovum
Pros: STI prevention (condoms only), no hormones, very effective if used well
Cons: user dependent

Combined oral contraceptive pill (COCP)

Description: tablet containing oestrogen and progesterone – taken for **21 days followed by a 7-day break.** (Guidelines now suggest more 'tailored' regimens involving less frequent and/or shorter hormone-free intervals (HFIs))
Primary MOA: suppresses ovulation
Pros: reliable, independent of sexual intercourse, helps to regulate bleeding and dysmenorrhoea
Cons: increased risks of deep vein thrombosis (DVT), stroke and breast cancer; missed pills; 9% failure rate in the first year with typical use
Contraindications: previous DVT, migraine with aura, cardiovascular disease, breast cancer
Missed pill rules (48 to <72 h since last pill was taken): always consult the guidelines, below is just a guide!

- **1 missed pill:** no extra precautions required, take pill as soon as remembered
- **2 or more missed pills:** take last pills as soon as remembered, condoms until pills have been taken for 7 consecutive days

Emergency contraception should be considered and condoms should be used until pills have been taken for 7 consecutive days, if:
- Unprotected sexual intercourse (UPSI) during the HFI **AND** late restarting following the HFI (≥9 days without an active pill)
- UPSI in the HFI or week 1 **AND** 2–7 pills are missed in week 1 after HFI
- >7 missed pills in any pill-taking week

NB: the combined transdermal patch and vaginal ring work in similar ways to COCPs and may be preferred by some women

Progesterone-only pill (POP)

Description: a tablet containing progesterone that is taken **daily (same time every day)**
Primary MOA: thickens the cervical mucus
Pros: reliable, independent of sexual intercourse, fewer contraindications than COCPs
Cons: irregular bleeding, missed pills
Contraindications: current breast cancer
Missed pill rules (if taken >12 h late or >3 h for some pills)

- **1 missed pill:** extra protection for 2 days
- Emergency contraception required if UPSI after missed pill

Long-acting Reversible Contraception

Progesterone implant – Nexplanon

Description: a small device implanted under the skin of the arm. Lasts for **3 years**
Primary MOA: preventing ovulation
Pros: very reliable, >99% effective, not user dependant, no delay in return to fertility
Cons: irregular, unpredictable bleeding, requires a procedure for inserting and removing

Progesterone injection

Description: IM or SC injection of progesterone given every **12–14 weeks**
Primary MOA: suppresses ovulation
Pros: very reliable
Cons: delay in return of fertility, osteoporosis, weight gain (particularly if <18 years of age and a BMI of >30 kg/m^2)

Levonorgestrel intrauterine system (IUS)

Description: progesterone-containing coil placed in the uterus for **3–5 years**

Primary MOA: prefertilisation effect (prevents blastocyst formation) and endometrium hostility

Pros: very reliable; low-level, localised hormone release; often amenorrhoeic

Cons: requires a procedure for inserting and removing, can introduce infection, missing threads

Contraindications: pelvic inflammatory disease (PID) acutely; cervical, breast or endometrial cancer

Intrauterine device (IUD) – copper coil

Description: copper coil placed in the uterus for up to **10 years**

Primary MOA: spermicidal and prevention of implantation

Pros: no hormones, very reliable

Cons: requires a procedure for inserting and removing, menorrhagia, dysmenorrhoea

Contraindications: PID – acute, cervical and endometrial cancer

Emergency Contraception

Oral medication or IUD to prevent pregnancy following UPSI. You should also check for STI risk and future contraceptive plans.

IUD: copper coil

- Always offer if eligible and advise that this device is the most effective method of emergency contraception
- Prevents fertilisation due to toxicity to the ovum and sperm
- Up to 120 h after UPSI OR up to 5 days after earliest likely ovulation date
  - To calculate: (shortest reported cycle −14) + 5
  - e.g., **28-day cycle:** subtract 14 = ovulation day (day 14). Add 5 days to **day 19**. Therefore, copper coil can be used up to day 19 of the cycle (where day 1 is the first day of menstruation)
- Not advised if symptomatic STI

Emergency hormonal contraception:

delays ovulation but INEFFECTIVE if ovulation has already occurred

- **Levonelle:** 1500 µg of levonorgestrel
  - High-dose progesterone inhibits/postpones ovulation
  - Up to **72 h** after UPSI
  - **Double dose** required if **BMI >26 kg/m²** or weight >70 kg

- **EllaOne:** 30 mg ulipristal acetate
- Selective progesterone-receptor modulator that delays ovulation
- Up to **120 h** after UPSI
- Wait 5 days before restarting POP or COCP – need extra protection
- NB: this should be avoided if POPs or COCPs have been used 7 days prior, as it may be less effective

EARLY PREGNANCY
Miscarriage

Definition: a spontaneous loss of pregnancy before 24 weeks gestation. May occur early (<13 weeks) or late (13–24 weeks). Types include:

- **Threatened:** viable pregnancy with vaginal bleeding
- **Incomplete:** non-viable pregnancy with vaginal bleeding and tissue present on USS
- **Missed:** non-viable pregnancy confirmed by USS with no vaginal bleeding
- **Inevitable:** non-viable pregnancy with vaginal bleeding and open os with tissue remaining
- **Complete:** all products of conception have been expelled, and bleeding has stopped
- **Recurrent:** three or more consecutive miscarriages with the same partner

Buzzwords:

- **Risk factors:** previous miscarriage, systemic lupus erythematous, antiphospholipid syndrome, clotting abnormalities, DM, uterine abnormalities, polycystic ovary syndrome (PCOS), STI, increasing maternal age
- **Presentation:** vaginal bleeding, lower abdominal pain

Investigations:

- **Urine β-hCG:** negative
- **Speculum examination:** to identify any tissue in the cervix
- **USS:** may show an empty gestational sac, no foetal heartbeat or a small crown-rump length for dates
  - TVUSS from 5.5 weeks gestation
  - Abdominal USS from 8 weeks gestation

Differentials: spotting, cervicitis, ectopic pregnancy, molar pregnancy

Management:

1. Discuss most appropriate management with patient
   - Expectant: watch and wait

- Medical: mifepristone and misoprostol
- Surgical: evacuation of retained products of conception
2. Anti-D given if mother is Rh negative and managed surgically
3. Repeat pregnancy test in 3 weeks and return if positive
4. If recurrent miscarriage, refer to specialist services

Ectopic Pregnancy

Definition: a pregnancy that implants outside of the uterine cavity, most commonly in the fallopian tube
Buzzwords:
- **Risk factors:** PID, previous ectopic, any uterine surgery, smoking, >35 years of age, IUD
- **Presentation:** 6–8 weeks, missed period, vaginal bleeding, abdominal pain, shoulder tip pain, shock

Investigations:
- **Urine β-hCG:** positive
- **Blood:** serum β-hCG and progesterone (to guide management) and group and save
- **TVUSS:** to identify the location and measure the size of the pregnancy
  - NB: if serum β-hCG >1500 IU/L and pregnancy is not located on USS, assume a pregnancy of unknown location
- Exploratory laparoscopy may be required
- If diagnostic uncertainty, repeat the serum β-hCG in 48 h. If it is between a 50% decrease and a 63% increase, it is likely an ectopic pregnancy

Differentials: molar pregnancy, ovarian torsion, appendicitis, PID
Management: dependent on the presentation and stage of pregnancy
Expectant management if: systemically well, tubal mass <3.5 cm, serum β-hCG <1500 IU/L
1. Repeat serum β-hCG levels twice weekly. >50% fall in 7 days is expected
2. Repeat USS in 1 week and expect a reduction in the adnexal mass
Medical management if: no signs of rupture, tubal mass <3.5 cm, serum β-hCG <5000 IU/L
1. Methotrexate (IM) (contraindications = immunodeficiency, anaemia, leucopoenia, breastfeeding)
2. Repeat serum β-hCG, FBC, U&Es and LFTs on days 1, 4 and 7
3. Repeat methotrexate if inadequate response
Surgical management if: significant pain and systemically unwell, tubal mass >3.5 cm, serum β-hCG >5000 IU/L

1. Laparoscopic salpingectomy
2. Anti-RhD if mother is Rh D negative
3. Home pregnancy test 3 weeks later

Molar Pregnancy

Definition: a spectrum of disease defined as gestational trophoblastic disease. There are multiple types:
- **Partial molar pregnancy:** a normal ovum is fertilised by two sperm resulting in 69 chromosomes. Foetus dies during weeks 8–9 of gestation
- **Complete molar pregnancy:** an enucleate ovum is fertilised by one sperm resulting in 23 chromosomes. No foetus
- **Malignant disease:** occurs as a result of the incomplete clearance of a molar pregnancy
  - Invasive: confined to the uterus
  - Choriocarcinoma: haematogenous spread
  - Placental site trophoblastic tumour

Buzzwords:
- **Risk factors:** N/A
- **Presentation:** irregular vaginal bleeding, large for dates, hyperemesis gravidarum, hyperthyroidism

Investigations:
- **USS:** 'snowstorm' appearance with increased vascularity
- **Histology:** to confirm type

Differentials: ectopic pregnancy, hyperemesis gravidarum, ovarian torsion, appendicitis
Management:
1. Surgical management required: suction curettage with histology
2. Referral to regional centre, chemotherapy may be required (more common if a complete mole)
3. Repeat serum β-hCG every 2 weeks
4. Wait for 6 months before trying to conceive again or follow advice given by regional centre

Termination

Definition: ending a pregnancy through a medical or surgical intervention. It may be performed for any of the below reasons (as per the 1967 Abortion Act):
- A – Continuing the pregnancy would involve risk to the life of the pregnant woman
- B – To prevent grave permanent injury to the physical or mental health of the mother
- **C – Pregnancy NOT exceeding 24 weeks and there is risk to the mother's physical or mental health**
- D – Pregnancy NOT exceeding 24 weeks and there is a risk to the other children of the mother

TABLE 15.8 Management Options for Abortion

Management Option	Description
Medical abortion (<10 weeks)	May be completed at home or in hospital 1. Oral mifepristone 2. Wait 24–48 h 3. Vaginal misoprostol
Medical abortion (10–24 weeks)	As above, however must occur at the hospital. May require repeat misoprostol
Medical abortion (>24 weeks)	Specialist centre management
Surgical abortion (<14 weeks)	1. Misoprostol PV/SL 2. Surgical-vacuum aspiration
Surgical abortion (14–24 weeks)	1. Misoprostol PV/SL 2. Surgical dilation and evacuation

- **E – Substantial risk that the child will be severely handicapped**

Clauses C and E are the most common reasons. The above conditions must be agreed upon by two registered medical practitioners.

Buzzwords:
- **Risk factors:** unplanned pregnancy, maternal health problems, congenital malformations, social problems
- **Presentation:** referral to a termination clinic

Investigations:
- **USS:** to confirm a live foetus
- **Bloods:** FBC, group and save, Rh status

Management: management should be completed within 2 weeks from the time of referral
- See Table 15.8 for management options
- Anti-Rh-D should be given to all Rh-negative females undergoing an abortion
- 2-week follow-up to ensure negative pregnancy test

Hyperemesis Gravidarum

Definition: prolonged and severe nausea and vomiting resulting in electrolyte imbalances and weight loss of >5% starting before 11 weeks of gestation. This is a diagnosis of exclusion.

Buzzwords:
- **Risk factors:** personal or family history, multiple gestation, obesity
- **Presentation:** nausea, vomiting, weight loss >5% (of pre-pregnancy weight), electrolyte disturbances, dehydration

Investigations:
- **Weight:** >5% weight loss from the pre-pregnancy weight
- **Urine dip:** to rule out a UTI and check for protein/ketones
- **Bloods:** deranged urea and electrolytes

Differentials: morning sickness, molar pregnancy, gastroenteritis

Management:
1. Reassurance that this condition should resolve by 16–20 weeks
2. If severe, try cyclizine, promethazine or prochlorperazine and review in a week
3. Metoclopramide or ondansetron may be tried for a maximum of 5 days

GYNAECOLOGICAL CONDITIONS

Polycystic Ovary Syndrome

Definition: an endocrine disorder that occurs at the time of puberty and is characterised by hyperandrogenism, polycystic ovaries and an increased incidence of glucose intolerance.

Buzzwords:
- **Risk factors:** familial, obesity
- **Presentation:** obesity, hirsutism, acne, oligomenorrhoea, infertility, dysmenorrhoea, alopecia, acanthosis nigricans

Investigations:
- Diagnostic tests (2/3 features present):
  - Total testosterone (raised), LH:FSH ratio (raised)
  - Day 21 progesterone (low in anovulatory cycles)
  - USS (>12 follicles in at least one ovary or ovarian volume >10 cm³)
- Other blood tests: prolactin, thyroid-stimulating hormone (TSH), fasting lipids

Differentials: obesity, hyperprolactinaemia, Cushing syndrome, hypogonadotrophic hypogonadism

Management: symptomatic management as no specific treatment
1. Promote healthy lifestyle and weight loss
2. Screen for T2DM, cardiovascular disease, obstructive sleep apnoea and low mood
3. Cyclical progestogen to induce withdrawal bleeds
4. Provide advice for management of hirsutism, acne and infertility

Endometriosis

Definition: oestrogen-receptive endometrial cells are found outside of the uterine cavity, resulting in cyclical symptoms. Common sites include the ovaries, uterosacral ligament and retro-uterine pouch. However, may be found anywhere (e.g., bladder, bowel, lungs).

Buzzwords:

- **Risk factors:** nulliparity, early menarche, family history, low BMI, white ethnicity
- **Presentation:** chronic pelvic pain (>6 months) and the **5 Ds = d**ysmenorrhoea**, d**yspareunia, **d**ysuria, **d**yschesia (painful bowel movements)**, d**isorders of menstruation (e.g., menorrhagia, irregular cycles). Also infertility, haematuria, adnexal tenderness

Investigations:

- **STI screen:** negative
- **Abdominal and pelvic USS:** cysts
- ***Laparoscopic visualisation of the pelvis*:** powder-burn lesions and chocolate cysts

Differentials: STIs, PCOS, adenomyosis, ovarian cysts, PID

Management:

1. Analgesia: paracetamol +/- NSAIDs
2. Hormonal: COCP, oral progestogen (medroxyprogesterone), Mirena coil
3. Surgical: if refractory to other methods
   a. Surgical ablation or excision of endometriotic lesions
   b. Radical hysterectomy
4. If infertility problems, consider IVF if not pregnant within 6 months of trying

Adenomyosis

Definition: a condition in which oestrogen-receptive endometrial cells are found within the muscular wall of the uterus

Buzzwords:

- **Risk factors:** family history, autoimmune conditions
- **Presentation:** cyclical symptoms, dysmenorrhoea, menorrhagia, feelings of heaviness in the pelvis

Investigations: often a clinical diagnosis once other causes have been excluded

- **TVUSS:** small cystic spaces within the myometrium
- **MRI:** endometrial tissue within the myometrium

Differentials: endometriosis, dysmenorrhoea, IBD, PID, ovarian cyst

Management: guided by symptoms and whether fertility needs to be preserved

1. Non-hormonal: mefenamic acid or NSAIDs
2. Hormonal: progesterone coil, COCP or other contraceptives
3. Surgical (permanently reverses fertility): uterine artery embolisation or hysterectomy

Pruritis Vulvae

Definition: itching of the vulva

Buzzwords:

- **Risk factors:** infections (e.g., candidiasis, trichomoniasis, bacterial vaginosis), pregnancy, atrophic vulvovaginitis, vulval cancer, lichen planus (glossy appearance) and lichen sclerosis (hypopigmentation), psoriasis
- **Presentation:** vaginal itching, soreness, vaginal bleeding, abnormal discharge

Investigations:

- **Vaginal swab:** test for infections
- **Skin biopsy:** if abnormal skin identified

Management:

1. Treat underlying cause
2. Refer if any additional concerns (e.g., malignancy)
3. Emollient and antihistamine + a low-potency steroid cream may be used for 2 weeks

Bartholin's Cyst/Abscess

Definition:

- **Bartholin gland:** small glands on each side of the vaginal vestibule which lubricate the vagina
- **Bartholin's cyst:** blockage of the duct resulting in a small, fluid-filled, epithelial cell–lined cavity
- **Bartholin's abscess:** infection of the cyst resulting in rapid development and inflammation at the site. This is most often caused by *Escherichia coli*

Buzzwords:

- **Risk factors:** reproductive age
- **Presentation:**
  - **Cyst:** focal vaginal swelling, worse after intercourse
  - **Abscess:** erythematous, indurated with a fluctuant centre

Investigations: clinical diagnosis

Management:

1. Conservative: warm bath and compresses to aid drainage
2. If abscess: antibiotics and incision and drainage may be required
3. If persistent or recurrent, surgical intervention:
   a. Marsupialisation
   b. Balloon catheter insertion

Fibroids

Definition: benign tumours (a.k.a., leiomyomas) that grow in uterine tissue (see Fig 15.10)

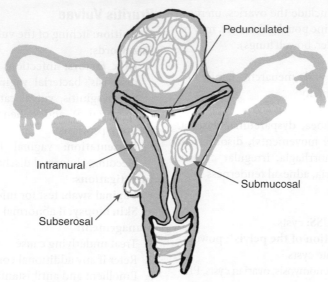

Pedunculated

Intramural

Submucosal

Subserosal

Fig 15.10 Types of Fibroids. (Illustrated by Hollie Blaber.)

Buzzwords:

- **Risk factors:** reproductive age, obesity, increasing age, Black ethnicity, family history, nulliparity
- **Presentation:** dysmenorrhoea, menorrhagia, IMB, dyspareunia, infertility, abdominal distension, mass effect symptoms (e.g., urinary retention and constipation)

Investigations:

- **USS:** to confirm the presence of fibroids
- **Endometrial biopsy** (if diagnostic uncertainty): no evidence of malignancy

Management: if asymptomatic – no management required

1. Medical management of menorrhagia:
   a. If no uterine distortion: hormonal coil (Mirena) may help
   b. If uterine distortion: tranexamic acid and NSAIDs
2. Other surgical management:
   a. Myomectomy
   b. Uterine artery embolisation
   c. Hysterectomy

Prolapse

Definition: descent of the uterus or other organs beyond their normal anatomical confines (see Fig 15.11).

Buzzwords:

- **Risk factors:** increasing age, childbirth, menopause, obesity, iatrogenic
- **Presentation:** dragging sensation, heaviness, urinary incontinence, sexual dysfunction, defecating issues

Investigations:

- Clinical diagnosis: vaginal examination to confirm which vaginal wall is affected

Differentials: stress incontinence, overactive bladder, obstructive defecation syndrome

Management:

1. Reassurance and conservative measures: weight loss and pelvic floor exercises
2. Topical vaginal oestrogen
3. Pessaries
4. Surgical repair may include:
   a. Anterior/posterior wall repair
   b. Vaginal hysterectomy
   c. Colpocleisis (closure of the vagina)

Menopause

Definition: the permanent cessation of menstruation due to loss of ovarian follicle activity, a fall in oestrogen and a rise in LH and FSH levels

- **Perimenopausal:** onset of irregular periods and vasomotor symptoms
- **Postmenopausal:** after the last period (determined retrospectively following 12 months of amenorrhoea)
- **Premature menopause:** menopause occurring before 40 years of age

Buzzwords:

- **Risk factors:** increasing age
- **Presentation:** irregular periods, vasomotor symptoms (e.g., hot flush, night sweats, sleep disturbances),

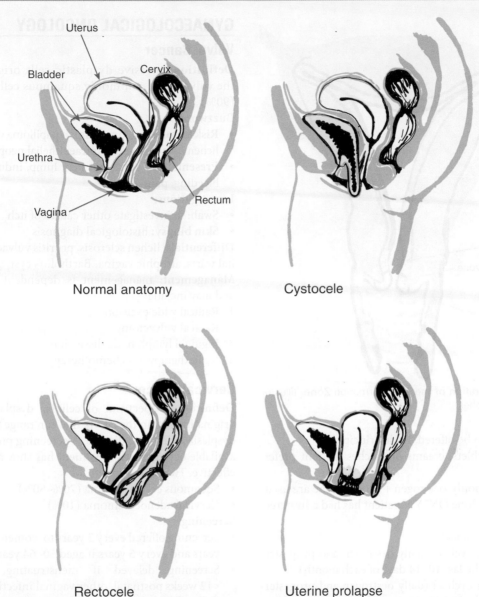

Normal anatomy — Uterus, Bladder, Cervix, Urethra, Vagina, Rectum

Cystocele

Rectocele

Uterine prolapse

Fig 15.11 Types of Prolapse. (Illustration by Hollie Blaber.)

urogenital problems (e.g., vaginal atrophy, dyspareunia, UTIs), decreased libido, osteoporosis

Investigations: usually a clinical diagnosis. To confirm diagnosis:

- **Serum FSH** (two samples, 4–6 weeks apart): raised
- **Anti-Mullerian hormone** (measures ovarian reserve): low
- **Blood:** ↓ oestradiol, ↑ LH, LFTs (should be checked prior to starting hormone replacement therapy (HRT))

Differentials: hypothyroidism, hyperthyroidism, pregnancy

Management: treatment offered for symptomatic management

1. Assess cardiovascular and osteoporosis risk (HRT is recommended until 50 years of age to reduce these risks)
2. Advise on lifestyle modifications to help cope with vasomotor symptoms and vaginal dryness
3. Selective serotonin reuptake inhibitors (SSRIs) may help with vasomotor symptoms

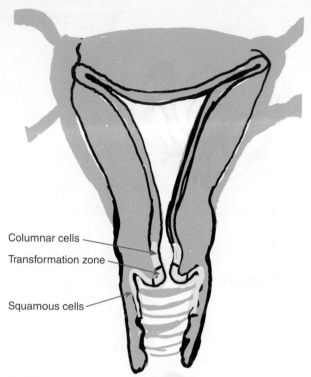

Columnar cells

Transformation zone

Squamous cells

Fig 15.12 Illustration of the Transformation Zone. (Illustration by Hollie Blaber.)

4. HRT should be offered. Basic principles:
- Given as tablets, creams or patches (patient preference)
- Most commonly, oestrogen + progesterone are used
- Oestrogen alone ONLY if patient has had a hysterectomy
- If perimenopausal
  - 1-month cyclical (daily oestrogen and progesterone for the last 10–14 days of each month)
  - 3-month cyclical (daily oestrogen and progesterone for the last 10–14 days of every 13 weeks)
- If postmenopausal
  - 3-month cyclical
  - Continuous combined (oestrogen and progesterone taken daily)
  - Tibolone may be given (must be postmenopausal >1 year)
- If early menopause
  - Sex steroid replacement and choice of combined HRT
- **Contraindications:** breast cancer or other oestrogen-dependent cancers, VTE risk, endometrial hyperplasia, deranged LFTs, recent myocardial infarction (MI)

GYNAECOLOGICAL ONCOLOGY

Vulval Cancer

Definition: invasive dysplastic cells originating on the vulva, most commonly squamous cell carcinoma (90%)

Buzzwords:
- **Risk factors:** smoking, human papilloma virus (HPV), lichen sclerosis, vulval intraepithelial neoplasia (VIN)
- **Presentation:** persistent itch, lump, indurated ulcer, bleeding, pain

Investigations:
- **Swab:** to investigate other causes of itch
- **Skin biopsy:** histological diagnosis

Differentials: lichen sclerosis, pruritis vulvae, VIN, genital warts, atrophic vagina, Bartholin's cyst

Management: management is dependent on staging and may include:
1. Radical wide excision
2. Radical vulvectomy
3. Inguinal lymph node dissection
4. Radiotherapy +/- chemotherapy

Cervical Cancer

Definition: a spectrum of cellular dysplasia in cells originating within the cervix that can range from a mild dysplasia to invasive disease. A screening programme is available because early treatment has shown to be very effective. Two main types:
- Squamous cell carcinoma (70%–80%)
- Cervical adenocarcinoma (10%)

Screening:
- Screening offered every 3 years to women aged 25–49 years and every 5 years if aged 50–64 years
- Screening delayed if menstruating, pregnant, <12 weeks postnatal, other vaginal infections
- Cells taken from the squamo-columnar junction (see Fig. 15.12) and tested for HPV 16/18.
- If positive: cytology is performed
  - Cytology normal: retest in 1 year
  - Cytology abnormal (see Table 15.9): refer for colposcopy (2 weeks if CIN II or CIN III, 6 weeks if CIN I)

Buzzwords:
- **Risk factors:** HPV 16/18, no Gardasil 9 vaccine, 25–49 years of age, multiple sexual partners, immunosuppression, smoking, increased oestrogen exposure, family history, non-attendance at screening
- **Presentation:** screening, postcoital bleeding, IMB, altered vaginal discharge, dyspareunia

TABLE 15.9 Grading of Cervical Cancer

Grade	Cytology	Histology	Management
CIN I	Mild dyskaryosis	Lower 1/3 of epithelium	May spontaneously regress
CIN II	Moderate dyskaryosis	Lower 2/3 of epithelium	Require LLETZ and 6-month follow-up
CIN III	Severe dyskaryosis	Full thickness of epithelium	

CIN, Cervical intraepithelial neoplasia; LLETZ, large loop excision of the transformation zone.

Investigations:

- **Cervical screening** (HPV testing +/- cytology): if detected during screening programme, send straight to colposcopy
- **Colposcopy**
  - Acetic acid: damaged cells appear white
  - Iodine: only taken up by normal cells
- **Large loop excision of the transformation zone** (LLETZ): histological confirmation of in situ or invasive
- Staging requires FBC, U&E, LFTs, chest X-ray (CXR), CT abdomen + pelvis, biopsy as above

Differentials: STI, ectropion, PID, vulval cancer, polyp, endometrial cancer

Management:

- **Prevention**: HPV vaccine – quadrivalent Gardasil (HPV 6, 11, 16, 18) for girls and boys aged 12–13 years.
- Dependent on staging (FIGO): see Table 15.10

Endometrial Cancer

Definition: a malignant neoplasm arising from the endometrium. The two most common types are:

- Endometroid (80%): including adenocarcinoma and mucinous adenocarcinoma
- Non-endometroid (20%): including serous carcinoma, clear cell or a mixed histology

Buzzwords:

- **Risk factors:** unopposed oestrogen (early menarche, nulliparity, HRT, COCP, PCOS, obesity, tamoxifen, liver cirrhosis), family history, hereditary nonpolyposis colorectal cancer (HNPCC), increasing age
- **Presentation:** PMB, IMB, endometrial hyperplasia

Investigations:

- **TVUSS:** endometrial thickness of >4 mm in a postmenopausal women is concerning

TABLE 15.10 FIGO Staging and Management of Cervical Cancer

FIGO Staging	Description	Management
0	CIN II or CIN III – in situ	LLETZ
Ia	Dysplastic cells limited to the cervix with only microscopic spread	Hysterectomy (family complete) OR LLETZ and bilateral pelvic lymph node dissection (to preserve fertility)
Ib	Dysplastic cells limited to the cervix with only microscopic spread	Radical hysterectomy OR Radical trachelectomy (only if fertility needs to be preserved)
II	Spread to uterus, parametrium and upper 2/3 vaginal wall	Chemoradiation is first line for advanced disease. Palliative care may be appropriate (see Palliative Care and Oncology in an Hour)
III	Spread to the pelvic side wall	
IV	Spread to adjacent organs (a) or distant metastases (b)	

CIN, Cervical intraepithelial neoplasm; LLETZ, large loop excision of the transformation zone.

- **Hysteroscopy and biopsy:** histological grading
- **Staging investigations**
  - **Blood:** FBC, U&E, LFTs
  - **CT chest, abdomen and pelvis (CAP)**
  - ***Surgical staging*** (see Table 15.11)

Differentials: endometrial hyperplasia, fibroids, polyp, cervical cancer

Management: see Table 15.11

TABLE 15.11 FIGO Staging and Management of Endometrial Cancer

FIGO Staging	Description	Management	Prognosis (5-year survival)
I	Limited to the body of the uterus	Total abdominal hysterectomy with bilateral salpingo-oophorectomy	85%
II	Limited to the uterus and cervix	Radical hysterectomy, bilateral lymph node dissection +/ para-aortic nodes. Pelvic washout and omental sampling. Radiotherapy	75%
III	Extension to the uterine serosa, peritoneal cavity and +/- lymph nodes (pelvic, then para-aortic)	As for stage II, with maximum tumour debulking. Radiotherapy and chemotherapy	45%
IV	Extension to adjacent organs and metastases		25%

TABLE 15.12 Interpretation of the Risk of Malignancy Index

Risk	Risk of Malignancy Index	Risk of Cancer
Low	<25	<3%
Medium	25–250	20%
High	>250	75%

Ovarian Cancer

Definition: a malignancy arising from ovarian tissue
- Epithelial (90%): serous adenocarcinoma, endometrioid adenocarcinoma, mucinous, clear cell
- Other (10%): germ cell tumours

Buzzwords:
- **Risk factors:** increasing age, increased ovulations (early menarche, late menopause, nulliparity, HRT, fertility treatment), endometriosis, cysts, radiotherapy, previous breast or ovarian cancer, smoking, obesity, BRCA1, BRCA2, HNPCC
- **Presentation:** insidious onset, bloating, indigestion, early satiety, abdominal pain, weight loss, mass effect (constipation, urinary frequency), ascites, palpable mass in pelvis

Investigations:
  If concerned about an ovarian malignancy, a risk of malignancy index should be calculated (see Table 15.12).
- **Menopausal state** (No = 1, Yes = 3)
- **Serum CA-125** (tumour marker)
- **Pelvic USS score (U)**

TABLE 15.13 FIGO Staging and Management of Ovarian Cancer

FIGO Staging	Description	Management	Prognosis (5-year survival)
I	Limited to ovaries	Surgery: total abdominal hysterectomy, Bilateral salpingo-oophorectomy, omentectomy, lymph node dissection. Adjuvant platinum-based chemotherapy	75%–90%
II	Limited to pelvis		45%–60%
III	Limited to abdomen	3 cycles of neoadjuvant platinum-based chemotherapy. Surgical resection as above. Palliative management may also be opted for	30%–40%
IV	Metastases		<20%

- 1 point for each: multilocular cyst, solid areas, metastases, ascites, bilateral cysts
- U = 0 (none of above)
- U = 1 (1 of above)
- U = 3 (2–5 of above)

Risk of malignancy index = menopausal status × USS score × CA-125 result. See Table 15.12 for interpretation

- 2-week-wait (2WW) referral if medium or high risk
- Serum β-hCG, alpha foetoprotein and lactate dehydrogenase (if under 40 years of age, to exclude germ cell tumours)
- **CA-125:** for monitoring disease

Management: See Table 15.13

THE ONE-LINE ROUND-UP!

Here are some key words to help you remember each condition/concept.

Condition/Concept	One-line Description
Miscarriage	Loss before 24 weeks
Ectopic pregnancy	Implantation outside the uterine cavity
Molar pregnancy	Snowstorm on USS
Termination	Medical vs surgical management
Hyperemesis gravidarum	Weight loss of >5%
PCOS	Hyperandrogenism, polycystic ovaries, anovulatory cycles
Endometriosis	Dysmenorrhoea, dyspareunia, dysuria, dyschezia, disorders of menstruation
Adenomyosis	Heaviness of the pelvis
Pruritis vulvae	Many different causes
Bartholin's cyst	Worse after intercourse
Bartholin's abscess	Indurated with fluctuant centre
Fibroids	Can cause mass effect
Prolapse	Dragging sensation and incontinence
Menopause	Permanent cessation of menstrual cycles
Vulval cancer	Usually squamous cell carcinoma
Cervical cancer	Screening 25–49 (3 yearly), 50–64 (5 yearly)
Endometrial cancer	Post-menopausal bleeding
Ovarian cancer	Risk of malignancy index

SEXUAL HEALTH

Key Concepts

Prevention:

- Sexual health history should be sought at key contact points (e.g., new registration, contraception consultation)

- Offer STI prevention advice/testing, particularly if <25 years of age, men who have sex with men (MSM), commercial sex workers, frequent partner changes, etc.
- Condom distribution schemes make protection readily available
- An appointment at a sexual health clinic should be available within 2 days or with an online testing service with self-sampling available
- Support for partner notification is given to ensure rapid treatment and to prevent reinfection
- Chlamydia screening is widely available and free to those 16–25 years of age

Prevention in higher risk groups, such as MSM and transgender women

- Discuss safer sex
- Offer hepatitis A and B vaccinations
- Gardasil HPV (6, 11, 16 and 18) vaccination if ≤45 years of age
- Offer pre-exposure prophylaxis (PrEP) if having unprotected anal intercourse
- Discuss post-exposure prophylaxis after sexual exposure (PEPSE) (condoms might break or not be used)
- Test annually for HIV and STIs and every 3 months if having condomless sex with new or casual partners

Chlamydia

Definition: an STI caused by *Chlamydia trachomatis*. The most common STI in the United Kingdom, usually asymptomatic

Buzzwords:

- **Risk factors:** unprotected sex, 15–24 years of age
- **Male presentation:** asymptomatic, urethral discharge, dysuria, rectal pain/discharge
- **Female presentation:** asymptomatic, vaginal discharge, dysuria, postcoital bleeding, lower abdominal pain, dyspareunia

Investigations:

- **Nucleic acid amplification test** (NAAT) detects *Chlamydia trachomatis* from the sites below:
  - **Vulvo-vaginal swab** (patients with a vagina)
  - **First-catch urine** (patients with penis, neo-penis, neo-vagina)
- Pharyngeal and rectal swabs as appropriate
- Window period of 2 weeks during which NAAT testing is inaccurate at detecting infections

Differentials: gonorrhoea, *Trichomonas vaginalis*, bacterial vaginosis (BV), *Candida albicans*

Management: Always check your local guidelines as antibiotics may change due to resistance.

1. Doxycycline 100 mg BD PO for 7 days, abstain from sex until treatment (of both patient and any partners) is completed
2. If pregnant: azithromycin 1 g then 500 mg OD for 2 days or erythromycin
3. Test of cure: only performed if pregnant or poor compliance. If <25 years of age, repeat at 3 months
4. Contact tracing: look-back period of 6 months (4 weeks if male with urethral symptoms)
5. If lymphogranuloma venereum (an invasive form of chlamydia resulting in tissue destruction and lymphadenopathy usually presenting as a rectal infection): requires 3/52 doxycycline

Gonorrhoea

Definition: an STI caused by the intracellular, Gram-negative diplococci, *Neisseria gonorrhoeae*. Infection rates are rapidly increasing (71% increase from 2015 to 2019)

Buzzwords:
- **Risk factors:** unprotected sex, MSM
- **Male presentation (90% men with urethral gonorrhoea will be symptomatic):** mucopurulent urethral discharge, dysuria, urethral irritation, rectal pain/discharge
- **Female presentation:** asymptomatic, vaginal discharge, dysuria, pelvic pain, postcoital bleeding

Investigations:
- **Microscopy** from urethral, rectal or endocervical swabs: intracellular Gram-negative diplococci
- **NAAT** (same sites as above): gonorrhoea detected
- **Culture:** for sensitivity testing (as increasing resistance) is mandatory

Differentials: chlamydia, trichomonas vaginalis, BV, *Candida albicans*

Management:
1. Ceftriaxone 1 g IM as a single dose, abstain from sex until 7 days after treatment (of both patient and any partners) is completed
2. Contract tracing (2 weeks if symptomatic, 3 months if asymptomatic)
3. Test of cure: repeat NAAT 14 days after completion of treatment
4. Disseminated gonorrhoea requires 7 days of ceftriaxone 1g IM/IV

Pelvic Inflammatory Disease (Females)

Definition: an ascending infection from the endocervix resulting in endometritis, salpingitis and oophoritis

Buzzwords:
- **Risk factors:** gonorrhoea, chlamydia, *Mycoplasma genitalium* (less common than chlamydia and usually does not cause disease; however, there is an increasing prevalence of antimicrobial resistance), IUD insertion
- **Presentation:** abdominal pain, vaginal discharge, abnormal bleeding, dyspareunia, fever, purulent cervical discharge, cervical motion and/or adnexal tenderness, RUQ pain (seen in Fitz-Hugh-Curtis syndrome)

Investigations:
- **Pregnancy test:** to rule out pregnancy
- **STI screen:** for chlamydia and gonorrhoea. However, the majority of PID cases are not caused by these organisms.
- **Blood:** ↑ CRP/WCC

Differentials: ectopic pregnancy, UTI, endometriosis, appendicitis, ovarian cyst torsion or rupture, functional pain

Management:
1. Outpatient therapy (if stable):
- 1 g ceftriaxone IM single dose AND
- 100 mg doxycycline PO BD for 14 days AND
- 400 mg metronidazole PO BD for 14 days
- OR metronidazole and ofloxacin (14 days) or moxifloxacin 400 mg OD 14 days
2. Inpatient therapy (if fever >38°C and evidence of abscess or peritonitis): IV until clinical improvement for 24 h
- 2 g ceftriaxone IV daily
- 100 mg doxycycline IV BD (or oral if tolerated)
THEN
- 100 mg doxycycline PO BD for 14 days
- 400 mg metronidazole PO BD for 14 days
3. Review at 72 h if moderate to severe or no improvement, review all at 2–4 weeks

Trichomonas Vaginalis

Definition: a flagellated protozoan that causes an infection transmitted through sexual intercourse

Buzzwords:
- **Risk factors:** unprotected sex, HIV
- **Male presentation:** asymptomatic, urethral discharge
- **Female presentation:** frothy, yellow discharge; malodour; vulval itching; strawberry cervix; vulvovaginitis, 10%–50% are asymptomatic

Investigations:
- **Microscopy** (posterior fornix or self-swab): mobile trichomonads
- **NAAT:** *Trichomonas vaginalis* identified

Differentials: gonorrhoea, chlamydia, BV, *Candida albicans*

Management:

1. Metronidazole, 2 g PO once OR 400 mg BD for 5–7 days, abstain from sex for 1 week and until partner(s) treated
2. Contact tracing from previous 4 weeks and treat partners
3. Test of cure only if recurrent symptoms

Bacterial Vaginosis

Definition: a fall in the number of *Lactobacilli*, with an increase in anaerobic bacteria and a raised vaginal pH (pH >4.5). Most common cause of abnormal vaginal discharge in women of child-bearing age. This condition is not an STI.

Buzzwords:

- **Risk factors:** vaginal douching, new sexual partner, smoking, STIs
- **Presentation:** offensive, fishy-smelling discharge; no itching or irritation; thin, homogenous discharge coating vaginal walls. Up to 50% are asymptomatic.

Investigations:

- **Gram-stained vaginal smear:** few or absent *Lactobacilli* (Gram-positive rods), increase in Gram-variable cocci/bacilli

Differentials: gonorrhoea, trichomonas, chlamydia, candidiasis

Management:

1. Avoid vaginal douching and soaps/shower gel in the genital area
2. Metronidazole 400 mg BD for 5–7 days or a 2g single dose
3. Intravaginal metronidazole gel (0.75%) OD for 5 days or intravaginal clindamycin (2%) cream OD for 7 days

Vulvo-vaginal Candidiasis

Definition: a yeast infection caused by *Candida* spp. (80%–89% are caused by *Candida albicans*). This condition is not an STI.

- Acute: single episode of vulvo-vaginal candidiasis (VVC)
- Recurrent: four episodes of VVC in 12 months

Buzzwords:

- **Risk factors:** DM, immunosuppression, pregnancy, recent antibiotics

- **Presentation:** vulval itch; non-offensive, curdy, white discharge; swelling; fissures

Investigations:

- **Microscopy from a high vaginal swab:** evidence of *Candida* spp. (Gram-positive spores/hyphae)
- **Culture** (if recurrent): sensitivity testing

Differentials: gonorrhoea, trichomonas vaginalis, chlamydia, BV

Management:

1. Good skin care: emollients recommended (avoid irritants such as perfumes and soaps)
2. Fluconazole 150 mg single dose PO (acute) or clotrimazole 500 mg pessary
3. If pregnant or breastfeeding: clotrimazole intravaginal pessary 500 mg for up to 7 nights
4. If recurrent: fluconazole given over 6 months. NB: fluconazole cannot be used in pregnancy

Genital Warts

Definition: benign lesions in the anogenital area caused by HPV. Most caused by HPV 6 and 11.

Buzzwords:

- **Risk factors:** unprotected sex, no HPV vaccine
- **Presentation:** asymptomatic; small, painless lumps; cauliflower-like

Investigations:

- Clinical diagnosis
- *Biopsy* (only if diagnostic uncertainty or lack of a response to treatment): histological confirmation

Differentials: pearly penile papules, molluscum contagiosum, penile cancer

Management:

1. STI screening
2. Podophyllotoxin or imiquimod. NB: these weaken condoms
3. Cryotherapy

Syphilis

Definition: a sexually transmitted infection caused by *Treponema pallidum* (a spirochete bacterium)

Buzzwords:

- **Risk factors:** MSM, recent increase in heterosexuals due to 'bridging' (i.e., bisexual men acquire the infection from other men and then transmit it to a female partner and thus into the heterosexual network), HIV, sub-Saharan Africa and other low- and middle-income countries

- **Presentation**
  - Often asymptomatic and only detected through screening (serology)
  - **Primary:** chancre, painless, indurated, local lymphadenopathy
  - **Secondary:** widespread mucocutaneous rash, condylomata lata, hepatitis, meningitis, deafness
  - Tertiary· cardiovascular syphilis, neurosyphilis (meningovascular (stroke), general paresis (dementia, psychosis)), tabes dorsalis, gait ataxia, paralysis, Argyll-Robertson pupils (accommodates but does not react to light), gummatous syphilis

Investigations:
- **Dark ground microscopy from ulcer:** spirochetes identified
- **PCR** from ulcer swab: treponemal (syphilis) DNA detected
- **Syphilis serology**
  - Enzyme immunoassay (EIA) and *Treponema pallidum* particle agglutination (TPPA): positive lifelong
  - IgM positive: likely to have a recent exposure
  - Rapid plasma reagin (RPR) titre: associated with the load of treponemal infection – used to monitor treatment effectiveness and to detect reinfection
- **STI screen** including HIV

Differentials: very extensive as presents in many ways! May include genital herpes, HIV, genital warts, viral exanthem, pityriasis rosea

Management:
- **Primary or secondary syphilis:** benzathine penicillin IM single dose (if penicillin allergic, give doxycycline)
- **Late latent, cardiovascular or gummatous:** benzathine penicillin IM once weekly for 3 weeks
- **Neurosyphilis:** 14 days of intramuscular procaine penicillin plus probenecid
- If neurological or cardiovascular involvement, give steroids
- Contact tracing: all patients with syphilis should have contact tracing. Look-back period depends on stage of infection
- Pregnant women in the United Kingdom are offered antenatal screening, all women with a positive syphilis serology should be treated unless a clear history of previous treatment and no suggestion of reinfection. Treatment is tailored to gestation and stage of infection
- Follow up at 3, 6 and 12 months (monitor changes in the RPR titre – a fourfold fall is consistent with effective treatment)

Genital Herpes

Definition: anogenital ulcerations caused by infections with either Herpes simplex virus (HSV)-1 (also causes oro-labial herpes) or HSV-2. (Do not confuse HPV (virus which causes genital warts) with HSV.)

Buzzwords:
- **Risk factors:** unprotected sex. ND. can occur in monogamous relationships
- **Presentation:** asymptomatic, multiple small blisters/ ulcers +/- scabs, **painful** ulcerations, inguinal lymphadenitis, systemic features, proctitis

Investigations:
- **HSV PCR from ulcer:** HSV identified
- Test for syphilis and HIV: common coinfections (consider testing for other STIs as appropriate)

Differentials: syphilis, trauma, VVC, UTIs (females), Behcet's disease

Management:
- Saline bathing, oral analgesia and topical anaesthetic (lignocaine ointment)
- Oral aciclovir for 5 days
- If recurrent (>6 cases per year), may offer suppressive antivirals (daily aciclovir)
- In pregnancy, the risk of transmission to the infant is low if the mother was previously infected (maternal antibodies): consider aciclovir suppression from 36 weeks. If primary infection, consider caesarean section

Human Immunodeficiency Virus (HIV)

Definition: a retrovirus that infects CD4-T cells, resulting in immunosuppression; may lead to acquired immunodeficiency syndrome (AIDS)

Buzzwords:
- **Risk factors:** MSM, Black African (50% of heterosexual males and females with HIV were born in countries with a high HIV prevalence), intravenous drug user, sex workers
- **Presentation:** broad spectrum, ranging from asymptomatic to severe illness (below is NOT an exhaustive list)
  - **Primary HIV infection:** fever, malaise, lethargy, sore throat, maculopapular rash, lymphadenopathy, arthralgias
  - **Long-standing HIV infection:** constitutional symptoms, opportunistic infections (e.g., *Pneumocystis jirovecii* pneumonia (formerly known as PCP), TB, cryptococcal meningitis, cerebral

toxoplasmosis), malignancies (e.g., lymphoma, Kaposi's sarcoma, cervical cancer), difficult-to-treat common skin conditions, oral candidiasis, oral hairy leucoplakia, aphthous ulcers, haematological abnormalities

Investigations:

- **HIV testing:** testing should be offered to those with significant risk factors and in areas of high prevalence. Testing should also be considered for patients with HIV indicator conditions, including STIs, hepatitis B or C, herpes zoster, malignant lymphoma, TB, bacterial pneumonia
- **Fourth-generation combined HIV Ab/Ag test:** positive (point of care tests also available)
- **CD4 count:** the risk of opportunistic infections increases as the CD4 count decreases.
- **Viral load:** if **undetectable, it is untransmissible** (U=U)
- **Hepatitis screening (B and C):** high risk of coinfection
- **Blood:** for monitoring and medications
- **STI screen**: chlamydia/ and syphilis

Differentials (for seroconversion): any flu-like illnesses, including syphilis, CMV, EBV, influenza

Management:

1. Referral to HIV specialist
2. Education and contract tracing
3. Treatment with antiretroviral therapy (ART). This is a rapidly evolving field and current guidelines should be used for specific regimens. A combination of at least two different classes should be used
4. Regular monitoring (aim for a CD4 level >350 cells/µL and a viral load of <50 copies)
5. Routine vaccinations offered
6. If CD4 count is <200 cells/µL, co-trimoxazole for prophylaxis against PCP

Prevention:

- **PEPSE:** given if considered high risk (e.g., if receptive anal or vaginal intercourse with HIV-positive, untreated individual). Twenty-eight days of tenofovir, emtricitabine and raltagrevir. Retested after 8–12 weeks
- **PrEP:** medication containing tenofovir and emtricitabine. Now available on NHS for MSM practicing unprotected anal intercourse and other high-risk groups to prevent transmission of HIV.
- **Treatment as prevention:** ART used to maintain an undetectable viral load, which prevents transmission of the disease

THE ONE-LINE ROUND-UP!

Here are some key words to help you remember each condition/concept.

Condition/Concept	One-line Description
Chlamydia	Asymptomatic
Gonorrhoea	Intracellular Gram-negative diplococci
PID	Cervical motion tenderness
Trichomonas vaginalis	Frothy yellow discharge
Bacterial vaginosis	Fishy discharge
Vulvovaginal candidiasis	White curdy discharge
Genital warts	Warty bumps
Syphilis	Painless ulcer
Genital herpes	Painful ulcer
HIV	Treatment as prevention, U=U

READING LIST: OBSTETRICS AND GYNAECOLOGY AND SEXUAL HEALTH IN AN HOUR

THE MENSTRUAL CYCLE

Collier, J. A. B., Longmore, J. M., & Amarakone, K. (2014). *Oxford handbook of clinical specialties*. Oxford University Press.

OBSTETRICS

NHS. *Pregnancy week-by-week*. Accessed April 2021. https://www.nhs.uk/pregnancy/week-by-week/.

Qureshi, H., Massey, E., Kirwan, D., Davies, T., Robson, S., White, J., Jones, J., & Allard, S. (2014). BCSH guideline for the use of anti–D immunoglobulin for the prevention of haemolytic disease of the fetus and newborn. *Transfusion Med*, 24, 8–20. https://doi.org/10.1111/tme.12091.

NICE. (2019). *CG62: Antenatal care for uncomplicated pregnancies*. Accessed April 2021. https://www.nice.org.uk/guidance/cg62/chapter/2-Research-recommendations.

NICE. (2019). *NG25: Preterm labour and birth*. Accessed April 2021. https://www.nice.org.uk/guidance/ng25/chapter/Recommendations#maternal-corticosteroids.

RCOG. (2015). *GTG37a: Reducing risk of venous thromboembolism during pregnancy and the puerperium*. Accessed April 2021. https://www.rcog.org.uk/globalassets/documents/guidelines/gtg-37a.pdf.

BNF. *Prescribing in pregnancy*. Accessed April 2021. https://bnf.nice.org.uk/guidance/prescribing-in-pregnancy.html.

Collier, J. A. B., Longmore, J. M., & Amarakone, K. (2014). *Oxford handbook of clinical specialties*. Oxford University Press.

Antenatal Conditions
Intrauterine Growth Restriction
RCOG. (2014). *GTG31: The investigations and management of the small-for-gestational-age fetus*. Accessed April 2021. https://www.rcog.org.uk/globalassets/documents/guidelines/gtg_31.pdf.

Gestation Diabetes Mellitus
NICE. (2015). *NG3: Diabetes in pregnancy: Management from preconception to the postnatal period*. Accessed April 2021. https://www.nice.org.uk/guidance/ng3/resources/diabetes-in-pregnancy-management-from-preconception-to-the-postnatal-period-pdf-51038446021.

Obstetric Cholestasis
RCOG. (2011). *GTG43: Obstetric cholestasis*. Accessed April 2021. https://www.rcog.org.uk/globalassets/documents/guidelines/gtg_43.pdf.

Gestational Hypertension
NICE. (2019). *NG133: Hypertension in pregnancy*. Accessed April 2021. https://www.nice.org.uk/guidance/ng133.

Preeclampsia
NICE. (2019). *NG133: Hypertension in pregnancy*. Accessed April 2021. https://www.nice.org.uk/guidance/ng133.

Antepartum Haemorrhage
RCOG. (2011). *GTG63: Antepartum haemorrhage*. Accessed April 2021. https://www.rcog.org.uk/globalassets/documents/guidelines/gtg_63.pdf.

Placenta Previa
RCOG. (2018). *GTG27a: Placenta praevia and placenta accreta: Diagnosis and management*. Accessed April 2021. https://obgyn.onlinelibrary.wiley.com/doi/pdf/10.1111/1471-0528.15306.

Vasa Previa
RCOG. (2011). *GTG63: Antepartum haemorrhage*. Accessed April 2021. https://www.rcog.org.uk/globalassets/documents/guidelines/gtg_63.pdf.

Placental Abruption
RCOG. (2011). *GTG63: Antepartum haemorrhage*. Accessed April 2021. https://www.rcog.org.uk/globalassets/documents/guidelines/gtg_63.pdf.

Labour
Normal Labour
NICE. (2017). *CG190: Intrapartum care for healthy women and babies*. Accessed April 2021. https://www.nice.org.uk/guidance/cg190.

Ayres-de-Campos, D., Spong, C. Y., & Chandraharan, E. (2015). FIGO consensus guidelines on intrapartum fetal monitoring: Cardiotocography. *International Journal of Gynecology & Obstetrics*, *131*, 13–24. https://doi.org/10.1016/j.ijgo.2015.06.020.
Collier, J. A. B., Longmore, J. M., & Amarakone, K. (2014). *Oxford handbook of clinical specialties*. Oxford University Press.

Induction of Labour
NICE. (2008). *CG70: Inducing labour*. Accessed April 2021. https://www.nice.org.uk/guidance/CG70.
NICE. (2015). *IPG528: Insertion of a double balloon catheter for induction of labour in pregnant women without previous caesarean section*. Accessed April 2021. https://www.nice.org.uk/guidance/ipg528/chapter/4-Efficacy.
BNF. *Oxytocin*. Accessed April 2021. https://bnf.nice.org.uk/drug/oxytocin.html.
Wormer, K. C., Bauer, A., & Williford, A. E. (2020). *Bishop score*. StatPearls. StatPearls Publishing. Accessed April 2021. https://www.ncbi.nlm.nih.gov/books/NBK470368/.

Fetal Distress
NICE. (2017). *CG190: Intrapartum care for healthy women and babies*. Accessed April 2021. https://www.nice.org.uk/guidance/cg190.

Breech
RCOG. (2017). *GTG20b: Management of breech presentation*. Accessed April 2021. https://obgyn.onlinelibrary.wiley.com/doi/full/10.1111/1471-0528.14465.

Operative/Instrumental Delivery
RCOG. (2020). *GTG26: Assisted vaginal birth*. Accessed April 2021. https://obgyn.onlinelibrary.wiley.com/doi/full/10.1111/1471-0528.16092.
NICE. (2019). *CG132: Caesarean section*. Accessed April 2021. https://www.nice.org.uk/guidance/cg132/chapter/1-Guidance#procedural-aspects-of-cs.

Preterm Labour
NICE. (2018). *DG33: Biomarker tests to help diagnose preterm labour in women with intact membranes*. Accessed April 2021. https://www.nice.org.uk/guidance/dg33/chapter/3-The-diagnostic-tests.
NICE. (2019). *NG25: Preterm labour and birth*. Accessed April 2021. https://www.nice.org.uk/guidance/ng25/chapter/Recommendations#diagnosing-preterm-prelabour-rupture-of-membranes-p-prom.

Premature Rupture of Membranes (PROM)
NICE. (2019). *NG25: Preterm labour and birth*. Accessed April 2021. https://www.nice.org.uk/guidance/ng25/chapter/Recommendations#diagnosing-preterm-prelabour-rupture-of-membranes-p-prom.

Cord Prolapse
RCOG. (2014). *GTG50: Umbilical cord prolapse*. Accessed April 2021. https://www.rcog.org.uk/globalassets/documents/guidelines/gtg-50-umbilicalcordprolapse-2014.pdf.

Postpartum Haemorrhage
RCOG. (2016). *GTG52: Prevention and management of postpartum haemorrhage*. Accessed April 2021. https://obgyn.onlinelibrary.wiley.com/doi/full/10.1111/1471-0528.14178.

Postpartum Mental Health
NICE. (2020). *CG192: Antenatal and postnatal mental health: Clinical management and service guidance*. Accessed April 2021. https://www.nice.org.uk/guidance/cg192.

Collier, J. A. B., Longmore, J. M., & Amarakone, K. (2014). *Oxford handbook of clinical specialties*. Oxford University Press.

GYNAECOLOGY
Contraception
FSRH. (2016). *UK medical eligibility criteria for contraceptive use*. Accessed April 2021. https://www.fsrh.org/standards-and-guidance/documents/ukmec-2016-digital-version/.

Long-acting Reversible Contraception (LARC)
FSRH CEU Guidance. (2020). *Recommended actions after incorrect use of combined hormonal contraception (e.g. late or missed pills, ring and patch)*. Accessed April 2021. https://www.fsrh.org/documents/fsrh-ceu-guidance-recommended-actions-after-incorrect-use-of/.

Emergency Contraception
FSRH Clinical Guideline. (2020). *Emergency contraception*. Accessed April 2021. https://www.fsrh.org/standards-and-guidance/documents/ceu-clinical-guidance-emergency-contraception-march-2017/.

Miscarriage
NICE. (2018). *CKS: Miscarriage*. Accessed April 2021. https://cks.nice.org.uk/topics/miscarriage/.

NICE. (2019). *NG126: Ectopic pregnancy and miscarriage: Diagnosis and initial management*. Accessed April 2021. https://www.nice.org.uk/guidance/ng126.

Ectopic Pregnancy
NICE. (2019). *NG126: Ectopic pregnancy and miscarriage: Diagnosis and initial management*. Accessed April 2021. https://www.nice.org.uk/guidance/ng126.

Molar Pregnancy
RCOG. (2020). *GTG38: The management of gestational trophoblastic disease*. Accessed April 2021. https://www.rcog.org.uk/en/guidelines-research-services/guidelines/gtg38/.

Termination
NICE. (2019). *NG140: Abortion care*. Accessed April 2021. https://www.nice.org.uk/guidance/ng140/resources/abortion-care-pdf-66141773098693.

Legislation.gov.uk. (1967). *Abortion Act 1967*. Accessed April 2021. https://www.legislation.gov.uk/ukpga/1967/87/contents.

Hyperemesis Gravidarum
RCOG. (2016). *GTG69: The management of nausea and vomiting of pregnancy and hyperemesis gravidarum*. Accessed April 2021. https://www.rcog.org.uk/globalassets/documents/guidelines/green-top-guidelines/gtg69-hyperemesis.pdf.

Polycystic Ovary Syndrome (PCOS)
RCOG. (2014). *GTG33: Long-term consequences of polycystic ovary syndrome*. Accessed April 2021. https://www.rcog.org.uk/en/guidelines-research-services/guidelines/gtg33/.

NICE. (2018). *CKS: Polycystic ovary syndrome*. Accessed April 2021. https://cks.nice.org.uk/polycystic-ovary-syndrome#!scenarioRecommendation:3.

Endometriosis
NICE. (2020). *CKS: Endometriosis*. Accessed April 2021. https://cks.nice.org.uk/endometriosis#!scenarioClarification:1.

Adenomyosis
NICE. (2020). *NG88: Heavy menstrual bleeding: assessment and management*. Accessed April 2021. https://www.nice.org.uk/guidance/ng88/chapter/Recommendations#investigations-for-the-cause-of-hmb.

Pruritis Vulvae
NICE. (2017). *CKS: Pruritis vulvae*. Accessed April 2021. https://cks.nice.org.uk/pruritus-vulvae#!diagnosisSub:2.

Bartholin's Cyst/Abscess
Patient info. (2016). *Bartholin's cyst and abscess*. Accessed April 2021. https://patient.info/doctor/bartholins-cyst-and-abscess-pro#ref-5.

NICE. (2009). *IPG323: Balloon catheter insertion for Bartholin's cyst or abscess*. Accessed April 2021. https://www.nice.org.uk/guidance/ipg323/resources/balloon-catheter-insertion-for-bartholins-cyst-or-abscess-pdf-1899867450616261.

Fibroids
NICE. (2018). *CKS: Menorrhagia*. Accessed April 2021. https://cks.nice.org.uk/menorrhagia#!scenario.

NICE. (2018). *CKS: Fibroids*. Accessed April 2021. https://cks.nice.org.uk/fibroids#!scenarioRecommendation.

Prolapse

NICE. (2019). *NG123: Urinary incontinence and pelvic organ prolapse in women: Management.* Accessed April 2021. https://www.nice.org.uk/guidance/ng123/chapter/Recommendations#assessing-pelvic-organ-prolapse.

Menopause

NICE. (2017). *CKS: Menopause.* Accessed April 2021. https://cks.nice.org.uk/menopause#!prescribingIntoSub.

GYNAE-ONCOLOGY
Vulval Cancer

RCOG. (2014). *Guidelines for the diagnosis and management of vulval carcinoma.* Accessed April 2021. https://www.rcog.org.uk/globalassets/documents/guidelines/vulvalcancerguideline.pdf.

Cervical Cancer

NICE. (2017). *CKS: Cervical screening.* Accessed April 2021. https://cks.nice.org.uk/topics/cervical-screening/.

NICE. (2017). *CKS: Cervical cancer and HPV.* Accessed April 2021. https://cks.nice.org.uk/topics/cervical-cancer-hpv/.

Endometrial Cancer

BGCS Guidelines. (2017). *Uterine cancer guideline.* Accessed April 2021. https://www.bgcs.org.uk/wp-content/uploads/2019/05/BGCS-Endometrial-Guidelines-2017.pdf.

NICE. (2021). *CKS: Gynaecological cancers – recognition and referral.* Accessed April 2021. https://cks.nice.org.uk/gynaecological-cancers-recognition-and-referral#!scenario.

Ovarian Cancer

NICE. (2021). *CKS: Gynaecological cancers – recognition and referral.* Accessed April 2021. https://cks.nice.org.uk/gynaecological-cancers-recognition-and-referral#!scenario.

BGCS. (2017). *Epithelial ovarian/fallopian tube/ primary peritoneal cancer guidelines: Recommendations for practice.* Accessed April 2021. https://www.bgcs.org.uk/wp-content/uploads/2019/05/BGCS-Guidelines-Ovarian-Guidelines-2017.pdf.

SEXUAL HEALTH
Key Concepts

NICE. (2019). *QS178: Sexual health.* Accessed April 2021. https://www.nice.org.uk/guidance/qs178/chapter/quality-statement-1-asking-people-about-their-sexual-history#quality-statement-1-asking-people-about-their-sexual-history.

Chlamydia

Nwokolo, N. C., Dragovic, B., Patel, S., Tong, C. Y., Barker, G., & Radcliffe, K. (2016). UK national guideline for the management of infection with Chlamydia trachomatis. *Int J STD AIDS, 27,* 251–267. https://doi.org/10.1177/0956462415615443

Gonorrhoea

BASHH. (2018). *Gonorrhoea.* Accessed April 2021. https://www.bashhguidelines.org/media/1238/gc-2018.pdf.

Public Health England. (2019). *Sexually transmitted infections and screening for chlamydia in England, 2019.* Accessed April 2021. https://assets.publishing.service.gov.uk/government/uploads/system/uploads/attachment_data/file/914184/STI_NCSP_report_2019.pdf.

Pelvic Inflammatory Disease (Females)

BASHH. (2019). *Pelvic inflammatory disease.* Accessed April 2021. https://www.bashhguidelines.org/current-guidelines/systemic-presentation-and-complications/pid-2019/.

Trichomonas Vaginalis

BASHH. (2014). *Trichomonas vaginalis.* Accessed April 2021. https://www.bashhguidelines.org/media/1042/tv_2014-ijstda.pdf.

Bacterial Vaginosis

BASHH. (2012). *Bacterial vaginosis.* Accessed April 2021. https://www.bashhguidelines.org/media/1041/bv-2012.pdf.

Vulvo-Vaginal Candidiasis (VVC)

BASHH. (2019). *Vulvovaginitis.* Accessed April 2021. https://www.bashhguidelines.org/media/1223/vvc-2019.pdf.

Genital Warts

BASHH. (2015). *Anogenital warts.* Accessed April 2021. https://www.bashhguidelines.org/current-guidelines/skin-conditions/anogenital-warts-2015/.

Syphilis

BASHH. (2019). *Syphilis.* Accessed April 2021. https://www.bashhguidelines.org/current-guidelines/all-guidelines/.

Genital Herpes

BASHH. (2015). *Anogenital herpes.* Accessed April 2021. https://www.bashhguidelines.org/current-guidelines/all-guidelines/.

Human Immunodeficiency Virus (HIV)

BHIVA. (2015). *Guidelines for the treatment of HIV-1-positive adults with antiretroviral therapy.* Accessed April 2021. https://www.bhiva.org/file/RVYKzFwyxpgiI/treatment-guidelines-2016-interim-update.pdf.

NICE. (2018). *CKS: HIV infection and AIDS.* Accessed April 2021. https://cks.nice.org.uk/hiv-infection-and-aids#!scenario:3.

BHIVA/BASHH. (2018). *Guideline on the use of HIV pre-exposure prophylaxis.* Accessed April 2021. https://www.bhiva.org/PrEP-guidelines.

Rodger, A. J., Cambiano, V., Bruun, T., et al. (2019). Risk of HIV transmission through condomless sex in serodifferent gay couples with the HIV-positive partner taking suppressive antiretroviral therapy (PARTNER): final results of a multicentre, prospective, observational study. *Lancet, 393*, 2428–2438. https://doi.org/10.1016/S0140-6736(19)30418-0

NICE. (2017). *QS157: HIV testing: Encouraging uptake.* Accessed April 2021. https://www.nice.org.uk/guidance/qs157/chapter/Quality-statement-3-HIV-indicator-conditions.

BASHH. (2021). *UK guideline for the use of HIV post-exposure prophylaxis.* Accessed April 2021. https://www.bashh-guidelines.org/media/1258/pep-2021.pdf.

16

Paediatrics in an Hour

Hannah Punter and Dan Magnus

Important topics covered in other chapters: epilepsy, meningitis, sepsis, epiglottitis

DEVELOPMENT, GROWTH AND PUBERTY

Developmental Delay

Definition: a condition in which the normal skills and behaviours acquired by a child are delayed
- **Median age:** age at which half of the standard population gains a milestone
- **Limit age:** two standard deviations from the mean age for reaching a milestone

Developmental delay may be global or in just one area. The four areas of development with key **limit ages** are shown in Table 16.1.

Buzzwords:
- **Causes:**
  - **Gross motor:** cerebral palsy, Duchenne's muscular dystrophy, spina bifida
  - **Fine motor:** visual impairment
  - **Speech and language:** hearing impairment, learning disability, cleft palate
  - **Social:** attention deficit hyperactivity disorder (ADHD), autism, attachment disorder
  - **Global:** genetic syndromes, cerebral palsy, congenital infections, hypoxic ischaemic encephalopathy, inborn errors of metabolism
  - **Developmental regression:** space-occupying lesion (SOL), infantile spasms, Rett syndrome, lysosomal storage disorders, child abuse

- **Presentation:** a failure to achieve any of the milestones listed in Table 16.1 by the specified age
  - **Gross motor:** asymmetrical motor skills in the first year of life
  - **Fine motor:** can't hold a bottle
  - **Speech and language:** no babbling, not talking yet, not responsive
  - **Social and emotional:** disinterested, doesn't make friends, concerns at nursery/school
  - **Global:** falling behind peers
  - **Developmental regression:** loss of previously gained milestones (this is always concerning!)

Investigations:
- **Developmental assessment:** some or all areas of development are delayed for the child's age
- **Neurological assessment:** focal neurology, reduced/increased tone
- **Vision/audiometry testing:** identify any visual or hearing impairments
- **Blood** (if concerned about infection or developmental regression): deranged thyroid function tests (TFTs), full blood count (FBC) (↑ WCC), ↑ CRP, liver function tests (LFTs) (↑ bilirubin)
- **Metabolic profile** (if developmental regression): inborn errors of metabolism
- **Karyotyping**
- **Electroencephalogram (EEG)** (if evidence of seizures)
- **MRI/CT brain** (if suspicion of an SOL)

Differentials: familial delay, social deprivation, child abuse or maltreatment

Management:

1. Identify and treat any reversible causes of developmental delay
2. Multidisciplinary (MDT) approach to addressing the medical, social and educational needs of the child

TABLE 16.1 Limit Ages for Different Areas of Development

Gross motor	Vision and fine motor
• Head control = 4 months • Sits unsupported = 9 months • Walks independently = 18 months	• Fix and follow = 3 months • Transfers objects = 9 months • Pincer grip = 12 months
Hearing, speech and language	**Social and emotional behaviour**
• Babbling = 7 months • One word = 1 year • Two words = 2 years • Three words = 3 years	• Smiles = 8 weeks • Symbolic play = 2–2.5 years • Interactive play = 3–3.5 years

Growth

Definitions:

- **Growth chart:** charts developed from national data showing the range of expected heights and weights of children at different ages. *Make sure you have familiarised yourself with what a growth chart looks like*
- **Centile:** a statistical term used to describe the distribution of data. If someone is in the 10th centile for height, 10% of the population are shorter than them.
- **Growth stage:** During childhood, the growth rate is dependent on the stage of growth (see Table 16.2). Faltering growth is an important sign that there may be an underlying problem.
- **Mid-parental height:** predicted final height based on the height of your parents
  - BOYS = ([father's height + mother's height] ÷ 2) + 7
  - GIRLS = ([father's height + mother's height] ÷ 2) −7
- **Growth velocity:** a measure of the rate of growth based on multiple measurements taken at least 6 months apart
- **Short stature:** height below the 2nd centile (see Table 16.3 for causes)

TABLE 16.2 Summary of the Growth Stages During Childhood and Disorders of Growth

Growth Stage	% of Final Height	Hormonal Control	Disorders
Foetal: rapid growth	30%	Insulin-like growth factor 2, insulin, human placental lactogen	Chromosomal abnormalities, antenatal infection
Infantile	15%	Good nutrition and thyroid	Cystic fibrosis, congenital heart problems, cleft palate, metabolic conditions
Childhood: slow and steady	40%	Insulin-like growth factor 1	Growth hormone deficiency, Turner syndrome
Pubertal: back length increases	15%	Testosterone and oestradiol	Precocious puberty – early fusion of the epiphyseal plates reduces the total height

TABLE 16.3 Possible Causes of Short and Tall Stature in Children

Causes of Short Stature	Causes of Tall Stature
• **Reduced calorific intake/increased calorific demand:** eating disorder, chronic illness, deprivation • **Endocrine:** growth hormone deficiency or insensitivity, hypothyroid, Cushing's disease • **Genetic:** Turner syndrome, Down syndrome, Noonan syndrome • **Skeletal:** rickets, skeletal dysplasia, scoliosis • **Other:** familial, intrauterine growth restriction, constitutional pubertal delay, chronic illness	• **Increased calorific intake:** obesity • **Endocrine:** hyperthyroidism, congenital adrenal hyperplasia (early growth spurt), excess growth hormone/sex steroids • **Genetic:** Klinefelter's syndrome (XXY), • **Skeletal:** Marfan syndrome, Ehlers-Danlos syndrome • **Other:** familial

- **Tall stature:** height above the 97th centile (see Table 16.3 for causes)

Faltering Growth

Definition: lower weight gain than expected for a child's age, previously referred to as failure to thrive. Considered if:

- Weight below the 2nd centile
- A fall across 2 centiles (or across 1 centile if the birth weight was below the 9th centile/across 3 centiles if the birth weight was above the 91st centile)

Buzzwords:

- **Risk factors:**
  - **Inadequate intake:** feeding difficulties (e.g., cleft palate), eating disorder, developmental delay, maltreatment
  - **Inadequate absorption:** gastro-oesophageal reflux disease (GORD), persistent vomiting, coeliac disease, inflammatory bowel disease (IBD), food allergies
  - **Excess energy expenditures:** cystic fibrosis (CF), cardiac conditions, metabolic conditions, malignancy, renal disease
- **Presentation:** falling weight, feeding difficulties, parental concern

Investigations:

- **Growth chart:** below 2nd centile or falling centiles
- **Food diary:** may show inadequate caloric intake
- **Blood** (if suspicion of an underlying cause): FBC, LFTs, CRP, TFTs, anti-TTG (results vary depending on the cause)

Differentials: prematurity, constitutional delay, familial short stature

Management:

1. Identify and treat the underlying cause
2. Increase intake +/- dietician referral
3. Regular review of growth

Obesity

Definition: body mass index (BMI) >98th centile for the child's height and age. This is an increasingly common problem in childhood and increases the risk of other comorbidities, including hypertension (HTN), hypercholesterolemia and obesity in adulthood.

Buzzwords:

- **Risk factors:** obese parents, sedentary lifestyle, social deprivation, steroids
- **Presentation:** increasing weight, overeating, bullying at school

Investigations: additional tests are often not required

- **Height and weight chart:** >98th centile for BMI
- **Bloods:** ↑ lipids, ↑ fasting glucose, deranged LFTs

Differentials: hypothyroidism, Prader-Willi syndrome, Cushing's syndrome

Management:

1. Assess for associated comorbidities, such as HTN, type 2 diabetes mellites (T2DM) and hypercholesterolaemia
2. Lifestyle modification and counselling
3. Encourage 60 min of moderate exercise daily
4. Orlistat. Consider a 6–12-month trial in children >12 years of age with evidence of comorbidities

Puberty

Definition: The process of sexual maturation resulting from gonadotrophins and sex hormones (see Endocrinology in an hour). The key stages of development for girls and boys are shown in Table 16.4. Common causes of precocious or delayed puberty are shown in Table 16.5.

CARDIOLOGY

Circulatory Changes at Birth

At birth, the cardiovascular system must change to divert blood to the lungs and away from the placenta (see Fig 16.1 and Table 16.6 for a summary of congenital cardiac conditions.). The changes that occur are:

TABLE 16.4	**Summary of Pubertal Development**			
	Average Age (Normal Range) (years)	**Order of Development**	**Precocious**	**Late**
Girls	11 (8–14)	1. Thelarche (breast development) 2. Pubic hair 3. Rapid growth 4. Menarche	Common (<8 years)	Concerning (>13 years with no thelarche or amenorrhea at 15)
Boys	12 (9–15)	1. Testicular enlargement 2. Pubic hair 3. Rapid growth	Concerning (<9 years)	Common (>14 years)

TABLE 16.5 Common Causes of Precocious and Delayed Puberty

Causes of Precocious Puberty	Causes of Delayed Puberty
Gonadotrophin dependent (80%): premature activation of the gonadal axis resulting in the normal sequence. Causes: • Intracranial tumour • Head injury **Gonadotrophin independent (20%):** excess sex steroids resulting in a dissonant sequence of development. Causes: • Congenital adrenal hyperplasia: prepubertal testes and large penis • Adrenal tumour: pubic hair before thelarche • Liver tumour (producing β-hCG): bilateral testicular enlargement	**Hypogonadotropic hypogonadism:** ↓ gonadotrophins. Causes: • Systemic disease • Intracranial tumour • Kallmann syndrome • Hypothyroidism **Hypergonadotropic hypogonadism:** normal gonadotrophins but no gonadal response. Causes: • Klinefelter's syndrome • Turner syndrome • Steroid hormone enzyme deficiencies • Acquired gonadal damage

• Inflation of the lungs lowers the pulmonary pressure because oxygen lowers the pulmonary vascular resistance

• Blood flow to the lungs increases and returns to left side of the heart, resulting in increasing pressures in the left side of the circulation and closure of the **foramen ovale.**

• Pressure changes and a drop in the level of the prostaglandins cause closure of the **ductus arteriosus.**

Patent Ductus Arteriosus

Definition: an acyanotic heart disease in which there is a failure of the ductus arteriosus to close, resulting in flow from the aorta to pulmonary artery.

Buzzwords:
• **Risk factors:** preterm birth, Down syndrome, maternal rubella, female
• **Presentation:** left-to-right shunt; continuous, machine-like murmur; collapsing pulse; heaving apical beat; failure to thrive; shortness of breath (SOB); apnoea

Investigations:
• **Electrocardiogram (ECG):** normal or left ventricular hypertrophy (LVH)
• **Chest x-ray (CXR):** normal or cardiomegaly and increased pulmonary vasculature
• ***ECHO*:** flow from the aorta into the pulmonary artery

Differentials: ventricular septal defect (VSD), atrioventricular septal defect (AVSD), aortic regurgitation

Management:
1. Indomethacin
2. Surgical closure with a coil or occlusion device if indomethacin is unsuccessful

Atrial Septal Defect

Definition: a defect in the septum between the atria (see Fig 16.2)

Buzzwords:
• **Risk factors:** female, maternal alcohol consumption
• **Presentation:** ejection systolic murmur at the upper left sternal edge (ULSE), widely split second heart sound, left-to-right shunt, acyanotic, recurrent chest infections, arrhythmias

Investigations:
• **ECG:** partial right bundle branch block
• **CXR:** cardiomegaly, enlarged pulmonary arteries, increased pulmonary vascular markings
• ***ECHO*:** blood flow between the atria

Differentials: VSD, AVSD, patent ductus arteriosus (PDA), pulmonary stenosis

Management:
1. Monitoring. Many ASDs close spontaneously
2. Cardiac catheterisation and occlusive device insertion

Ventricular Septal Defect

Definition: a defect in the septum between the ventricles (see Fig 16.3)
• Small VSD (<3 mm)
• Large VSD (>3 mm)

Buzzwords:
• **Risk factors:** Down syndrome, Edwards syndrome (trisomy 18), maternal alcohol consumption
• **Presentation:** asymptomatic (if small), loud pansystolic murmur at lower left sternal edge, heart failure, recurrent chest infections, hepatomegaly, acyanotic

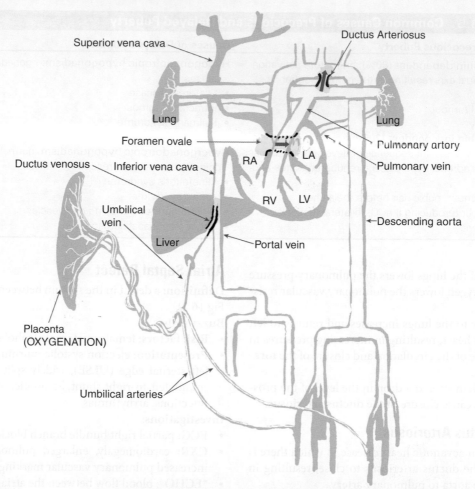

Fig 16.1 Foetal Circulation (Illustrated by Dr Hollie Blaber)

TABLE 16.6 Summary of Paediatric Congenital Cardiac Conditions

	Acyanotic	Cyanotic	Mixed	Obstructive
Presentation	Breathless	Hypoxic	Breathless and hypoxic	Cardiovascular collapse
Problem	Left to right shunt –poor perfusion but good oxygenation	Right to left shunt – poor oxygenation	Mixing between right and left circulation	Severe obstruction to flow
Conditions	Patent ductus arteriosus Atrial septal defect Ventricular septal defect	Tetralogy of Fallot Transposition of the great arteries Eisenmenger's syndrome	Atrioventricular septal defect	Coarctation of the aorta

- **Eisenmenger's syndrome**: increased pulmonary pressures cause a thickening of the pulmonary arteries and an increase in right-sided pressures. This results in a right-to-left shunt and cyanosis.

Investigations:
- **ECG:** bilateral hypertrophy
- **CXR:** cardiomegaly, enlarged pulmonary arteries
- **ECHO:** blood flow between the ventricles

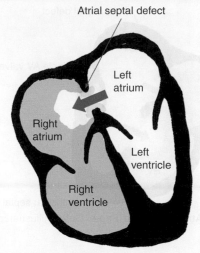

Fig 16.2 Atrial Septal Defect (Illustrated by Hollie Blaber)

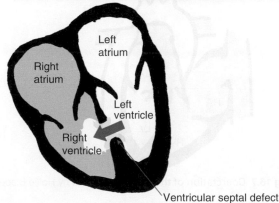

Fig 16.3 Ventricular Septal Defect (Illustrated by Hollie Blaber)

Differentials: ASD, AVSD, PDA, pulmonary stenosis

Management:
1. Manage heart failure (diuretics and captopril)
2. Surgery to prevent Eisenmenger's syndrome
3. There is poor prognosis if Eisenmenger's syndrome develops, and the patient may require a heart/lung transplant.

Tetralogy of Fallot

Definition: a cyanotic heart disease with four key features (see Fig 16.4):
- Large VSD
- Overriding aorta
- Pulmonary stenosis
- Right ventricular hypertrophy (RVH)

Buzzwords:
- **Risk factors:** DiGeorge syndrome, 22q11 microdeletion syndrome, Down syndrome
- **Presentation:** cyanosis, hypercapnic spells, clubbing, loud harsh systolic ejection murmur

Investigations:
- ***ECHO*:** pulmonary stenosis, flow between ventricles, RVH, overriding aorta
- **CXR:** boot-shaped heart

Differentials: AVSD, transposition of the great arteries (TGA)

Management:
1. Prostaglandin infusion: The patient is dependent on the patency of the ductus arteriosus and this prevents its closure.
2. Surgery at 6 months to repair the VSD and perform a pulmonary valve repair/replacement

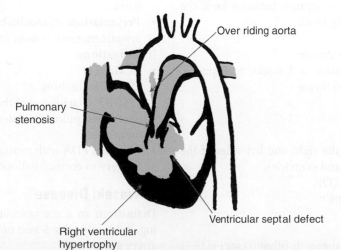

Fig 16.4 Tetralogy of Fallot (Illustrated by Hollie Blaber)

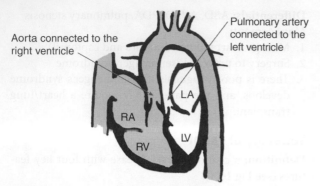

Fig 16.5 Transposition of the Great Arteries (Illustrated by Hollie Blaber)

Transposition of the Great Arteries

Definition: the aorta is connected to the right ventricle, and the pulmonary artery is connected to the left ventricle (see Fig 16.5)

Buzzwords:
- **Risk factors:** rubella, maternal age >40 years
- **Presentation:** cyanotic on day 2

Investigations:
- ***ECHO*:** flow from the right ventricle into the aorta and flow from the left ventricle into the pulmonary artery
- **CXR:** egg-shaped heart

Differentials: AVSD, Tetralogy of Fallot (TOF), coarctation

Management:
1. Prostaglandin infusion
2. Arterial-switch surgical procedure

Atrioventricular Septal Defect

Definition: a defect in the septum between both the atria and ventricles (see Fig 16.6).

Buzzwords:
- **Risk factors:** Down syndrome
- **Presentation:** heart failure at 3 weeks, tachypnoea, hepatomegaly, failure to thrive

Investigations:
- **ECG:** normal
- **CXR:** normal
- **ECHO:** flow between the right and left sides of the heart in both the atria and ventricles.

Differentials: large VSD, TOF

Management: surgical repair

Coarctation

Definition: a narrowing of the aortic isthmus (see Fig 16.7)

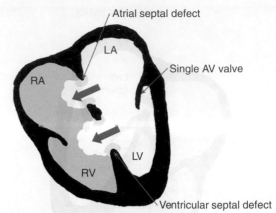

Fig 16.6 Atrioventricular Septal Defect (Illustrated by Hollie Blaber)

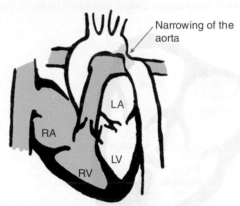

Fig 16.7 Coarctation of the Aorta (Illustrated by Hollie Blaber)

Buzzwords:
- **Risk factors:** Turner syndrome, bicuspid aortic valve
- **Presentation:** cyanosis, brachio-femoral delay, end systolic murmur, loss of femoral artery pulse, HTN

Investigations:
- **ECG:** LVH
- **CXR:** rib notching
- ***ECHO*:** narrowing of the thoracic aorta

Differentials: pulmonary stenosis, aortic stenosis

Management:
1. Maintain PDA with prostaglandins
2. Surgery to correct: balloon dilation or angioplasty

Kawasaki Disease

Definition: an acute vasculitis most commonly affecting children under 5 years of age. Can cause coronary artery aneurysms

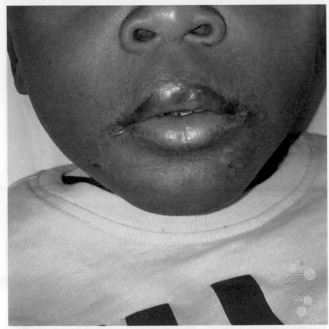

Fig 16.8 Cheilitis of the Lips in Darker Skin (From *SKINDEEP.*)

Buzzwords:
- **Risk factors:** ethnicity (e.g., Japanese, Korean, Taiwanese), familial, male, <5 years of age
- **Presentation**:

  First phase: fever lasting at least 5 days + four or more of:
  - Bilateral conjunctivitis
  - Inflammation of the mucous membranes leading to a sore throat, cheilitis (see Figs 16.8 and 16.9(A)), strawberry tongue (see Fig 16.9(B))
  - Lymphadenopathy
  - Redness and swelling of the hands/feet
  - Polymorphic rash

  Second phase: 2–3 weeks after the fever:
  - Peeling of the polymorphic rash
  - Abdominal pain, diarrhoea, vomiting
  - Joint pain

Investigations: clinical diagnosis
- **ECG:** tachycardia
- **Bloods:** ↑ CRP, ↑ ESR, ↓ Hb ↑ platelets, ↓ albumin, ↑ ALT
- **ECHO:** coronary artery aneurysms

Differentials: viral exanthems, conjunctivitis, sepsis, Stevens-Johnson syndrome, drug reaction, paediatric multisystem inflammatory syndrome

Management:
1. Aspirin
2. Intravenous immunoglobulin

RESPIRATORY

Signs of respiratory distress include:
- Tachypnoea
- Intercostal/subcostal/suprasternal/sternal recession
- Paradoxical breathing
- Tracheal tug (+/- head bobbing)
- Nasal flaring
- Grunting
- Stridor
- Wheeze

Infant Respiratory Distress Syndrome

Definition: inadequate surfactant production in the lungs leads to reduced lung compliance and an increased work of breathing

Buzzwords:
- **Risk factors:** premature birth
- **Presentation:** respiratory distress

Investigations:
- **Pulse oximetry:** aim for 91%–95% in preterm babies
- **CXR:** small lung volumes with ground glass opacity, air bronchogram

Differentials: transient tachypnoea of the newborn (TTN), meconium aspiration, pneumonia, pneumothorax (see Table 16.7)

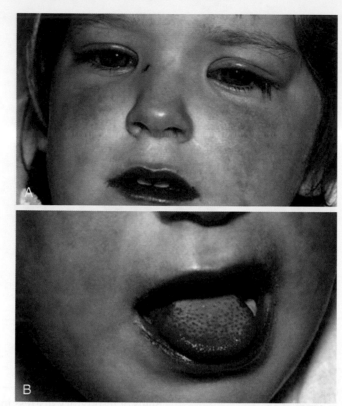

Fig 16.9 (A) Cheilitis of the Lips in Lighter Skin; (B) Strawberry Tongue (From Torok, K., et al. (2012). *Rheumatology*. In Zitelli, B.J., et al., eds. Zitelli and Davis' atlas of pediatric physical diagnosis, (6th ed.). Saunders, pp. 259-298, Fig 7-70.)

Management:

- **Prevention:** glucocorticoids given to mother if 24–34 weeks gestation and in preterm labour
- **Treatment:** oxygen, continuous positive airway pressure (CPAP), surfactant given via endotracheal (ET) tube

Transient Tachypnoea of the Newborn

Definition: excess fluid in the lungs resulting in a reduced lung compliance and increased airway resistance

Buzzwords:

- **Risk factors:** following caesarean delivery
- **Presentation:** respiratory distress, recovery within 2–5 days

Investigations:

- **Pulse oximetry:** low saturations
- **CXR:** large lung volumes and interstitial oedema

Differentials: meconium aspiration, pneumonia, infant respiratory distress syndrome (IRDS), tracheoesophageal fistula, pneumothorax

TABLE 16.7   Other Causes of Respiratory Distress at Birth

Condition	Buzzword
Meconium aspiration syndrome	Meconium passed in labour **CXR:** hyperinflation
Persistent pulmonary hypertension of the newborn	Cyanosis **ECHO:** high pulmonary pressures
Pneumonia	Premature rupture of membranes Sepsis
Pneumothorax	Transillumination
Tracheoesophageal fistula	Respiratory distress when feeding
Diaphragmatic hernia	**CXR:** abdominal organs in chest

Abbreviations: CXR, chest x-ray; ECHO, echocardiogram.

Management:

1. Oxygen
2. CPAP
3. Recovery should be seen within a few days of birth

Laryngomalacia

Definition: a congenital laryngeal abnormality resulting in laryngeal collapse during inspiration
Buzzwords:

- **Risk factors:** male, neurological abnormality
- **Presentation:** stridor, 2/52 old, feeding difficulties, apnoea

Investigations:

- **Flexible laryngoscopy:** direct visualisation of the supraglottic tissues collapsing with inspiration

Differentials: vocal cord palsy, laryngeal cleft, subglottic stenosis
Management:

1. Conservative (if mild). 80% resolve by 18–20 months
2. Endoscopic supraglottoplasty (if severe)
3. Tracheostomy if all other treatments fail

Bronchiolitis

Definition: a viral-induced inflammation of the bronchioles
Buzzwords:

- **Risk factors:** <2 years of age, prematurity, smoke exposure, congenital heart disease
- **Presentation:** tachypnoea, poor feeding, increased work of breathing

Investigations:

- **Nasopharyngeal aspirate for polymerase chain reaction (PCR):** may show *Respiratory syncytial virus* (RSV), *Parainfluenza*, *Adenovirus* or *Rhinovirus*
- **CXR** (if severe): hyperinflation, atelectasis

Differentials: pneumonia, croup, CF
Management:

1. Fluids, feeding support, humidified O_2 to maintain an adequate oxygen saturation (usually >92%)
2. Palivizumab if: chronic lung disease, long-term ventilation, cardiac disease, severe combined immunodeficiency
3. Discharge if feeding at 2/3rds of baseline and adequate oxygen saturations are maintained for 8 h.

Atopic Asthma

Definition: a chronic inflammatory condition of the airways. The airways are hyperresponsive and constrict easily in response to a wide range of stimuli. A diagnosis of asthma can be made from 5 years of age. Prior to this, children with wheezing may be considered to have:

- **Viral-induced wheeze (6 month–5 years of age):** wheezing associated with a respiratory tract infection

- **Transient early wheezing (<3 years):** multiple episodes of wheezing before age 3 and then stopping. Usually, no associated atopy

Buzzwords:

- **Risk factors:** atopy (or family history of atopy)
- **Presentation:** SOB, wheeze, cough, diurnal variation

Investigations: no single test for asthma, rather a combination of history and tests that support the diagnosis. If the child is under the age of 5 years and there is a clinical suspicion of asthma, treat the symptoms and review regularly. The investigations below should be completed once the patient turns 5 years of age if there are ongoing symptoms:

- **Symptom diary:** to identify triggers
- **Peak flow:** diurnal variability, variability >20%
- **Spirometry with bronchodilator reversibility test:** obstructive lung disease pattern (FEV1/FVC <70%) with an improvement by at least 12% after bronchodilator use
- **Fractional exhaled nitric oxide** (if diagnostic uncertainty): >35 ppb

Differentials: viral-induced wheeze, allergies, CF
Management: for acute management see Respiratory in an Hour.
Chronic management (NICE guideline 2019 >5 years of age):

1. Short-acting beta agonist (SABA)
2. SABA + very low–dose inhaled corticosteroid (ICS)
3. SABA + very low–dose ICS + leukotriene-receptor antagonist (LTRA)*
4. SABA + very low–dose ICS + long-acting beta agonist (LABA) and STOP LTRA
5. SABA + maintenance and reliever therapy (MART)
6. If still not controlled, refer to specialist

*In the BTS guidelines, a LABA or LTRA can be added at this stage
An assessment of symptom control is used to guide management. If the symptoms are not controlled, the next step is tried. Symptoms are not controlled if:

- SABA use 3 times per week
- Symptoms 3 times per week
- Night-time symptoms
- One severe asthma attack in last 2 years

Other important aspects of management: inhaler technique, vaccinations, self-management plan, parental smoking cessation if applicable, follow-up with an asthma nurse

Croup

Definition: a lower respiratory tract infection (LRTI) commonly caused by *Parainfluenza* resulting in a barking cough. It can be classified as mild, moderate or severe.

Buzzwords:
- **Risk factors:** *Parainfluenza* infection at 6 months–6 years of age
- **Presentation:**
  - Mild: barking cough (worse at night), coryza, low-grade fever, hoarse voice
  - Moderate: symptoms as in mild + stridor and sternal recession
  - Severe: symptoms as in moderate + agitation and lethargy

Investigations:
- Clinical diagnosis
- Do not try to inspect the throat

Differentials: bacterial tracheitis, epiglottitis, upper airway foreign body, retropharyngeal abscess, pneumonia, whooping cough

Management:
1. Admit if features of moderate/severe disease, requiring oxygen or in a high-risk category (e.g., immunosuppressed, chronic lung disease, congenital heart disease)
2. Oral dexamethasone
3. Paracetamol/ibuprofen
4. If hospital admission is not required, careful safety netting advice must be given

Bacterial Tracheitis

Definition: inflammation of the trachea caused by a bacterial infection, most commonly following a viral upper airway infection. Causative organisms include *Staphylococcus aureus, Streptococcus pneumonia, Streptococcus pyogenes, Moraxella catarrhalis* and *Haemophilus influenza type B.*

Buzzwords:
- **Risk factors:** recent viral illness, immunocompromise, long-term tracheostomy
- **Presentation:** prodromal symptoms, mucopurulent secretions, stridor, high fever, lethargy, cyanosis (drooling and tripoding are more commonly seen with epiglottitis)

Investigations:
- Investigations may prompt distress and clinical deterioration

- Do not examine the throat
- **Blood cultures** (ONLY once the airway has been secured): identify specific organism
- **Blood:** ↑ CRP, ↑ ESR, ↑ WCC
- **Xray:** tracheal narrowing (lateral neck film), evidence of pneumonia

Differentials: epiglottitis (this is now less common due to vaccination – see ENT and Ophthalmology in an hour for more information), croup, whooping cough, pneumonia, upper airway foreign body, retropharyngeal abscess, angioedema

Management: This is an emergency because it may compromise the airway.
1. Airway control (usually gas induction in theatre with senior anaesthetics and ENT support)
2. Broad antibiotic coverage
3. Inhaled dexamethasone does NOT result in clinical improvement

Whooping Cough

Definition: a LRTI caused by *Bordetella pertussis* resulting in a persistent cough

Buzzwords:
- **Risk factors:** unvaccinated
- **Presentation:**
  - Catarrhal phase (week 1): coryza
  - Paroxysmal phase (weeks 2–7): cough and inspiratory whoop
  - Convalescent phase (months): resolving symptoms

Investigations:
- Clinical diagnosis
- **Nasal swab for cultures/PCR:** *Bordetella pertussis*
- **Blood:** FBC (↑↑ lymphocytes)

Differentials: other LRTIs, croup, asthma

Management:
1. Admit to hospital if acutely unwell
2. Macrolide (azithromycin or clarithromycin if <1 year of age) if within 21 days of cough onset
3. Vaccination catch-up program if applicable
4. Prophylactic antibiotics for close contacts if high risk of infection or transmission. (e.g., unimmunised infants, pregnant females, healthcare workers)
5. Notify Public Health England (PHE)

Community-acquired Pneumonia

Definition: a community-acquired infection in which the alveoli become filled with microorganisms (see Table 16.8), fluid and inflammatory cells

TABLE 16.8 Common Causative Organisms of Pneumonia by Age

Age	Common Organisms	Viral
Birth–3 weeks	*Escherichia coli*, Group B *Streptococcus, Listeria monocytogenes*	
3 weeks–3 months	*Chlamydia trachomatis, Streptococcus pneumoniae*	*Adenovirus, Respiratory syncytial virus, Influenza, Parainfluenza*
4 months–5 years	*Streptococcus pneumoniae, Chlamydia pneumoniae, Mycoplasma pneumoniae, Haemophilus influenza* B	*Adenovirus, Respiratory syncytial virus, Influenza, Parainfluenza*
5 years–adolescence	*Streptococcus pneumoniae, Chlamydia pneumoniae, Mycoplasma pneumoniae, Haemophilus influenza* B	

Buzzwords:
- **Risk factors**: male, prematurity, <5 years of age
- **Presentation**:
  - Fever, SOB, cough, wheeze, chest pain, abdominal pain, headache
  - **Severe infection**: saturations <92%, RR >60 rpm, cyanotic, drowsy, temperature >39°C

Investigations: if managed in the community, no investigations are required
- **Blood**: FBC (↑ WCC), ↑ CRP, +/-lactate (↑)
- **CXR**: consolidation (repeat CXR is not routinely required in children)
- **Blood cultures**: may identify the organism
- **Nasopharyngeal swab**: may identify the organism
- **COVID/flu swab**: if clinical concern

Differentials: bronchiolitis, LRTI, CF

Management:
1. If managing at home, advice given to manage the fever, prevent dehydration and identify deterioration
2. Admit if evidence of severe infection or significant empyema/effusion
3. Oxygen to maintain saturations >92%
4. IV fluids if required
5. Antibiotics as per hospital guidelines

Cystic Fibrosis

Definition: an autosomal-recessive condition resulting in malfunctioning cystic fibrosis transmembrane conductance regulator (CFTR) channels. Mutations most commonly affect *delta F508* on chromosome 7.

Buzzwords:
- **Risk factors**: family history (1-in-4 chance if both parents are carriers)
- **Presentation**:
  - **Newborn**: newborn screening, meconium ileus

- **Infancy**: jaundice, faltering growth, steatorrhoea, recurrent chest infections
- **Child**: bronchiectasis, rectal prolapse, nasal polyps, sinusitis
- **Adolescent**: diabetes mellitus (DM), infertility, portal hypertension, cirrhosis

Investigations:
- **Preconception screening** (if high risk)
- **Heel prick**: elevated immunoreactive trypsinogen (IRT)
- **Sweat test**: chloride >60 mmol/L. Pilocarpine is applied to the skin, sweating is then stimulated with a low-voltage current and collected. Chloride levels in sweat are then analysed.
- **Genetic testing** (if a raised IRT or positive sweat test): specific genetic mutation identified

Differentials: primary ciliary dyskinesia, coeliac disease

Management:
1. MDT approach
2. Physiotherapy to improve mucus clearance
3. Increased calories
4. Fat-soluble vitamin (e.g., A, D, E and K) supplements
5. Saline nebulisers
6. Ivacaftor/lumacaftor (if *F508del*)

GASTROENTEROLOGY AND GENERAL SURGERY

Functional/Recurrent Abdominal Pain

Definition: a common childhood condition of unknown cause resulting in sufficient abdominal pain to disrupt normal activities for more than 3 months

Buzzwords:
- **Risk factors**: constipation, anxiety, irritable bowel syndrome (IBS), abdominal migraine

- **Presentation:** chronic abdominal pain for >3 months, missing school, headaches, absence of worrying features

Investigations:

- **Symptom diary:** trend or triggers identified
- **Urine MC&S** (if suspicion of UTI): + nitrites, + leukocytes
- **Blood** (if ongoing problem): TFTs and coeliac screen

Differentials: IBS, IBD, coeliac disease, food intolerance, abdominal migraine

Management: reassurance

Constipation

Definition: decreased frequency of bowel movements. Average frequency:

- 0–1 year of age: 2–4 soft stools/day
- >1 year of age: from 3 stools/day to 3 stools/week

Buzzwords:

- **Risk factors:** impaired mobility, neurodevelopmental disorder, dehydration
- **Presentation:** straining, pain on passing stool, poor appetite, rabbit droppings, abdominal pain
  - **Red flags:** ribbon stool, leg weakness, failure to pass meconium, abdominal distension, anal abnormalities

Investigations: none required if no concerning features. Refer to secondary care if there are red-flag features

Differentials: Hirschsprung disease, spina bifida, hypothyroidism, hypercalcaemia, perianal fissure

Management:

1. Conservative: reassurance, keep active, encourage hydration
2. If impacted: Macrogol at increasing doses
3. Stimulant laxative (e.g., senna) if required
4. Maintenance laxative: half the compaction dose, continue until a few weeks of normal stools

Hirschsprung Disease

Definition: a congenital partial or complete absence of ganglionic cells in the myenteric plexus of the bowel, most commonly affecting the rectum/sigmoid colon

Buzzwords:

- **Risk factors:** male, Down syndrome
- **Presentation:** delayed meconium, abdominal distension, chronic constipation, enterocolitis

Investigations:

- **Blood test** (if generally unwell): ↑ WCC (if enterocolitis)

TABLE 16.9   Differentials for Diarrhoea

Acute	Chronic
• Viral gastroenteritis (e.g., *Norovirus*, *Rotavirus*) • Bacterial gastroenteritis	• Cow's milk allergy • Lactose intolerance • Toddler diarrhoea • Coeliac disease[a] • Inflammatory bowel disease[a] • Irritable bowel syndrome[a]

[a]Condition is covered in Gastroenterology in an hour

- **Abdominal x-ray (AXR):** may show obstruction or distension
- **Anorectal manometry:** failure of reflex relaxation of the sphincters
- ***Rectal biopsy*** **(DIAGNOSTIC):** absence of ganglionic cells in the myenteric plexus

Differentials: constipation

Management:

1. Bowel washouts/laxatives
2. Surgical resection of the aganglionic section of bowel

Diarrhoea

Definition: passage of three of more loose or liquid stools per day

Differentials: see Table 16.9

Viral Gastroenteritis

Definition: a gastrointestinal infection most commonly caused by *Norovirus* or *Rotavirus*.

Buzzwords:

- **Risk factors:** contact with an infected individual, nonvaccinated (*Rotavirus*)
- **Presentation:** watery diarrhoea, projectile vomiting, 1–2 days (*Norovirus*), 3–8 days (*Rotavirus*)

Investigations:

- Clinical diagnosis – investigations usually not required
- **Stool sample for MC&S** (required if: recent travel, no better by day 7, diagnostic uncertainty, suspected septicaemia, blood or mucus in the stool, immunocompromise): to identify the specific organism

Differentials: see Table 16.9

Management:

1. Oral hydration (usually a self-limiting condition)
2. Admit for rehydration if acutely unwell/haemodynamically unstable
3. Infection control measures: school exclusion for 48 h and good hand hygiene

Cow's Milk Allergy

Definition: an immune-mediated reaction against proteins that are present in cow's milk. Two types:
- **IgE mediated**: presents immediately after cow milk ingestion
- **Non-IgE mediated:** delayed presentation

Buzzwords:
- **Risk factors:** male, known food allergy, atopic conditions, family history
- **Presentation:**
  - **IgE:** diarrhoea, pruritis, oedema, rapid onset, abdominal pain +/- angio-oedema
  - **Non-IgE:** diarrhoea (bloody or mucus), GORD, colicky, perianal redness

Investigations: clinical diagnosis – no investigations required
- **Allergy testing** (if suspecting IgE mediated): may be associated with other allergies

Differentials: See Table 16.9

Management:
1. Referral to a paediatric dietician
2. Cow milk–free diet for child/mother (if breastfeeding) for at least 6 months (or until child is 9–12 months of age) followed by a slow reintroduction of cow's milk
3. If concerns of IgE mediated: consider referral to allergy specialist

Toddler Diarrhoea

Definition: a benign condition in toddlers leading to diarrhoea caused by a rapid transit time through the gut

Buzzwords:
- **Risk factors:** toddler, fruit juice, low-fat diet, male
- **Presentation:** food pieces in stool, chronic diarrhoea

Investigations: none required if maintaining a good weight

Differentials: See Table 16.9

Management: increased fat intake and a low-fibre diet

Gastroesophageal Reflux Disease

Definition: a weakness of the lower oesophageal sphincter resulting in leakage of gastric contents into the oesophagus

Buzzwords:
- **Risk factors**: neurodevelopmental disorder, duodenal atresia, prematurity, hiatus hernia, obesity
- **Presentation**: vomiting after feeding, failure to thrive (if severe), feeding difficulties, pneumonia

Investigations: usually not necessary but required if severe or persistent
- **24-h pH impedance monitoring:** frequently the pH is <4
- **Endoscopy:** may see oesophagitis

Differentials: colic, pyloric stenosis, intestinal obstruction

Management:
1. Reassurance, add Gaviscon to feeds, 30° head elevation after feeding
2. Ranitidine or omeprazole if severe

Neonatal Jaundice

Definition: a blood bilirubin level of >80 micromol/L. Causes:
- **Pathological:**
  - <24 h: haemolysis, rhesus disease, ABO incompatibility, spherocytosis
  - Persistent (>2 weeks): biliary atresia, congenital hypothyroidism
- **Physiological:** 2 days–2 weeks after birth. Most often seen in breastfed babies

Buzzwords:
- **Risk factors:** Asian, low birth weight, prematurity, breastfeeding
- **Presentation:** jaundice, yellow sclera, poor weight gain

Investigations:
- **Transcutaneous bilirubinometer:** >250 micromol/L, check serum bilirubin
- **Serum bilirubin:** plot on a treatment-threshold graph to guide treatment (see Fig 16.10)
- Blood tests to determine the cause may include a **direct Coombs test, blood grouping, full blood count and blood film.**

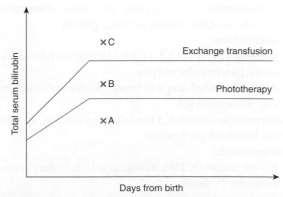

Fig 16.10 Illustration of the Thresholds for Treatment of Neonatal Jaundice.

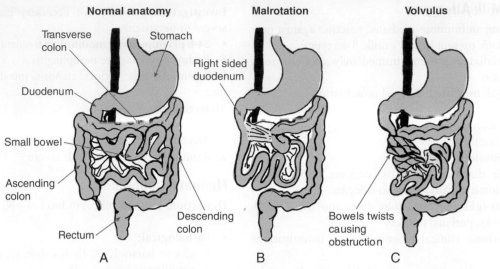

Fig 16.11 (A) Normal Anatomy, (B) Malrotation, (C) Volvulus. (Illustrated by Hollie Blaber)

Management:
1. Monitor if below the treatment threshold (see Fig 16.10(A))
2. Phototherapy: if above the threshold for phototherapy (see Fig 16.10(B)). Recheck bilirubin levels every 6–12 h. Eye protection.
3. Exchange transfusion: if above the threshold (see Fig 16.10(C)). Measure bilirubin after 2 h of therapy.
4. Manage any underlying causes of pathological jaundice

Necrotising Enterocolitis

Definition: an inflammation of the intestines resulting in necrosis and perforation
Buzzwords:
- **Risk factors:** prematurity, formula fed
- **Presentation:** poor feeding, abdominal distension, bloody stool, increasing gastric aspirates
Investigations:
- **Bloods:** FBC (↑WCC), ↑CRP, ↑lactate, metabolic acidosis, baseline electrolytes
- **AXR:** distended loops of bowel, bowel-wall thickening, intramural gas
Differentials: volvulus, Hirschsprung disease, spontaneous intestinal perforation
Management:
1. Nil by mouth (NBM), nasogastric (NG) tube decompression, IV fluids
2. Total parenteral nutrition
3. IV antibiotics
4. Surgery required if perforation is suspected

Malrotation

Definition: a congenital condition in which bowel rotation is incomplete, increasing the risk of a volvulus (see Fig 16.11)
Buzzwords:
- **Risk factors:** days 1–3 of life
- **Presentation**:
  - Malrotation with volvulus: bilious vomiting, colicky pain
  - Malrotation with vascular compromise: acutely unwell, bilious vomiting, acidotic, peritonitic
  - May be associated with gastroschisis or omphalocele in which the abdominal cavity doesn't fully close (see Table 16.10)
Investigations:
- **Plain AXR:** distension
- ***Upper GI contrast study*:** right-sided duodenum
Differentials: obstruction, volvulus, duodenal atresia, pyloric stenosis
Management: Ladd's procedure

Duodenal Atresia

Definition: a congenital absence or narrowing of the duodenum
Buzzwords:
- **Risk factors:** Down syndrome, polyhydramnios, first week of life
- **Presentation**: bilious vomiting, poor feeding, polyhydramnios

TABLE 16.10 Key Features of Gastroschisis and Omphalocele

	Gastroschisis	Omphalocele
Key feature	No protective membrane	Protective membrane
Risk factors	Often an isolated condition	Associated with many genetic abnormalities
Management	Fluid resuscitation and nasogastric tube decompression	
	URGENT surgery or coverage required	Elective repair and conservative management (urgent repair required if sack is ruptured)

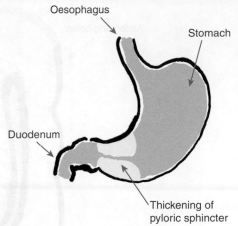

Fig 16.13 Pyloric Stenosis (Illustrated by Hollie Blaber)

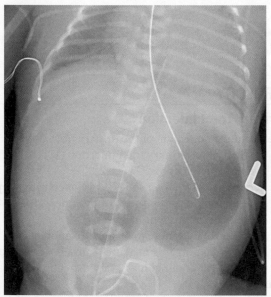

Fig 16.12 'Double Bubble' Sign on Abdominal X-ray (From Flynn-O'Brien, K.T., Rice-Townsend, S., Ledbetter, D.J. (2018). *71 Structural Anomalies of the Gastrointestinal Tract.* In Avery's Diseases of the Newborn. Elsevier)

Investigations:
- **AXR:** Double bubble sign (see Fig 16.12)

Differentials: pyloric stenosis, intussusception, malrotation

Management:
1. Fluids and NG decompression
2. Surgical repair

Pyloric Stenosis

Definition: an idiopathic thickening of the pyloric sphincter (see Fig 16.13)

Buzzwords:
- **Risk factors:** family history, age 2–8 weeks
- **Presentation:** projectile vomiting, weight loss, olive-shaped mass in the right upper quadrant, hypochloraemic metabolic alkalosis

Investigations:
- **Test feed:** gastric peristalsis, projectile vomiting
- **Blood:** ↓ chloride, metabolic alkalosis
- ***USS*:** thickening of the pyloric muscle

Differentials: GORD, intussusception, malrotation, food allergy

Management:
1. NBM, NG tube decompression, IV fluids
2. Pyloromyotomy

Intussusception

Definition: an invagination of the proximal bowel into the distal part (see Fig 16.14)

Buzzwords:
- **Risk factors:** Meckel's diverticulum, polyps, Peutz-Jeghers syndrome, male, 3 months–2 years of age
- **Presentation:** intermittent abdominal pain, feed refusal, sausage-shaped mass, red currant jelly stool, abdominal distension

Investigations:
- **USS:** doughnut or target sign

Differentials: appendicitis, pyloric stenosis, gastroenteritis, UTI

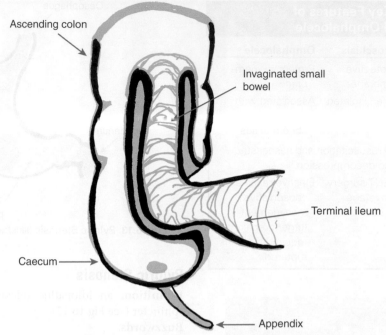

Ascending colon

Invaginated small bowel

Terminal ileum

Caecum

Appendix

Fig 16.14 Intussusception (Illustrated by Hollie Blaber)

Management:
1. NBM, NG tube decompression, IV fluids
2. Air enema
3. Laparotomy required if shock, evidence of perforation or the above methods have failed

Mesenteric Adenitis

Definition: an inflammation of the mesenteric lymph nodes
Buzzwords:
- **Risk factors:** recent viral infection
- **Presentation:** presentation is similar to appendicitis with abdominal pain, nausea, anorexia
Investigation:
- **Bloods:** usually normal (if ↑ WCC and ↑ CRP may suggest appendicitis)
Differentials: appendicitis, ectopic pregnancy
Management:
1. Conservative
2. If appendicitis is suspected, laparoscopy to confirm the diagnosis. Visualisation of mesenteric nodes is diagnostic. Appendix is removed (see General Surgery in an Hour).

UROLOGY

Urinary Tract Infection

Definition: an infection of the urinary tract
- **Cystitis:** lower urinary tract infection (UTI)
- **Pyelonephritis:** upper UTI
- **Recurrent UTI:** an episode of pyelonephritis + episode of cystitis, ≥2 episodes of pyelonephritis or ≥3 episodes of cystitis within a year
- **Atypical UTI:** a failure to respond to antibiotics in 48 h, non-*E. coli* organism, acutely unwell, sepsis, poor urine flow, abdominal mass, raised creatinine

Buzzwords:
- **Risk factors:** female, horseshoe kidney, renal tract abnormalities, vesicoureteric reflux, <1 year of age, sexual abuse
- **Presentation:**
  - **Infants:** fever, vomiting, lethargy, irritability, foul-smelling urine, septicaemia
  - **Children:** dysuria, frequency, urgency, loin tenderness, secondary enuresis

Investigations:
- **'Clean-catch' urine dip:** nitrite and leukocyte positive (nitrite is often negative in children)

- ***Urine MC&S***: >100 WBC/microlitre and growth of specific organisms
- **Blood** (if systemically unwell): ↑ WCC, ↑ CRP
- **USS:** to identify structural abnormalities within the urinary tract
  - URGENT if: atypical or <6 months of age and recurring
  - Within 6 weeks if: >6 months of age and recurring, <6 months
- **Dimercaptosuccinic acid (DMSA) scan** (if recurrent or atypical infection <3 years): identifies renal scarring (NB. must wait 2 months after UTI)
- **Micturating cystourethrogram (MCUG)** (if <1 year or family history of vesicoureteric reflux): to identify vesicoureteric reflux

Differentials: appendicitis, gastroenteritis, urethritis

Management:

- Admit to hospital if <3 months of age (will require IV antibiotics) or clinically unstable
- **Acute pyelonephritis (>3 months of age):** cefalexin or co-amoxiclav PO for 7–10 days
- **Cystitis (>3 months of age):** trimethoprim or nitrofurantoin PO for 3 days
- **Recurrent:** consider prophylactic antibiotics (nitro or trimethoprim), review in 6 months
- Safety netting, analgesia and hydration

Vesicoureteric Reflux

Definition: a congenital condition in which the ureters have ineffective valves. This condition may lead to intra-renal reflux, damage to the kidneys and recurrent UTIs (see Fig 16.15).

Buzzwords:

- **Risk factors:** female, male (if a newborn), family history, other renal/urinary tract abnormalities
- **Presentation:** recurrent UTI, fever

Investigations:

- See above for UTI investigations
- ***MCUG*:** to visualise reflux into the ureters (see Fig 16.16)

Differentials: UTI

Management:

1. Treat any associated UTIs to reduce renal scarring
2. Surgical management is NOT recommended.

Enuresis

Definition:

- **Primary enuresis:** bladder control has not yet been attained (common)
- **Secondary enuresis:** relapse after becoming continent of urine for at least 6 months

Buzzwords:

- **Risk factors:** emotional hardship (e.g., new school, bullying, family disruption), UTI, constipation, polyuria

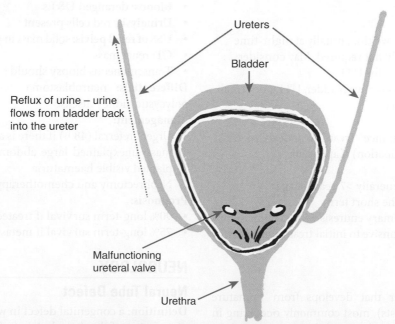

Fig 16.15 Vesicoureteric Reflux. (Illustrated by Hollie Blaber.)

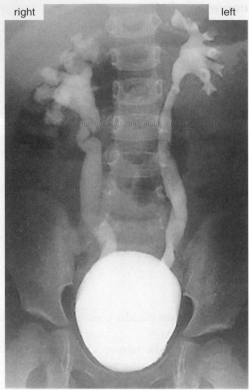

right   left

Fig 16.16 Micturating Cystourethrogram Showing Bilateral Vesicoureteric Reflux (From Lissauer, T., Lissauer, T. (2018). *19 Kidney and urinary tract disorders.* In Illustrated Textbook of Paediatrics. Elsevier.)

- **Presentation:** bed-wetting, usually at night-time
Investigations: usually not required. May consider:
- **Urinalysis:** to assess for UTI
Differentials: DM, overactive bladder, UTI, abnormalities of the urinary tract
Management:
1. Advice and reassurance. Treat the underlying cause (e.g., UTI or constipation) if applicable
2. Reward system
3. Enuresis alarm (generally >7 years of age)
4. Desmopressin in the short term
5. If secondary or primary enuresis with daytime symptoms and not responsive to initial treatment, refer for secondary care

Neuroblastoma

Definition: a cancer that develops from immature nerve cells (neuroblasts), most commonly occurring in the adrenal glands (see Fig 16.17). Can occur anywhere along the sympathetic chain.

Buzzword:
- **Risk factors:** family history
- **Presentation:** palpable abdominal mass, failure to thrive, vomiting, bruising
Investigations:
- **Urinalysis:** catecholamines present
- **USS abdomen/CT scan:** heterogeneous mass
- ***Biopsy*:** histological confirmation
Differentials: Wilms' tumour, leukaemia
Management:
1. Urgent referral (48 h) if there is a palpable abdominal mass or unexplained large abdominal organ
2. Chemotherapy and surgical resection
Prognosis: dependent on the tumour type at diagnosis:
- Low risk: 95% 5-year survival
- Intermediate risk: 90%–95% 5-year survival
- High risk: 40%–50% 5-year survival

Wilms' Tumour (Nephroblastoma)

Definition: a mesodermal tumour found in the primitive renal tubules and mesenchymal cells (see Fig 16.18)
Buzzword:
- **Risk factors:** Edwards syndrome, hereditary, 2–5 years of age
- **Presentation:** asymmetrical abdominal mass, haematuria, UTI
Investigations:
- **Bloods:** deranged U&Es
- **Urinalysis:** red cells present
- **USS of renal pelvis:** solid mass in the kidneys, not cystic
- **CT:** renal mass
- Transcutaneous biopsy should be AVOIDED
Differentials: neuroblastoma, renal cell carcinoma, polycystic kidney disease
Management:
1. Urgent referral (48 h) if there is a palpable abdominal mass, unexplained large abdominal organ or unexplained visible haematuria
2. Nephrectomy and chemotherapy
Prognosis:
- 90% long-term survival if treated
- 75% long-term survival if metastatic disease

NEUROLOGY

Neural Tube Defect

Definition: a congenital defect in which there is incomplete fusion of the neural plate to form the neural tube (see Fig 16.19)

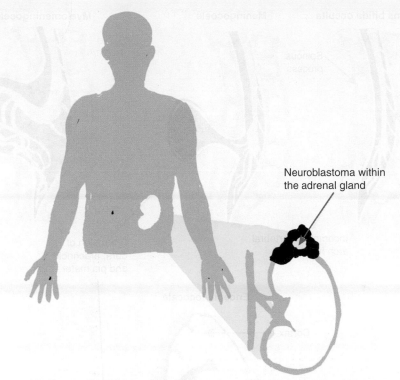

Neuroblastoma within the adrenal gland

Fig 16.17 Illustration of a Neuroblastoma. (Illustrated by Hollie Blaber.)

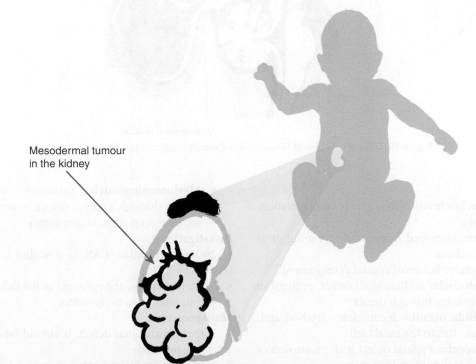

Mesodermal tumour in the kidney

Fig 16.18 Wilms' Tumour. (Illustrated by Hollie Blaber.)

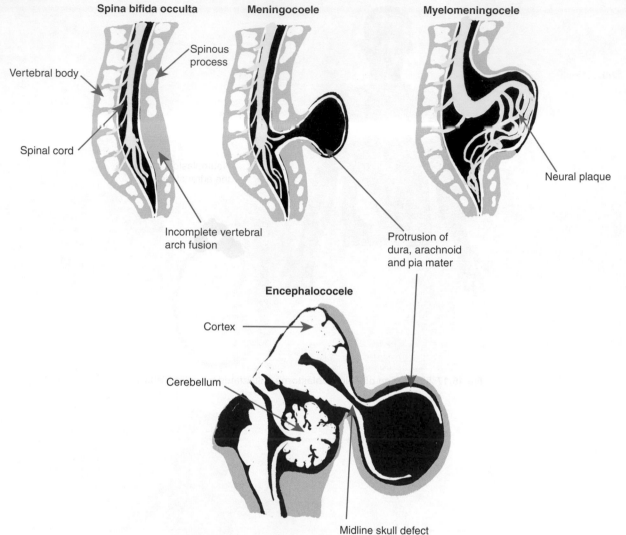

Fig 16.19 Different Types of Neural Tube Defects (Illustrated by Hollie Blaber)

Buzzwords:
- **Risk factors:** low levels of folic acid in early gestation, family history
- **Presentation:** identified in prenatal screening or at the newborn check
  - **Anencephaly:** failure of cranial development
  - **Encephalocoele:** midline skull defect, protrusion of the meninges through defect
  - **Spina bifida occulta:** incomplete vertebral arch fusion, hair tuft in the natal cleft
  - **Meningocoele:** a spinal defect with protrusion of the dura, arachnoid and pia mater
  - **Myelomeningocoele:** protrusion of a neural plaque through a spinal defect, neurological deficit, hydrocephalus, incontinence

Investigations:
- **20-week gestation USS:** to visualise a neural tube defect
- **MRI:** to visualise the contents of the defect
- **CT:** to establish a bony defect

Management:
1. If there is an open defect, it should be covered and closed promptly
2. MDT assessment/symptom management

Prevention: folic acid supplementation in the first trimester of pregnancy

Cerebral Palsy

Definition: a permanent, nonprogressive disorder of movement caused by a brain injury before the age of 2 years. The three main types are spastic, dyskinetic and ataxic. This condition is graded according to gross motor function (see Table 16.11 and Fig 16.20).

Buzzwords:

- **Risk factors:** see Table 16.12

TABLE 16.11 **Levels of Gross Motor Functional Impairment**	
Gross Motor Function	**Description**
Level I	Walks without limitation
Level II	Walks with limitation
Level III	Walks with handheld mobility device
Level IV	Self-mobility, motorised chair
Level V	Manual wheelchair

- **Presentation:** abnormal posture, delayed motor milestones, feeding difficulties, GORD, handedness at 12 months, abnormal gait
  - **Spastic:** velocity-dependent, increased tone, brisk reflexes
  - **Dyskinetic:** floppiness, poor truncal control, chorea (irregular, sudden, nonrepetitive movements), athetosis (slow, writhing movements), dystonia (twisting motion due to antagonistic muscles simultaneously contracting)
  - **Ataxic:** poor balance, tremor, hypotonia
  - **Complications:** hearing problems, sleep disturbances, aspiration, epilepsy, incontinence, osteoporosis, hydrocephalus

Investigations:

- **MRI:** to establish a cause

Differentials: brain tumour, spinal muscular atrophy, muscular dystrophy

Management:

1. MDT approach: physiotherapy, occupational therapy, SALT
2. Orthoses: to enhance function and reduce pain

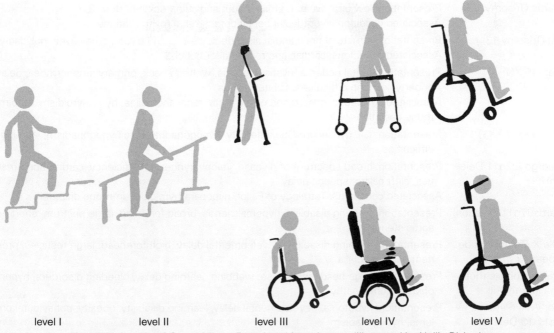

| level I | level II | level III | level IV | level V |

Fig 16.20 Levels of Gross Motor Functional Impairment (Illustrated by Hollie Blaber)

TABLE 16.12 Causes of Cerebral Palsy

Antenatal (80%)	Perinatal (10%)	Postnatal (10%)
Prematurity	Hypoxic ischaemic encephalopathy	Hyperbilirubin-emia
Multiple births		
Chorioamnionitis	Birth trauma	Interventricular haemorrhage
Thyroid disease	Placental abruption	
TORCH[a]	Post-maturity	Seizures
Teratogen exposure	Prolonged obstructed labour	Sepsis
		Respiratory distress
		Meningitis
		Sepsis
		Non-accidental injury

[a]Antenatal infection with *Toxoplasmosis*, Other organisms (*Treponema pallidum, Parvovirus, Varicella-zoster virus*), *Rubella, Cytomegalovirus, Herpes simplex virus*)

3. Medications: botulinum toxin (injected for spasticity), baclofen
4. Deep brain stimulation

Febrile Convulsions

Definition: a seizure associated with a fever in the absence of another pathology

Buzzwords:

- **Risk factors:** 6 months–6 years of age, family history, roseola
- **Presentation:** fever, viral infection, convulsions, <1-min tonic-clonic seizure

Investigations: based on the presumed cause of the fever. No investigations required specifically for the seizure

Differentials: meningitis, epilepsy (see Neurology in an hour), other intracranial pathology (e.g., tumour, trauma)

TABLE 16.13 Key Features of Common Genetic Disorders

Condition (Genetics)	Buzzwords
Down Syndrome (Trisomy 21)	Presentation: hypotonia, flat occiput, single palmar crease, macroglossia, developmental delay, learning difficulties, short stature Associated conditions: atrioventricular septal defect, ventricular septal defect, duodenal atresia, leukaemia, cataracts, hearing impairment, atlantoaxial instability, early-onset Alzheimer's disease, leukaemia, obstructive sleep apnoea
Edwards (Trisomy 18)	Presentation: low birth weight, small mouth and chin, rocker-bottom feet Associated conditions: ventricular septal defect, renal malformations
Patau (Trisomy 13)	Presentation: structural brain and scalp defect, cleft lip and palate, small eyes, polydactyly Associated conditions: cardiac and renal malformations
Turner (45 XO)	Presentation: foetal oedema, cystic hygroma, webbed neck, primary amenorrhoea, delayed puberty, learning difficulties, cubitus valgus Associated conditions: coarctation of the aorta, renal anomalies, hypothyroidism, autoimmune conditions
Klinefelter (47 XXY)	Presentation: tall, gynaecomastia, infertility, hypogonadotrophic hypogonadism, learning difficulties
Di George (22q11 Deletion)	Presentation: broad spectrum of disease, velopharyngeal insufficiency, cardiac abnormalities, cleft palate, speech delay Associated conditions: Tetralogy of Fallot, hypoparathyroidism, immune disorders
Williams (7q11 Deletion)	Presentation: learning disability, hypercalcaemia, broad forehead, large philtrum, short nose, aortic stenosis
Fragile X (Tri-nucleotide Repeat)	Presentation: learning disability, developmental delay, high forehead, large testicles, prominent ears, echolalia
Noonan (Multiple mutations identified)	Presentation: large head, short nose, webbing, learning delay, bleeding disorders, hypertrophic cardiomyopathy
Prader-Willi (Paternal 15q11-13 Deletion)	Presentation: hypotonia, developmental delay, learning disability, obesity, behavioural problems, hypogonadism
Angelman's Syndrome (Maternal 15q11-13 Deletion)	Presentation: developmental delay, severe speech delay, fair hair, smiley, epilepsy, sleeping disorders

Management:
1. Manage the underlying illness
2. Parental education
3. Rescue meds (buccal midazolam) ONLY if a complex seizure and lives far from the hospital
4. Treatment for status epilepticus as per Advanced Paediatric Life Support if a prolonged seizure

GENETIC DISORDERS

See Table 16.13. Management of these conditions requires an MDT approach focused on enabling the child to reach their developmental potential and supporting the family.

INFECTIOUS DISEASE

Measles (1st Disease)

Definition: infection caused by *Morbillivirus* (*Paramyxovirus* family)

Buzzwords:
- **Risk factors:** no vaccinations
- **Presentation:** cough, coryza, morbilliform rash (see Figs 16.21 & 16.22), Koplick spots (see Fig 16.23) and fever

- **Complications:** encephalitis, subacute sclerosing panencephalitis, pneumonia

Investigations: clinical diagnosis

Differentials: scarlet fever, mumps, rubella, roseola, erythema infectiosum

Management:
1. Supportive
2. Ribavirin if immunocompromised
3. Notify PHE

Prevention: measles, mumps and rubella (MMR) vaccination

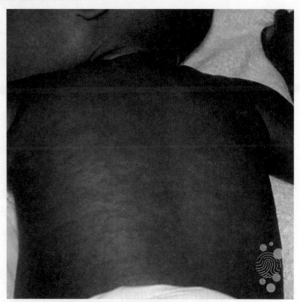

Fig 16.22 Measles in Darker Skin. (From SKINDEEP.)

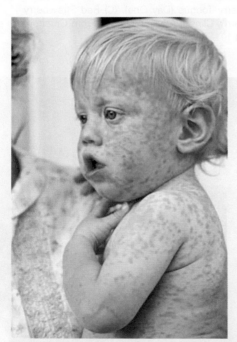

Fig 16.21 Measles in Lighter Skin (From Seethala, R., Takhar, S.S. (2018). *Chapter 122 Viruses*. In Rosen's Emergency Medicine: Concepts and Clinical Practice. Elsevier.)

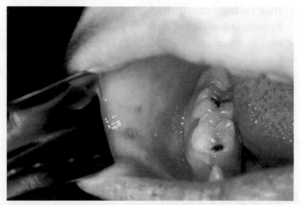

Fig 16.23 Koplick Spots. (From Seethala, R., Takhar, S.S. (2018). *Chapter 122 Viruses*. In Rosen's Emergency Medicine: Concepts and Clinical Practice. Elsevier.)

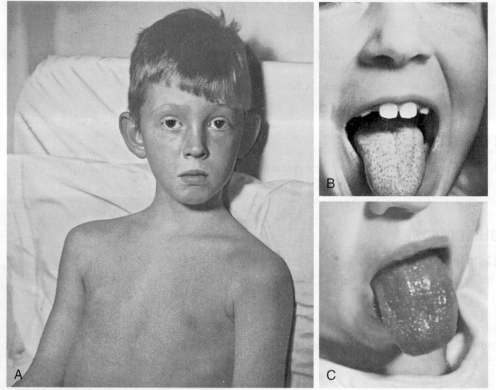

Fig 16.24 (A) Scarlet Fever in Lighter Skin, (B) White Strawberry Tongue (Day One), (C) Red Strawberry Tongue (Day Three) (From Ferri, F.F. (2021). Scarlet Fever. In Ferri's Clinical Advisor. Elsevier.From Gershon, A.A., et al. (2002). Krugman's infectious diseases of children, ed 11. Philadelphia. Mosby.)

Scarlet Fever (2nd Disease)

Definition: infection caused by *Streptococcus pyogenes*
Buzzwords:
- **Risk factors**: strep throat
- **Presentation**: sandpaper rash, sore throat, strawberry tongue (see Figs 16.24 & 16.25), fever
- **Complications:** rheumatic fever

Investigations: clinical diagnosis
Management:
1. Phenoxymethylpenicillin (Pen V). Azithromycin if penicillin allergy
2. Advise about supportive care and to avoid nursery/school for at least 24 h after starting antibiotics
3. Notify PHE

Rubella (3rd Disease)

Definition: an infection caused by *Rubivirus* (a.k.a., German measles)

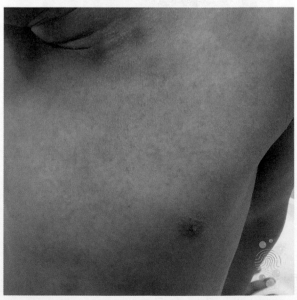

Fig 16.25 Scarlet Fever in Darker Skin (From SKINDEEP.)

Buzzwords:
- **Risk factors**: no vaccinations, infective contact
- **Presentation**: 'blueberry muffin' maculopapular rash (face and neck then across body) (see Figs 16.26 & 16.27), lymphadenopathy, headache, malaise, myalgia
- **Complications**: arthritis, encephalitis, myocarditis, congenital rubella syndrome, thrombocytopenia

Investigations: clinical diagnosis
Management:
1. Supportive

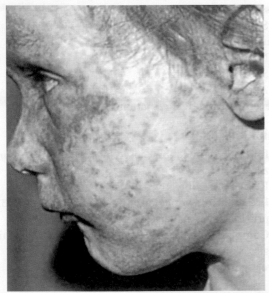

Fig 16.26 Rubella in Lighter Skin (From Ferri, F.F. (2021). Rubella. In Ferri's Clinical Advisor. Elsevier.)

2. Notify PHE
3. Identify infective contacts – females <20 weeks pregnant at greatest risk

Prevention: MMR vaccine

Erythema Infectiosum (5th Disease)

Definition: an infection caused by *Parvovirus* B19
Buzzwords:
- **Risk factors**: N/A
- **Presentation**: 'slapped cheek' rash (see Fig 16.28), malaise, headache, myalgia, low-grade fever
- **Complications**: aplastic crisis, hydrops fetalis (if pregnant woman infected)

Investigations: clinical diagnosis
Management:
1. Supportive
2. No need to stay off school/work as not contagious once the rash develops
3. Contacts should be identified and advice given

Roseola (6th Disease)

Definition: an infection caused by *Human herpesvirus* 6&7 (HHV 6&7)
Buzzwords:
- **Risk factors**: <3 years of age
- **Presentation**: high fever followed by a maculopapular rash (see Figs 16.29 & 16.30), rhinitis, irritability
- **Complications**: febrile convulsion, aseptic meningitis, encephalitis

Investigations: clinical diagnosis
Management: supportive

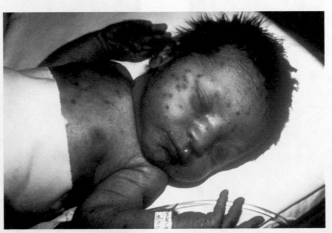

Fig 16.27 Rubella in Darker Skin (From Rochester, C.K., Adams D.J. (2022). *12 Rubella*. In Netter's Infectious Diseases. Elsevier.)

Mumps

Definition: a viral infection caused by the single-stranded RNA virus, *Paramyxovirus*, which is spread through respiratory droplets

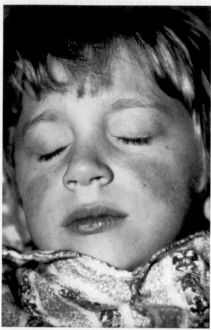

Fig 16.28 'Slapped Cheek' Appearance (From Brown, K.E. (2019). 43 Parvoviruses B19 infection; erythema infectiosum. In Medical Microbiology. Elsevier.)

Buzzwords:
- **Risk factors:** no vaccinations, immunosuppression
- **Presentations:** low-grade fever, myalgia, headache, joint pain, painful bilateral parotid swelling (hamster cheek)
- **Complications:** aseptic meningitis, encephalitis, orchitis/oophoritis (if postpubertal), transient hearing loss, pancreatitis

Differentials: Epstein-Barr virus, bacterial parotitis, parotid duct obstruction

Investigations: usually a clinical diagnosis, but the diagnosis should be confirmed
- **Salivary IgM:** confirms mumps

Management:
1. Notify PHE
2. Supportive management
3. Avoid school/work for 5 days following symptoms

Prevention: MMR vaccination

Chicken Pox

Definition: an infection caused by *Varicella-zoster virus*

Buzzwords:
- **Risk factors:** infective contacts, <10 years of age
- **Presentation:** vesicular rash (see Figs 16.31 & 16.32), pruritis, fever, malaise, crusting within 5 days
- **Complications:** meningoencephalitis, scarring, shingles, skin infections, acute cerebellar ataxia

Investigations: clinical diagnosis

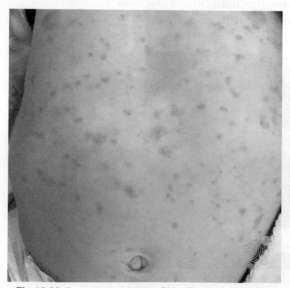

Fig 16.29 Roseola in Lighter Skin (From SKINDEEP.)

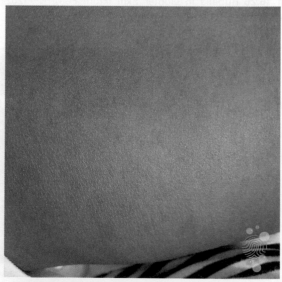

Fig 16.30 Roseola in Darker Skin. (From SKINDEEP.)

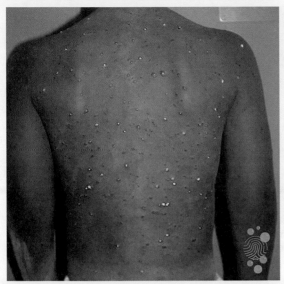

Fig 16.31 Chicken Pox in Darker Skin (From SKINDEEP.)

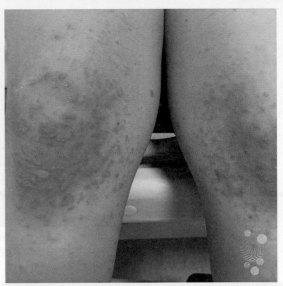

Fig 16.33 Hand, Foot and Mouth Disease in Lighter Skin (From SKINDEEP.)

Hand, Foot and Mouth

Definition: a viral infection most commonly caused by *Coxsackievirus* A16

Buzzwords:

- **Risk factors:** infective contact
- **Presentation:** malaise, anorexia, cough, fever, oral ulceration, macules and papules on the hands and feet (see Figs 16.33 & 16.34)
- **Complications:** dehydration due to mouth soreness, aseptic meningitis (rare)

Investigations: clinical diagnosis

Management:

1. Supportive: encourage oral intake and soft diet
2. No time off school/nursery required to reduce spread
3. Transmission reduction through good hand hygiene

CHILD PROTECTION

Child Maltreatment

Definition: all forms of maltreatment resulting in potential or actual harm to a child

- **Physical:** causing physical harm
- **Emotional:** persistent emotional maltreatment causing adverse effects on development
- **Sexual:** involving a child in sexual activities including active and passive exposure
- **Neglect:** a persistent inability to meet a child's needs causing adverse effects on child development

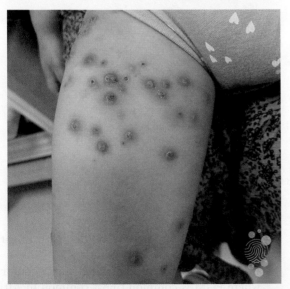

Fig 16.32 Chicken Pox in Lighter Skin (From SKINDEEP.)

Differentials: HSV, hand, foot and mouth disease, scabies, guttate psoriasis

Management:

1. Supportive
2. Avoid scratching spots
3. Remain off school/work until lesions are crusted
4. Acyclovir if severe and within 24 h of lesions appearing

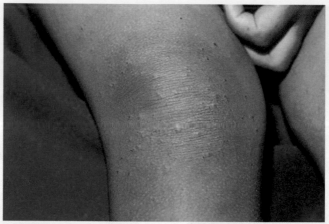

Fig 16.34 Hand Foot and Mouth Disease in Darker Skin (From Paller, A.S., Mancini, A.J. (2016). Chapter: 16 Exanthematous Diseases of Childhood. In Hurwitz Clinical Pediatric Dermatology. Elsevier.)

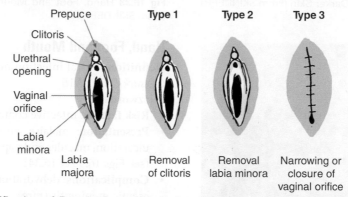

Fig 16.35 Classification of Female Genital Mutilation Areas removed are highlighted in yellow. Type 4 encompasses all other harmful procedures not performed for medical purposes (Illustrated by Hollie Blaber)

- **Fabricated/induced illness:** misrepresentation of a child as being unwell
- **Female genital mutilation (FGM):** removal or injury to any part of a female's genitals for nonmedical purposes. This is a criminal offence and must be reported to the police (see Fig 16.35).

Buzzwords:
- **Risk factors:**
  - **Social factors:** poverty, intrafamilial abuse, poor housing
  - **Parental factors:** substance misuse, mental health, learning difficulties, history of violence or abuse, refusal to engage with services
  - **Child factors:** physical/mental disability, in care system
  - **FGM:** family history, originating from a country where FGM is common (most common in African countries)
- **Presentation:** see below for individual types
  - **Physical:** torn frenulum, rib fractures, multiple fractures, fractures in a nonmobile child, handprint bruise, bruise of soft areas (see Fig 16.36), burns on hands and feet, bite marks
  - **Shaken baby syndrome:** subdural haemorrhage, cerebral oedema, retinal haemorrhage

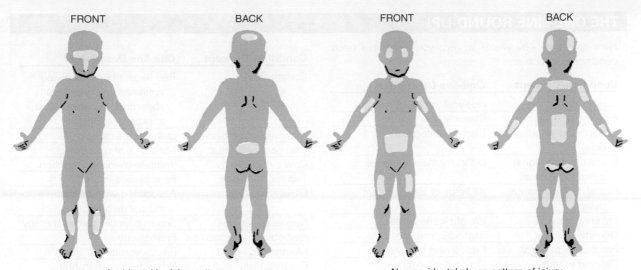

FRONT　　　　BACK　　　　FRONT　　　　BACK

Accidental bruising pattern　　　　Non-accidental abuse pattern of injury

Fig 16.36 Body Maps Showing Classic Bruising Patterns in Accidental and Nonaccidental Injuries (Illustrated by Hollie Blaber)

- **Emotional:** apathetic, delayed development, violent, fearful, secondary enuresis, nonattendance, self-harm, depression, inappropriate child/carer interaction
- **Sexual:** persistent UTI, sexually transmitted infection, pregnancy, vaginal bleeding, anal bruising, anal bleeding, sexualised behaviours, self-harm
- **Neglect:** missed appointments, ravenous, dirty clothes, unwashed, unsupervised at home, drug and alcohol abuse, poor dentition
- **Fabricated:** unclear diagnosis, significant clinical uncertainty, multiple opinions sought, unexpected wheelchair use
- **FGM:** unexpected school absence, genital pain, recurrent UTIs, resistance to intimate examination

Investigations:
- **Immediate CT +/- MRI** (if brain injury suspected): brain haemorrhage

- **Full skeletal survey** (if <30 months of age): to identify any new or healing bony injuries
- **Coagulation test:** extensive bruising may be due to an underlying haematological condition

Differentials: bleeding disorder, behavioural problems

Management:
1. Treat any associated medical conditions appropriately
2. If concerned, get senior advice and follow local safeguarding policy
3. Meticulous OBJECTIVE notes (including a body map, see Fig 16.36) must be taken throughout
4. If FGM is present, you must report to the police
5. If a referral is required, gain consent from the parents or young person unless this will put them at immediate danger
6. Consider the immediate safety of the child and other children at home

THE ONE-LINE ROUND-UP!

Here are some key words to help you remember each condition/concept.

Condition/Concept	One-line Description
Gross motor delay	Not walking by 18 months
Fine motor delay	Check vision
Speech and language delay	Check hearing
Social and emotional behavioural delay	Difficulty making friends
Global developmental delay	All fields of development
Faltering growth	Weight <2nd centile
Obesity	BMI >98th centile
Precocious puberty	Concerning in boys
Delayed puberty	Concerning in girls
PDA	Continuous machine-like murmur
ASD	Systolic ejection ULSE
VSD	Heart failure
TOF	Large VSD, overriding aorta, pulmonary stenosis, right ventricular hypertrophy
TGA	Egg-shaped heart
AVSD	Surgical repair required
Coarctation	Brachio-femoral delay
Kawasaki disease	Aspirin, coronary artery aneurysm
IRDS	Inadequate surfactant
TTN	Excess fluid in the lungs
Laryngomalacia	Stridor
Bronchiolitis	Viral-induced inflammation
Asthma	Diurnal variability
Croup	Barking cough
Bacterial tracheitis	Emergency! High risk of airway obstruction
Whooping cough	Persistent cough
Cystic fibrosis	Autosomal recessive CFTR-channel mutation
Functional/recurrent abdominal pain	Symptom diary

Condition/Concept	One-line Description
Constipation	Red flags: ribbon stool, leg weakness, no meconium, abdominal distension and anal abnormalities
Hirschsprung disease	Delayed meconium
Viral gastroenteritis	Norovirus or rotavirus
Cow's milk allergy	Immune-mediated reaction
Toddler diarrhoea	Food pieces in stool
GORD	Associated with neurodevelopmental disorders
Neonatal jaundice	Serum bilirubin guides therapy
Necrotising enterocolitis	Prematurity
Malrotation	Bilious vomit
Gastroschisis	No protective membrane
Omphalocele	Protective membrane intact
Duodenal atresia	Double bubble
Pyloric stenosis	Projectile vomit
Intussusception	Red currant jelly stool and target sign
Mesenteric adenitis	Appendicitis mimic
UTI	May need USS, DMSA or MCUG
Vesicoureteric reflux	Recurrent UTIs
Enuresis	Desmopressin for short-term fix
Neuroblastoma	Catecholamines
Wilms' tumour	Haematuria
Cerebral palsy	MDT approach
Febrile convulsions	Viral infection
Neural tube defect	Folate replacement
Measles	Koplick spots
Scarlet fever	Sandpaper rash, strawberry tongue
Rubella	Lymphadenopathy
Erythema infectiosum	Slapped cheek
Roseola	Febrile convulsions
Mumps	Parotid swelling
Chicken pox	Vesicular rash
Hand foot and mouth	Coxsackie A16
Child maltreatment	Body maps and objective documentation

READING LIST: PAEDIATRICS IN AN HOUR

Development, Growth and Puberty

Developmental Delay

Dosman, C. F., Andrews, D., & Goulden, K. J. (2012). Evidence-based milestone ages as a framework for developmental surveillance. *Paediatr Child Health*, *17*, 561–568. https://doi.org/10.1093/pch/17.10.561.

Longmore, J. M., Amarakone, K., & Collier, J. A. B. (2013). *Oxford handbook of clinical specialties* (8th ed.). Oxford University Press.

Lissauer, T., & Carroll, W. (2017). *Illustrated textbook of paediatrics* (5th ed.). Elsevier Science.

Growth

BMJ Best Practice. (2021). *Assessment of short stature.* Accessed April 2021. https://bestpractice.bmj.com/topics/en-gb/749/diagnosis-approach#referencePop27.

Kumar, S. (2013). Tall stature in children: Differential diagnosis and management. *Int J Pediatr Endocrinol* (Suppl. 1). https://doi.org/10.1186/1687-9856-2013-S1-P53.

Lissauer, T., & Carroll, W. (2017). *Illustrated textbook of paediatrics* (5th ed.). Elsevier Science.

Faltering Growth (Previously Referred to as Failure to Thrive)

NICE. (2018). *CKS: Faltering growth.* Accessed April 2021. https://cks.nice.org.uk/faltering-growth#!topicSummary.

Obesity

NICE. (2014). *CG189: Obesity: identification, assessment and management.* Accessed April 2021. https://www.nice.org.uk/guidance/cg189.

Puberty

Patient info. (2015). *Precocious puberty.* Accessed April 2021. https://patient.info/doctor/precocious-puberty-pro.

Patient info. (2015). *Delayed puberty.* Accessed April 2021. https://patient.info/doctor/delayed-puberty#nav-1.

Lissauer, T., & Carroll, W. (2017). *Illustrated textbook of paediatrics* (5th ed.). Elsevier Science.

Cardiology

Circulatory Changes at Birth

Lissauer, T., & Carroll, W. (2017). *Illustrated textbook of paediatrics* (5th ed.). Elsevier Science.

Patent Ductus Arteriosus

Longmore, J. M., Amarakone, K., & Collier, J. A. B. (2013). *Oxford handbook of clinical specialties* (8th ed.). Oxford University Press.

Atrial Septal Defect

Patient info. (2015). *Atrial septal defect.* Accessed April 2021. https://patient.info/doctor/atrial-septal-defect-pro.

Ventricular Septal Defect

Patient info. (2014). *Eisenmenger's syndrome.* Accessed April 2021. https://patient.info/doctor/eisenmengers-syndrome#nav-3.

Patient info. (2015). *Ventricular septal defect.* Accessed April 2021. https://patient.info/doctor/ventricular-septal-defect-pro.

Tetralogy of Fallot

Centers for Disease Control and Prevention. (2020). *Tetralogy of Fallot.* Accessed April 2021. https://www.cdc.gov/ncbddd/heartdefects/tetralogyoffallot.html.

Patient info. (2014). *Fallot's tetralogy.* Accessed April 2021. https://patient.info/doctor/fallots-tetralogy.

BMJ Best Practice. (2020). *Tetralogy of Fallot.* Accessed April 2021. https://bestpractice.bmj.com/topics/en-gb/701/management-approach.

Transposition of the Great Arteries

Warnes, C. A. (2006). Transposition of the great arteries. *Circulation*, *114*, 2699–2709. https://doi.org/10.1161/CIRCULATIONAHA.105.592352.

Lissauer, T., & Carroll, W. (2017). *Illustrated textbook of paediatrics* (5th ed.). Elsevier Science.

AVSD

Lissauer, T., & Carroll, W. (2017). *Illustrated textbook of paediatrics* (5th ed.). Elsevier Science.

Coarctation

Lissauer, T., & Carroll, W. (2017). *Illustrated textbook of paediatrics* (5th ed.). Elsevier Science.

BMJ Best Practice. (2018). *Aortic coarctation.* Accessed April 2021. https://bestpractice.bmj.com/topics/en-gb/698.

Kawasaki Disease

NHS. (2018). *Kawasaki disease.* Accessed April 2021. https://www.nhs.uk/conditions/kawasaki-disease/.

McCrindle, B. W., Rowley, A. H., Newburger, J. W., et al. (2017). Diagnosis, treatment, and long-term management of Kawasaki Disease: A scientific statement for health professionals from the American Heart Association. *Circulation*, *135*, e927–e999. https://doi.org/10.1161/CIR.0000000000000484.

NICE. (2019). *NG143: Fever in under 5s: assessment and initial management.* Accessed April 2021. https://www.nice.org.uk/guidance/ng143.

National Organization for Rare Disorders. (2009). *Kawasaki disease.* Accessed April 2021. https://rarediseases.org/rare-diseases/kawasaki-disease/.

Respiratory

Infant Respiratory Distress Syndrome

Patient info. (2016). *Infant respiratory distress syndrome.* Accessed April 2021. https://patient.info/doctor/infant-respiratory-distress-syndrome.

Transient Tachypnoea of the Newborn

Jha, K., Nassar, G. N., & Makker, K. (2020). *Transient tachypnea of the newborn.* StatPearls. StatPearls Publishing. Accessed April 2021. https://www.ncbi.nlm.nih.gov/books/NBK537354/.

Lissauer, T., & Carroll, W. (2017). *Illustrated textbook of paediatrics* (5th ed.). Elsevier Science.

Laryngomalacia

Dobbie, A. M., & White, D. R. (2013). Laryngomalacia. *Pediatr Clin North Am, 60,* 893–902. https://doi.org/10.1016/j.pcl.2013.04.013.

Bronchiolitis

NICE. (2015). *NG9: Bronchiolitis in children: diagnosis and management.* Accessed April 2021. https://www.nice.org.uk/guidance/ng9

Atopic Asthma

BTS/SIGN. (2019). *British guideline on the management of asthma.* Accessed April 2021. https://www.brit-thoracic.org.uk/quality-improvement/guidelines/asthma/.

NICE. (2021). *NG80: Asthma: Diagnosis, monitoring and chronic asthma management.* Accessed April 2021. https://www.nice.org.uk/guidance/ng80/chapter/Recommendations#principles-of-pharmacological-treatment.

NICE. (2020). *CKS: Cough.* Accessed April 2021. https://cks.nice.org.uk/cough-acute-with-chest-signs-in-children#!scenario.

Croup

NICE. (2019). *CKS: Croup.* Accessed April 2021. https://cks.nice.org.uk/topics/croup/management/management/.

Bacterial Tracheitis

Burton, L. V., & Silberman, M. (2021). *Bacterial tracheitis.* StatPearls. StatPearls Publishing. Accessed April 2021. https://www.ncbi.nlm.nih.gov/books/NBK470240/.

Whooping Cough

NICE. (2018). *CKS: Whooping cough.* Accessed April 2021. https://cks.nice.org.uk/topics/whooping-cough/.

Community-acquired Pneumonia

BTS. (2011). *British Thoracic Society (BTS) guidelines for the management of community acquired pneumonia in children.* Accessed April 2021. https://thorax.bmj.com/content/66/Suppl_2/ii1.

NICE. (2019). *NG143: Fever in under 5s: Assessment and initial management.* Accessed April 2021. https://www.nice.org.uk/guidance/ng143.

Stuckey-Schrock, K., Hayes, B. L., & George, C. M. (2012). Community-acquired pneumonia in children. *Am Fam Physician, 86,* 661–667.

Cystic Fibrosis

NICE. (2017). *NG78: Cystic fibrosis: Diagnosis and management.* Accessed April 2021. https://www.nice.org.uk/guidance/ng78.

Gastroenterology and General Surgery

Functional/Recurrent Abdominal Pain

Patient info. (2017). *Recurrent abdominal pain in children.* Accessed April 2021. https://patient.info/doctor/recurrent-abdominal-pain-in-children-pro.

Constipation

NICE. (2019). *CKS: Constipation.* Accessed April 2021. https://cks.nice.org.uk/constipation-in-children#!diagnosisSub.

NICE. (2017). *CG99: Constipation in children and people: diagnosis and management.* Accessed April 2021. https://www.nice.org.uk/guidance/cg99/chapter/1-Guidance#history-taking-and-physical-examination.

Hirschsprung Disease

Patient info. (2014). *Hirschsprung's disease.* Accessed April 2021. https://patient.info/doctor/hirschsprungs-disease-pro.

NICE. (2017). *CG99: Constipation in children and people: diagnosis and management.* Accessed April 2021. https://www.nice.org.uk/guidance/cg99/chapter/1-Guidance#history-taking-and-physical-examination.

GOSH. (2020). *Hirschsprung's disease.* Accessed April 2021. https://www.gosh.nhs.uk/conditions-and-treatments/conditions-we-treat/hirschsprungs-disease.

Diarrhoea

NICE. (2009). *CG84: Diarrhoea and vomiting caused by gastroenteritis in under 5s: Diagnosis and management.* Accessed April 2021. https://www.nice.org.uk/guidance/cg84.

Viral Gastroenteritis

NICE. (2020). *CKS: Child gastroenteritis.* Accessed April 2021. https://cks.nice.org.uk/topics/gastroenteritis/management/child-gastroenteritis/.

Cow's Milk Allergy

NICE. (2019). *CKS: Cow's milk allergy in children.* Accessed April 2021. https://cks.nice.org.uk/topics/cows-milk-allergy-in-children/.

Toddler Diarrhoea

Patient info. (2018). *Toddler's diarrhoea.* Accessed April 2021. https://patient.info/childrens-health/acute-diarrhoea-in-children/toddlers-diarrhoea.

Gastroesophageal Reflux Disease

NICE. (2020). *CKS: Management of gastro-oesophageal reflux disease in children.* Accessed April 2021. https://cks.nice.org.uk/topics/gord-in-children/management/management/.

Neonatal Jaundice

NICE. (2016). *CG98: Jaundice in newborn babies under 28 days.* Accessed April 2021. https://www.nice.org.uk/guidance/cg98.

Necrotising Enterocolitis

Lissauer, T., & Carroll, W. (2017). *Illustrated textbook of paediatrics* (5th ed.). Elsevier Science.

Gregory, K. E., Deforge, C. E., Natale, K. M., Phillips, M., & Van Marter, L. J. (2011). Necrotizing enterocolitis in the premature infant: neonatal nursing assessment, disease pathogenesis, and clinical presentation. *Adv Neonatal Care*, 11, 155–166. https://doi.org/10.1097/ANC.0b013e-31821baaf4.

Malrotation

Patient info. (2015). *Volvulus and midgut malrotations*. Accessed April 2021. https://patient.info/doctor/volvulus-and-midgut-malrotations.

BMJ Best Practice. (2018). *Omphalocele and gastroschisis*. Accessed April 2021. https://bestpractice.bmj.com/topics/en-gb/1158.

Duodenal Atresia

Sigmon, D. F., Eovaldi, B. J., & Cohen, H. L. (2021). *Duodenal atresia and stenosis*. StatPearls. StatPearls Publishing. Accessed April 2021. https://www.ncbi.nlm.nih.gov/books/NBK470548/.

Pyloric Stenosis

Lissauer, T., & Carroll, W. (2017). *Illustrated textbook of paediatrics* (5th ed.). Elsevier Science.

Intussusception

Patient info. (2016). *Intussusception in children*. Accessed April 2021. https://patient.info/doctor/intussusception-in-children.

Mesenteric Adenitis

NIC E. (2020). *CKS: Appendicitis*. Accessed April 2021. https://cks.nice.org.uk/topics/appendicitis/diagnosis/differential-diagnosis/.

Lissauer, T., & Carroll, W. (2017). *Illustrated textbook of paediatrics* (5th ed.). Elsevier Science.

Urology

Urinary Tract Infection

NICE. (2019). *CKS: Urinary tract infection in children*. Accessed April 2021. https://cks.nice.org.uk/topics/urinary-tract-infection-children/management/uti-in-children/.

Vesicoureteric Reflux

NICE. (2018). *CG54: Urinary tract infection in under 16s: diagnosis and management*. https://www.nice.org.uk/guidance/cg54/chapter/Recommendations#surgical-intervention.

NIH NIDDK. (2018). *Vesicoureteral reflux*. Accessed April 2021. https://www.niddk.nih.gov/health-information/urologic-diseases/hydronephrosis-newborns/vesicoureteral-reflux.

Enuresis

NICE. (2020). *CKS: Bedwetting (enuresis)*. Accessed April 2021. https://cks.nice.org.uk/bedwetting-enuresis.

Neuroblastoma

NICE. (2021). *CKS: Childhood cancers – recognition and referral*. Accessed April 2021. https://cks.nice.org.uk/childhood-cancers-recognition-and-referral#!scenarioRecommendation:4.

Patient info. (2015). *Neuroblastomas*. Accessed April 2021. https://patient.info/doctor/neuroblastomas.

Cancer.net. (2021). *Neuroblastoma – childhood: Statistics*. Accessed April 2021. https://www.cancer.net/cancer-types/neuroblastoma-childhood/statistics.

Wilms' Tumour (Nephroblastoma)

NICE. (2021). *CKS: Childhood cancers – recognition and referral*. Accessed April 2021. https://cks.nice.org.uk/childhood-cancers-recognition-and-referral#!scenarioRecommendation:4.

Patient info. (2016). *Wilms' tumour*. Accessed April 2021. https://patient.info/doctor/wilms-tumour-pro.

Neurology

Neural Tube Defects

Patient info. (2014). *Neural tube defects*. Accessed April 2021. https://patient.info/doctor/neural-tube-defects#nav-2.

Cerebral Palsy

NICE. (2017). *NG62: Cerebral palsy in under 25s: Assessment and management*. Accessed April 2021. https://www.nice.org.uk/guidance/ng62.

Rosenbaum, P. L., Palisano, R. J., Bartlett, D. J., Galuppi, B. E., & Russell, D. J. (2008). Development of the Gross Motor Function Classification System for cerebral palsy. *Dev Med Child Neurol*, 50, 249–253.

Lissauer, T., & Carroll, W. (2017). *Illustrated textbook of paediatrics* (5th ed.). Elsevier Science.

Febrile Convulsions

NICE. (2018). *CKS: Febrile seizure*. Accessed April 2021. https://cks.nice.org.uk/topics/febrile-seizure/.

Patient info. (2020). *Reflexic anoxic seizures*. Accessed April 2021. https://patient.info/doctor/reflexic-anoxic-seizures.

Lissauer, T., & Carroll, W. (2017). *Illustrated textbook of paediatrics* (5th ed.). Elsevier Science.

Genetic Disorders

NICE. (2020). *CKS: Learning disabilities*. Accessed April 2021. https://cks.nice.org.uk/learning-disabilities#!background Sub:2.

Patient info. (2016). *Down's syndrome*. Accessed April 2021. https://patient.info/doctor/downs-syndrome-trisomy-21.

Public Health England. (2018). *NHS fetal anomaly screening programme handbook*. Accessed April 2021. https://assets.publishing.service.gov.uk/government/uploads/system/uploads/attachment_data/file/749742/NHS_fetal_anomaly_screening_programme_handbook_FINAL1.2_18.10.18. pdf.

Patient info. (2014). *22q11.2 Deletion syndrome.* Accessed April 2021. https://patient.info/doctor/22q112-deletion-syndrome.

Patient info. (2014). *Angelman's syndrome.* Accessed April 2021. https://patient.info/doctor/angelmans-syndrome.

Patient info. (2015). *Edwards' syndrome.* Accessed April 2021. https://patient.info/doctor/edwards-syndrome-trisomy-18-pro.

Patient info. (2015). *Turner syndrome.* Accessed April 2021. https://patient.info/doctor/turner-syndrome-pro.

Patient info. (2015). *Klinefelter's syndrome.* Accessed April 2021. https://patient.info/doctor/klinefelters-syndrome-pro.

Patient info. (2015). *Infantile hypercalcaemia – Williams' syndrome.* Accessed April 2021. https://patient.info/doctor/infantile-hypercalcaemia-williams-syndrome.

Patient info. (2015). *Fragile X syndrome.* Accessed April 2021. https://patient.info/doctor/fragile-x-syndrome.

Patient info. (2015). *Prader-Willi syndrome.* Accessed April 2021. https://patient.info/doctor/prader-willi-syndrome-pro.

Patient info. (2016). *Noonan's syndrome.* Accessed April 2021. https://patient.info/doctor/noonans-syndrome.

Patient info. (2016). *Patau's syndrome.* Accessed April 2021. https://patient.info/doctor/pataus-syndrome-trisomy-13.

Lissauer, T., & Carroll, W. (2017). *Illustrated textbook of paediatrics* (5th ed.). Elsevier Science.

Infectious Disease

Measles

NICE. (2018). *CKS: Measles.* Accessed April 2021. https://cks.nice.org.uk/topics/measles/background-information/prevalence/.

Scarlet Fever

NICE. (2020). *CKS: Scarlet fever.* Accessed April 2021. https://cks.nice.org.uk/topics/scarlet-fever/diagnosis/diagnosis/.

Rubella

NICE. (2018). *CKS: Rubella.* Accessed April 2021. https://cks.nice.org.uk/topics/rubella/background-information/cause/.

Erythema Infectiosum

NICE. (2017). *CKS: Parvovirus B19 infection.* Accessed April 2021. https://cks.nice.org.uk/topics/parvovirus-b19-infection/.

Roseola

Dermnet, N. Z. (2015). *Roseola.* Accessed April 2021. https://dermnetnz.org/topics/roseola/.

Mumps

Gov.uk. (2013). *Mumps: The Green Book* Chapter 23. Accessed April 2021. https://www.gov.uk/government/publications/mumps-the-green-book-chapter-23.

BMJ Best Practice. (2021). *Mumps.* Accessed April 2021. https://bestpractice.bmj.com/topics/en-gb/1037/references.

NICE. (2018). *CKS: Mumps.* Accessed April 2021. https://cks.nice.org.uk/topics/mumps/diagnosis/differential-diagnosis/.

Chicken Pox

NICE. (2018). *CKS: Chickenpox.* Accessed April 2021. https://cks.nice.org.uk/chickenpox#!scenario.

Hand, Foot and Mouth

NICE. (2020). *CKS: Hand foot and mouth disease.* Accessed April 2021. https://cks.nice.org.uk/hand-foot-and-mouth-disease#!scenario.

Child Protection

Child Maltreatment

NICE. (2019). *QS179: Child abuse and neglect.* Accessed April 2021. https://www.nice.org.uk/guidance/qs179.

WHO. Eliminating female genital mutilation – An interagency statement. https://apps.who.int/iris/bitstream/handle/10665/43839/9789241596442_eng.pdf;jsessionid=C-C3A612F5A433B09947E6651DD9D2EE3?sequence=1. Accessed April 2021.

NHS. (2019). *FGM.* Accessed April 2021. https://www.nhs.uk/conditions/female-genital-mutilation-fgm/.

Palliative Care and Oncology in an Hour

Hannah Punter, Thomas Bird, and Laura Cochran

ONCOLOGY

Epidemiology and Definitions

Definitions:
- **Metaplasia:** conversion from one cell type to another, predisposing a tissue to neoplastic changes
- **Dysplasia:** the presence of abnormal cells, may occur prior to neoplastic changes
- **Hyperplasia:** an increase in the number of cells within a tissue or organ
- **Carcinoma:** a cancer that begins in the epithelium
- **Adenocarcinoma:** a type of carcinoma originating from glandular cells
- **Sarcoma:** a cancer that begins in the connective tissues
- **Leukaemia:** a blood cancer that begins in the bone marrow
- **Lymphoma:** a cancer that usually begins in the lymphatic system and affects lymphocytes
- **Metastasis:** when a cancer spreads to another part of the body

Most common cancers:
- Breast (15%)
- Prostate (13%)
- Lung (13%)
- Bowel (11%)

Cancer screening programs:
- Breast screening: mammograms for females every 3 years from 50–70 years of age
- Cervical screening: a cervical smear for females every 3 years from 25–49 years of age, then every 5 years from 50–64 years of age
- Bowel cancer: a home-testing kit (faecal immunochemical test) of a faecal sample every 2 years from 60–74 years of age

Grading

A histological assessment of a cancer to predict how the cancer cells will grow. The higher the grade, the more likely the cancer will grow and spread rapidly (see Fig 17.1).

TNM Staging

The most commonly used staging system for cancers. The stage describes the size of the tumour and how far it has spread. This information is important for treatment planning and estimating prognosis (see Table 17.1 and Fig 17.2).

Tumour Markers

Definition: biomarkers in the blood, urine or stool that are produced by specific types of cancer cells.
Clinical uses:
- To monitor disease progression/response to therapy
- May help to identify if a cancer is present but should not be used without other diagnostic tests (see Table 17.2)

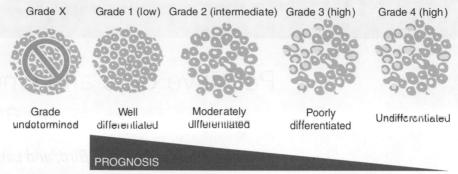

Fig 17.1 **Histological Grading of Cancer.** (Illustrated by Hollie Blaber.)

TABLE 17.1	**TNM Staging Summary**	
TNM STAGING		
T = tumour size	Tx	Tumour cannot be measured
	T0	Original tumour cannot be identified
	T1–T4	Describes the size of the tumour, specific to each cancer type
N = nodes	Nx	Node cannot be measured
	N0	No evidence of tumour in nodes
	N1–N3	Evidence of tumour in nearby or distant nodes
M = metastasis	Mx	Metastasis not investigated
	M0	No evidence of metastasis
	M1	Tumour has spread to other parts of the body

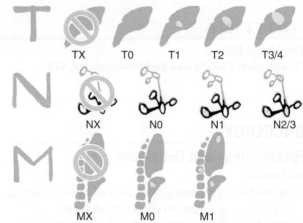

Fig 17.2 **TNM Cancer Staging.** (Illustrated by Hollie Blaber.)

TABLE 17.2	**Tumour Markers**
Tumour Marker	**Type of Cancer**
Alpha fetoprotein (AFP)	Germ cell (testicular), hepatocellular
Beta-human chorionic gonadotrophin (β-hCG)	Germ cell (testicular and ovarian)/gestational trophoblastic disease
Cancer antigen 125 (Ca 125)	Ovarian
Cancer antigen 15-3 (Ca 15-3)	Breast
Cancer antigen 19-9 (Ca 19-9)	Pancreatic/biliary
Carcinoembryonic antigen (CEA)	Bowel
Lactate dehydrogenase (LDH)	Lymphoma, melanoma, testicular
Prostate-specific antigen (PSA)	Prostate

Treatment Modalities

Many different therapies are available for treating cancer. Treatment plans are made by a multidisciplinary team (MDT), which includes surgeons/physicians, oncologists, radiologists, pathologists and other specialists, and often combines multiple treatment modalities. The aim of a therapy largely depends on the stage of the cancer but also may vary from patient to patient depending on their fitness, comorbidities and/or wishes. The aim of the therapy may be:

- **Radical**: to cure the disease
- **Palliative**: to manage the symptoms and potentially extend the length of life

In addition to the main treatment modality (e.g., surgery), further therapies may be given as:

- **Adjuvant:** given **following** a radical treatment to reduce recurrences
- **Neoadjuvant:** given **before** a radical treatment to shrink the tumour size and/or reduce recurrences

Below is an overview of the different treatment modalities available.

Surgery

Definition: a surgical intervention to remove diseased tissue or relieve symptoms caused by a mass effect.

Aims of therapy:

- **Biopsy and staging:** surgery (often laparoscopic) can be performed to identify tumours and stage them, often with a tissue biopsy
- **Radical management:** resection of a tumour with a curative intent (e.g., a bowel resection)
- **Reconstruction:** surgical reconstruction of an affected tissue (e.g., a breast reconstruction)
- **Palliative:** to manage symptoms (e.g., stent insertion, defunctioning stoma placement)

Side effects:

- Surgical risks: infection, bleeding, damage to surrounding structures
- Incomplete resection

Chemotherapy

Definition: cytotoxic drugs that preferentially destroy replicating cells. Since tumour cells grow and divide more rapidly than most cells in the body, chemotherapy drugs affect cancer cells more than other cells. Treatment is usually given in cycles.

Aims of therapy:

- **Curative:** chemotherapy alone (often multi-drug) can be curative for a few types of cancers (e.g., testicular, lymphoma)
- **Adjuvant:** to reduce the risk of recurrence and increase the chance of a cure
- **Neoadjuvant:** to help shrink a tumour prior to resection and/or to reduce the risk of recurrence
- **Palliative:** to help improve cancer-related symptoms and potentially extend the length of life

Side effects: depend on the exact drugs used but can include nausea, vomiting, hair loss, mucositis, myelosuppression, neuropathy, cardiotoxicity, infertility, neutropenic sepsis

Radiotherapy

Definition: ionising radiation targeted at cancerous cells and causing DNA damage and cell death. Normal cells may also be affected by radiation but have a greater capacity for repair.

- **Gray:** a unit of measurement of absorbed radiation
- **Fraction:** a single treatment (e.g., 20 Gray in 5 fractions: 4Gy × 5 treatments)

Types:

- **External beam** (e.g., spinal cord compression): a machine outside the body generates beams of radiation that are precisely targeted at the tumour
- **Brachytherapy** (e.g., brachytherapy for prostate cancer): small pieces of radioactive material are inserted into the tumour to deliver localised radiation
- **Molecular radiotherapy** (e.g., I^{131} in thyroid cancer): radioactive isotopes are given (either orally or IV) and are preferentially taken up by tumour cells, delivering localised radiation

Aims of therapy:

- **Curative:** usually given at high doses over a longer time course
- **Palliative:** usually given at lower doses over a shorter time course to minimise side effects and the number of hospital visits

Side effects: depend on the site of the body being treated and the dose given. Can include fatigue, skin changes, nausea and mucositis

Hormone Therapy

Definition: drugs that mimic or block the actions of certain hormones that some cancer cells rely on to grow. This approach is most commonly used in breast (e.g., tamoxifen) and prostate (e.g., bicalutamide) cancers.

Aims of therapy:

- **Adjuvant:** often used alongside other therapies to prevent recurrence
- **Palliative:** to help improve cancer-related symptoms and potentially extend the length of life

Side effects: depend on the drug used but can include fatigue, headaches, nausea, hot flushes, increased osteoporosis risk

Targeted Therapy

Definition: drugs that target specific mutations in cancer cells. These drugs only affect cells that express the target and therefore are more specific than chemotherapy or radiotherapy, potentially resulting in fewer side effects.

Types:

- **Small molecules:** these agents are small enough to enter cells and prevent tumour growth through several mechanisms, including angiogenesis inhibition (preventing blood vessel formation) and growth-signal blocking.
- **Monoclonal antibodies:** molecules that specifically attach to the outside of cells and that may block signalling to prevent cell division, label cells for destruction by the immune system or locally deliver a cytotoxic drug

Aims of therapy:

- **Adjuvant:** often used in combination with other therapies to prevent recurrence (e.g., trastuzumab for breast cancer)
- **Palliative:** either used alone or in combination with cytotoxic chemotherapy

Side effects: depend on the drug used but can include diarrhoea, mucositis hepatitis, hypertension, rash

Immunotherapy

Definition: therapies that make use of the immune system to attack cancer cells. Cancer cells often survive because they are not easily recognised by our own immune cells. Immunotherapy aims to increase the immune system's ability to recognise and destroy cancerous cells.

Types:

- **Monoclonal antibody:** antibodies specific to cancers cells act as labels, enhancing the immune system's ability to detect cancer cells
- **Chimeric antigen receptor T-cell:** a highly specialised treatment that involves retraining the patient's own immune cells in a lab to target specific tumour cells. T cells are then replicated and reintroduced into the patient's blood stream (e.g., used for B cell acute lymphoblastic leukaemia)

Aims of therapy:

- **Adjuvant:** often used alongside other therapies to prevent recurrence (e.g., pembrolizumab for malignant melanoma)
- **Palliative:** either used alone or in combination with cytotoxic chemotherapy

Side effects:

- Muscle cramps, rash, fever, aches
- Autoimmune related: thyroiditis, colitis, pneumonitis, hepatitis, rash, etc.

TABLE 17.3   Most Common Sites of Metastasis

Metastatic Site	Common Primary
Bone (LP Thomas Knows Best)	Lung Prostate Thyroid Kidney Breast
Brain (Bad Stuff Kills Glia)	Breast Skin Kidney Gastrointestinal
Liver (Cancer Sometimes Penetrates Benign Liver)	Colon Stomach Pancreas Breast Lung
Lung	Renal cell carcinoma – "cannonball mets" Head and neck cancer
Peritoneum	Gastrointestinal Gynaecological

ONCOLOGICAL CONDITIONS AND EMERGENCIES

Metastases

Definition: a secondary malignant growth distant from the primary site. Cancer cells most commonly spread through the bloodstream and lymphatic system, with different primary cancers having characteristic metastatic sites (see Table 17.3).

Buzzwords:

- **Risk factor:** high-grade tumour, advanced-stage cancer
- **Presentation** (depends on the site):
  - **Systemic:** weight loss, fatigue, night sweats, decreased appetite, lymphadenopathy
  - **Bone:** pathological fractures, bony pain, night pain, thoracic back pain
  - **Brain:** visual changes, behavioural changes, seizures, limb weakness, headache, vomiting
  - **Liver:** jaundice, right upper quadrant liver capsule pain
  - **Lung:** shortness of breath (SOB), cough, pleuritic pain, haemoptysis
  - **Peritoneum:** ascites, pelvic mass

Investigations: if the primary site is known, further investigations should be balanced with how they might impact further treatments.

If at first presentation, investigations should aim at identifying the primary site. The order of investigations may be affected by the presentation.

- **CT chest/abdomen/pelvis (CAP):** evidence of malignancy. May guide further investigations depending on the locations of lesions
- **Biopsy:** histology to determine the cancer type. May be achieved through colonoscopy, endoscopy, bronchoscopy, radiology-guided biopsy or surgical excision
- **Blood:** may show hypercalcaemia, ↑ LDH, ↑ tumour markers
- **Myeloma screen** (if evidence of lytic bone lesions): ↑ calcium, ↑ ESR, ↑ paraproteins, Bence Jones proteins

Management:

- Metastatic disease is a poor prognostic sign and usually means the disease is incurable. A primary tumour site MDT discussion is required to guide further management (usually chemotherapy/targeted therapy/immunotherapy)
- Palliative care should be considered early to ensure patient comfort

Cancer of Unknown Primary

Definition:

- **Cancer of unknown primary:** following many tests, still unable to classify the cancer type. A biopsy usually shows very poor differentiation, making identification of the primary cancer type difficult. This is a poor prognostic sign.
- **Malignancy of unknown origin:** evidence of malignancy is seen on CT imaging; however, further tests (e.g., biopsy) to confirm the primary site are not carried out. This may occur if identifying the primary site would not impact the management plan (e.g., if the patient is not well enough to receive treatment).

Buzzwords:

- **Risk factors:** N/A
- **Presentation:** weight loss, fatigue, bone pain, spinal cord compression

Investigations:

- Extensive tests as described above (see Metastases) are completed, and the primary tumour site is still unclear
- **Biopsy:** unable to determine the cancer type from biopsy

Management:

1. Assessment by the primary team for cancer of unknown primary
2. An MDT discussion is required, and the treatment is guided by the investigation results and the patient's prognostic factors
3. Chemotherapy may be offered

Neutropenic Sepsis

Definition: temperature >38°C and neutrophils <0.5 × 10^9/L. Also treat as neutropenic sepsis if patient has a normal temperature but other signs of sepsis.

Buzzwords:

- **Risk factors:** chemotherapy 7–10 days prior
- **Presentation:** fever, fatigue, abdominal pain, generally unwell, sepsis, shock

Investigations: *SHOULD NOT DELAY MANAGEMENT*

- **Sepsis blood tests:** ↓ WCC (<0.5 × 10^9/L), ↑ lactate, ↑ CRP
- **Blood cultures:** bacteraemia
- **Urinalysis and mid-stream specimen of urine:** positive for leukocytes and nitrites if a urinary source
- **Chest X-ray (CXR):** consolidation if a chest source
- Other investigations to identify a source are guided by the symptoms and may include stool sample/swabs/lumbar puncture (LP)/central-line cultures

Differentials: sepsis, drug reaction

Management:

1. Piperacillin with tazobactam (Tazocin) 4.5 g IV QDS within 1 h if neutropenic sepsis is suspected. This is usually 1st line, however it is important to check the local guidelines and if the patient has a penicillin allergy!
2. Sepsis 6 management (see Emergency Medicine in an Hour)

Hypercalcemia of Malignancy

Definition: a serum-adjusted calcium of >**2.6 mmol/L** in the presence of a malignancy. This is a poor prognostic sign.

Buzzwords:

- **Risk factors:** myeloma, known bone metastases, breast/lung/prostate cancer
- **Presentation:** dehydration, polydipsia, polyuria, bone pain, fatigue, nausea, vomiting, anorexia, seizures, coma

Investigations:

- **Blood:** serum-adjusted calcium >2.6 mmol/L, ↓ parathyroid hormone

- **Electrocardiogram:** short QT (see Renal and Chemical Pathology in an Hour)

Differentials: other causes of hypercalcaemia (e.g., primary hyperparathyroidism)

Management:

1. 24 h IV rehydration
2. IV bisphosphonates: 4 mg IV zoledronic acid
3. Recheck calcium in 3 days. Consider repeating step 2 if calcium >3 mmol/L

Spinal Cord Compression

Definition: pressure on the spinal cord resulting in neurological dysfunction as a result of a tumour or vertebral collapse secondary to metastases. Can also affect the cauda equina.

Buzzwords:

- **Risk factors:** myeloma, bone metastases (lung, prostate, thyroid, kidney, breast)
- **Signs and symptoms:** focal neurological findings, sensory changes, saddle anaesthesia, back pain, progressive symptoms, incontinence

Investigations:

- **Whole-spine MRI:** to identify the site and number of lesions

Differentials: disc herniation, vertebral fracture, spinal abscess

Management:

1. Dexamethasone 16 mg stat, then dexamethasone 8 mg BD
2. Nurse patient flat until stability of the spine has been established
3. Referral to neurosurgical team and discuss with an acute oncologist to determine most appropriate management strategy, which may include:
   a. Surgery: if spinal instability, single-level metastasis
   b. Radiotherapy: if metastasis at multiple levels, poor prognosis
   c. Chemotherapy: ONLY for lymphoma, testicular cancer and small cell lung cancer

Malignant Bowel Obstruction

Definition: a bowel obstruction resulting from a malignancy.

Buzzwords:

- **Risk factors:** bowel cancer, ovarian cancer (due to peritoneal spread)
- **Presentation:** distension, absolute constipation, no flatus, nausea, vomiting

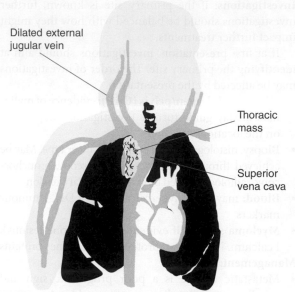

Fig 17.3 Diagram of a Superior Vena Cava Obstruction. (Illustrated by Hollie Blaber.)

Investigations:

- **Abdominal X-ray (AXR):** dilated bowel loops
- **CT** (only if it will guide management): malignancy, bowel wall thickening, air-fluid level

Differentials: acute bowel obstruction from another cause (e.g., adhesions), constipation

Management:

1. NG tube placement and IV fluids
2. If for active management, refer for a surgical review (see General Surgery in an Hour)
3. Dependent on the extent of the obstruction:
   a. If a partial obstruction: metoclopramide
   b. If a complete obstruction: a stent or stoma may be offered to alleviate symptoms

Superior Vena Cava Obstruction

Definition: obstruction of the superior vena cava, often as a result of a mediastinal mass (see Fig 17.3).

Buzzwords:

- **Risk factors:** lung cancer, lymphoma, thyroid cancer
- **Presentation:** SOB, arm swelling, Pemberton's sign (red face when raising arms above the head), distended neck veins, positional headache

Investigations:

- **CXR:** widened mediastinum

- **CT scan**: mediastinal mass, thrombosis, lymphadenopathy

Differentials: pulmonary embolism, cardiac tamponade, constrictive pericarditis

Management:

1. Sit patient up, oxygen therapy
2. Consider 16 mg dexamethasone
3. Referral to vascular surgery for possible stent insertion
4. Offer chemotherapy or radiotherapy depending on the type of malignancy

Tumour Lysis Syndrome

Definition: metabolic and electrolyte abnormalities, including hyperuricemia, hyperkalaemia, hyperphosphatemia and hypocalcaemia, which result from the release of cellular components into the blood after rapid death (lysis) of malignant cells.

Buzzwords:

- **Risk factors**: high tumour turnover (e.g., after cytotoxic therapy, lymphoma, leukaemia, Burkitt's lymphoma), poor clearance (e.g., chronic kidney disease), large tumour burden
- **Presentation:** arrhythmias, seizure, organ failure, hyperkalaemia, hyperphosphatemia, hyperuricaemia, hypocalcaemia, tetany, overload

Investigations:

- **Blood:** ↑ urea, ↑ potassium, ↑ phosphate, ↓ calcium

Differentials: isolated electrolyte disturbance

Management: prevention is best!

It is important to identify patients at high risk of tumour lysis. These patients should be well hydrated prior to chemotherapy and should have their electrolytes monitored. They may also be treated prophylactically with allopurinol.

1. Rehydration therapy
2. Electrolyte correction
3. Haemodialysis if required (see Renal and Chemical Pathology in an Hour)

Catastrophic Bleed

Definition: a large bleed resulting from the erosion of a vessel. May present as haemoptysis, haematemesis, rectal (PR) bleeding or surface bleeding

Buzzwords:

- **Risk factors:** lung cancer, bowel cancer, stomach cancer, throat cancer, head and neck cancer, varices
- **Presentation:** haemoptysis, haematemesis, PR bleeding

Investigations: patients receiving end-of-life care should be managed conservatively and made comfortable. If an intervention is indicated, the investigations below should be completed.

- **Blood:** group & save, crossmatch
- **Imaging:** oesophagogastroduodenoscopy/colonoscopy

Differentials: N/A

Management:

- Nonpalliative patients: see condition-specific chapters
- Terminal event in palliative patients:
  1. Anticipate and prepare patient if the event is likely to occur
  2. Review medications (anticoagulants and antiplatelets held)
  3. Dark towels
  4. Midazolam 10 mg IM

PALLIATIVE CARE

Palliative care: a holistic approach to caring for patients with any life-limiting conditions. Prioritises good symptom control and multidisciplinary support for the patient and family throughout the illness and into bereavement.

End of life: refers to the last year of life

Dying: refers to the last days of life

Recognising the Dying Patient

Recognising a dying patient is a difficult but important skill for all doctors. Some important points to consider:

- Would you be surprised if this patient died during this admission/in the next year?
- Has the patient deteriorated over months, weeks, days or hours? (This can be helpful in estimating how long a patient will survive (e.g., deterioration over days may suggest the patient has days to live))
- Has the patient continued to deteriorate despite medical treatment?
- Is there evidence of irreversible organ damage?
- Signs that a patient is actively dying (i.e., last hours or days) include semi-unconsciousness, minimal/no oral intake, irregular/faint pulse, restlessness/agitation, irregular breathing pattern

If the above signs suggest that a patient is actively dying, a senior clinical review should be undertaken followed by conversations with the patient, family and palliative care team as soon as possible. This allows a care plan to be put into place for the patient's last days of life.

TABLE 17.4 **Anticipatory Medicines**

Anticipatory Medicine	Examples
Pain relief	Morphine sulphate IR (2.5–5 mg SC PRN hourly) OR oxycodone IR (1–2.5 mg SC PRN hourly) NB: if already on regular analgesia, the PRN dose should be 1/6th of total 24-h dose
Anti-dyspnoea	Morphine IR (1–2.5 mg SC PRN hourly)
Anti-agitation	Midazolam (2.5–5 mg SC PRN, max dose depends on renal function) If at risk of sudden terminal event (e.g., haemorrhage), prescribe 5–10 mg IM stat with a clear indication when to give
Anti-secretory	Hyoscine butylbromide (20 mg SC PRN, max 120 mg/24 h) OR Glycopyrronium (200 micrograms SC PRN)
Anti-sickness	Haloperidol (0.5–1.5 mg SC PRN max 10 mg/24 h) OR Domperidone (10 mg PO/PEG/NG PRN max TDS) OR Ondansetron (4–8 mg SC/IV PRN max BD) OR Cyclizine OR levomepromazine Avoid haloperidol/levomepromazine in Parkinson's/Lewy body dementia

IM, Intramuscular; IR, immediate release *IV*, intravenous; *NG*, nasogastric; *PEG*, percutaneous endoscopic gastrostomy; *PO*, oral; *PRN*, as required; *SC*, subcutaneous; TDS, to be taken three times daily.

Anticipatory Medications

Anticipatory medications (a.k.a., 'just in case meds') should be prescribed for all patients who are dying or are expected to deteriorate in the coming days/weeks. The medications should be prescribed subcutaneously PRN. If more than one dose is required within 24 h, consider starting a syringe pump. Local guidelines should be used, and, if the patient has any renal or liver impairment, you should contact your palliative care team. As a guide, see Table 17.4 for some commonly used anticipatory medications.

Pain

Key concepts (an example case is available in the appendix)
- Follow the World Health Organization (WHO) analgesic ladder (see Fig 17.4). Principles are:
  - By the clock
  - By the mouth
  - By the ladder
- Continuous pain needs continuous pain relief
- If required, opioid pain relief should be a sixth of the total daily requirement
- Laxatives and anti-sickness medications should always be prescribed with opiates
- Monitor renal function. If the eGFR is <30, avoid morphine and use oxycodone
- Continually assess pain and alter doses accordingly
- If switching between different analgesics, ensure equivalent doses are given (see Table 17.5)
- Adjuvant drugs are drugs with a primary indication other than pain that have been found to have analgesic properties for some conditions. For example:
  - If pain is not controlled or there is **neuropathic pain**, consider adjuncts such as amitriptyline or pregabalin
  - Metastatic pain may respond well to **steroids**
- Monitor for evidence of opioid toxicity and manage appropriately (see Table 17.6)

Equivalence tables

When converting between analgesics, it is important to know the equivalent dose. In an exam, an equivalence table should be given. Some common ones you should remember are:
- PO codeine → PO morphine = divide codeine dose by 10 for PO morphine
- PO morphine → IV/SC/IM morphine = divide PO morphine dose by 2 for IV/IM/SC morphine

NB: the route affects the dosing.

How to use the equivalence table

An example: 60 mg morphine SC to oxycodone PO

1. Select the appropriate rows from the table (e.g., morphine SC (5 mg), oxycodone PO (6.6 mg))
2. **'Divide by itself'**: e.g., 60 mg (the dose we want to convert) ÷ 5 mg (morphine SC dose in the equivalence table) = 12
3. **'Multiply by what you want'**: e.g., 12 (from the previous step) × 6.6 mg (oxycodone PO in the equivalence table) = 79.2 mg (round this up to 80 mg)
4. Therefore **60 mg morphine SC = 80 mg oxycodone PO**

e.g., 240 mg codeine is equivalent to 24 mg morphine PO or 12 mg morphine SC

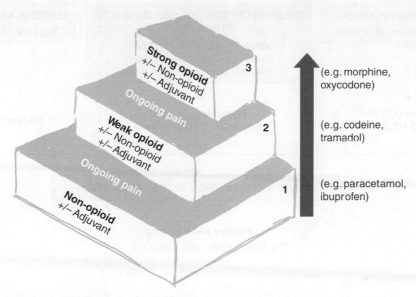

Fig 17.4 World Health Organization Analgesic Ladder. (Illustrated by Hollie Blaber.)

Strong opioid
+/– Non-opioid
+/– Adjuvant
3 (e.g. morphine, oxycodone)

Ongoing pain

Weak opioid
+/– Non-opioid
+/– Adjuvant
2 (e.g. codeine, tramadol)

Ongoing pain

Non-opioid
+/– Adjuvant
1 (e.g. paracetamol, ibuprofen)

TABLE 17.5	**Equivalent Doses**
Analgesic and Route	**Equivalent Doses**
Codeine: PO	100 mg
Tramadol: PO	100 mg
Diamorphine: IM, IV, SC	3 mg
Morphine: PO	10 mg
Morphine: IM, IV, SC	5 mg
Oxycodone: PO	6.6 mg

IM, Intramuscular; *IV,* intravenous; *PO,* oral; *SC,* subcutaneous.

TABLE 17.6	**Opioid Side Effects**
Dose independent	Constipation
	Nausea and vomiting
Dose dependent	Drowsiness
	Confusion
	Hallucinations[a]
	Myoclonus[a]
	Vivid dreams[a]

[a]Associated with signs of toxicity

When converting to patches (e.g., fentanyl or buprenorphine patch), you should check the equivalence tables in the British National Formulary (BNF).

Opioid toxicity

Management if there is evidence of opioid toxicity:

- Ask for help from the palliative care team early if you are concerned about toxicity
- **Pain controlled and toxic:** reduce the dose of analgesia
- **Pain uncontrolled and toxic:** check renal function. Assess the patient for reversible problems (e.g., a fever can cause increased absorption from a fentanyl patch, deranged LFTs/dehydration can affect sensitivity to opioids). Consider switching to oxycodone.

Chronic Pain

Definition: pain that has been present for more than 12 weeks and beyond the expected duration of wound healing. Often neuropathic.

Buzzwords:

- **Risk factors:** arthritis, diabetes, vascular disease, surgery, previous complex injury/amputation, chemotherapy, shingles, disc disease, drug/alcohol dependence
- **Presentation:** pain >12-week duration – possibly depression, distress, disability, opioid addiction, loss of livelihood. May see hyperalgesia/allodynia

Investigations:

- Clinical diagnosis
- Consider imaging for occult fractures/disc disease/nerve impingement
- Diagnostic nerve blocks can show the responsible nerve
- Screen for psychosocial factors

Differentials: drug-seeking behaviour is a diagnosis of exclusion

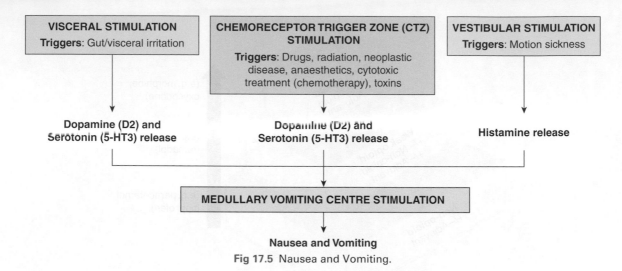

Fig 17.5 Nausea and Vomiting.

Management:

1. Specialist referral if pain is poorly controlled
2. Pharmacological: see the WHO analgesic ladder (Fig 17.4)
3. Neuropathic pain management:
   - Paracetamol ± nonsteroidal antiinflammatory drug trial for all
   - Common first line: amitriptyline/pregabalin, alone or in combination
   - Gabapentin, not with pregabalin
   - Duloxetine: diabetic neuropathy
   - Topical: lidocaine patch/capsaicin
   - Opioid: often less effective. Short/medium-term use recommended only. Tramadol can be used for exacerbations.
   - Trigeminal neuralgia: carbamazepine is first line
4. Nerve blocks, epidurals, intra-articular steroids
5. Non-pharmacological:
   - Exercise
   - Psychological interventions (e.g., cognitive behavioural therapy)
   - Nerve stimulator (TENS)

Constipation

Laxatives should always be co-prescribed with opiates. Stool charts should be kept, and doses should be adjusted accordingly.

Commonly used laxatives for opioid-induced constipation:

- **Senna:** stimulant

- **Docusate sodium:** stool softener
- **Glycerol suppository:** stool softener
- **Lactulose:** osmotic
- **Macrogols:** osmotic

A complete list of laxatives can be found in the appendix.

Nausea and Vomiting

Nausea and vomiting are common symptoms in palliative care. Many conditions can cause nausea and vomiting, and they are also a common side effect of many drugs, including opiates. When picking an antiemetic, it is important to consider the cause of the nausea and vomiting (see Fig 17.5).

Choosing the right antiemetic:

1. Manage reversible causes of nausea and vomiting (e.g., hypercalcaemia, drug side effects)
2. Consider if the most likely cause is **central** (e.g., chemotherapy, radiation, neoplasia, drug induced) or **peripheral** (e.g., gut irritation)
3. If a central cause, trial:
   a. Cyclizine 50 mg PO/IV TDS
   b. Ondansetron 8 mg PO/IV BD (contraindicated (CI) if QT prolongation) – most commonly for emetogenic chemotherapy/radiotherapy
   c. If secondary to brain metastases, dexamethasone can be effective
4. If a peripheral cause, try:
   a. Metoclopramide 10 mg PO/IV/SC TDS (CI in Parkinson's disease and complete bowel obstruction)

5. If in the last days of life, try (these are both quite sedating and therefore avoided unless in last days of life):
   a. Haloperidol 2.5–10 mg/24 h SC (CI in Parkinson's disease and patients with long QT)
   b. Levomepromazine: 5–25 mg/24 h SC
6. Reassess and consider using a different antiemetic or adding an additional one if symptoms are not controlled
7. If the patient has ongoing, difficult-to-control symptoms, seek help from the palliative care team

Breathlessness

Definition: a sensation of being unable to catch your breath. The cause is often multifactorial.
Buzzwords:
- **Risk factors:** end of life, cardiac failure, respiratory failure, anxiety
- **Presentation:** breathlessness, agitation

Investigations: often not required if the cause of breathlessness is known
- **CXR** (if new-onset or worsening SOB): to guide symptom management

Management:
- Treat reversible causes (e.g., if a new pleural effusion, a pleural tap may relieve breathlessness). Chemotherapy or radiotherapy to relieve symptoms may be considered for some cancer patients.
- Discuss breathing techniques and place in a cool, well-ventilated room
- Anti-dyspnoea medications as above
- Anxiolytics may be used in some cases

Dry Mouth

Definition: a common problem at the end of life causing pain and discomfort. May occur from dehydration, medication side effects or radiotherapy and may lead to a *Candida* infection
Buzzwords:
- **Risk factors:** radiotherapy, cyclizine, antimuscarinics
- **Presentation:** mouth pain, dry mucus membranes, white coating, cracked tongue

Investigations: nil indicated
Management: good mouth care and oral hygiene whilst treating the cause
- **Dry mouth:** chewing gum or false saliva
- **Nonspecific:** chlorhexidine

- **Oral candidiasis:** nystatin 100,000 units QDS. Remove dentures and treat these separately until the infection is treated
- **Oesophageal candidiasis:** fluconazole 50 mg OD
- **Cancer related:** call head and neck cancer team

CONFIRMING DEATH AND DEATH CERTIFICATION

Confirming Death

1. Confirm the identity of the patient
2. Assess the patient for 5 min
3. Confirm:
   - No motor response to voice or pain
   - No circulation (absence of pulse and heart sounds)
   - No respiratory effort
   - Corneal reflex absent
   - Pupils fixed and dilated
   - Check for a pacemaker
4. Document each step, the results, and the time of confirmed death (this is when you have finished your assessment, not when you were told they had died)
5. Sign and print your full name, grade, registration number and contact number

Death Certification

When completing a death certificate:
- The coroner should be informed if:
  - Death within 24 h of admission to the hospital
  - Unknown cause
  - During or following an operation
  - An accident is linked to the death
  - Suspicious circumstances
  - Suicide
  - Industrial-related disease
  - Not seen by a doctor in the 14 days prior to death
  - Detained under Mental Health Act (MHA)
  - In prison or recently released
- **Cause of death**
  - 1a: immediate terminal event
  - 1b: condition leading to 1a
  - 1c: condition leading to 1b
  - 2: significant comorbidities

These should be causes and not modes of death.

THE ONE-LINE ROUND-UP!

Here are some key words to help you remember each condition/concept!

Condition/Concept	One-line Description
Grading	Histology
Staging	The size and spread
Chemotherapy	Multiple = curative, single = palliative
Radiotherapy	Common adjuvant
Targeted therapy	Specific small molecules
Immunotherapy	Autoimmune side effects
Cancer of unknown primary	Many tests, poor prognosis
Metastasis	Bone, brain, liver, lung
Neutropenic sepsis	Golden-hour antibiotics
SVCO	Dexamethasone
Hypercalcaemia of malignancy	Rehydration
Spinal cord compression	Full spine MRI and dexamethasone
Tumour lysis syndrome	Electrolyte abnormality
Pain management	PRN = total daily requirement ÷ 6
Anticipatory medications	Analgesia, antiemetics, antisecretory, anxiolytics
Confirming death	5 min and make sure to document
Certifying death	Do you need to inform the coroner?

READING LIST: PALLIATIVE CARE AND ONCOLOGY IN AN HOUR

Epidemiology And Definitions

Cancer Research UK. (2017). *Cancer incidence for common cancers*. https://www.cancerresearchuk.org/health-professional/cancer-statistics/incidence/common-cancers-compared#heading-Zero. [Accessed February 2021].

GOV. UK. (2015). *Breast screening: Programme overview*. https://www.gov.uk/guidance/breast-screening-programme-overview. [Accessed February 2021].

GOV. UK. (2019). *Cervical screening: Programme overview*. https://www.gov.uk/guidance/cervical-screening-programme-overview. [Accessed February 2021].

GOV. UK. (2019). *Bowel cancer screening: Programme overview*. https://www.gov.uk/guidance/bowel-cancer-screening-programme-overview. [Accessed February 2021].

Grading

National Cancer Institute. (2013). *Tumour grade*. https://www.cancer.gov/about-cancer/diagnosis-staging/prognosis/tumor-grade-fact-sheet. [Accessed February 2021].

TNM Staging

National Cancer Institute. (2015). *Cancer staging*. https://www.cancer.gov/about-cancer/diagnosis-staging/staging. [Accessed February 2021].

Tumour Markers

Patient info. (2015). *Tumour markers*. https://patient.info/doctor/tumour-markers. [Accessed February 2021].

Surgery

National Cancer Institute. (2015). *Surgery to treat cancer*. https://www.cancer.gov/about-cancer/treatment/types/surgery. [Accessed February 2021].

Chemotherapy

National Cancer Institute. (2015). *Chemotherapy to treat cancer*. https://www.cancer.gov/about-cancer/treatment/types/chemotherapy. [Accessed February 2021].

Radiotherapy

National Cancer Institute. (2019). *Radiation therapy to treat cancer*. https://www.cancer.gov/about-cancer/treatment/types/radiation-therapy#:~:text=Radiation%20therapy%20(also%20called%20radiotherapy,your%20teeth%20or%20broken%20bones. [Accessed February 2021].

Hormone Therapy

National Cancer Institute. (2020). *Hormone therapy to treat cancer*. https://www.cancer.gov/about-cancer/treatment/types/hormone-therapy. [Accessed February 2021].

Targeted Therapy

National Cancer Institute. (2020). *Targeted therapy to treat cancer*. https://www.cancer.gov/about-cancer/treatment/types/targeted-therapies. [Accessed February 2021].

Immunotherapy

National Cancer Institute. (2019). *Immunotherapy to treat cancer*. https://www.cancer.gov/about-cancer/treatment/types/immunotherapy. [Accessed February 2021].

Oncological Conditions and Emergencies
Metastases

National Cancer Institute. (2017). *Metastatic cancer*. https://www.cancer.gov/types/metastatic-cancer. [Accessed February 2021].

Cancer of Unknown Primary

NICE. (2010). *CG104: Metastatic malignant disease of unknown primary origin in adults: Diagnosis and management*. https://www.nice.org.uk/guidance/cg104. [Accessed Feb 2021].

Neutropenic Sepsis

NICE. (2012). *CG151: Neutropenic sepsis: Prevention and management in people with cancer.* https://www.nice.org.uk/guidance/cg151 [Accessed Feb 2021].

Hypercalcemia of Malignancy

NICE. (2019). *CKS: Hypercalcaemia.* https://cks.nice.org.uk/topics/hypercalcaemia/ [Accessed Feb 2021].

Spinal Cord Compression

NICE. (2008). *CG75: Metastatic spinal cord compression in adults: Risk assessment, diagnosis and management.* https://www.nice.org.uk/guidance/cg75. [Accessed Feb 2021].

Malignant Bowel Obstruction

NICE. (2020). *NG151: Colorectal cancer.* https://www.nice.org.uk/guidance/ng151 [Accessed Feb 2021].

Greater Manchester Health and Social Care Partnership. (2019). *Palliative care pain & symptom control guidelines for adults.* https://www.england.nhs.uk/north-west/wp-content/uploads/sites/48/2020/01/Palliative-Care-Pain-and-Symptom-Control-Guidelines.pdf.

Superior Vena Cava Obstruction

NICE. (2004). *IPG79: Stent placement for vena caval obstruction.* https://www.nice.org.uk/guidance/ipg79. [Accessed Feb 2021].

Tumour Lysis Syndrome

Jones, G. L., Will, A., Jackson, G. H., Webb, N. J., Rule, S., & British Committee for Standards in Haematology. (2015). Guidelines for the management of tumour lysis syndrome in adults and children with haematological malignancies on behalf of the British Committee for Standards in Haematology. *British Journal of Haematology, 169,* 661–671. https://doi.org/10.1111/bjh.13403.

Catastrophic Bleed

Scottish Palliative Care Guidelines. (2020). *Bleeding.* https://www.palliativecareguidelines.scot.nhs.uk/guidelines/palliative-emergencies/bleeding.aspx.

Anticipatory Medications

NICE. (2020). *CKS: Palliative care – general issues.* https://cks.nice.org.uk/palliative-care-general-issues#!scenario:1. [Accessed June 2020].

Pain

BNF. (2020). *Prescribing in palliative care.* https://bnf.nice.org.uk/guidance/prescribing-in-palliative-care.html. [Accessed June 2020].

NICE. (2016). *CKS: Palliative cancer care – pain.* https://cks.nice.org.uk/palliative-cancer-care-pain. [Accessed June 2020].

Chronic Pain

NICE. (2020). *BNF. Treatment summary: Pain, chronic.* https://bnf.nice.org.uk/treatment-summary/pain-chronic.html [Accessed Feb 2021].

SIGN. (2019). *Guideline 136. Management of chronic pain.* https://www.sign.ac.uk/our-guidelines/management-of-chronic-pain/. [Accessed Feb 2021].

HEE e-LFH. (2020). *Anaesthesia eLA, core training, multi-modal analgesia.* portal.e-lfh.org.uk. [Accessed 20 November 2020].

Nausea and Vomiting

BNF. (2020). *Prescribing in palliative care.* https://bnf.nice.org.uk/guidance/prescribing-in-palliative-care.html. [Accessed June 2020].

Breathlessness

NICE. (2020). *CKS: Palliative care – dyspnoea.* https://cks.nice.org.uk/palliative-care-dyspnoea. [Accessed June 2020].

Dry Mouth

BNF. (2020). *Prescribing on palliative care.* https://bnf.nice.org.uk/guidance/prescribing-in-palliative-care.html. [Accessed June 2020].

NICE. (2018). *CKS: Palliative care – oral.* https://cks.nice.org.uk/palliative-care-oral#!scenario:2. [Accessed June 2020].

Confirming Death and Death Certification
Confirming Death

AOMRC. (2008). *A code of practice for the diagnosis and confirmation of death.* https://www.aomrc.org.uk/wp-content/uploads/2016/04/Code_Practice_Confirmation_Diagnosis_Death_1008-4.pdf. [Accessed June 2020].

Death Certification

Gov.UK. (2018). *Completing a medical certificate of cause of death (MCCD).* https://www.gov.uk/government/publications/guidance-notes-for-completing-a-medical-certificate-of-cause-of-death.

18

Psychiatry in an Hour

Frankie Mayes, Nicola Taylor and Joanne Davies

Psychiatric emergencies, including lithium toxicity, neuroleptic malignant syndrome and serotonin syndrome, are covered in Emergency Medicine in an Hour.

MOOD DISORDERS

Depression

Definition: two of the three core symptoms are present on most days for at least 2 weeks and are associated with at least two further cognitive, biological, physical and/or psychotic symptoms. Classified as:

- **Mild:** two core symptoms + two other symptoms
- **Moderate:** two core symptoms + three other symptoms
- **Severe:** three core symptoms + ≥four symptoms
- **Severe with psychosis:** three core symptoms + ≥four symptoms + psychosis

Buzzwords:

- **Risk factors:** >65 years of age, physical chronic comorbidities (e.g., diabetes mellitus, chronic obstructive pulmonary disease (COPD), multiple sclerosis (MS), pain syndromes), female, adverse childhood experiences, medications (e.g., propranolol, corticosteroids, oral contraceptives, isotretinoin), postnatal, psychosocial events (e.g., family breakdown, unemployment, lower socioeconomic status, social isolation), personal or family history of depression

- **Presentation:**
  - **Core symptoms:**
    - Anhedonia (a lack of interest in things that were previously enjoyed)
    - Low mood
    - Anergia (low energy)
  - **Other symptoms:**
    - **Cognitive:** feelings of worthlessness/hopelessness/guilt, decreased memory/concentration, increased irritation, suicidal ideation or intent, Beck's triad (negative thoughts about themselves, the world, the future)
    - **Biological:** altered sleep (e.g., insomnia, early-morning rising), altered appetite with possible resultant changes in weight, decreased libido, diurnal variation in mood
    - **Physical:** constipation, anergia, aches and pains, dysmenorrhea, agitation or slowing of movements
    - **Psychotic:** auditory hallucinations and delusions (hypochondriacal, guilt, persecutory, nihilistic)

Investigations: clinical diagnosis

- **Rating scales:** Beck's
- **Questionnaires:** Patient Health Questionnaire (PHQ)-9 (mild = score of 5–9; moderate = score of 10–14; moderate to severe = score of 15–19; severe = score of >20), Hospital Anxiety and Depression Scale

(HADS), Beck Depression Inventory (BDI)-II, Edinburgh Postnatal Depression Scale, Geriatric Depression Scale
- **Blood:** vitamin B12 and folic acid, since patients with depression have been found to have deficiencies in these compared with non-sufferers; however, not diagnostic

Differentials:
- **Physical:** hypothyroidism, head injury, Cushing's disease, obstructive sleep apnoea syndrome
- **Other:** normal sadness, bereavement (numbness, overwhelming 'pangs of grief', abnormal if prolonged (>6 months)), adjustment disorder (a state of emotional disturbance arising in the period of adaptation following a stressful event), bipolar affective disorder (BPAD)/schizoaffective disorder/schizophrenia, substance misuse, dementia
- Consider appropriate investigations if the history is suggestive of an underlying organic pathology

Management: escalation is dependent on severity
- **All: SUICIDE RISK** and safeguarding concerns
- **Mild: watchful waiting.** Supportive interventions (e.g., self-help guides, computerised cognitive behavioural therapy (CBT), physical activity programmes), psychotherapy (e.g., CBT or interpersonal psychotherapy). Antidepressants are not recommended at this stage
- **Moderate:**
  - Antidepressant (selective serotonin reuptake inhibitors (SSRIs)) for 6 months after resolution of symptoms if the first presentation or for 2 years after resolution of symptoms if the second presentation. Lifelong if there are multiple presentations
  - Psychotherapy (CBT or interpersonal therapy)
- **Severe:** optimisation of antidepressant medications with psychiatric input, consider hospitalisation and antipsychotics if exhibiting psychotic symptoms, consideration of electroconvulsive therapy (ECT) by psychiatrist

Prognosis:
- 50% of patients will experience another episode in their lifetime.
- Up to 15% of people with a major depressive episode will commit suicide.
- Severe depression with psychotic features has a worse prognosis.

Bipolar Affective Disorder

Definition: a mood disorder characterised by fluctuating episodes of mania and depression (or mixed episodes) without an identifiable external cause, including substance misuse, physical medical conditions (e.g., hyperthyroidism, infection) or medications (e.g., antidepressants, corticosteroids). For diagnosis, a specialist review and a history of at least two episodes, one of which was characterised by mania or hypomania, is required.

Buzzwords:
- **Risk factors:** family history, age <20 years, early life stress, childhood abuse, emotional neglect, medication or substance abuse
- **Presentation:**
  - **Mania without psychosis:** symptoms present for >1 week
    - Elevated mood
    - Increased energy: overactivity, pressured speech, racing thoughts, decreased need for sleep, increased sexual activity
    - Attention cannot be sustained
    - Inflated self-esteem: grandiose ideas
    - Reckless behaviour (may be associated with significant risk)
    - Loss of social inhibition and overfamiliarity
  - **Mania with psychosis:** as above, but also with psychosis (delusions and/or hallucinations)
  - **Hypomania:** a less severe form of mania. Symptoms present for <1 week without interfering with life

Investigations:
- **Questionnaires:** Primary Care Evaluation of Mental Disorders (PRIME- MD), Mood Disorder Questionnaire, Bipolarity Index
- **CT/MRI:** not routinely ordered unless there is an atypical presentation of new-onset disease or if considering an organic pathology
- **Prior to starting lithium:** baseline blood tests (e.g., liver function tests (LFTs), U&E, thyroid function tests (TFTs)), pregnancy test, electrocardiogram (ECG)

Differentials: schizophrenia/schizoaffective disorder, cyclothymia, organic causes (e.g., drug induced, dementia, delirium)

Management:
- Consider admission
- **Stop precipitating factors:** antidepressants, steroids, recreational drugs

- **Mood stabilizers** (with input from psychiatrist)
  - Lithium (weekly then 3/12 monitoring of U&E and TFTs at 12-h post-dose)
  - Sodium valproate (avoid in females of childbearing age)
  - Carbamazepine (can cause toxicity, induces liver enzymes)
- **Antipsychotics:** olanzapine, quetiapine, risperidone, haloperidol (atypicals > typicals)
- Consider a short course of benzodiazepines to assist with sedation
- **Long term:** relapses are likely; therefore, consider an ongoing combination of a mood stabiliser with or without an antidepressant. Do not give ONLY an antidepressant
- **Psychological**
  - CBT: recognition of remission and the skills to avoid relapse
  - Structured psychoeducational programmes
  - Social interventions: family education and support

Prognosis: the majority of patients have multiple episodes throughout their lifetimes and will require long-term follow-up.

PSYCHOTIC DISORDERS

Psychosis

Definition: psychosis is a term used to describe symptoms that cause a person to perceive and interpret things around them differently than other people ('losing touch with reality'). Symptoms may include:

- **Positive symptoms:**
  - **Hallucinations:** a perception (in any modality but most commonly auditory, visual or tactile) in the absence of a stimulus
  - **Delusions:** a fixed, false belief that is held despite rational evidence and is not explained by the cultural, religious or educational background of the patient (see Table 18.1)
  - **Thought disturbance:** disordered thoughts, behaviour and/or speech
- **Negative symptoms** (mnemonic 4 As)
  - **Avolition:** decreased motivation
  - **Anhedonia:** a lack of pleasure in activities that were previously enjoyed

TABLE 18.1 Types of Delusions

Delusion	Description
Capgras syndrome ('imposter syndrome')	A belief that someone they know has been replaced by someone else
Fregoli syndrome	A belief that a stranger is actually someone they know 'in disguise'
Cotard's syndrome	A nihilistic delusion in which the patient sees themselves as rotting or dead
De Clerambault syndrome	A belief that someone of high social standing, such as a celebrity or politician, is infatuated or in love with them
Folie a deux	One psychotic patient's ideas are shared with another, usually a subservient or codependent close family member or friend
Grandiose delusions	A belief that they have more power or importance than in reality
Hypochondrial delusions	Excessive worry due to the belief that they have a serious medical condition, such as cancer
Infestation delusion	A belief that they have become infested
Persecutory delusions	A belief that an organization or individual has the intention of harming or killing them

- **Affect:** blunted, decreased ability to express emotions and abnormal behaviour
- **Asocial behaviour**

Causes include:

- Mental health disorder (e.g., schizophrenia, severe depression, BPAD)
- Drug induced
- Organic disease (e.g., head injury, dementia)

Buzzwords:

- **Presentation:** Hallucinations, delusions, thought disturbance, negative symptoms

Investigations: clinical diagnosis

Differentials: see causes

Management: depends on the cause – see relevant section

Prognosis: patients are more likely to be involved in substance misuse and have a higher rate of self-harm and suicide

Schizophrenia

Definition: schizophrenia, the most common psychotic disorder, is characterised by psychosis in the absence of an organic disease or drug-induced aetiology. **Schizoaffective disorder** is a condition in which elements of a mood disorder (e.g., depression or mania) and elements of schizophrenia are present simultaneously

Buzzwords:

- **Risk factors:** first-degree relatives, obstetric complications, substance abuse, lower socioeconomic background, stressful life events, urban life and migration
- **Presentation:** dependent on the type of schizophrenia:
  - **Paranoid schizophrenia (most common):** mainly positive symptoms. Speech, affect and volition are not usually affected.
  - **Hebephrenic schizophrenia ('disorganised schizophrenia'):** positive symptoms are brief, and negative symptoms develop quickly. Disorganised thoughts, behaviour and speech. Age of onset between 15–25 years
  - **Catatonic schizophrenia (rare):** sudden and limited movement, fluctuating between periods of hyperactivity and periods of being very still
  - **Undifferentiated schizophrenia:** symptoms of different types of schizophrenia are present and cannot be categorised into one subtype alone
  - **Residual schizophrenia:** a history of psychosis but now experiencing only negative symptoms
  - **Simple schizophrenia (rare):** mainly negative symptoms with rare positive symptoms

Investigations: clinical diagnosis based on International Classification of Disease (ICD)-10 criteria:

- Symptoms present for at least 1 month
- One of the following symptoms:
  - Schneider's first-rank symptoms:
    - **Delusional perception:** a true perception to which the patient attributes false meaning (e.g., the sun is shining, hence I must be the chosen one)
    - **Auditory hallucinations:** commenting, third person

- **Thought:** echo, insertion, withdrawal, broadcasting
- **Passivity phenomenon:** actions/emotions controlled by an external source
- Persistent bizarre delusions
- Or two of the following symptoms:
- Persistent hallucinations of any form
- Catatonic behaviour
- Negative symptoms
- Significant behavioural changes
- Breaks in the train of thought leading to incoherent speech or neologisms (invented words)
- Additional tests to exclude differentials should be considered

Differentials:

- Organic disease (e.g., delirium, thyroid dysfunction, dementia, brain tumour, temporal lobe epilepsy, head injury, CNS infection, electrolyte disturbances)
- Substance induced (e.g., alcohol, stimulants (e.g., amphetamines/cocaine), cannabis, hallucinogens, steroids, antihistamines)
- Other disorders characterised by psychosis (e.g., mood disorders with psychotic features, schizoaffective disorder, delusional disorder, acute/transient psychotic disorder)

Management:

- Consider admission
- **Antipsychotics:** the drug of choice is dependent on the patient and its side effects. Generally, a second-generation drug is trialled during the first instance
  - Typical or first-generation antipsychotics: haloperidol, zuclopenthixol (extrapyramidal side effects, see Table 18.3 for further information)
  - Atypical or second-generation antipsychotics: risperidone, quetiapine, olanzapine, aripiprazole (side effects include metabolic disturbances and cardiovascular complications, see Table 18.3 for further information)
  - Clozapine can be considered if the patient has been inadequately treated after trialling at least two other antipsychotics, one of which was a second-generation agent
  - Depot administration can be considered if there is a high risk of noncompliance

- **Psychological therapies**, including CBT for psychosis, family therapy and psychoeducation, are a key component of long-term management

Prognosis:
- 80% of patients respond well to treatment in the first year, and 20% will remain relapse-free for the next 5 years. However, the majority will experience recurrent relapses.
- Poor prognosis is associated with being male, having negative symptoms, family history, lower socioeconomic status, substance abuse and insidious onset.

ANXIETY AND STRESS-RELATED DISORDERS

Generalised Anxiety Disorder

Definition: chronic excessive worrying disproportionate to the true risk. The intensity of symptoms may vary but must be present for at least 6 months, causing distress and having an impact on the quality of life. Often coexists with depression.

Buzzwords:
- **Risk factors:** female, family history, poor early attachments, history of abuse
- **Presentation:** continuous and generalised worry; may present as nervousness, fatigue, headaches, sweating, dizziness, trembling, palpitations, poor concentration, an inability to sleep

Investigations: a clinical diagnosis of generalised anxiety is based on the following ICD-10 criteria:
- Generalised, excessive worry for ≥6 months
- At least four symptoms out of the following (one from each category):
  - **Autonomic arousal symptoms:** palpitations, sweating, trembling, dry mouth
  - **Symptoms concerning the chest and abdomen:** shortness of breath (SOB), choking, chest pain/discomfort, abdominal pain/discomfort
  - **Symptoms concerning the brain and mind:** dizziness, derealisation (a feeling that objects are not real), depersonalisation (a feeling that one is not really here), fear of passing out or dying
  - **General symptoms:** hot flushes or chills, numbness
  - **Symptoms of tension:** muscle tension, restlessness, feeling on edge, feeling a lump in the throat

- **Other nonspecific symptoms:** an exaggerated response to minor stimuli, difficulty concentrating, irritability, difficulty sleeping
- Not due to another mental health disorder
- Not due to another medical condition or substance misuse (request tests accordingly)

Differentials: hyperthyroidism, substance abuse, excess caffeine, depression, dementia, schizophrenia

Management:
- Basic counselling, mindfulness, sleep-hygiene education and self-help tools
- CBT
- Pharmacological
  - First-line treatment is with an SSRI
  - Alternative: serotonin-norepinephrine reuptake inhibitor (SNRI)
  - If not tolerated or effective, consider pregabalin
  - Benzodiazepines can be used in a crisis for short periods of time.

Prognosis: usually improves by the age 50 years

Panic Attacks

Definition: an unpredictable acute attack of extreme anxiety that is not triggered by a specific stimulant

Buzzwords:
- **Risk factors:** family history, external life stressors, associated mental health conditions, including anxiety and mood disorders
- **Presentation:** breathing difficulties, tingling, dizziness, chest tightness, palpitations

Investigations: the clinical diagnosis of panic disorder is based on the following ICD-10 criteria:
- Recurrent, unpredictable acute attacks of extreme anxiety with a varying frequency
- A discrete episode that starts suddenly, reaches a crescendo within minutes and lasts for a couple of minutes
- At least four of the following symptoms (one from each category):
  - **Autonomic arousal symptoms:** palpitations, sweating, trembling, dry mouth
  - **Symptoms concerning the chest and abdomen:** SOB, choking, chest pain/discomfort, abdominal pain/discomfort
  - **Symptoms concerning the brain and mind:** dizziness, derealisation (a feeling that objects are not real), depersonalisation (a feeling that one is not really here), a fear of passing out or dying

- **General symptoms:** hot flushes or chills, numbness
- **Symptoms of tension:** muscle tension, restlessness, feeling on the edge, feeling a lump in the throat
  - **Other nonspecific symptoms:** an exaggerated response to minor stimuli, difficulty concentrating, irritability, difficulty sleeping
- Not caused by other mental health disorders, medical conditions or drugs

Differentials: other anxiety disorders, substance misuse or withdrawal, mood disorders, medical conditions presenting with similar symptoms (e.g., Cushing's, hyperthyroidism, hypoglycaemia, hypoparathyroidism, phaeochromocytoma, anaemia, arrythmias, myocardial infarction (MI), COPD, asthma)

Management:
- Acute: reassurance and benzodiazepine use (short term only)
- Ongoing: CBT +/− SSRI, self-help. SNRIs as an alternative.

Prognosis: if left untreated, panic attacks can be chronic and disabling.

Phobic Anxiety Disorders

Definition: a group of disorders characterised by an irrational fear of a specific object, situation or person that the patient tries to avoid. The three most common types include:
- **Agoraphobia:** fear of open and confined places, accompanied by an overwhelming need to return home
- **Social phobia:** a fear of criticism or scrutiny from others, often occurring in adolescence and self-medicated with alcohol and drugs
- **Specific phobias:** a fear of a highly specific situation or stimulant (e.g., the sight of blood), usually develops in childhood. Can be treated with exposure therapy

Buzzwords:
- **Risk factors:** acute traumatic events, anxiety, mood disorders, first-degree relatives
- **Presentation:** specific situations or objects cause anxiety and panic attack–like symptoms

Investigations: clinical diagnosis

Differentials: anxiety, panic disorder, post-traumatic stress disorder (PTSD)

Management:
- CBT +/− exposure therapy
- Can consider a benzodiazepine in the short term if symptoms interfere with daily activities

Prognosis: variable course, exposure therapy is thought to be effective but may need to be revisited if symptoms relapse

Post-traumatic Stress Disorder

Definition: the development of symptoms after having experienced or witnessed a traumatic event, such as abuse, violence, serious injury, threatened death or following military service. The patient relives these experiences through intrusive thoughts, dreams or flashbacks. An **acute stress reaction** occurs in response to a specific, overwhelmingly stressful event. This reaction occurs shortly after the event, lasts hours to days and involves dissociation followed by a combination of anxiety, numbness and confusion.

Buzzwords:
- **Risk factors:** experiencing or witnessing a serious incident (e.g., natural disaster, terrorist attack, violence), combat exposure, low social support, previous mental health issues, history of substance abuse
- **Presentation:** reliving the trauma through flashbacks, intrusive thoughts or nightmares; avoidance of certain triggering situations (e.g., conversations, activities, places or people); increased arousal (e.g., hypervigilance, startled responses, uncontrolled outbursts of anger/irritability); difficulty concentrating. Symptoms present for over 1 month.

Investigations: a clinical diagnosis based on the following ICD-10 criteria:
- Exposure to a stressful event or situation
- Reliving the event/situation through flashbacks or nightmares or experiencing distress when similar situations are encountered
- Avoidance of similar events
- An inability to fully recall events or increased arousal (e.g., hypervigilance, startled responses, uncontrolled outbursts of anger/irritability)
- Symptoms present within 6 months of a stressful event
- **Questionnaire:** PTSD Checklist DSM-5

Differentials: anxiety, depression, adjustment disorder (a state of emotional disturbance usually impacting daily life and arising after a significant life stressor), psychotic disorders, substance-induced disorders

Management:
- Trauma-focused CBT
- Antidepressants (SSRI)
- Eye movement desensitization and reprocessing

Prognosis: around half of patients experience a reduction in symptom severity within the first year. Recovery is often better if the event was singular with no lasting secondary problems (e.g., ongoing legal action).

Obsessive-Compulsive Disorder

Definition: anxiety produces recurrent, unwanted, intrusive thoughts or impulses relieved by ritualistic behaviours, such as counting, checking or cleaning. Patients recognize their thoughts as their own. Symptoms are chronic, time-consuming and greatly impact the patient's life.

Buzzwords:
- **Risk factors:** family history, paediatric autoimmune neuropsychiatric disorders associated with a streptococcal infection, pregnancy, male
- **Presentation: obsessions** (thoughts, ideas, images) and **compulsions** (acts) appear purposeless to the patient and disrupt their day-to-day activities

Investigation: a clinical diagnosis based on the following ICD-10 criteria:
- Obsessions and/or compulsions on most days for at least 2 weeks
- Obsessions/compulsions are self-originating (not imposed by an external force), repetitive and unpleasant. The patient tries to resist them but fails on at least one occasion, even though carrying out the obsession/compulsion is not pleasurable
- Obsessions/compulsions interfere with the patient's quality of life
- Not caused by other mental health disorders, conditions or drugs
- **Yale-Brown Obsessive-Compulsive Scale:** to determine the severity (not ICD-10 criteria)

Differentials: anxiety disorder, depression, schizophrenia

Management:
- CBT with exposure and response prevention behavioural therapy
- +/− SSRI

Prognosis: the course is chronic, often relapsing in times of stress.

MEDICALLY UNEXPLAINED SYMPTOMS

Somatisation Disorder (Somatic Symptom Disorder)

Definition: the patient experiences multiple physical symptoms that often have no demonstrable organic pathology but cause significant psychological distress and impairment. If any physical disorder is present, it does not explain the nature or extent of the symptoms or the patient's preoccupation with the symptoms. The patient experiences excessive thoughts, feelings or behaviours related to the physical symptoms. This disorder may be explained by psychological distress that is unconsciously manifesting as somatic symptoms.

Example: a patient may genuinely experience chronic abdominal pain and various other physical symptoms with no evidence of a structural pathology. The patient may repeatedly present to doctors and experience high levels of distress related to their symptoms.

Buzzwords:
- **Risk factors:** a history of abuse (physical or sexual), female, early-life difficulties
- **Presentation:** symptoms may be distractable. The patient's notes are often voluminous, reports are multiple, histrionic and often affecting different systems of the body over 2 years, with investigations offering little reassurance.

Investigation: clinical diagnosis
- Physical causes should be considered and excluded

Differentials: anxiety, schizophrenia, BPAD, MS

Management:
- Symptom control
- Avoiding unnecessary investigations and procedures
- Regular psychiatric appointments

Dissociative (Conversion) Disorder

Definition: patients experience disconnection with others around them and their environment and/or a loss of control/function of bodily movements. Often precipitated by psychological distress.
- **Dissociative amnesia** (previously hysteria): dissociative amnesia is the most common form. Can be localised, generalised or selective

- **Dissociative motor disorder:** a loss of the ability to move a whole or part of a limb
- **Dissociative convulsions:** may mimic epileptic seizures, consciousness often maintained
- **Depersonalization-derealization disorder:** depersonalisation is when a patient experiences a detachment from themselves or parts of their body. Patients do not lose touch with reality. Derealization is when the detachment is from the environment. These can occur separately or simultaneously.
- **Dissociative identity disorder:** the patient has multiple personalities.

Buzzwords:
- **Risk factors:** childhood trauma, abuse and/or neglect
- **Presentation:** varies greatly, there may also be memory gaps, distinct changes in personality

Investigations: a clinical diagnosis but ensure a complete assessment of differentials

Differentials: head injury, substance abuse

Management:
- Psychotherapy

Factitious Disorder

Definition: symptoms are deliberately invented with no clear incentive. In factitious disorder, the symptoms are consciously feigned but the motivation is sometimes unconscious, although there is often a desire to assume the sick role. Munchausen syndrome is an extreme form of factitious disorder (also known as Munchausen's by proxy), in which the patient invents symptoms for another person in their care.

Example: patients have been known to inflict harm to themselves, such as introducing faeces into wounds or lines with the intent of causing infection. The act is deliberate, though there is no clear incentive.

Buzzwords:
- **Risk factors:**
  - **Factitious disorder:** female, healthcare employment such as nursing, Cluster B personality disorders
  - **Munchausen disorder:** male, 40–50 years of age, antisocial personality traits
- **Presentation:** long history of unexplained, inconsistent, exaggerated presentations at several different medical centres. Symptoms are often unwitnessed or unsubstantiated in comparison with test results.

Investigations: clinical diagnosis

Differentials: anxiety and depression, hypochondriasis, schizophrenia, delusional disorder

Management:
- Multidisciplinary team (MDT) approach with a primary care provider
- Treat objective findings
- Psychological therapy

Malingering

Definition: malingering disorder is similar to factitious disorder; however, there is an external gain, such as a financial incentive or avoiding prison. It is a conscious act.

Example: a person faking back pain to avoid work and gain financial benefit.

Buzzwords:
- **Risk factors:** antisocial personality disorder
- **Presentation:** dependent on the symptoms portrayed. Injuries may appear self-inflicted, poorly described or over-inflated, with discrepancies between the reported and objective findings. The patient will not take unnecessary risks, such as an investigatory surgery.

Investigations: clinical diagnosis

Management:
- MDT approach
- Support and focus on emotional impact

PERSONALITY DISORDERS

Definition: a personality disorder is pervasive (in all areas of life), persistent (present from adolescence onwards) and pathological (impairing function).

For a personality disorder to be diagnosed, ICD-10 criteria state that it must interfere with a patient's relationships, be enduring and pervasive, must have an onset during childhood, and must cause distress in occupational and social situations.

Buzzwords:
- **Risk factors:** childhood trauma, such as physical, emotional or sexual abuse; continual stress; exposure to alcohol in the antenatal period; poor early attachments
- **Presentation (DSM criteria):**
  - **CLUSTER A:** odd or eccentric
    - **Paranoid:** suspicious, bears grudges, jealous, self-important, conspiracy theories

- **Schizoid:** anhedonic, indifference to praise or criticism, emotionally cold
- **Schizotypal:** magical thinking, anhedonic, emotionally cold
- **CLUSTER B:** dramatic, erratic or emotional
  - **Emotionally unstable:** affect instability, explosive behaviour and inability to consider consequences of actions, repetitive self-harm
  - **Histrionic:** inappropriate and dramatic, attention-seeking behaviour; often racy or seductive
  - **Narcissistic (not included in ICD-10):** arrogant, manipulative, high self-worth, envious of others, lacks empathy
  - **Antisocial:** conduct disorder before 15 years of age with a previous antisocial act or arrest, lies often
- **CLUSTER C:** anxious and avoidant
  - **Anankastic/obsessive:** minimal pleasurable activities, task- and work-focussed, rigid stubbornness regarding adherence to rules and morals
  - **Anxious:** fears of rejection, abandonment or criticism and, therefore, avoids social interactions, only getting involved if sure of acceptance with a strong desire to be liked
  - **Dependent:** fears abandonment and 'clings' to caregiver, helpless when alone, requires constant reassurance

Investigations: a clinical diagnosis based on the following ICD-10 criteria:

- Interferes with relationships, enduring and pervasive, onset during childhood, causes distress in occupational and social situations

Differentials: mood or anxiety disorders, substance abuse

Management:

- The main indication for medication in patients with personality disorders is to treat comorbid mental illnesses, substance abuse and short-term management of a crisis.
- There are therapeutic options:
  - **Cluster A:** therapy focusses on improving communication and relationships. Antipsychotics, antidepressants and substance abuse therapy should be considered.
  - **Cluster B:** therapy also focusses on communication and relationships with others, also consider

substance abuse therapy. Dialectical behavioural therapy (DBT) is often useful for this cluster. Disorders such as borderline and antisocial personality disorders may benefit from psychodynamic psychotherapy.

- **Cluster C:** therapy focusing on improving communication, social skills and relationships. This cluster also benefits from psychotherapy and consideration of comorbid substance abuse therapy.

SELF-HARM, SUICIDE AND SUBSTANCE ABUSE

Deliberate Self-harm

Definition: the intentional infliction of injury or suffering for a variety of reasons, including but not limited to overwhelming emotions, regaining control, an inability to cope and communicating a message. The term encompasses suicide attempts with little or no intent.

Buzzwords:

- **Risk factors:** age (peaks during adolescence for females and late 20s for males); family history; stressful life situations such as neglect, physical, emotional or sexual abuse; bullying; comorbid physical and mental health difficulties; substance misuse; lower socioeconomic status
- **Presentation:** very variable depending on the injury type and extent of the injury. Of those presenting to a hospital, the majority are overdoses followed by cutting. Many do not seek medical assistance

Investigations: clinical diagnosis

Management:

- Examine and treat any physical injuries
- Thorough history, including intent, psychosocial risks, protective factors and any safe-guarding concerns
- Consider the Mental Capacity Act and Mental Health Act
- Prevent further access to methods of self-harm
- Offer support to the patient and caregivers if appropriate, include a MDT with primary care and specialist mental health teams, including children and adolescent mental health service (CAMHS), if appropriate

Prognosis:

- 10% require admission
- 30% require ongoing community input
- Repeated episodes of self-harm are common
- There is an increased risk of suicide

Suicide

Definition: an intentionally self-inflicted death
Buzzwords:
- **Risk factors:**
  - **Comorbidities:** mental health disorders such as depression, previous self-harm and substance abuse
  - **Gender:** males account for around 75% of suicides and tend to complete suicide by more violent means such as hanging and suffocation. Previously, females tended to complete suicide by overdosing; however, recent patterns suggest an increase in hanging
  - **Age:** there are two peaks for suicide completion, the first in those 45–54 years of age and the second in those over age 80. Suicide is the most common cause of death in males <35 years of age
  - **Occupation:** employment is a protective factor; however, some occupations, such as veterinarians, have higher rates
- **Presentation:** dependent on the attempt
Investigations: clinical diagnosis
Management:
- Thorough history, risk assessment and safety plan
- Treat physical injuries
- Psychiatric assessment
- Consider the need for ongoing community support
Prognosis: multiple attempts increase the risk of completion

Substance Abuse

Definition: the inappropriate use of a substance resulting in harm to one's physical, social or mental health and leading to a dependency syndrome
Buzzwords:
- **Risk factors:** difficulties in childhood, including aggressive behaviour and neglect; lower socioeconomic status; peer use and exposure
- **Presentation:** varies depending on the substance abused. May present with out-of-character behaviour or a gradual change over time, drug-seeking behaviour, acute intoxication, psychosis and withdrawal symptoms if not in use. Physical signs may include injection marks or complications like hepatitis or HIV.

Investigations:
- Toxicology screen is dependent on the substance suspected
- Clinical diagnosis may be appropriate from the history
Management: specific to the substance and the physical, social and mental health complications caused. May require inpatient detox

EATING DISORDERS

Anorexia Nervosa

Definition: deliberate weight loss by restricting intake due to a distorted body image and fear of gaining weight with a body mass index (BMI) of <17.5 kg/m². **Refeeding syndrome** is a complication associated with treating a patient with severely reduced oral intake. Refeeding syndrome leads to electrolyte imbalances (e.g., hypokalaemia, hypomagnesaemia and hypophosphataemia), with these electrolytes moving intracellularly during the transition from fat to carbohydrate metabolism during refeeding.
Buzzwords:
- **Risk factors:** family history, female, adolescence, low self-esteem, sociocultural pressures, childhood abuse, obsessive personality traits, parental overprotection, occupation (e.g., athlete, dancer, model)
- **Presentation:** low BMI, may present with physical complications like amenorrhoea, cold intolerance, lanugo hair, hypotension, bradycardia, arrhythmias, osteoporosis
Investigations:
- **BMI:** <17.5 kg/m²
- **Squat test:** proximal myopathy
- **Bloods:** may show pancytopenia, anaemia, leucopenia or thrombocytopaenia, deranged TFTs/U&E/LFTs, deranged creatine kinase (CK), deranged glucose
- **ECG:** bradycardia, arrhythmias, prolonged QT
- **DEXA scan:** reduced bone density
Differentials: hyperthyroidism, malignancy, Addison's disease, bulimia, psychosis (food is poisoned)
Management:
- Family therapy and engagement
- Treatment of comorbid psychiatric illness
- Weekly weight management, eating plan and monitoring for refeeding syndrome

- Psychotherapy: motivational interviewing, family therapy, interpersonal therapy, CBT
- Admit as inpatient if: BMI <13 kg/m², serious physical complications, high suicide risk

Prognosis: one-third of patients recover, one-third of patients improve and one-third of patients develop lifelong complications. High mortality due to both medical complications and suicide.

Bulimia Nervosa

Definition: repeated bouts of binging on food followed by purging (e.g., vomiting or laxative abuse, excessive exercise, fasting) associated with feelings of guilt, shame and body image distortion. BMI of >17.5 kg/m².

Buzzwords:

- **Risk factors:** female, personality disorder, history of abuse, history of depression, alcoholism or another eating disorder
- **Presentation:** weight may be within the normal range, episodes of purging, preoccupation with body image, dental erosion, parotid hypertrophy, Russell's sign, arrhythmias, menstrual irregularities

Investigations:

- **Blood:** deranged U&E (especially K⁺, Mg²⁺), creatinine and CK
- **ECG** (if electrolyte deficiency): QTc or arrhythmias

Differentials: Other eating disorders

Management:

- Treat medical complications and comorbid psychiatric conditions
- CBT
- Nutritional and meal support
- SSRI: fluoxetine increases impulse control

Prognosis: lower mortality rate than with anorexia nervosa (AN)

PAEDIATRIC PSYCHIATRY

Attention Deficit Hyperactivity Disorder

Definition: hyperactivity, inattention and impulsivity presenting by the age of 6 years and in two or more environments, including school, home and social situations.

Buzzwords:

- **Risk factors:** male, family history, low birth weight, maternal nicotine use during pregnancy

- **Presentation:** an inability to concentrate, stay still or focus on a task; may appear as if ignoring instructions or not listening; often distracted with apparent forgetfulness. The child may talk excessively, fidget or have tics

Investigations:

- Clinical diagnosis of attention-deficit hyperactivity disorder (ADHD) guided by:
  - Questionnaires: Connor's rating scale
  - Classroom observation or teacher report
  - Educational psychology assessments

Differentials: hearing impairment, low IQ, behavioural disorders

Management:

- Support for teachers and family
- Behavioural therapy
- Pharmacological: stimulants such as methylphenidate, dexamphetamine

Prognosis: symptoms tend to decrease during adolescence. Patients are more likely to have conduct disorder or behavioural disorders.

Autism-spectrum Disorder

Definition: a lifelong neurodevelopmental spectrum condition defined by limited interests, an inability to perceive others' emotions, behaviours restricted to routine, and repetition and communication abnormalities.

Buzzwords:

- **Risk factors:** obstetric complications, perinatal infections such as rubella, family history
- **Presentation:** child is perceived as 'different' by peers, displays limited social interactions, imagination with certain fixations, limited interests and activity choices with a need for routine

Investigations:

- Hearing, speech and language assessments: likely delayed
- Assess IQ

Differentials: deafness, Asperger's, learning difficulties, neglect

Management:

- Support for the family
- Speech and language therapy
- Manage comorbid conditions such as epilepsy
- Pharmacological (rare): antipsychotics or mood stabilisers

LAW

Mental Capacity Act (2005)

Definition:

- A person is considered to have mental capacity until proven otherwise, and all practicable steps to enable an informed decision must have been taken. An unwise decision does not mean the patient lacks capacity
- If acting on the patient's behalf, it must be in their best interest and the least restrictive approach
- Capacity is determined for a specific decision
- **Gillick competence:** considers whether a child <16 years of age has the capacity to consent to investigations, examinations, procedures or treatments

To assess capacity: four criteria must be fulfilled to have capacity:

- **Understand** the information presented (may have to be written or spoken or presented via a translator)
- **Weigh** the information provided and be capable of considering the pros and cons without external influence
- **Retain** the information
- **Communicate** their decision

Mental Health Act

Definition: legislation that relates to the assessment, treatment and rights of people with mental disorders. Allows for the compulsory detention of those who are mentally ill

Section 2:

- Compulsory detention in the hospital for an assessment (+/− treatment) **lasting up to 28 days**, recommended by two doctors (one of whom is ideally previously known to the patient and one who must be 'Section 12 approved'), as well as an approved mental health professional (AMHP)
- Patient can appeal within 14 days
- Cannot be renewed
- Diagnosis does not have to be decided
- Patient **can be treated** against their will

Section 3:

- Compulsory detention in a hospital for up to **6 months**, recommended by **two doctors** and an AMPH who agree that community management is unsuitable
- Patients can appeal in the first 6 months
- Can be renewed for a further 6 months and then annually

- The category of mental illness must be decided
- Patient **can be treated** against their will

Section 4:

- **72-h order** for urgent admission when a Section 2 application would be too slow, AMHP and **one doctor** are required, a second doctor must then assess within 72 h
- **Assessment only**, no treatment
- Can be converted to a Section 2 or 3

Section 5(2):

- Detention of a patient who is already in the **hospital** (A&E is not a ward so cannot be detained here)
- Used as a holding power but cannot be used to give treatment
- **72 h**, during which a formal mental health act (MHA) assessment can be completed

Section 5(4):

- **Nurses** holding power – can detain patients for up to **6 h**
- Within these 6 h, the patient must be assessed by a doctor

Section 135:

- Police may enter **patient premises** and remove a person to a place of safety if accompanied by a doctor or AMHP with a warrant from a Magistrates' Court
- **Up to 24 h** (can be extended by 12 h), within which time the patient should have an MHA assessment (two doctors (at least one of which is Section 12 approved) and an AMHP)
- **No treatment** without patient consent (unless patient does not have capacity)

Section 136:

- Police can remove a person to a place of safety from a **public space** if the Police believe they are mentally unwell
- **Up to 24 h** (can be extended by 12 h), within which time they should have an MHA assessment (two doctors (at least one of which is Section 12 approved) and an AMHP)
- **No treatment** without patient consent (unless patient does not have capacity)

COMMON MEDICATIONS

Antidepressents

Generally work by increasing serotonin and noradrenaline and sometimes dopamine. See Table 18.2 for more information.

TABLE 18.2 Summary of Antidepressants

	Selective Serotonin Reuptake Inhibitor (SSRI)	Serotonin and Noradrenalin Reuptake Inhibitor (SNRI)	Noradrenergic and Specific Serotonin antidepressant (NASSAs)	Tricyclic Antidepressant (TCA)
Examples	Fluoxetine, Sertraline, Citalopram, Paroxetine	Venlafaxine, Duloxetine	Mirtazapine	Amitriptyline, Nortriptyline, Clomipramine
Mechanism of Action	Inhibit neuronal reuptake of serotonin, increasing serotonin in the synaptic cleft	Increase serotonin and noradrenaline in the synaptic cleft	Antagonist of inhibitory pre-synaptic alpha2 adrenoceptors	Block a wide array of receptors preventing uptake
Indications	Depression, generalized anxiety disorder, panic disorder, post-traumatic stress disorder, obsessive-compulsive disorder Fluoxetine is used in children. Sertraline is preferred in patients with ischemic heart disease	Depression, Venlafaxine can be used in post-traumatic stress disorder	Used in depression if first-line options aren't effective or not tolerated	Moderate to severe depression, especially if neuropathic pain is contributing
Interactions	These medications each carry a theoretical risk of serotonin syndrome if they are used with other antidepressants (e.g., monoamine oxidase inhibitors) or serotonergic agents (such as tramadol)			
Side effects	Nausea/vomiting, appetite/weight change, hyponatraemia and lowering of the seizure threshold. Insomnia, anxiety, agitation, headache, sweating. Citalopram can cause dose-dependent QT interval propagation	Similar to SSRIs but due to actions on noradrenaline, also causes constipation, hypertension and raises cholesterol	Sedation and increased appetite, which can be useful. Can also cause GI upset. Use with caution in renal and hepatic impairment	Increased risk of arrythmias (overdose), tachycardia, blurred vision, dry mouth, lethargy and overflow incontinence

Antipsychotics

See Table 18.3 for more information

TABLE 18.3 Summary of 1st and 2nd generation Antipsychotics

	First Generation/Typical	Second Generation/Atypical
Examples	Chlorpromazine, Haloperidol, Zuclopenthixol, Flupentixol	Olanzapine, Risperidone, Quetiapine, Clozapine (see below for more information)
Mechanism of action	Specific D2 dopamine antagonism	Partial D2 dopamine antagonism, 5HT2A antagonism
Indications	Can be used in psychosis such as with schizophrenia and also as a mood stabiliser for bipolar disorder, particularly in mania/hypomania	
Interactions	Medications prolonging the QT interval (e.g., amiodarone and macrolide antibiotics)	Dopamine-blocking antiemetics and drugs that prolong the QT interval
Side effects	Extrapyramidal side effects, drowsiness, hypotension, QT prolongation, erectile dysfunction and hyperprolactinemia	Extrapyramidal side effects can occur with less frequency than with typical antipsychotics. Other side effects include weight gain and a predisposition to diabetes (especially for olanzapine and quetiapine), hyperprolactinemia and QT prolongation

Extrapyramidal Side Effects

- Movement disorder caused by antipsychotics. Includes slurring speech, akathisia (may take weeks to develop) and dystonia, which occurs quickly after the initiation of the medication and can be treated with IM procyclidine 5–10 mg. Longer term side effects include pseudo-parkinsonism (e.g., tremor, rigidity, bradykinesia), which requires a lower dose or a change in the antipsychotic.

Clozapine

- Must be monitored
- Used when other antipsychotics have been ineffective (must have trialled at least two) and the patient is considered treatment resistant
- Started slowly and titrated up. If doses are missed for 48 h need to restart titration
- Side effects: neutropenia and agranulocytosis; therefore, monthly blood tests are needed
- Levels are affected by smoking and caffeine

INTERVENTIONS

Cognitive Behavioural Therapy

Definition: goal-orientated therapy focusing on the relationships between thoughts, behaviours, physical sensations and emotions, and how these perceptions can be consciously challenged and therefore altered. The focus is predominately on the present.

Indication: anxiety disorders, depression, obsessive-compulsive disorder (OCD), bipolar disorders, eating disorders, schizophrenia, substance abuse

Interpersonal Therapy

Definition: therapy focusing on the relationships the patient has with other people

Indication: depression

Psychodynamic Therapy

Definition: therapy focusing on the patient's unconscious thoughts and feelings, recognising them and bringing them into consciousness to increase self-awareness

Indication: depression, grief, somatic disorders

Electroconvulsive Therapy

Definition: the induction of generalised seizures under sedation in a controlled environment via electrodes placed over both hemispheres

Indication: severe, treatment-resistant depression is the most common indication, especially if the patient is highly suicidal with self-neglect. Other indications include BPAD and catatonia.

THE ONE-LINE ROUND-UP!

Here are some key words to help you remember each condition/concept.

Condition/Concept	One-line Description
Depression	Low mood, anergia, anhedonia
Bipolar affective disorder	Fluctuating mania/depression
Psychosis	Positive and negative symptoms
Schizophrenia	Psychotic disorder, delusions, hallucinations
GAD	Excessive worry, distress, palpitations
Panic attack	Unpredictable, acute, extreme anxiety
Phobic anxiety disorder	Irrational fear to specific trigger
PTSD	Re-experiencing trauma, flashbacks, nightmares, intrusive thoughts
OCD	Intrusive, recurrent, unwanted thoughts, ritualistic behaviour
Somatisation disorder	Unconscious symptom production, no physiological cause
Dissociative disorder	Disconnection, depersonalisation, dissociation
Factitious disorder	Deliberate symptom invention, no clear incentive
Malingering	Deliberate symptom invention, clear incentive
Personality disorders	Pervasive, persistent, pathological
Deliberate self-harm	Reduce risk of further self-harm
Suicide	Risk assessment
Substance abuse	Toxicology may be required
Anorexia nervosa	Restrictive intake, distorted body image, BMI <17.5 kg/m²
Bulimia nervosa	Binging and purging, normal body weight
ADHD	Hyperactivity, impulsivity, inattention
Autism	Limited interests, restricted behaviours, inability to read emotions

Contraindications:

- Known intracranial pathology, such as a space-occupying lesion or recent bleed/aneurysm
- Recent MI or arrhythmia
- Stroke

Side effects:

- Risks associated with the anaesthetic and airway complications
- Memory loss (retrograde and anterograde)
- Confusion
- Headaches

READING LIST: PSYCHIATRY IN AN HOUR

Mood Disorders
Depression
BMJ Best Practice. (2019). *Depression in adults*. https://best-practice.bmj.com/topics/en-gb/55. Accessed Nov 2020.

Baldwin, A., Hjelde, N., Goumalatsou, C., & Myers, G. (2016). *Oxford handbook of clinical specialities* (10th ed.). Oxford University Press.

NICE. (2020). *CKS: Depression*. https://cks.nice.org.uk/topics/depression/. Accessed Nov 2020.

Azam, M., Qureshi, M., & Kinnair, D. (2016). *Psychiatry: A clinical handbook*. Scion.

Bipolar Affective Disorder
BMJ Best Practice. (2019). *Bipolar disorder in adults*. https://bestpractice.bmj.com/topics/en-gb/488. Accessed Nov 2020.

Baldwin, A., Hjelde, N., Goumalatsou, C., & Myers, G. (2016). *Oxford handbook of clinical specialities* (10th ed.). Oxford University Press.

NICE. (2020). *CKS: Bipolar disorder*. https://cks.nice.org.uk/topics/bipolar-disorder/. Accessed Nov 2020.

Psychotic Disorders
Psychosis
NICE. (2020). *CKS: Psychosis and schizophrenia*. https://cks.nice.org.uk/topics/psychosis-schizophrenia/. Accessed Jan 2021.

NHS. *Psychosis*. http://www.nhsinform.scot/illnesses-and-conditions/mental-health/psychosis. Accessed Jan 2021.

The ICD-10 classification of mental and behavioural disorders. [ebook]. https://www.who.int/classifications/icd/en/bluebook.pdf. Accessed Nov 2020.

Baldwin, A., Hjelde, N., Goumalatsou, C., & Myers, G. (2016). *Oxford handbook of clinical specialities* (10th ed.). Oxford University Press.

NHS. (2021). *Symptoms – Psychosis*. https://www.nhs.uk/conditions/psychosis/symptoms/. Accessed Nov 2020.

NHS. (2021). *Health anxiety*. https://www.nhs.uk/conditions/health-anxiety/. Accessed November 2020.

Azam, M., Qureshi, M., & Kinnair, D. (2016). *Psychiatry: a clinical handbook*. Scion.

Schizophrenia
BMJ Best Practice. (2019). *Schizophrenia*. https://bestpractice.bmj.com/topics/en-gb/406. Accessed Nov 2020.

Baldwin, A., Hjelde, N., Goumalatsou, C., & Myers, G. (2016). *Oxford handbook of clinical specialities* (10th ed.). Oxford University Press.

NICE. (2020). *CKS: Psychosis and schizophrenia*. https://cks.nice.org.uk/topics/psychosis-schizophrenia/. Accessed Jan 2021.

BNF. (2020). *Psychoses and related disorders | Treatment summary | BNF content published by NICE*. https://bnf.nice.org.uk/treatment-summary/psychoses-and-related-disorders.html. Accessed Nov 2020.

The ICD-10 classification of mental and behavioural disorders. [ebook]. https://www.who.int/classifications/icd/en/bluebook.pdf. Accessed Nov 2020.

Mental Health UK. (2020). *Mental Health UK - Forward Together*. https://mentalhealth-uk.org/. Accessed Nov 2020.

Azam, M., Qureshi, M., & Kinnair, D. (2016). *Psychiatry: A clinical handbook*. Scion.

Anxiety (and Stress-related) Disorders
Generalised Anxiety Disorder
BMJ Best Practice. (2019). *Generalised anxiety disorder*. https://bestpractice.bmj.com/topics/en-gb/120. Accessed Nov 2020.

Baldwin, A., Hjelde, N., Goumalatsou, C., & Myers, G. (2016). *Oxford handbook of clinical specialities* (10th ed.). Oxford University Press.

NICE. (2017). *CKS: Generalised anxiety disorder*. https://cks.nice.org.uk/topics/generalized-anxiety-disorder/. Accessed Nov 2020.

Barton, S., Karner, C., Salih, F., Baldwin, D. S., & Edwards, S. J. (2014). Clinical effectiveness of interventions for treatment-resistant anxiety in older people: A systematic review. *Health Technol Assess*, 18, 1–59. Appendix 1, Diagnostic criteria for anxiety disorders set out in DSM-IV and ICD-10 classification systems. https://www.ncbi.nlm.nih.gov/books/NBK262332/.

Panic Attacks
Barton, S., Karner, C., Salih, F., Baldwin, D. S., & Edwards, S. J. (2014). Clinical effectiveness of interventions for treatment-resistant anxiety in older people: A systematic review. *Health Technol Assess*, 18, 1–59. Appendix 1, Diagnostic criteria for anxiety disorders set out in DSM-IV and ICD-10 classification systems. https://www.ncbi.nlm.nih.gov/books/NBK262332/.

BMJ Best Practice. (2021). *Panic disorders – Symptoms, diagnosis and treatment*. BMJ Best Practice. https://bestpractice.bmj.com/topics/en-gb/121/treatment-algorithm. Accessed Nov 2020.

Phobic Anxiety Disorder

The ICD-10 classification of mental and behavioural disorders. [ebook]. https://www.who.int/classifications/icd/en/bluebook.pdf. Accessed Nov 2020.

Bestpractice.bmj.com. *Phobias – Symptoms, diagnosis and treatment.* BMJ Best Practice. https://bestpractice.bmj.com/topics/en-gb/693/investigations. Accessed Nov 2020.

Obsessive Compulsive Disorder

BMJ Best Practice. (2018). *Obsessive-compulsive disorder.* https://bestpractice.bmj.com/topics/en-gb/362. Accessed Nov 2020.

Baldwin, A., Hjelde, N., Goumalatsou, C., & Myers, G. (2016). *Oxford handbook of clinical specialities* (10th ed.). Oxford University Press.

NICE. (2018). *CKS: Obsessive-compulsive disorder.* https://cks.nice.org.uk/topics/obsessive-compulsive-disorder/. Accessed Nov 2020.

Barton, S., Karner, C., Salih, F., Baldwin, D. S., & Edwards, S. J. (2014). Clinical effectiveness of interventions for treatment-resistant anxiety in older people: A systematic review. *Health Technol Assess, 18,* 1–59. *Appendix 1, Diagnostic criteria for anxiety disorders set out in DSM-IV and ICD-10 classification systems.* https://www.ncbi.nlm.nih.gov/books/NBK262332/.

Post-traumatic Stress Disorder

BMJ Best Practice. (2019). *Posttraumatic stress disorder.* https://bestpractice.bmj.com/topics/en-gb/430. Accessed Nov 2020.

Baldwin, A., Hjelde, N., Goumalatsou, C., & Myers, G. (2016). *Oxford handbook of clinical specialities* (10th ed.). Oxford University Press.

NICE. (2020). *CKS: Post traumatic stress disorder.* https://cks.nice.org.uk/topics/post-traumatic-stress-disorder/. Accessed Nov 2020.

Barton, S., Karner, C., Salih, F., Baldwin, D. S., & Edwards, S. J. (2014). Clinical effectiveness of interventions for treatment-resistant anxiety in older people: A systematic review. *Health Technol Assess, 18,* 1–59. *Appendix 1, Diagnostic criteria for anxiety disorders set out in DSM-IV and ICD-10 classification systems.* https://www.ncbi.nlm.nih.gov/books/NBK262332/.

Ehlers, A., Harvey, A., & Bryant, R. (2012). Acute stress reactions. In *New Oxford textbook of psychiatry.* Oxford University Press.

Medically Unexplained Symptoms
Somatisation Disorder (Somatic Symptom Disorder)

Psychiatry.org. *What is somatic symptom disorder?* https://www.psychiatry.org/patients-families/somatic-symptom-disorder/what-is-somatic-symptom-disorder. Accessed December 2020.

Baldwin, A., Hjelde, N., Goumalatsou, C., & Myers, G. (2016). *Oxford handbook of clinical specialities* (10th ed.). Oxford University Press.

Dissociative (Conversion) Disorders

BMJ Best Practice. (2018). *Conversion and somatic symptom disorders.* https://bestpractice.bmj.com/topics/en-gb/989?q=Conversion%20disorders&c=suggested. Accessed Nov 2020.

NHS. (2020). *Dissociative disorders.* https://www.nhs.uk/conditions/dissociative-disorders/. Accessed Dec 2020.

Psychiatry.org. (2018). *What are dissociative disorders?.* https://www.psychiatry.org/patients-families/dissociative-disorders/what-are-dissociative-disorders. Accessed Dec 2020.

Factitious Disorder

BMJ Best Practice. (2019). *Factitious disorder.* https://bestpractice.bmj.com/topics/en-gb/695. Accessed Nov 2020.

Malingering

The ICD-10 classification of mental and behavioural disorders. [ebook]. https://www.who.int/classifications/icd/en/bluebook.pdf. Accessed Nov 2020.

BMJ Best Practice. (2019). *Factitious disorder.* https://bestpractice.bmj.com/topics/en-gb/695. Accessed Nov 2020.

The ICD-10 classification of mental and behavioural disorders. [ebook]. https://www.who.int/classifications/icd/en/bluebook.pdf. Accessed Nov 2020.

Baldwin, A., Hjelde, N., Goumalatsou, C., & Myers, G. (2016). *Oxford handbook of clinical specialities* (10th ed.). Oxford University Press.

BMJ Best Practice. (2019). *Personality disorders – Symptoms, diagnosis and treatment.* https://bestpractice.bmj.com/topics/en-gb/489. Accessed Dec 2020.

Self-harm and Suicide
Deliberate Self-harm

Mind.org.uk. (2020). *What is self-harm?.* https://www.mind.org.uk/information-support/types-of-mental-health-problems/self-harm/about-self-harm/. Accessed March 2020.

NICE. (2020). *CKS: Self-harm.* https://cks.nice.org.uk/topics/self-harm/. Accessed March 2021.

Baldwin, A., Hjelde, N., Goumalatsou, C., & Myers, G. (2016). *Oxford handbook of clinical specialities* (10th ed.). Oxford University Press.

Suicide

BMJ Best Practice. (2020). *Suicide risk mitigation.* https://bestpractice.bmj.com/topics/en-gb/3000095-. Accessed March 2021.

Baldwin, A., Hjelde, N., Goumalatsou, C., & Myers, G. (2016). *Oxford handbook of clinical specialities* (10th ed.). Oxford University Press.

Office for National Statistics UK Government. (2020). *Suicides in England and Wales: 2019 registrations.* https://www.ons.gov.uk/peoplepopulationandcommunity/birthsdeathsandmarriages/deaths/bulletins/suicidesintheunitedkingdom/2019registrations. Accessed March 2021.

Substance Abuse

NICE. (2017). *CKS: Poisoning or overdose.* https://cks.nice.org.uk/topics/poisoning or overdose/. Accessed February 2021.

National Institute on Drug Abuse. *What are risk factors and protective factors?* https://www.drugabuse.gov/publications/preventing-drug-use-among-children-adolescents/chapter-1-risk-factors-protective-factors/what-are-risk-factors. Accessed March 2020.

Baldwin, A., Hjelde, N., Goumalatsou, C., & Myers, G. (2016). *Oxford handbook of clinical specialities* (10th ed.). Oxford University Press.

Eating Disorders
Anorexia Nervosa

BMJ Best Practice. (2018). *Anorexia nervosa.* https://bestpractice.bmj.com/topics/en-gb/440. Accessed Nov 2020.

Baldwin, A., Hjelde, N., Goumalatsou, C., & Myers, G. (2016). *Oxford handbook of clinical specialities* (10th ed.). Oxford University Press.

NICE. (2019). *CKS: Eating disorders.* https://cks.nice.org.uk/topics/eating-disorders/. Accessed Nov 2020.

Bulimia Nervosa

BMJ Best Practice. (2020). *Bulimia nervosa.* https://bestpractice.bmj.com/topics/en-gb/441. Accessed Nov 2020.

Baldwin, A., Hjelde, N., Goumalatsou, C., & Myers, G. (2016). *Oxford handbook of clinical specialities* (10th ed.). Oxford University Press.

NICE. (2019). *CKS: Eating disorders.* https://cks.nice.org.uk/topics/eating-disorders/. Accessed Nov 2020.

Paediatric Psychiatry
Attention Deficit Hyperactivity Disorder (ADHD)

BMJ Best Practice. (2020). *Attention deficit hyperactivity disorder in adults.* https://bestpractice.bmj.com/topics/en-gb/814. Accessed Nov 2020.

Baldwin, A., Hjelde, N., Goumalatsou, C., & Myers, G. (2016). *Oxford handbook of clinical specialities* (10th ed.). Oxford University Press.

Autism Spectrum Disorder

BMJ Best Practice. (2018). *Autism spectrum disorder.* https://bestpractice.bmj.com/topics/en-gb/379. Accessed Nov 2020.

Baldwin, A., Hjelde, N., Goumalatsou, C., & Myers, G. (2016). *Oxford handbook of clinical specialities* (10th ed.). Oxford University Press.

NICE. (2019). *CKS: Autism in adults.* https://cks.nice.org.uk/topics/autism-in-adults/. Accessed Nov 2020.

Law
Mental Capacity Act (2005)

Baldwin, A., Hjelde, N., Goumalatsou, C., & Myers, G. (2016). *Oxford handbook of clinical specialities* (10th ed.). Oxford University Press.

Legislation.gov.uk. *Mental Capacity Act 2005.* https://www.legislation.gov.uk/ukpga/2005/9/contents. Accessed Dec 2020.

NHS. (2019). *Consent to treatment - children and young people.* https://www.nhs.uk/conditions/consent-to-treatment/children/. Accessed Dec 2020.

Mental Health Act

Baldwin, A., Hjelde, N., Goumalatsou, C., & Myers, G. (2016). *Oxford handbook of clinical specialities* (10th ed.). Oxford University Press.

Department of Health UK Government. (2015). *Mental Health Act 1983: Code of practice.* https://assets.publishing.service.gov.uk/government/uploads/system/uploads/attachment_data/file/435512/MHA_Code_of_Practice.PDF. Accessed Dec 2020.

Legislation.gov.uk. *Mental Health Act 1983.* https://www.legislation.gov.uk/ukpga/1983/20/section/136. Accessed Dec 2020.

Legislation.gov.uk. *Mental Health Act 1983.* https://. www.legislation.gov.uk/ukpga/1983/20/section/135. Accessed Dec 2020.

Common Medications

Hitchings, A., Lonsdale, D., Burrage, D., & Baker, E. *The top 100 drugs.* Churchill Livingstone Elsevier Ltd.

NICE. (2020). *BNF British National Formulary.* https://bnf.nice.org.uk/. Accessed Dec 2020.

Baldwin, A., Hjelde, N., Goumalatsou, C., & Myers, G. (2016). *Oxford handbook of clinical specialities* (10th ed.). Oxford University Press.

Interventions

Baldwin, A., Hjelde, N., Goumalatsou, C., & Myers, G. (2016). *Oxford handbook of clinical specialities* (10th ed.). Oxford University Press.

NHS. (2022). *Types of talking therapies.* https://www.nhs.uk/conditions/stress-anxiety-depression/types-of-therapy/. Accessed Dec 2020.

NICE. (2009). *Guidance on the use of electroconvulsive therapy.* NICE. https://www.nice.org.uk/guidance/ta59/chapter/1-Guidance. Accessed Dec 2020.

19

Radiology in an Hour

Gregory Oxenham and Sanjay Gandhi

OUTLINE

INTRODUCTION TO RADIOLOGY

In this chapter, we have included approaches to interpreting chest X-rays (CXRs), abdominal X-rays (AXRs) and certain computed tomography (CT)-diagnosed conditions to reflect the level of knowledge expected in final-year students. Many radiological studies will be interpreted by expert radiologists or sonographers and, for that reason, magnetic resonance imaging (MRI), positron emission tomography (PET) and ultrasonography is not included in this chapter. Indications for these imaging studies are found in the relevant chapters.

Interpreting chest radiographs is a commonplace activity, and a systematic approach will aid you when confronted with the more complicated films. You should develop your own approach; however, if you don't have one, here is one to try. As you read through, refer to the normal CXR (see Fig. 19.1) to ensure you understand the anatomy and, most importantly, what is *normal*. Check your anatomy with the line drawing (Fig. 19.2).

A SYSTEMATIC APPROACH (PATIENT A-E)

Patient and quality:

- **Right patient? Right image?** Looking at the wrong X-ray is a quick way to make the wrong diagnosis.
- **PA or AP?** The heart and mediastinum can look bigger from the AP view.
- Is the patient **supine or erect?** X-rays taken in unwell patients may be supine. Fluid shifts upwards from the bases, and pneumothoraces can move anteriorly and be missed.
- Is the **entire lung** from the apices to the costophrenic (CP) angle included?
- **Exposure:** is the whole image too white or too black?
- **Inspiration:** can you see 5–7 anterior ribs? Poor inspiration can mimic lower lobe consolidation/collapse because the vessels are crowded together.
- **Rotation:** do the clavicular heads look symmetrical around the spine?

A – Airway:

- **Trachea – central?** Pushed to one side because of an effusion or pneumothorax (PTX)?
- Is there an endotracheal tube (ETT) and is it in the right place?

B – Breathing:

- Are the **hila** a normal size? The left should be higher or at the same level. The hila can be enlarged due to lymphadenopathy, sarcoidosis or pulmonary arterial hypertension (PAH). Bilateral hilar lymphadenopathy occurs secondary to sarcoid, lymphoma and tuberculosis (TB).
- **Lung markings:** are they seen from the apex to the base? Is there a PTX? Are the pleura crisply defined or irregular?
- **Opacification:**
  - **Nodules and masses:** could it be neoplasia, infection, granuloma, atrioventricular malformation (AVM), embolus or metastasis?

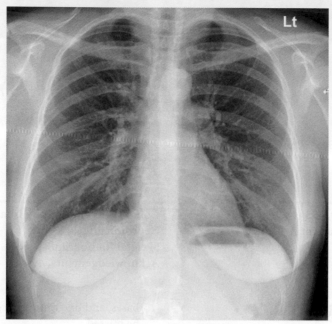

Fig 19.1 Normal Erect PA Film.

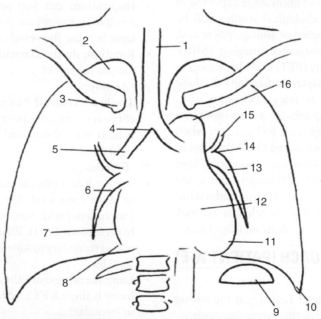

Fig. 19.2 Line Diagram of a Normal Chest X-ray . Answers: 1. Trachea, 2. Right lung apex, 3. Clavicle, 4. Carina, 5. Right main bronchus, 6. Right lower lobe pulmonary artery, 7. Right atrium, 8. Right cardio-phrenic angle, 9. Gastric air bubble, 10. Costophrenic angle, 11. Left ventricle, 12. Descending thoracic aorta, 13. Left lower lobe pulmonary artery, 14. Left hilum, 15. Left upper lobe pulmonary vein, 16. Aortic arch

- **'Miliary' opacification:** widely distributed micro-nodules. May be TB, sarcoid, metastases (thyroid/melanoma)
- **Consolidation:** something filling up the airspaces, often with poorly defined margins and usually no volume loss. Is it pus (pneumonia), blood (haemorrhage), water (heart/renal/liver failure) or cells (lymphoma, carcinoma)?
- **Collapse:** opacification with features of volume loss. Are the hila/trachea being pulled towards the opacification?

C – Cardiac:

- Is the heart a **normal size?**
- Sternal wires/valve replacement/pacemaker wires/coronary stents?
- Can you see the **heart border clearly?** *Loss of the left/right heart border can infer adjacent collapse or consolidation*

D – Diaphragm and CP angles:

- Can you see the **whole diaphragm?** An obscured hemidiaphragm can mean a lower lobe consolidation
- Can you see the **CP angles?**
- Is there **air under the diaphragm?** May indicate a bowel perforation
- Is there an **effusion?** Is it on one side or both? Unilateral pleural effusions should prompt a search for a malignancy.

E – Extras and extrathoracic:

- **Lines:**
  - Nasogastric tube (NGT) in the right place?
  - ETT in the right place?
  - Central/PICC lines in the right place?
  - Chest drain in the right place?
- **Bones:** a broken rib, clavicle, humerus or dislocated shoulder?
- **Soft tissue:** surgical emphysema from a chest drain? *The absence of a breast shadow in patients who have undergone a mastectomy will cause asymmetrical opacification.*
- **Abdomen:** free gas/pneumoperitoneum? Evidence of dilated bowel loops? Hiatus hernia with a bubble behind the heart?
- **Medical equipment:** is the patient attached to oxygen or electrocardiogram (ECG) electrodes?

CHEST RADIOGRAPHS

Figs 19.3-19.20 are examples of some common chest radiographs. **Try to spot what's happening before looking at the description!**

For further information about these following conditions, see Respiratory Medicine in an Hour unless otherwise specified.

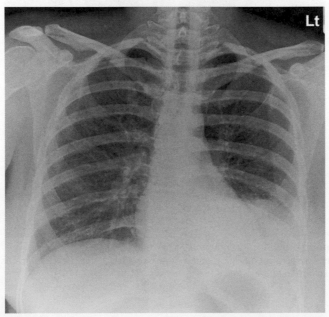

Fig. 19.3 Left Lower Zone Consolidation. Increased density is obscuring the left heart border and hemidiaphragm. Other considerations: A follow-up CXR in 6/52 is usually required to assess for resolution and check for an underlying mass.

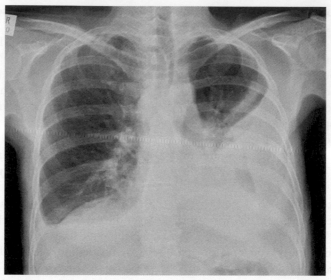

Fig. 19.4 Large Left and Small Right Pleural Effusions. Other considerations: Is it bilateral or unilateral? Bilateral effusions are most commonly related to cardiac/renal/liver failure. Unilateral effusions are most commonly related to a malignancy or infection. In trauma, a flattened effusion can imply air in the pleural space (i.e., a hemopneumothorax).

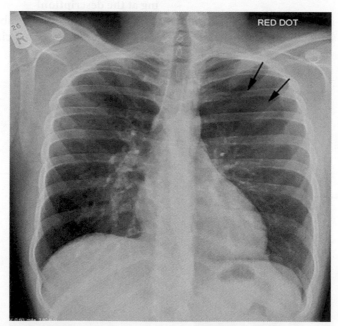

Fig. 19.5 Left Pneumothorax. *Arrows* show the visible lung edge.
Other considerations: Observe for deviation of the mediastinum/trachea, which indicates a tension pneumothorax (PTX). Also exclude fractures.

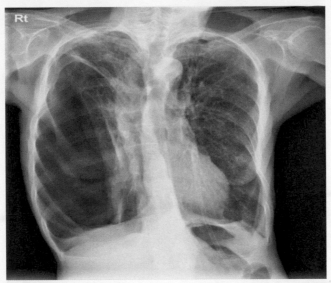

Fig. 19.6 Tension Pneumothorax on the Right Side, Displacing the Trachea and Mediastinum to the Left. The ipsilateral (right) hemidiaphragm is depressed. Other considerations: Immediate management is required. If a tension PTX is suspected it should be treated prior to a CXR. Repeat CXRs are required after placement of a chest drain to ensure correct placement and after removal to ensure the PTX hasn't reoccurred.

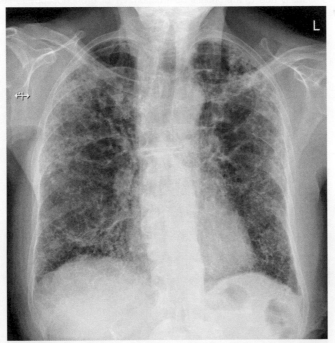

Fig. 19.7 Interstitial Fibrosis.
Other considerations: The definitive investigation is a CT of the chest in combination with spirometry.

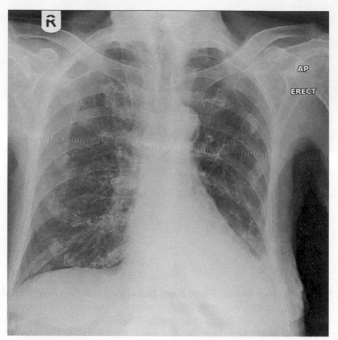

Fig. 19.8 Left Lower Lobe Collapse.
Note the increased density behind the heart, the depressed left hilum and the loss of the silhouette of the left hemidiaphragm.
Other considerations: Usually due to a bronchial obstruction. CT or bronchoscopy to search for the cause, often cancer.

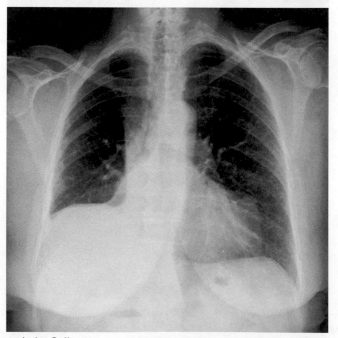

Fig. 19.9 Right Lower Lobe Collapse.
Note the increased density behind the right heart, the depressed right hilum and the loss of the right hemidiaphragm silhouette.
Other considerations: A foreign body is one cause of this type of collapse, which is most likely to become lodged in right-sided bronchi.

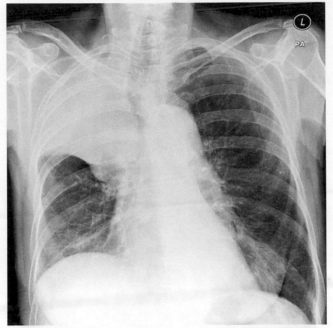

Fig. 19.10 Right Upper Lobe Collapse. The trachea is pulled **towards** the opacity.

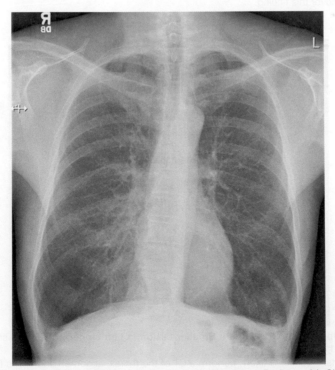

Fig. 19.11 Hyperinflation with Flattening of the Hemidiaphragms in a Patient with Chronic Obstructive Pulmonary Disease.

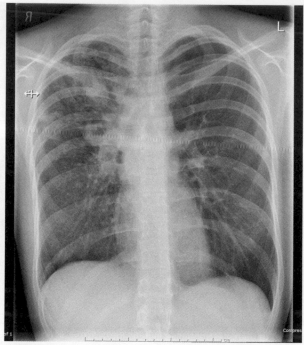

Fig. 19.12 Cavitating Pulmonary Tuberculosis with Lymphadenopathy.
Other considerations: See Infectious Diseases in an Hour. Will require immediate airborne isolation as an inpatient if you discover this finding.

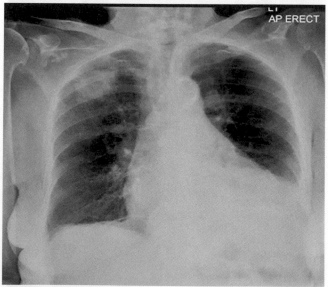

Fig. 19.13 Right Upper Lobe Mass and a Smaller Lesion in Left Upper Zone. Also shows a left pleural effusion and hiatus hernia.
Other considerations: If cancer is likely, perform a CT of the thorax, abdomen and pelvis (TAP), and possibly FDG-PET for staging, bronchoscopy and biopsy, a bone scan and CT imaging of the head (CTH) if there are concerns about cerebral metastasis.

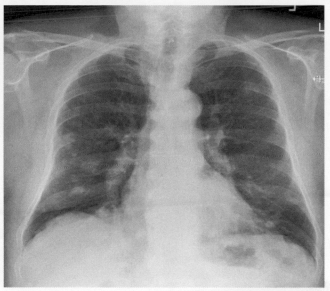

Fig. 19.14 Pulmonary Metastases. Bilateral nodules in a patient with rectal carcinoma.

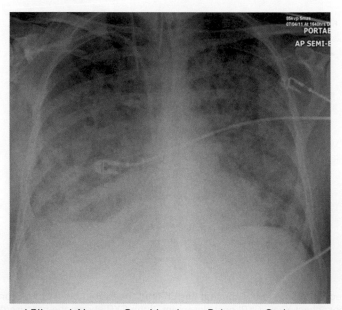

Fig. 19.15 Widespread Bilateral Airspace Opacities due to Pulmonary Oedema.
Other considerations: will likely need an echocardiogram (ECHO) to assess cardiac function (see Cardiology in an Hour for further information).

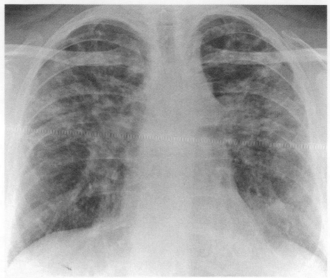

Fig. 19.16 Sarcoidosis.
Bilateral hilar enlargement with reticulonodular shadowing.
Other considerations: bilateral hilar lymphadenopathy – biopsy is often required for a diagnosis of sarcoid, consider acid-fast bacillus staining for tuberculosis, CT chest if concerns about malignancy,

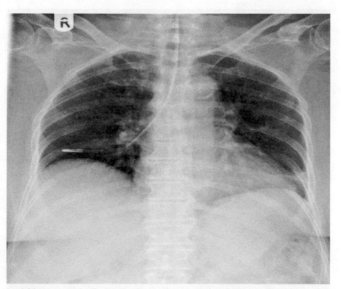

Fig. 19.17 Misdirected Nasogastric Tube that has Entered the Right Lower Lobe Bronchus.
Other considerations: chest X-ray (CXR) post-placement. If the CXR shows the nasogastric tube in the lung, immediately remove it, resite the nasogastric tube and repeat the CXR.

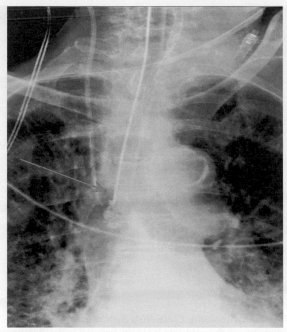

Fig. 19.18 Endotracheal Tube in the Right Main Bronchus *(arrow).*
The tube should be withdrawn by approximately 3 cm. Satisfactory placement of the right internal jugular line.

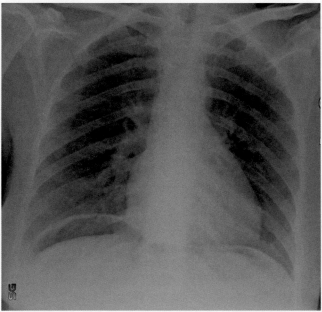

Fig. 19.19 Pneumoperitoneum. Erect chest x-ray showing free gas under the diaphragm.
Other considerations: if there is evidence of a perforation, should proceed to a CTAP with contrast. Patients presenting acutely unwell with evidence of a perforation should proceed straight to a CTAP without a CXR. Remember that free air persists in the abdomen for 4–5 days postoperatively.

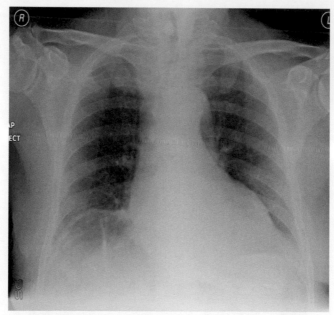

Fig. 19.20 Mimicking Pneumoperitoneum, *Chilaiditi's Syndrome.*
Colonic loop below the diaphragm on the right side (note the haustral folds). A correctly sited nasogastric tube with the tip below the left diaphragm.

ABDOMINAL RADIOGRAPHS

See Figs 19.21-19.31 for examples of some common abdominal radiographs. **Try to spot what's happening before looking at the description!**

For further information about these conditions, see General Surgery in an Hour unless otherwise specified.

Introduction

These are rarely diagnostic and have limited indications:
- Suspicion of obstruction
- To look for toxic megacolon in inflammatory bowel disease (IBD) flares
- Kidney, ureter, bladder (KUB) x-rays to monitor renal stones (CT-KUB is often the first-line investigation)
- Evaluation of a radiopaque foreign body (FB) to assess positioning and monitor for passage/complications
- Evaluation of radiopaque lines/tubes

Bowel Gas Patterns

The pattern depends on the volume of faeces and gas in the bowel as well as the position of the bowel at the time the image was taken. Normal findings (see Fig 19.21):
- **Stomach:** an air-fluid level can often be seen in an erect film (a.k.a., a gastric bubble)
- **Small bowel:** usually central but may dip into the pelvis. It is normal to not have bowel gas here, as the content is usually fluid. Distended if the width is >3 cm
- **Large bowel:** more common to see because there is more intraluminal gas. Hepatic and splenic flexures are usually fixed in the upper quadrants, while the caecum is often visible in the right lower quadrant (RLQ). The caecum is distended if >9 cm, and the large bowel distal to the caecum is distended if >6 cm

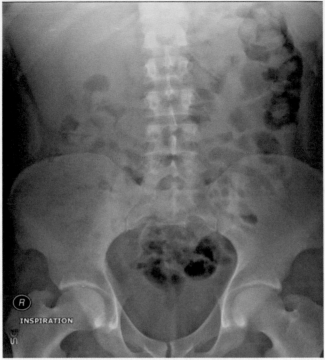

Fig. 19.21 Normal Bowel Gas Distribution.

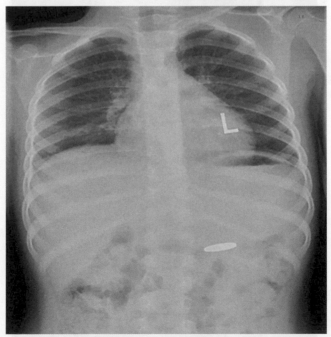

Fig. 19.22 Foreign Body (a Coin) in the Stomach. The side marker (L) lies outside the body!
Other considerations: Work out which coin it is! Bigger coins are much less likely to pass the pylorus and may
need endoscopy for retrieval.

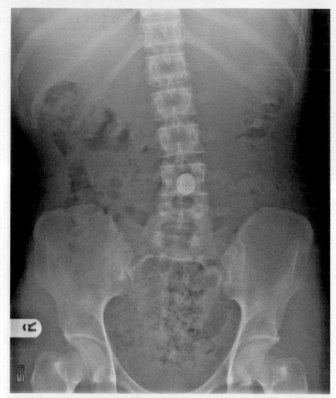

Fig. 19.23 Two Swallowed Razor Blades (one in the left upper quadrant and another in the pelvis) and a Button. Other considerations: Take-home message – if you spot one abnormality, look for the next one!

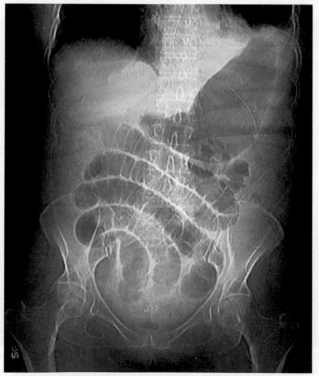

Fig. 19.24 Dilated Small Bowel in the Centre of the Abdomen. Note the valvulae conniventes crossing the entire lumen.
Other considerations: most commonly (80%) caused by adhesions (hernias are the second-most common cause). NGT placement, nil by mouth (NBM) and IV fluids are the initial management steps.

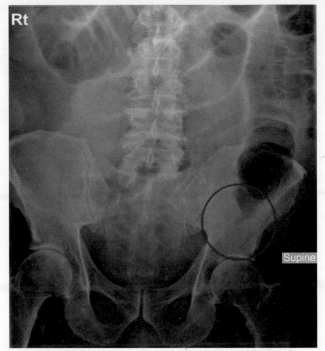

Fig. 19.25 Large Bowel Obstruction. Dilated peripheral loops of bowel with haustra. The cut-off point *(circle)* is at the sigmoid, and there is no gas in the rectum.
Other considerations: most commonly due to cancer. Hartmann's procedure is performed in an emergency. You may see a small bowel obstruction (SBO) and large bowel obstruction (LBO) together in cases in which the ileocecal valve is incompetent, with the large bowel decompressing into the small bowel.

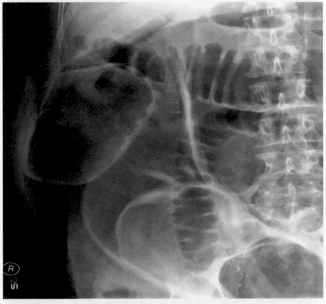

Fig. 19.26 Pneumoperitoneum.
Rigler's sign: gas outlining the inner and outer walls of the bowel gives a 'ghost-like' appearance. The falciform ligament is shown in the right upper quadrant *(arrows)*.
Other considerations: The most common cause of free gas is a peptic ulcer perforation.

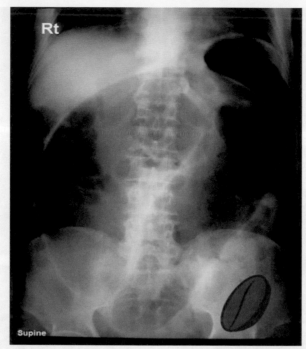

Fig. 19.27 'Coffee-bean Sign' in a Sigmoid Volvulus.

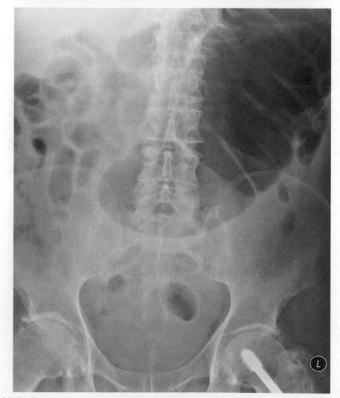

Fig. 19.28 Caecal Volvulus.

Other considerations: Haustral markings are often preserved in a caecal volvulus compared with a sigmoid volvulus. The dilated bowel (>9 cm) is usually aligned along a line between the left upper quadrant (LUQ) and right lower quadrant (RLQ).

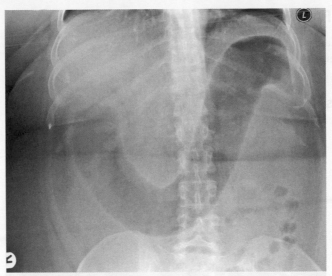

Fig. 19.29 Colitis. Wall thickening, loss of haustral markings and a 'lead pipe' appearance.
Other considerations: Colitis can be compatible with infective, inflammatory or ischaemic aetiologies. Assess for toxic megacolon.

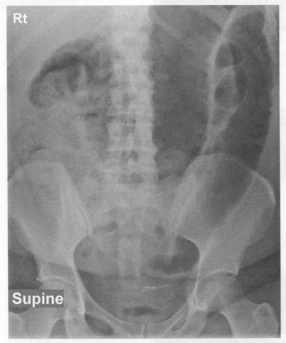

Fig. 19.30 Toxic Megacolon (Dilation >6 cm). Severe colitis can lead to a loss of muscular tone in the bowel and severe dilation.
Other considerations: Dilation of >6 cm greatly increases the risk of a perforation in patients with colitis.

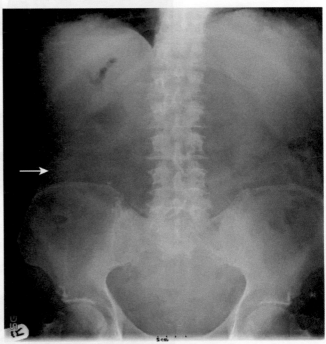

Fig. 19.31 Gallstone Ileus.
Gas in the biliary tree with a calcified gallstone *(arrow)*. Clinically, the patient was believed to have a bowel obstruction; however, this diagnosis is not clear based on the image because the bowel is filled with fluid rather than gas.
Other considerations: The most common site of an obstruction is the terminal ileum.

COMPUTED TOMOGRAPHY IMAGING

See Figs 19.32-19.44 for examples of some CT imaging. **Try to spot what's happening before looking at the description!**

Respiratory Conditions

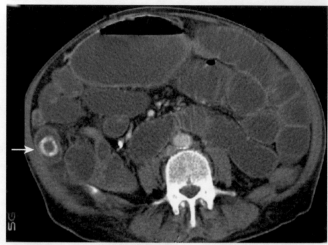

Fig. 19.32 Computed Tomography Imaging of the Same Patient as in Fig 19.31. The gallstone *(arrow)* is causing a small bowel obstruction (note the fluid-filled bowel loops).

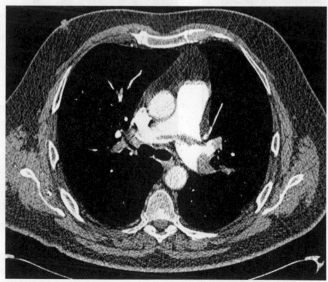

Fig. 19.33 Pulmonary Embolism.
A saddle embolus (grey filling defect) straddles the bifurcation of the right and left pulmonary arteries. There are further filling defects seen in the branch vessels (see Emergency Medicine in an Hour).

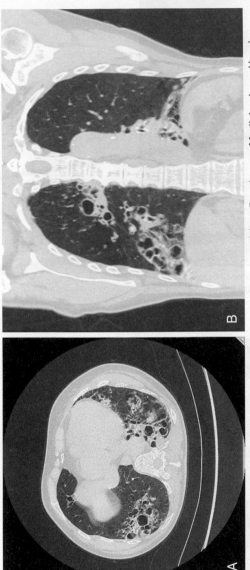

Fig. 19.34 (A and B) Bronchiectasis (axial and coronal images) (see Respiratory Medicine in an Hour).

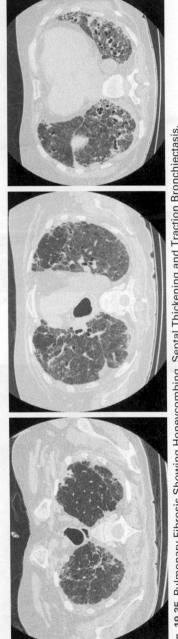

Fig. 19.35 Pulmonary Fibrosis Showing Honeycombing, Septal Thickening and Traction Bronchiectasis. The three axial images are progressing from superior to inferior (see Respiratory Medicine in an Hour).

Thoracic Trauma

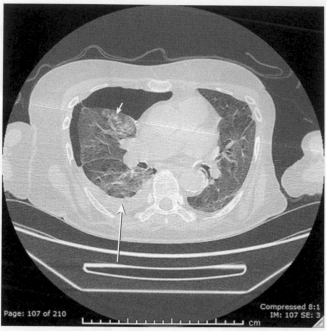

Fig. 19.36 Blunt Thoracic Trauma with a Moderate Right Pneumothorax.
Opacities within the right lung parenchyma *(small arrow)* caused by either collapse of the lung or contusions (or a bit of both). Right pleural effusion consistent with a haemothorax *(large arrow)*.

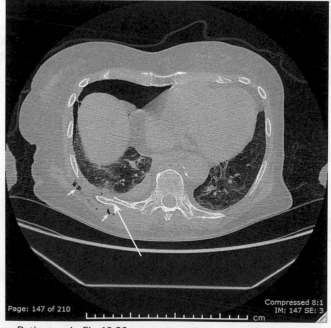

Fig. 19.37 The Same Patient as in Fig 19.36.
More inferiorly, there are several displaced rib fractures *(large arrow)* and several locules of surgical emphysema *(small arrows)*.

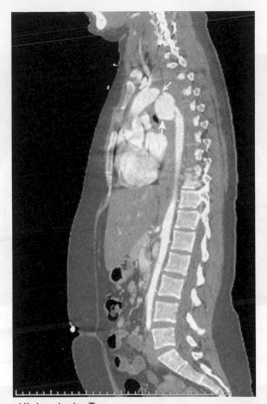

Fig. 19.38 Aortic Injury in a High-velocity Trauma.
There is a dissection flap that appears to be occluding the vessel lumen (*small arrow*); however, contrast is passing distally, suggesting that this occlusion is not complete. Immediately distal to the dissection flap is a pseudoaneurysm (*large arrow*). The vessel is dilated here because of an injury to the vessel wall. This vessel is at high risk of rupture if it is not stented.
Other considerations: The three most common sites of aortic injury are locations where the vessel can move less freely, such as at the aortic root, the attachment of the ligamentum arteriosum (as in this case) and at the diaphragm.

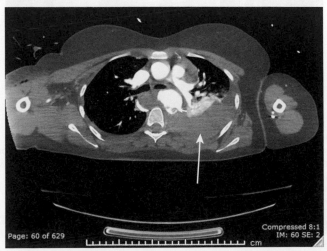

Fig. 19.39 The Same Patient as in Fig 19.38. Dissection flap (small arrow).
Large left pleural fluid collection (*large arrow*) consistent with a haemorrhage (haemothorax).

Abdominal Trauma

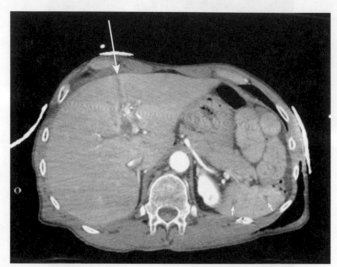

Fig 19.40 A Laceration through the Left Lobe of the Liver *(large arrow),* with Further Small Lacerations in the Spleen *(small arrows).*

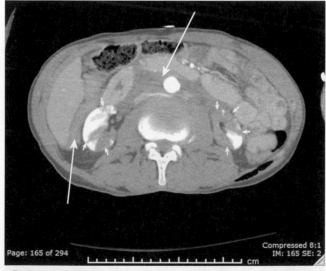

Fig 19.41 The Same Patient as in Fig 19.40.
Multiple hypoattenuating areas in both kidneys *(small arrows),* representing a combination of lacerations and infarctions secondary to a renal artery injury. There is also intermediate-density fluid within the abdomen consistent with a haematoma *(large arrows).*

Abdominal Aortic Aneurysm

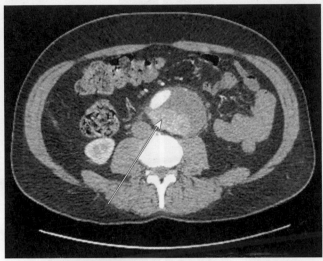

Fig 19.42 Large Infrarenal Abdominal Aortic Aneurysm.
No blood is seen within the abdominal cavity to suggest a rupture; however, contrast is entering the thrombosed aneurysmal sac *(arrow).*

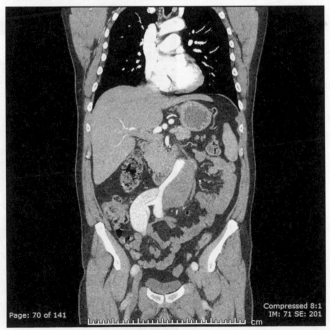

Fig 19.43 The Same Patient as in Fig 19.42 (Coronal Section).

Ischaemic Bowel

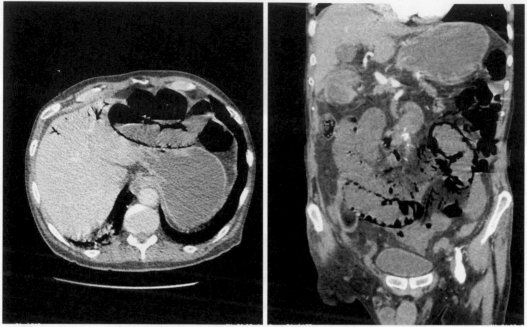

Fig 19.44 Non-enhancing Bowel Wall with Mural Gas. Gas is also seen in hepatic venous radicals.

NEUROIMAGING

See Figs 19.45-19.58 for examples of neuroimaging. **Try to spot what's happening before looking at the description!**

For further information about these conditions, see Neurology and Neurosurgery in an Hour, unless otherwise specified.

Stroke Imaging

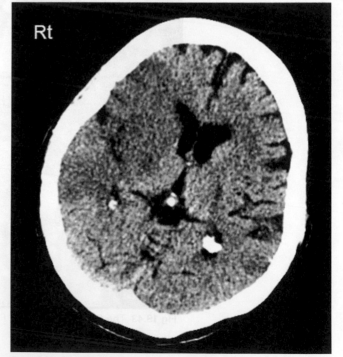

Fig 19.45 Ischaemic Stroke. A well-defined area of low density is seen in the right frontoparietal area. Appearances are consistent with a right middle cerebral artery infarction.

Other considerations: In an acute stroke, CT imaging is often initially normal because it takes time for CT changes to develop.

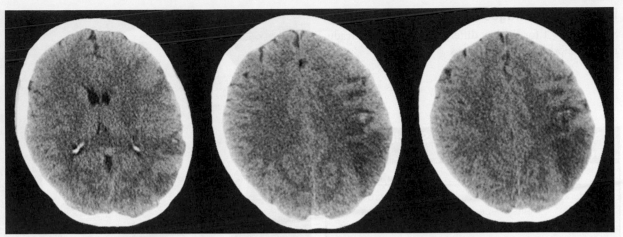

Fig 19.46 Haemorrhagic Stroke.
Large area of low attenuation (dark) encompassing the left parietal and temporal regions, which is consistent with an infarct with a mass effect on the lateral ventricle. A small focus of high attenuation (bright) is seen within the area of the infarct, which is typical of a haemorrhage, as clearly shown by a white arrow in Fig 19.47.

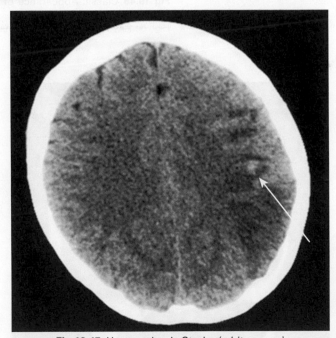

Fig 19.47 Haemorrhagic Stroke *(white arrow)*.

Brain Haemorrhages

See Table 19.1 for the key differences between Extradural and Subdural haemorrhages.

TABLE 19.1   **Extradural vs Subdural Haemorrhages**

	Shape	Boundaries
Extradural	Usually biconvex/lens-shaped	Does not cross skull sutures
Subdural	Usually crescent-shaped	Does not cross the midline

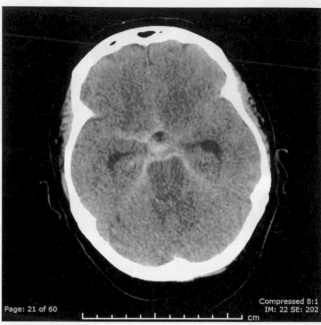

Fig 19.48 Classic Appearance of an Acute Subarachnoid Haemorrhage.
High density within the basal cisterns forming a star-shaped pattern.

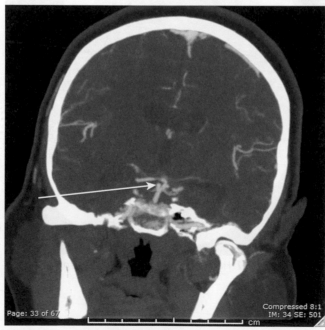

Fig 19.49 CT Angiography. A basilar tip aneurysm *(arrow)* was the source of haemorrhage.

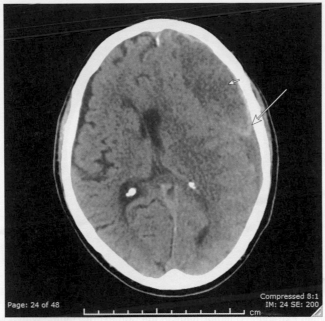

Fig 19.50 Large Left Subdural Haematoma with a Midline Shift.
The haematoma is heterogenous with high-density blood *(large arrow)* and low-density blood *(small arrow)*, indicating both acute and subacute blood within the haematoma.

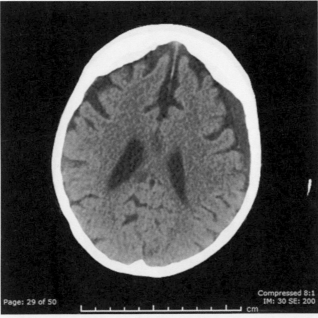

Fig 19.51 Chronic Subdural Haematoma on the Left.
Over time the density decreases and it can look similar to cerebrospinal fluid, as in this patient.

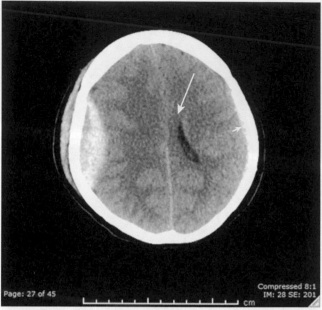

Fig 19.52 A Right-sided Extradural Haemorrhage in the Context of Trauma with a Midline Shift *(large arrow)* and Contralateral Acute Subdural Haemorrhage *(small arrow).*

Meningioma

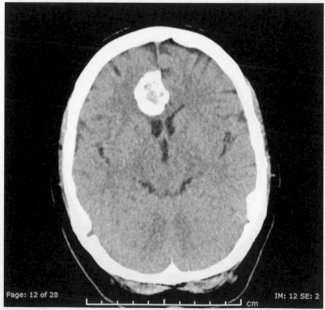

Fig 19.53 CT Imaging Showing a Durally Based Calcified Meningioma.
Other considerations: Meningiomas can occur anywhere there are meninges. While these growths are benign, their rapid growth can cause local compression, an elevated intracranial pressure (ICP) and consequent neurological symptoms.

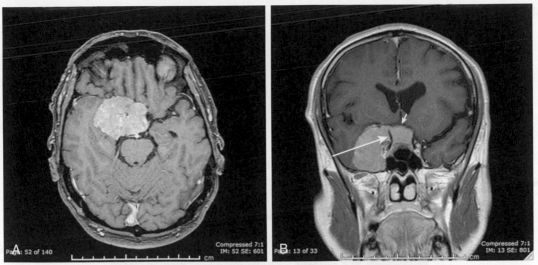

Fig 19.54 Contrast-enhanced MRI Showing **(A)** A Large Meningioma in the Right Cavernous Sinus.
(B) The tumour is causing a mass effect on the temporal lobe and effacement of the cavernous sinus,
encasing the right internal carotid artery *(large arrow)* and elevating the optic chiasm *(small arrow)*.
Other considerations: This patient presented with visual impairment. Consider a cavernous sinus pathology
in patients with CN III–VI involvement.

Pituitary Tumour

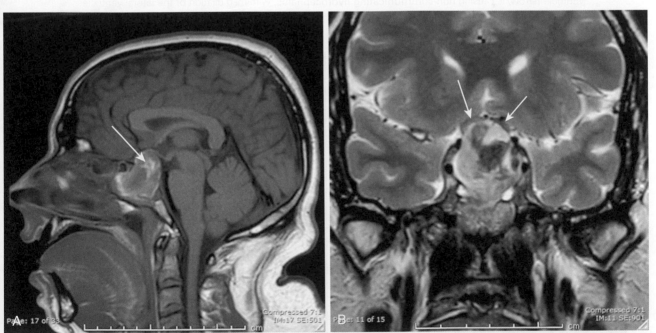

Fig 19.55 MRI of the Head. **(A)** A large pituitary mass is extending into the suprasellar cistern. The T1 hyperintensity shows a high signal in the mass *(arrow)* consistent with a haemorrhage, representing pituitary apoplexy.
(B) The mass is displacing the optic chiasm superiorly *(arrows)*.
Other considerations: This patient presented with **bitemporal hemianopia.** The most common cause is compression of the chiasm by a tumour.

Acoustic Neuroma

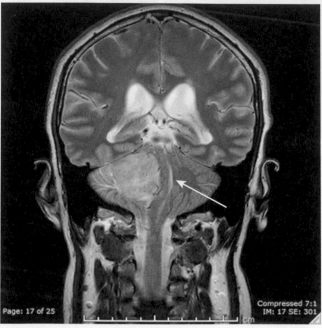

Fig 19.56 MRI of the Head.
A heterogenous mass is arising from the right internal auditory meatus. Compression of the pons and 4th ventricle *(arrow)* is causing **non-communicating hydrocephalus,** with mild dilation of the lateral ventricles.

Glioma

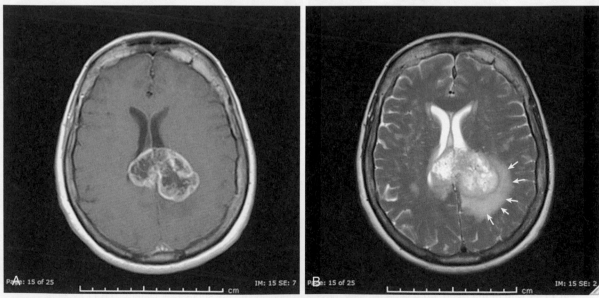

Fig 19.57 Glioma on MRI of the Head with Contrast. (A) T1 showing a large lesion crossing the midline and (B) T2 showing oedema *(arrows)*, which is likely a combination of vasogenic oedema and tumour infiltration.

Other considerations: High-grade astrocytomas are also known as glioblastomas multiforme (GBMs), which are the most common primary intracranial neoplasm in adults (see Neurosurgery in an Hour).

Multiple Sclerosis

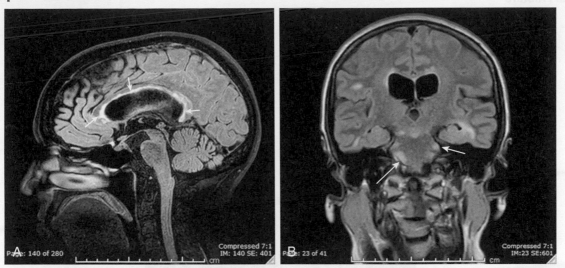

Fig 19.58 MRI of the Head (FLAIR). (A) There are high-signal lesions at the callosal-septal interface *(arrows)*, which is one of the most specific locations for multiple sclerosis (see Neurology in an Hour). (B) Lesions are also seen in the brainstem *(arrows)*.

SKELETAL RADIOGRAPHS

See Figs 19.59-19.83 for examples of some skeletal radiographs. For further information about these conditions, see Trauma and Orthopaedics in an Hour.

Fractures and Trauma
Colles' Fracture

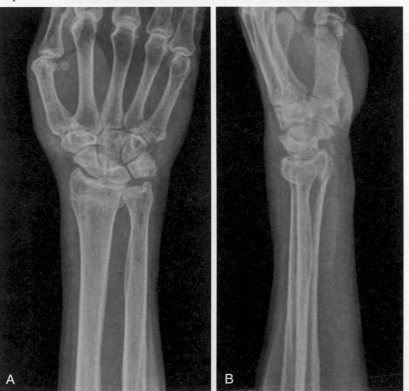

Fig 19.59 (A) Colles' fracture (anteroposterior view) and (B) Colles' fracture (lateral view) with dorsal displacement.

Smith Fracture

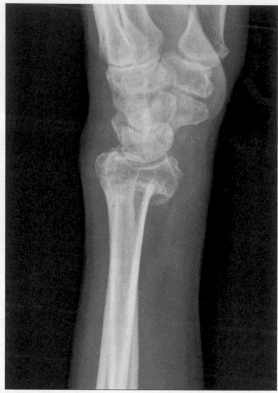

Fig 19.60 Smiths' Fracture (lateral view) with Volar Displacement.

Scaphoid Fracture

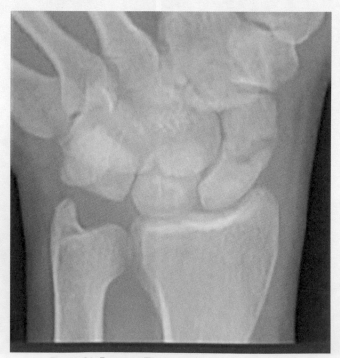

Fig 19.61 Fracture Through the Scaphoid Waist.

Shoulder Dislocation

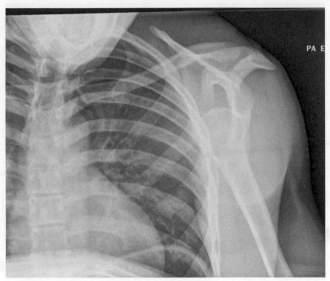

Fig 19.62 Anterior Shoulder Dislocation.
The humeral head is lying anterior and medial to the glenoid fossa.

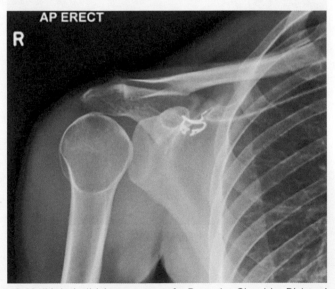

Fig 19.63 'Light bulb' Appearance of a Posterior Shoulder Dislocation.

Hip Fractures

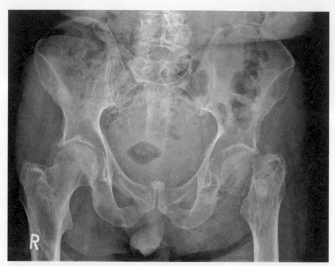

Fig 19.64 Left Intracapsular Neck of Femur Fracture.

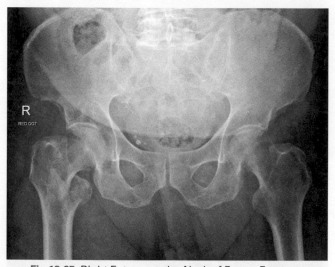

Fig 19.65 Right Extracapsular Neck of Femur Fracture.

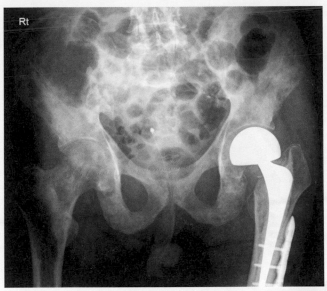

Fig 19.66 Left Hemiarthroplasty.

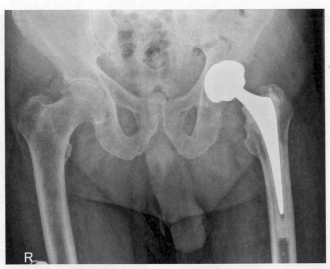

Fig 19.67 Left Total Hip Replacement.

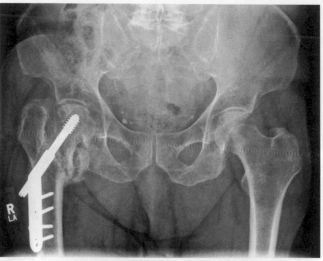

Fig 19.68 Right Dynamic Hip Screw.

Hip Dislocation

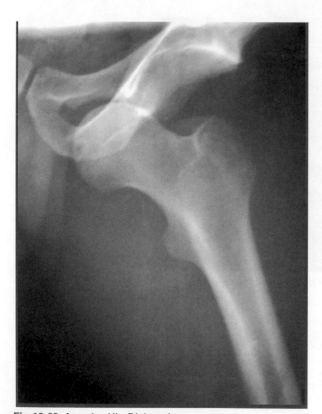

Fig 19.69 Anterior Hip Dislocation.
There is loss of Shenton's line, and the femoral head is inferior to the acetabulum. The lesser trochanter is more visible because of external rotation.

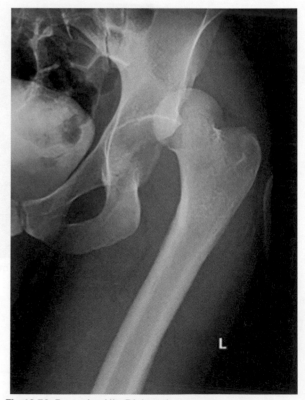

Fig 19.70 Posterior Hip Dislocation.
The femoral head is displaced posteriorly, superior and lateral to the acetabulum. Because the hip is internally rotated, the lesser trochanter is obscured on the AP view.

Trimalleolar Fracture

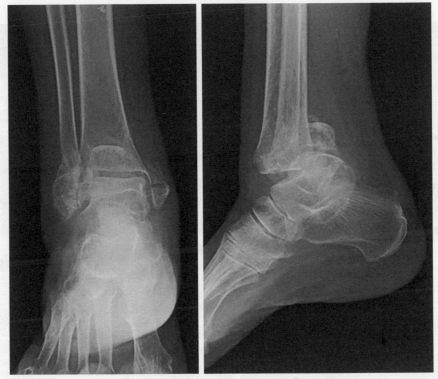

Fig 19.71 Comminuted Tri-Malleolar Fracture.

Lipohaemarthrosis

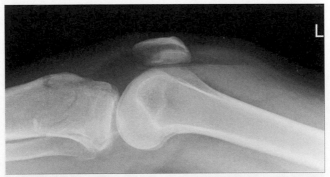

Fig 19.72 Fat-fluid Level (Haemarthrosis) in the Suprapatellar Region.
Other considerations: Finding a lipohaemarthrosis should prompt a search for a fracture. Note the proximal tibial fracture here.

Benign Bone and Cartilage Tumours
Osteoid Osteoma

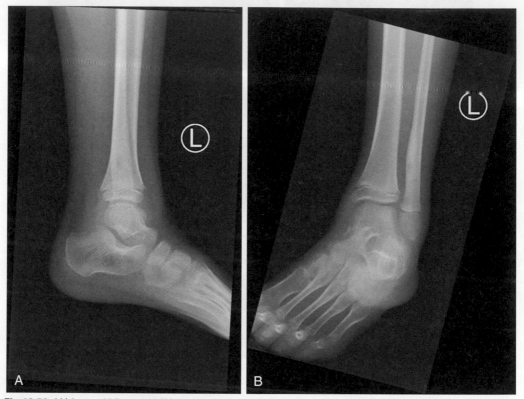

Fig 19.73 (A) Lateral View and (B) AP View of an Osteoid Osteoma in the Left Distal Fibula.
The lesion is a well-defined lucent lesion in the distal fibula with surrounding sclerosis and cortical and periosteal thickening.

Osteoblastoma

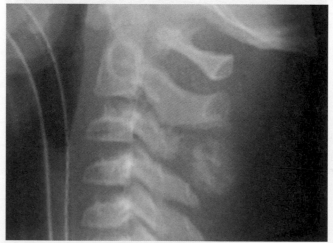

Fig 19.74 Lateral Radiograph of the Spine Showing a Possible Osteoblastoma on a Spinous Process.

Giant Cell Tumour

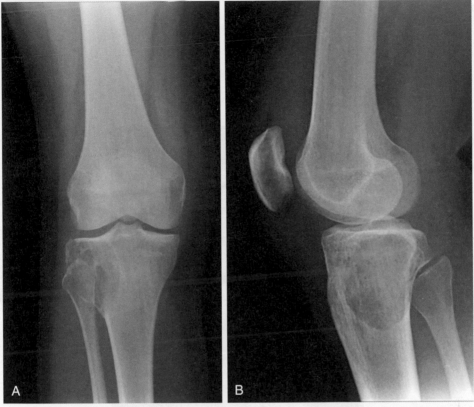

Fig 19.75 (A) AP View and (B) Lateral View of a Giant Cell Tumour.
The lesion is a well-defined, multiloculated, expansile lesion with a narrow zone of transition in the proximal tibia. Note the pathological fracture through the lesion.

Osteochondroma

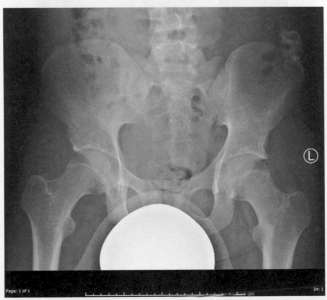

Fig 19.76 Plain AP Film Depicts an Atypical Osteochondroma Arising from the Left Iliac Bone.

Malignant Bone and Cartilage Tumours
Ewing Sarcoma

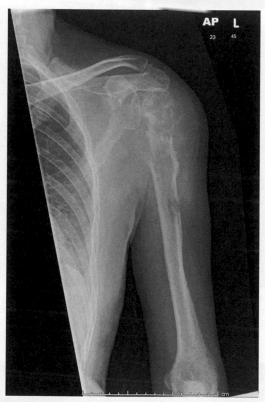

Fig 19.77 Ewing Sarcoma.
Extensive 'moth-eaten' appearance of the left proximal humerus. Sometimes seen as an 'onion skin' appearance.

Osteosarcoma

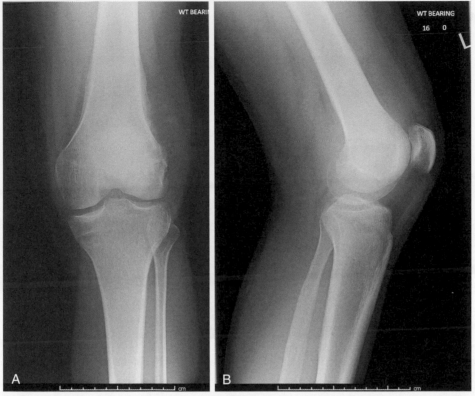

Fig 19.78 (A) AP View and (B) Lateral View of an Osteosarcoma of the Left Knee.
There is a periosteal reaction in the distal femur along with extraosseous soft tissue and osteoid mineralisation in the soft tissues.

Chondrosarcoma

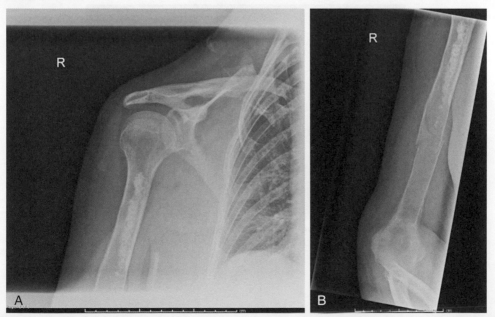

Fig 19.79 (A) Left Humeral Chondroid Calcification (Chondrosarcoma) and (B) A Midshaft Pathological Fracture in the Same Patient.

Paediatric Orthopaedic Conditions
Developmental Dysplasia Of The Hip

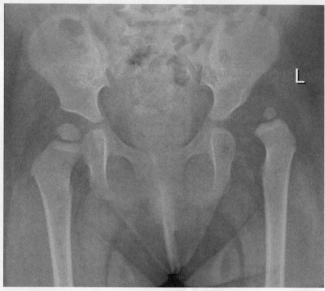

Fig 19.80 Developmental Dysplasia of the Hip.
Superolateral displacement of the left femoral epiphysis. The femoral head is not contained within the acetabulum.

Legg-Calve-Perthes Disease

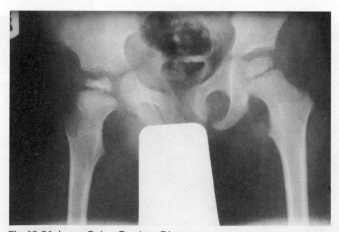

Fig 19.81 Legg-Calve-Perthes Disease.
Sclerosis and partial collapse of the head of the right femur.

Slipped Upper Femoral Epiphysis (SUFE)

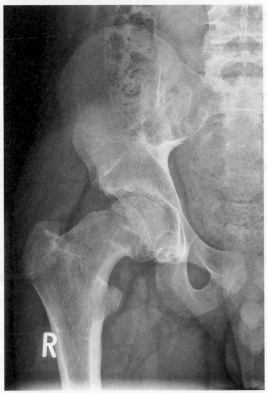

Fig 19.82 AP View Showing a Slipped Upper Femoral Epiphysis on the Right Hip.

Osgood-Schlatter Disease

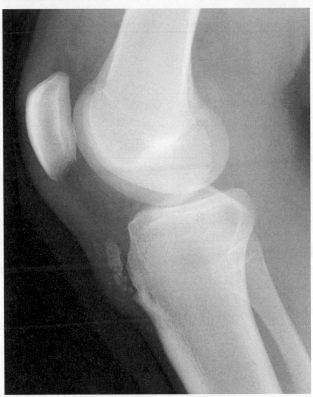

Fig 19.83 Osgood-Schlatter Disease.
Lateral knee radiograph showing fragmentation at the tibial tuberosity.

THE ONE-LINE ROUND-UP!

Here are some key words to help you remember each condition/concept.

Condition/Concept	*One-line Description*
Plain films	
Consolidation	*Opacification – follow-up CXR in 6/52*
Pleural effusion	*Meniscus and rounding of the CP angles*
Pneumothorax	*Loss of lung markings around the peripheries*
Tension pneumothorax	*Loss of lung markings and tracheal deviation away*
Interstitial fibrosis	*Hazy opacification with a poorly defined diaphragm*
LLL collapse	*Sail sign*
RLL collapse	*Loss of right hemidiaphragm silhouette*

Condition/Concept	*One-line Description*
RUL collapse	*Opacity with trachea pulled towards*
Pulmonary TB	*Apical opacities with lymphadenopathy*
Pulmonary metastases	*Multiple bilateral nodules*
Cardiac failure	*ABCDE*
Sarcoidosis	*Bilateral hilar enlargement with reticulonodular shadowing*
NG tube	*Bisects the carina, sits to the left below the diaphragm*
ET tube	*Tip should lie just above the carina*
Pneumoperitoneum	*Air below the diaphragm**** don't miss this one!*
Foreign bodies	*If you spot one, look for others*

continued

THE ONE-LINE ROUND-UP!—cont'd

Condition/Concept	One-line Description
Bowel obstruction	Remember 3 cm, 6 cm, 9 cm (small bowel, large bowel, caecum) as maximum diameters
Small bowel obstruction	Central, valvulae conniventes fully cross the lumen
Large bowel obstruction	Peripheral, haustra cross 2/3 of lumen
Sigmoid volvulus	Coffee bean sign
Caecal volvulus	Foetus sign
Colitis	Wall thickening, thumb printing and lead pipe
Toxic megacolon	IBD, colon >6 cm
CT scans and MRIs	
Pulmonary embolism	Look for filling defects
Bronchiectasis	Signet ring and tree in bud
Pulmonary fibrosis	Honeycombing
Thoracic trauma	Look for pneumothorax (black), haemothorax, contusions and rib fractures
Aortic injury	Most likely at the aortic root, ligamentum arteriosum and diaphragm
Abdominal trauma	Look for bleeding (intermediate density fluid), lacerations and hypoattenuation
AAA	>3 cm, any false lumen?
Ischaemic bowel	Mural gas in non-enhancing bowel
Subarachnoid haemorrhage	Star shape (hyperdensity in the cisterns)
Subdural haemorrhage	Crescenteric (white = acute, dark = chronic), doesn't cross the midline
Extradural haemorrhage	Lens shape (biconvex), doesn't cross suture lines
Meningioma	Arise from the meninges
Pituitary tumour	Mass may compress the optic chiasm (bitemporal hemianopia)
Acoustic neuroma	Mass from the internal auditory meatus

Condition/Concept	One-line Description
Glioma	Ring-enhancing lesion with oedema
MS	High signal at the callosal-septal interface
Skeletal radiographs – always get two views!	
Colles' fracture	Dinner fork – impaction and dorsal angulation
Smith fracture	Volar angulation
Scaphoid fracture	Risk of avascular necrosis
Anterior shoulder dislocation	Humeral head anterior and medial to glenoid fossa
Posterior shoulder dislocation	Light bulb
Intracapsular NOF fracture	Shenton's line is broken, subcapital, transcervical and basicervical
Extracapsular NOF fracture	Shenton's line is broken, trochanteric and subtrochanteric
Anterior hip dislocation	Shenton's line is broken
Posterior hip dislocation	Femoral head posterior, superior and lateral to acetabulum
Tri-malleolar fracture	Unstable, lateral, medial and posterior affected
Lipohaemarthrosis	Look for the fracture!
Osteoid osteoma	Well-defined lucent lesion
Osteoblastoma	Small lytic lesion surrounded by sclerosis
Giant cell tumour	Soap bubble appearance
Osteochondroma	Mushroom appearance
Ewing sarcoma	Onion skin
Osteosarcoma	Sunburst and Codman's triangle
Chondrosarcoma	Moth eaten
DDH	Femoral head not in the acetabulum
Legg-Calve-Perthes	Collapse of the femoral head
SUFE	Femoral epiphysis slips down (think of a melting ice-cream cone)
Osgood-Schlatter disease	Fragmentation of the tibial tuberosity

ACKNOWLEDGEMENTS

We would like to extend our immense gratitude to Professor Gandhi, Dr Jacob Whitworth, Dr Simranjeet Kaur and their Radiology departments for provision of the images in this chapter.

READING LIST: RADIOLOGY IN AN HOUR

Gandhi, S., Whitworth, J. & Kaur, S. Images and interpretations provided by expert co-authors.

Di Muzio, B. & Weerakkody, Y. *Idiopathic pulmonary fibrosis*. Radiopaedia. https://radiopaedia.org/articles/idiopathic-pulmonary-fibrosis?lang=us. [Accessed December 2020].

Hacking, C., Jones, J., et al. *Lobar collapse (summary)*. Radiopaedia. https://radiopaedia.org/articles/lobar-collapse-summary?lang=us. [Accessed December 2020].

Bell, D., Knipe, H., et al. *COVID-19 (summary)*. Radiopaedia. https://radiopaedia.org/articles/covid-19-summary?lang=us. [Accessed December 2020].

Hacking, C., Jones, J., et al. *Abdominal x-ray (summary)*. Radiopaedia. https://radiopaedia.org/articles/lobar-collapse-summary?lang=us. [Accessed March 2021].

El-Feky, M., Clopton, D., et al. *Toxic megacolon*. Radiopaedia. https://radiopaedia.org/articles/toxic-megacolon?lang=us. [Accessed March 2021].

Rasuli, B., Jones, J., et al. *l. Pneumoperitoneum*. Radiopaedia. https://radiopaedia.org/articles/pneumoperitoneum. [Accessed February 2021].

Saber, M., Gaillaird, F., et al. *Cecal volvulus*. Radiopaedia. https://radiopaedia.org/articles/caecal-volvulus?lang=us. [Accessed January 2021].

20

Renal Medicine and Chemical Pathology in an Hour

Mark Lam, Gregory Oxenham, Simon Satchell,
Berenice Aguirrezabala Armbruster and Judith Fox

OUTLINE

RENAL MEDICINE

ANATOMY

See Figs 20.1-20.2 for a reminder of the important anatomy.

INFECTIONS

Urinary Tract Infections

Definition: an infection that can affect the kidneys, bladder or urethra. Most common causative organisms include *Escherichia coli*, *Staphylococcus saprophyticus* (young and sexually active or elderly and immunocompromised), *Proteus mirabilis* (male or renal tract abnormality). Key terminology includes:

- **Bacteriuria:** the presence of bacteria in the urine
- **Urinary tract infection (UTI):** a diagnosis based on signs, symptoms and significant bacteriuria
- **Lower UTI:** an infection of the bladder (cystitis)
- **Upper UTI:** an infection of the ureters and kidneys (pyelitis and pyelonephritis, respectively)

- **Uncomplicated UTI:** caused by typical pathogens in a patient with a normal urinary tract and kidney function and with no predisposing comorbidities
- **Complicated UTI:** an increased likelihood of complications due to anatomical, functional or pharmacological factors predisposing to persistent infections, recurrent infections or treatment failure
- **Recurrent UTI:** ≥2 episodes of UTI in 6 months or ≥3 episodes in 1 year. Can be a relapse (same strain of an organism) or a reinfection (due to a different organism)
- **Catheter-associated UTI (CAUTI):** infection in the presence of a long-term catheter or urinary catheter placed within the previous 48 h

Buzzwords:

- **Risk factors:** previous UTI, recent instrumentation of the renal tract, renal tract abnormalities, benign prostatic enlargement (BPE), antibiotic use, sexual activity, new sexual partner, catheter, urinary calculi
- **Presentation:**
  - **Key diagnostic symptoms:** dysuria, nocturia, cloudy urine

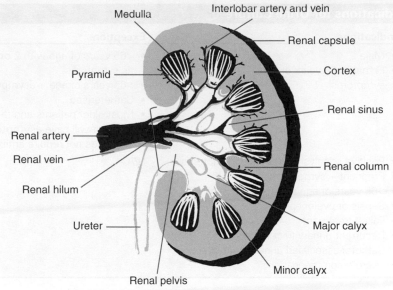

Fig 20.1 **Gross Renal Anatomy.** (Illustrated by Hollie Blaber.)

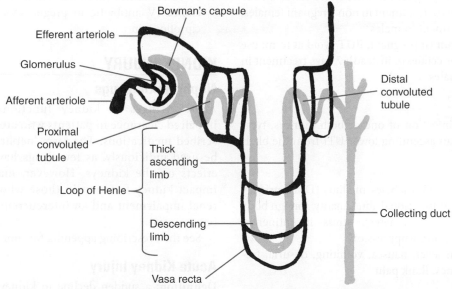

Fig 20.2 **Nephron Anatomy.** (Illustrated by Hollie Blaber.)

- **Other:** increased frequency, urgency, suprapubic pain, haematuria, delirium (especially in elderly patients)

Investigations:

- **Urinalysis** (all males and females <65 years of age + urinary tract symptoms): ↑ nitrites or ↑ leukocytes
- **Urine MC&S** (see Table 20.1): identification of organisms

- **Blood:** ↑ WCC, ↑ CRP
- **Blood cultures** (if systemically unwell): identification of the organism

Differentials: pyelonephritis, renal colic, prostatitis, urethritis

Management:

1. **Nitrofurantoin or trimethoprim** (or amoxicillin if a CAUTI and cultures show susceptibility): all

TABLE 20.1	Indications for Urine Culture	
Investigation	**Indications**	**Exceptions**
Urinalysis	• Male • Female <65 years of age + urinary tract symptoms	• <65 years of age with **2 out of 3** key diagnostic symptoms • >65 years of age + asymptomatic • Catheterised. • Most older patients and those with a urinary catheter will have asymptomatic **bacteriuria.** This does not require antibiotics.
Urine MC&S	• Positive urinalysis and urinary symptoms • Pregnant + symptomatic • >65 years of age and symptomatic • Sepsis or pyelonephritis • Failed treatment • Recurrent urinary tract infections • Catheter-associated urinary tract infection • Micro recommendation	N/A

males and non-pregnant females with a lower UTI or CAUTI, 3 days of treatment in non-pregnant females, 7 days of treatment in males

2. **Nitrofurantoin** (if pregnant, BUT avoid at term; use amoxicillin or cefalexin instead): 7 days treatment in pregnant females

Pyelonephritis

Definition: an infection of one or both kidneys, typically caused by an ascending lower UTI from the bladder

Buzzwords:

• **Risk factors:** UTI, diabetes mellitus (DM), urinary tract structural/functional abnormality, foreign body (e.g., urolithiasis, catheter), stress incontinence, pregnancy, immunosuppression

• **Presentation:** fever, nausea, vomiting, dysuria, frequency, urgency, flank pain

Investigations:

• **Urinalysis:** ↑ nitrites or ↑ leukocytes

• **Urine MC&S:** identification of an organism (see UTI risk factors)

• **Blood:** ↑ WCC, ↑ CRP, ↑ creatinine and urea

• **Blood cultures:** identification of the organism

Differentials: renal colic, lower UTI, pelvic inflammatory disease, lower respiratory tract infection

Management:

1. PO cefalexin (also first line in pregnancy), co-amoxiclav (if cultures show susceptibility), trimethoprim (if cultures show susceptibility) or ciprofloxacin

2. IV co-amoxiclav (in combination), cefuroxime (first-choice IV antibiotic in pregnancy), ceftriaxone or ciprofloxacin

KIDNEY INJURY

Nephrotoxic Drugs

Acute changes in kidney function can lead to impaired clearance in patients who are regularly prescribed medications. The term 'nephrotoxic' should be used judiciously, as few drugs have direct toxic effects on the kidneys. However, many drugs can impact kidney function in those who have existing renal impairment and an intercurrent disease states (e.g., sepsis).

See the Prescribing appendix for more information.

Acute Kidney Injury

Definition: a sudden decline in kidney function over hours to days. The most common cause of acute kidney injury (AKI) is **acute tubular necrosis** (ATN), resulting from either hypoperfusion or a toxic injury to tubular cells. According to the Kidney Disease: Improving Global Outcomes (KDIGO) criteria, AKI is defined as any of the following:

• An increase in the serum creatinine* by **≥26.5 μmol/L** within 48 h

• An increase in the serum creatinine* by **≥1.5 times** the baseline within 7 days

• Urine output **<0.5 mL/kg/h** for 6 h

TABLE 20.2 Kidney Disease: Improving Global Outcomes (KDIGO) Acute Kidney Injury Criteria

Stage	Serum creatinine	Urine output
1	1.5–1.9 × baseline (7 days) **or** ≥26 µmol/L increase (48 h)	<0.5 mL/kg/h for >6 h
2	2.0–2.9 × baseline (7 days)	<0.5 mL/kg/h for >12 h
3	3.0 × baseline **or** Increase in serum creatinine to ≥354 µmol/L **or** On renal replacement therapy **or** <18 years of age and a decrease in the eGFR to <35 mL/min per 1.73 m²	<0.3 mL/kg/h for 24 h **or** anuria for 12 h

*From the baseline serum creatinine (lowest value over last 3 months or the last 6–12 months if the patient does not have chronic kidney disease (CKD)).

Several different classification systems have been used to grade the severity of AKI, including the **RIFLE** and **AKIN** criteria. The most recent KDIGO criteria amalgamate elements of both (see Table 20.2).

Buzzwords:
- **Risk factors:**
  - **Pre-renal**: hypovolaemia, cardiac failure, sepsis, angiotensin-converting enzyme inhibitor (ACEi) or nonsteroidal anti-inflammatory drugs (NSAIDs), renal artery stenosis
  - **Renal**: atherosclerosis, thromboembolic disease, vasculitides, disseminated intravascular coagulation (DIC), glomerulonephritis, acute interstitial nephritis (AIN), nephrotoxics (see Prescribing appendix), rhabdomyolysis
  - **Post-renal**: obstructive uropathy (e.g., stones, malignancy, strictures, BPE)
- **Presentation:** signs of dehydration (e.g., reduced capillary refill time, dry mucous membranes, oliguria, orthostatic hypotension, confusion), nausea, vomiting, fluid overload (pedal oedema, shortness of breath (SOB), orthopnoea, ↑ jugular venous pressure (JVP)), arthralgia, rashes, fever, loin-to-groin pain, lower urinary tract symptoms (LUTS), palpable bladder

Investigations:
- **Urinalysis +/− MC&S:** ↑ nitrites or ↑ leukocytes (UTI), proteinuria and haematuria (glomerular disease), muddy brown casts (ATN)
- **Blood:** ↑ urea and creatinine, ↓ eGFR, ↑ K⁺, ↑ WCC and CRP (infection)
- **VBG:** acidosis, ↑ lactate
- **Blood culture** (if infection is suspected)

- **Bladder scan + ultrasound (US) of the renal tract:** +/− retention/hydronephrosis

Differentials: CKD, hepatorenal syndrome, increased muscle mass, medication-induced side effects

Management:
1. ABCDE assessment and resuscitation
2. Care bundle: **MNEMONIC = STOP**
   - **S**epsis: septic screen and sepsis six
   - **T**oxins: identify and stop nephrotoxics
   - **O**ptimise volume status and blood pressure (BP): IV crystalloid, consider loop diuretics for overload, consider referral to the critical care or renal team
   - **P**revent harm: treat reversible causes (e.g., relief of a urinary tract obstruction), treat life-threatening complications (hyperkalaemia and acidosis; see Chemical Pathology), review and modify medication doses due to AKI
3. Referral to one or more of:
   - **Renal:** stage 3 AKI, AKI of any stage that is not improving, suspected vasculitis, underlying systemic inflammatory cause, indication for dialysis (see below)
   - **Urology:** obstruction on ultrasound scan (USS)
   - **Critical care:** multiorgan failure, haemodynamically unstable and requiring inotropic support
4. Consider renal replacement therapy (RRT) acutely if unresponsive to medical management (see Renal Replacement Therapy)

Chronic Kidney Disease

Definition: abnormalities of kidney structure or function present for >3 months with associated health implications. CKD is classified based on the underlying cause, GFR category and albuminuria category. Symptoms are

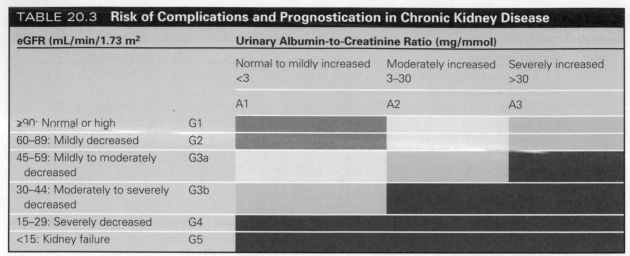

TABLE 20.3 **Risk of Complications and Prognostication in Chronic Kidney Disease**

eGFR (mL/min/1.73 m²)		Urinary Albumin-to-Creatinine Ratio (mg/mmol)		
		Normal to mildly increased <3	Moderately increased 3–30	Severely increased >30
		A1	A2	A3
≥90: Normal or high	G1			
60–89: Mildly decreased	G2			
45–59: Mildly to moderately decreased	G3a			
30–44: Moderately to severely decreased	G3b			
15–29: Severely decreased	G4			
<15: Kidney failure	G5			

Green = low risk (if no other markers of kidney disease, no chronic kidney disease); Yellow = moderately increased risk; Orange = high risk; Red = very high risk.

rare with CKD3, they may develop with CKD4 but are only usually marked in CKD5.

Buzzwords:

- **Risk factors:** hypertension (HTN), DM, glomerular disease, previous AKI, nephrotoxic drugs, obstructive uropathy, multisystem disease (e.g., SLE, vasculitis, myeloma), family history, cardiovascular disease (CVD), obesity with metabolic syndrome
- **Presentation:** often asymptomatic, lethargy, itchy, cramps at night, bone pain, loss of appetite, weight loss, change in urine output (e.g., polyuria, oliguria, anuria), ammonia breath, peripheral oedema, anaemia, gout, yellow skin, uraemic flap

Investigations:

- **Blood:**
  - ***Diagnosis*:** eGFR <60 mL/min/1.73 m² and/or ACR >3 mg/mmol for 3 months
  - **HbA1c** (to rule out DM)
  - **Myeloma screen** (particularly if anaemic and/or hypercalcaemic, bone pain)
- **Blood pressure** (to rule out HTN)
- **Urinalysis +/− urine MC&S:** haematuria (urological cancer), ↑ nitrites or leukocytes (UTI)
- **US renal tract** (particularly if suspected urolithiasis, obstruction or family history of polycystic kidney disease (PKD))
- **Monitoring:** eGFR and urinary albumin-to-creatinine ratio (ACR) predicts the risk of complications and can prognosticate in CKD (see Table 20.3),

Hb, calcium, phosphate and parathyroid hormone (PTH) (if eGFR <60), lipid profile (all patients)

Differentials: obstructive uropathy, nephrotic syndrome, glomerulonephritis

Management:

- Lifestyle advice and modifications
- Management of risk factors and comorbidities of CKD
- Long-term monitoring of disease progression
- Specialist referral and input for rapidly progressive and end-stage disease

Management of end stage disease

1. Reduce or stop nephrotoxic drugs as needed
2. BP control: aim for a systolic blood pressure (SBP) of <140 mm Hg (130 if the ACR is ≥70 mg/mmol) and a diastolic blood pressure (DBP) of <90 mm Hg (<80 if the ACR is ≥70 mg/mmol). Treat with an ACEi or angiotensin-receptor blocker (ARB) if:
   - Diabetic and ACR of ≥3 mg/mmol
   - Hypertensive and ACR of ≥30 mg/mmol
   - ACR >70 mg/mmol (independent of CVD)
   - Otherwise, follow the NICE HTN guidelines (see Cardiology and ECGs in an Hour)
3. Statin
4. Antiplatelet drug: consider offering in CKD for secondary prevention of CVD
5. Treat complications:
   - Anaemia: iron therapy or an erythropoiesis-stimulating agent (e.g., epoetin alfa)

TABLE 20.4 Acute Indications for Renal Replacement Therapy

	Acute Indications
A	**A**cidosis or **A**nuria: pH <7.15, absolute anuria for 12 h
E	**E**lectrolytes: refractory hyperkalaemia >6.5 mmol/L
I	**I**ntoxication: Remember the mnemonic SLIME for drugs and toxins (**S**alicylates, **L**ithium, **I**sopropanolol, **M**ethanol, **E**thylene glycol)
O	**O**verload, multiple **O**rgan failure or **O**liguria: refractory to diuresis, U/O <0.3 mL/kg for 24 h
U	**U**raemia: generally, if levels >30–35mmol/L (not strict criteria) with signs of uraemia (e.g., pericarditis, neuropathy, bleeding, encephalopathy)

- Hyperkalaemia: acute management (see Chemical Pathology), ↓ potassium diet, potassium-binding resins and acidosis correction (oral sodium bicarbonate)
- Oedema: fluid restriction and high-dose loop diuretics
- Hypocalcaemia: dietary supplements and alfacalcidol or calcitriol
- Hyperphosphataemia: dietary restriction and phosphate binders
- Hyperparathyroidism: alfacalcidol, calcimimetics or surgery

6. Renal Replacement Therapy (RRT): usually when the GFR is <10 and/or there is refractory fluid overload, hyperkalaemia, uraemia, anorexia or lethargy

Renal Replacement Therapy

Indications for RRT may be acute (see Table 20.4 - mnemonic AEIOU) or due to CKD (see above)

Types of RRT (see Table 20.5):

TABLE 20.5 Continuous Renal Replacement Therapy (CRRT) vs Intermittent Haemodialysis (HD) vs Peritoneal Dialysis (PD)

Modality	Length of treatment	Access	Pros	Cons
CRRT	Continuous	CVC – (see Anaesthetics and Critical Care in an Hour) (VasCath)	• More haemodynamic stability • Can remove large volumes of fluid • Relatively easy to start • Can be started acutely	• Constant attachment to the machine • Risk of placing CVC • Requires continuous blood flow – patient must be anticoagulated • Slow correction of electrolytes
Intermittent haemodialysis	3–5 h per session, usually 3×/week	Commonly AV fistula or tunnelled dialysis CVC	• Quicker correction of urea/electrolytes • Intermittent treatment – can be done as outpatient	• More haemodynamic instability • Requires more expertise to set up and manage • Patients have stricter fluid restrictions • Risk of infection with CVC
PD	CAPD – dialysate changes 3–5×/day APD – automated whilst asleep	Permanent tube inserted into abdomen	• Can be mobile while dialysing • Patients can manage their own dialysate exchanges • Often better satisfaction	• Risk of peritonitis • May have to transfer to intermittent haemodialysis eventually due to peritoneal sclerosis • Weight gain due to glucose in dialysate

APD, Automated peritoneal dialysis; AV, Arteriovenous; CAPD, continuous ambulatory peritoneal dialysis; CVC, central venous catheter; CRRT, continuous renal replacement therapy; PD, peritoneal dialysis.

- **Continuous renal replacement therapies (CRRT):** includes continuous haemofiltration/continuous haemodiafiltration usually in an intensive care setting. Continuous veno-venous haemofiltration is the most common modality used acutely
- **Intermittent haemodialysis (IHD):** most common modality in outpatient settings for CKD
- **Peritoneal dialysis (PD):** the peritoneum is used as a semipermeable membrane for the removal of solutes
  - Continuous ambulatory PD (CAPD): the dialysate is infused multiple times each day by the patient
  - Automated PD (APD): a pump circulates the dialysate, typically when asleep

How is waste removed:

- **Haemofiltration:** the patient's blood is passed through a semipermeable membrane at high pressure to remove fluids and solutes. A balanced crystalloid replaces the removed fluid and blood returns to the patient (see Fig 20.3).
- **Haemodialysis:** the patient's blood is passed over a semipermeable membrane that separates it from dialysis fluid travelling in the opposite direction. The dialysis fluid sets up an osmotic gradient, and fluids/solutes move from the patients' blood into the dialysis fluid. The dialysis fluid is then discarded, and the blood is returned to the patient (see Fig 20.4).
- **Peritoneal dialysis:** works similarly, except that the semipermeable membrane is the patient's own peritoneum

Renal Transplantation

Transplant offers better long-term outcomes than dialysis in terms of both the quality and quantity of life. However, assessing patients and donors for transplantation is a lengthy process.

Important factors to screen for prior to transplantation include:

- **Cardiovascular risk:** CVD is a major cause of death in transplant recipients because CKD is a significant risk factor for the development of coronary artery disease (CAD) and cerebrovascular disease. Usually requires aggressive modification

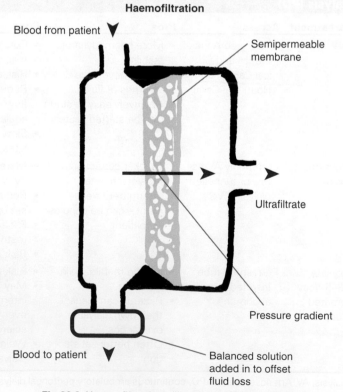

Haemofiltration

Blood from patient

Semipermeable membrane

Ultrafiltrate

Pressure gradient

Blood to patient

Balanced solution added in to offset fluid loss

Fig 20.3 Haemofiltration. (Illustrated by Hollie Blaber.)

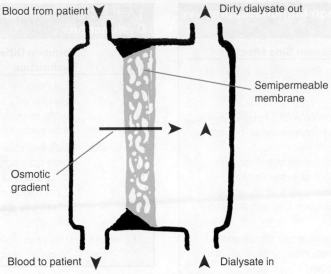

Fig 20.4 Haemodialysis. (Illustrated by Hollie Blaber.)

of risk factors. Consideration is given to treatment of systolic dysfunction, medical management of CAD and angiography +/− stenting/CABG prior to transplantation.

- **Malignancy:** immunosuppression for transplantation is associated with an increased risk of cancer (recurrence and de novo). Most wait for a 2–5-year cancer-free interval prior to transplantation. Increased risk of non-melanoma skin cancer and lymphoma in recipients.
- **Infection risk:** immunosuppression also increases the risk of infection. Prior to transplantation, patients (and donors) are assessed for Epstein-Barr virus (EBV), cytomegalovirus (CMV), hepatitis B (HBV), hepatitis C (HCV) and human immunodeficiency virus (HIV). There is also a risk of reactivation of latent tuberculosis (TB) in at-risk individuals. CMV is a significant cause of graft failure.

Surgical placement: incision in the left lower quadrant (LLQ) or right lower quadrant (RLQ), the kidney is placed in the extraperitoneal iliac fossa and the vessels/ureter are then anastomosed to the iliac vein/artery and bladder, respectively. The native kidneys are usually left in place (see Fig 20.5).

Types of graft:

- **Isograft:** a graft from a genetically identical human (i.e., from an identical twin). Typically, no rejection occurs

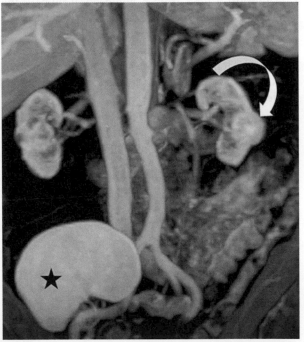

Fig 20.5 Renal Cell Carcinoma in the Left Native Kidney *(arrow)* and a Transplanted Kidney in the Right Lower Quadrant *(star).* (With permission from Low, G., Jaremko, J. L., Lomas, D. J. (2015). Extravascular complications following abdominal organ transplantation (Fig. 16). *Clinical Radiology* Publisher: Elsevier. *Copyright © 2015 The Royal College of Radiologists. Published by Elsevier Ltd. All rights reserved.)*

TABLE 20.6 Common Immunosuppressive Medications

Drug	Common Side Effects
Corticosteroids (maintenance and acute rejection)	See Endocrinology in an Hour
Calcineurin inhibitors: ciclosporin and tacrolimus (maintenance)	Nephrotoxicity, hyperkalaemia, hypomagnesomia, hypertension, diabetes *Ciclosporin*: eye discomfort, gingival hyperplasia *Tacrolimus*: tremor, increased infection risk, altered sensation
Mycophenolate (maintenance)	Bone marrow suppression, oesophagitis, gastritis, diarrhoea

TABLE 20.7 Differentials for Graft Dysfunction

Time	Common Differentials for Graft Dysfunction
Week 1	Acute tubular necrosis, hyperacute rejection (usually a donor-specific antibody), urologic obstruction or urine leak, renal artery/vein thrombosis
<12 weeks	Calcineurin toxicity, acute rejection, volume contraction, renal artery stenosis/thrombosis, obstruction, pyelonephritis, *Cytomegalovirus* infection, recurrence of primary disease (e.g., glomerulonephritis)
>12 weeks	Renal vessel stenosis, acute/chronic rejection, recurrence of primary disease

- **Allograft:** a graft from a nonidentical human, the primary source for renal transplants (cadaveric or living kidney donors). Risk of rejection

Immunosuppression: Required in almost all transplant recipients. All immunosuppressives confer an increased risk of infection to some extent. Common medications are described in Table 20.6

Graft dysfunction: refers to any impairments in graft function. The differentials are wide (see Table 20.7). Early graft dysfunction often impairs long-term graft survival.

Rejection: a specific cause of graft dysfunction caused by an immune response to a transplanted kidney. Defined histologically and can be hyperacute, acute or chronic. The two main types are:

1. Antibody mediated (humoral): circulating donor-specific antibodies
2. T-cell mediated: infiltration of predominantly CD4/CD8 cells into the graft

GLOMERULAR DISEASE

Significant overlap exists between the categories of primary glomerular diseases, and various classification systems are used. However, one pragmatic approach is to categorise these disorders according to their predominant characteristics at presentation:

- With nephrotic syndrome
- With glomerular haematuria
- With AKI

With Nephrotic Syndrome

Definition: a syndrome consisting of:

1. Proteinuria
   a. Adults: >3.5 g/24 h **or** urine protein-to-creatinine ratio (PCR) of >300 mg/mmol
   b. Children: >2 g/24 h **or** urine PCR of >200 mg/mmol
2. Hypoalbuminaemia (<30 g/L)
3. Generalised oedema (worse in the morning, periorbital, ankle and lower limb, abdominal and genital)
4. Hyperlipidaemia

The most common glomerular diseases presenting with nephrotic syndrome include:

- Minimal change disease (MCD)
- Focal segmental glomerulosclerosis (FSGS)
- Membranous nephropathy (MN)

Buzzwords:

- **Risk factors:** DM, HBV, HIV, malignancy, gold salts, penicillin, autoimmune (e.g., systemic lupus erythematosus (SLE))
- **Presentation:** frothy urine, periorbital oedema, peripheral oedema
  - **MCD:** 2–8 or 25–50 years of age, steroid responsive with a likelihood of relapse
  - **FSGS:** 15–30 years of age, idiopathic (primary) or associated with a condition (secondary) (e.g., obesity, DM, HTN)
  - **MN:** 50–60 years of age. The majority are idiopathic, rarely associated with conditions (e.g.,

malignancy, autoimmune) or medications (e.g., NSAIDs, penicillamine, gold)

Investigations:
- **Urinalysis**: proteinuria
- **Urine PCR**: >300 mg/mmol in adults, >200 mg/mmol in children
- **Blood**: hypoalbuminaemia, hyperlipidaemia
- ***Kidney biopsy*** (NB: generally not required in children)

Differentials: conditions as above, diabetic kidney disease (DKD), amyloidosis, hypertensive kidney disease (proteinuria but not usually in the 'nephrotic range')

Management:
- **First line for MCD and FSGS**: oral prednisolone
- **First line for MN**: tacrolimus, cyclophosphamide or rituximab, or depending upon risk stratification

With Haematuria

Definition: the presence of red blood cells (RBCs) in the urine, which can be macroscopic (visible) or microscopic (non-visible). Causes can be divided into glomerular and non-glomerular (see Urology in an Hour). Typically, the presence of RBC casts and dysmorphic RBCs on microscopy are strongly suggestive of a glomerular pathology. The most common causes include:
- Thin basement membrane disease
- IgA nephropathy
- Alport syndrome

Buzzwords:
- **Risk factors**: family history, chronic infections (e.g., HBV/HCV), autoimmune (e.g., SLE), paraproteinaemias
- **Presentation**:
  - **Thin basement membrane disease**: asymptomatic, microscopic haematuria
  - **IgA nephropathy**: young adult, 1–2 **DAYS** post-upper respiratory tract infection (URTI), gastrointestinal (GI) infection or strenuous exercise, may have episodic gross haematuria, often asymptomatic, microscopic haematuria. May have significant proteinuria
  - **Alport syndrome**: asymptomatic gross haematuria in infancy, nephritic/nephrotic syndrome, sensorineural deafness, retinopathy. (**Remember**: can't pee, can't see, can't hear a bee)

Investigations:
- **Urinalysis**: nephritic sediment (microhaematuria, proteinuria, pyuria)
- **Blood**: ↑ urea and creatinine, ↑ CRP

- ***Kidney biopsy***
- ***Next-generation sequencing***: used in Alport syndrome

Differentials: conditions as above, urolithiasis, bladder cancer, renal cancer

Management:
- **Thin basement membrane disease**: benign disease course usually requiring no active treatment. CKD management if symptomatic as needed
- **IgA nephropathy**: CKD management, immunosuppression (if rapid progression and crescents on biopsy)
- **Alport syndrome**: CKD management

With Acute Kidney Injury

Definition: in certain glomerulonephritides, patients can present with AKI and, in certain cases, can rapidly progress to end-stage renal failure. The two main conditions are:
- Post-streptococcal glomerulonephritis (PSGN)
- Rapidly progressive glomerulonephritis (RPGN)

Buzzwords:
- **Risk factors**: group A *Streptococcus*, URTI, autoimmune conditions, HBV, HCV, HIV monoclonal gammopathy
- **Presentation**:
  - **PSGN**: 3–12 years of age, 1–2 **WEEKS** post-pharyngitis/tonsillitis infection, cola-coloured urine
  - **RPGN**: often systemic/constitutional symptoms, oliguria, haemoptysis (pulmonary-renal syndrome). Three subtypes:
    - Type 1: anti-glomerular basement membrane (GBM) disease (also known as Goodpasture syndrome)
    - Type 2: immune complex–mediated secondary to other disorders (e.g., SLE)
    - Type 3: associated with a vasculitis (e.g., microscopic polyangiitis, Churg-Strauss syndrome, granulomatosis with polyangiitis)

Investigations:
- **Urinalysis**: haematuria, proteinuria
- **Blood**:
  - ↓ C3 and ↑ antistreptolysin O and anti-DNase B (PSGN)
  - ↑ Anti-GBM antibody (Goodpasture's)
  - ↑ p-ANCA (microscopic polyangiitis)
  - ↑ c-ANCA (granulomatosis with polyangiitis)
  - ↑ ANA and anti-DS DNA (SLE)
- ***Renal biopsy***

Differentials: IgA nephropathy, FSGS, MN, HSP, urolithiasis, haemolytic uraemic syndrome (HUS)
Management:
- **PSGN:** usually self-limiting, supportive
- **RPGN:** cyclophosphamide (or rituximab if associated vasculitis) and steroids +/− plasmapheresis (if Goodpasture's)

RENAL MANIFESTATIONS OF SYSTEMIC DISEASE

Several systemic conditions can commonly present with renal manifestations. These include:
- DKD
- Hypertensive kidney disease
- Hepatorenal syndrome (HRS)
- Lupus nephritis (see also Rheumatology in an Hour)
- Amyloidosis
- Vasculitides (see Glomerular disease and Rheumatology in an Hour)
- Monoclonal gammopathy of renal significance (MGRS)

Diabetic Kidney Disease

Definition: classical presentation of established DM with albuminuria and a progressive reduction in the GFR in the absence of another renal disease. However, DKD with minimal or absent albuminuria is increasingly being recognised.
Buzzwords:
- **Risk factors:** type 1 or type 2 DM for >10 years
- **Presentation:** poor diabetes control (polyuria, polydipsia, peripheral neuropathy, retinopathy), proteinuria, peripheral oedema
Investigations:
- **Urinalysis:** ↑ glucose and proteinuria
- **Urinary ACR:** albuminuria >3 mg/mmol. NB: not all patients with DKD present with this
- **Blood:** ↑ HbA1c, ↑ creatinine, ↓ eGFR
- **US kidneys** (if an alternative cause of renal impairment suspected): normal or large kidneys
Differentials: hypertensive kidney disease, glomerular diseases
Management:
1. CKD management (lifestyle modifications, BP control, statin therapy, etc.)
2. Optimise diabetic control (see Endocrinology in an Hour)

Hypertensive Kidney Disease

Definition: renal impairment (or nephrosclerosis) secondary to high blood pressure. The clinical diagnosis of nephrosclerosis is one of exclusion.
Buzzwords:
- **Risk factors:** poorly controlled HTN
- **Presentation:** majority are asymptomatic (see the Hypertension and CKD sections)
Investigations:
- **BP monitoring:** HTN
- **Urinalysis:** mild proteinuria and microscopic haematuria
- **Blood:** ↑ creatinine, ↑ urea, ↓ eGFR
Differentials: DKD, glomerular diseases
Management: CKD management

Hepatorenal Syndrome

Definition: impaired renal functioning in the presence of chronic liver dysfunction (cirrhosis with ascites) that is unresponsive to diuretic withdrawal in the absence of other causes of renal failure (e.g., shock, hypovolaemia, nephrotoxics or structural kidney injury). Classified into two types:
- HRS-AKI
- HRS-NAKI (non-AKI). This is further subdivided into HRS-acute kidney disease if eGFR is <60 mL/min/1.73 m^2 for <3 months or HRS-CKD if >3 months
Buzzwords:
- **Risk factors:** spontaneous bacterial peritonitis (SBP), GI bleeding, concurrent infections, hyponatraemia
- **Presentation:** ascites, jaundice, bleeding disorders, signs of AKI or CKD
Investigations:
- **Urinalysis + urine osmolarity:** absence of heavy proteinuria (<500 mg/day), low urinary sodium, urine osmolarity > plasma osmolarity
- **Blood cultures** (if suspected underlying infection)
- **US renal tract:** no evidence of obstruction
- **Ascitic fluid culture** (if suspected SBP)
Differentials: prerenal, renal or postrenal AKI causes (see AKI section), glomerular diseases
Management:
1. Human albumin solution (HAS) and terlipressin
2. RRT (for patients unresponsive to vasoconstrictor therapy) if there is a reasonable expectation of improvement in liver disease
3. Liver transplantation

Lupus Nephritis

Definition: a glomerulonephritis caused by SLE involving immune complex deposition in glomeruli

Buzzwords:

- **Risk factors:** family history, ethnicity (twice as common in Black than White patients), male
- **Presentation:** systemic manifestations of SLE (see Rheumatology in an Hour), nephrotic- or nephritic-syndrome clinical picture

Investigations:

- **Urinalysis:** proteinuria
- **Bloods:** ↑ creatinine, ↓ eGFR, ANA ↑, anti-DS DNA ↑, ↓ C3 and C4 levels
- ***Kidney biopsy*** (determine the pathological class and severity)

Differentials: glomerular diseases

Management:

1. CKD management
2. Hydroxychloroquine
3. Immunosuppression: glucocorticoids, mycophenolate mofetil, cyclophosphamide, rituximab

Amyloidosis

Definition: extracellular deposition of abnormal fibril-forming proteins. Subtypes of amyloidosis include:

- Amyloid light-chain (AL): most common, secondary to plasma cell dyscrasias (e.g., multiple myeloma)
- Reactive (AA): secondary to chronic inflammatory, chronic infectious disease and/or malignancy

Buzzwords:

- **Risk factors:** family history (*transthyretin* gene mutation), 50–65 years of age, chronic inflammatory diseases (e.g., inflammatory bowel disease (IBD), rheumatoid arthritis (RA), SLE), infection (e.g., TB, osteomyelitis, intravenous drug use (IVDU)), malignancy (e.g., renal cell carcinoma, lymphomas), haemodialysis
- **Presentation:** nephrotic syndrome, restrictive cardiomyopathy, heart block, macroglossia, autonomic neuropathy, GI malabsorption

Investigations:

- **Urinalysis:** proteinuria, positive Bence-Jones proteins
- **Blood:** ↑ ESR and CRP (reactive)
- **Serum protein electrophoresis:** positive free light chain
- **Serum immunoglobulin free light chain assay:** abnormal kappa-to-lambda ratio

- ***Renal biopsy*** (abdominal fat or rectal mucosa can also be considered) with **Congo red stain***: amyloid deposits show apple-green birefringence under polarised light

Differentials: MM, MGUS, WM, hypertrophic cardiomyopathy, glomerular diseases

Management:

- **AL:** treat as for myeloma (combination chemotherapy with dexamethasone), lenalidomide or bortezomib (if a rapid response is required (e.g., renal impairment, cardiac involvement, fluid retention, severe hypoalbuminaemia)), referral to haematology and likely a bone marrow biopsy
- **AA:** correction of the underlying cause

Monoclonal Gammopathy of Renal Significance (MGRS)

Definition: renal deposition of monoclonal immunoglobulin or its components, secondary to a B cell or plasma cell lymphoproliferative disease in the absence of tumour complications and a need for immediate treatment

Buzzwords:

- **Risk factors:** MM, MGUS, WM, MBL, CLL, MBL, B-cell lymphoproliferative disorders, amyloidosis
- **Presentation:** variable depending on the underlying condition but can have features of nephrotic syndrome, HTN, haematuria or AKI

Investigations:

- **Urinalysis:** proteinuria, haematuria
- **Urinary ACR:** >3 mg/mmol
- **Blood:** ↓ GFR, ↑ creatinine, ↑ urea; HCO_3^-, Cl^-, PO_4^-, uric acid, glucose (Fanconi syndrome screen)
- **Serum protein electrophoresis:** presence of monoclonal protein
- **Serum immunoglobulin free light chain assay:** abnormal kappa-to-lambda ratio
- ***Kidney biopsy*:** identification of MGRS lesion
- ***Bone marrow biopsy*:** identification of an underlying monoclonal gammopathy

Differentials: glomerular diseases, lupus nephritis

Management:

1. CKD management
2. Treat underlying condition (see Haematology in an Hour)

RENAL TUBULAR DISORDERS

Renal tubules possess an important role in electrolyte reabsorption, fluid balance and acid-base homeostasis.

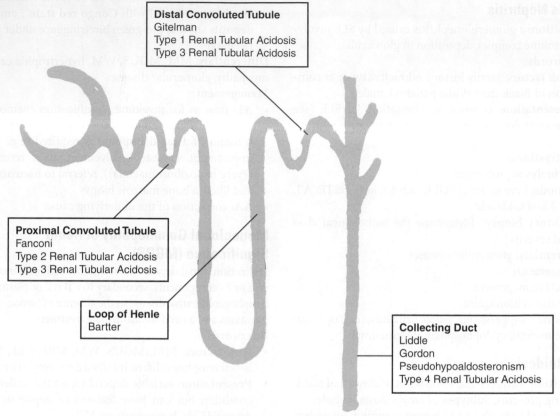

Distal Convoluted Tubule
Gitelman
Type 1 Renal Tubular Acidosis
Type 3 Renal Tubular Acidosis

Proximal Convoluted Tubule
Fanconi
Type 2 Renal Tubular Acidosis
Type 3 Renal Tubular Acidosis

Loop of Henle
Bartter

Collecting Duct
Liddle
Gordon
Pseudohypoaldosteronism
Type 4 Renal Tubular Acidosis

Fig 20.6 Common Renal Tubular Disorders. (Illustrated by Hollie Blaber.)

Renal tubular disorders are a group of conditions presenting with either a generalised dysfunction (e.g., proximal convoluted tubule defect in Fanconi syndrome) or genetic mutations of specific cotransporters or ion channels (e.g., Na-K-2Cl co-transporter in Bartter, NaCl symporter in Gitelman, ENaC in Liddle syndrome) (Fig 20.6). The latter conditions are beyond the scope of this textbook. Fanconi syndrome can be associated with the development of **renal tubular acidosis** (see below), although this can also occur in isolation.

Renal Tubular Acidosis

Definition: disorders characterized by impaired H^+ secretion or HCO_3^- reabsorption in the absence of, or out of proportion to, an impairment in the GFR. The four main types are:

- **Type 1** (distal renal tubular acidosis (RTA)): failure of H^+ secretion
- **Type 2** (proximal RTA): failure of reabsorption of filtered HCO_3^-. This commonly occurs as part of

Fanconi syndrome, which is characterised by excessive urinary excretion of HCO_3^-, K^+, Ca^{2+}, PO_4^-, amino acids, glucose and uric acid.
- **Type 3:** combination of Type 1 and Type 2 (extremely rare)
- **Type 4:** aldosterone deficiency or resistance

Buzzwords:
- **Risk factors:**
  - **Type 1:** autoimmune conditions (e.g., SLE, Sjögren's), hyperparathyroidism, obstructive uropathy, chronic UTIs
  - **Type 2:** Wilson's disease, glycogen storage disorders, cystinosis, tetracyclines, tenofovir, lead poisoning, multiple myeloma, MGUS
  - **Type 3:** carbonic anhydrase deficiency
  - **Type 4:** DM, Addison's disease, CAH, NSAIDs, ACEi, beta blockers, potassium-sparing diuretics, glomerulonephritis
- **Presentation:**
  - **Type 1:** asymptomatic, failure to thrive in children, hyperventilation, muscle weakness, cardiac

arrhythmias, bone pain, history of renal calculi or nephrocalcinosis
- **Type 2:** polyuria, polydipsia, muscle weakness, rickets, osteomalacia, growth failure
- **Type 3:** conductive hearing loss and visual impairment
- **Type 4:** usually asymptomatic, hyperkalaemia, hyperchloraemic metabolic acidosis

Investigations:
- **Blood:** $\downarrow HCO_3^-$, $\leftrightarrow Na^+$, $\downarrow K^+$ (type 1, 2 and 3), $\uparrow K^+$ (type 4)
- **Blood gas:** hyperchloraemic metabolic acidosis, normal anion gap
- ***Urinary pH*:**
  - Hypokalaemia and pH >5.3 (Type 1)
  - Hypokalaemia and pH <5.3 (Type 2)
  - Hypokalaemia and pH >5.3 (Type 3)
  - Hyperkalaemia and pH <5.3 (Type 4)
- Further investigations guided by the type of RTA

Differentials: GI causes of HCO_3^- loss (e.g., diarrhoea), iatrogenic acid loading

Management:
1. Bicarbonate +/- potassium replacement (types 1, 2 and 3)
2. Fludrocortisone + potassium restriction (type 4)

OTHER RENAL CONDITIONS

Interstitial Nephritis

Definition: kidney inflammation localised to the renal tubulo-interstitial space (the area between the kidney surrounding the renal tubules). This can be acute or chronic.

Buzzwords:
- **Risk factors:**
  - **Acute:** drug hypersensitivity (e.g., NSAIDs, beta lactam antibiotics (e.g., penicillins), cephalosporins, carbapenems, PPIs, diuretics), infection (e.g., *Streptococcus*, *Pneumococcus*, *Staphylococcus*, EBV)
  - **Chronic:** NSAID use, infection (e.g., TB, pyelonephritis), autoimmune (e.g., sarcoid, Sjögren's syndrome), lead, cadmium, myeloma, Alport syndrome
- **Presentation:**
  - **Acute:** non-oliguric AKI, fever, maculopapular rash and eosinophilia ('classic triad' – only seen

in roughly 10% of cases), oedema and nephrotic syndrome (occasionally seen with NSAIDs)
  - **Chronic:** 30–70 years of age, long-term analgesic use for pain, history of peptic ulcer disease, flank pain, haematuria

Investigations:
- **Urinalysis:** non-nephrotic proteinuria (NSAIDs can produce nephrotic syndrome), sterile pyuria
- **Blood:** $\uparrow$ urea and creatinine, $\uparrow$ eosinophils
- **US:** enlarged echogenic kidneys
- ***Kidney biopsy*** (if the patient is not responsive to a discontinuation of medication, unclear diagnosis or if steroid treatment is being considered)

Differentials: acute glomerulonephritis, ATN, pyelonephritis, DKD

Management:
1. Discontinue medication
2. Oral prednisolone +/- diuretic (if signs of fluid retention) +/- dialysis (if severe AKI or unresponsive to treatment)
3. CKD management as appropriate

Renal Artery Stenosis

Definition: renal hypoperfusion caused by diseases in the arterial supply to the kidney, commonly due to atherosclerosis or fibromuscular dysplasia (FMD).

Buzzwords:
- **Risk factors:** CVD, DM, smoking, hyperlipidaemia, vasculitides, aberrant renal artery anatomy
- **Presentation:** HTN (can present as resistant or malignant), <30 years of age (FMD), >55 years of age (atherosclerosis), symptoms of AKI, flash pulmonary oedema, abdominal bruit

Investigations:
- **Urinalysis:** usually normal
- **Blood:** $\leftrightarrow$ or $\uparrow$ creatinine, $\downarrow$ or $\leftrightarrow K^+$, $\uparrow$ cholesterol and LDL, $\downarrow$ HDL
- **Duplex ultrasound:** reduced renal artery diameter
- ***CT angiography*** (if CrCl >60 mL/min) or **MR angiography** (if CrCl >30 mL/min): atherosclerotic calcifications, 'string of beads appearance' (FMD), aneurysms (vasculitides), thrombus, extrinsic compression by the crus of the diaphragm or the psoas muscle

Differentials: essential HTN, hypertensive kidney disease, glomerular diseases, renal artery embolism, DKD

Management:

1. Control HTN (ACEi or ARB can be considered in unilateral disease, but NB may cause AKI and contraindicated in bilateral renal artery disease), statin and antiplatelet therapy (if risk factors)
2. Balloon angioplasty +/− stenting (FMD). Consider in atherosclerotic stenosis if:
   - >60% stenosis and symptomatic
   - Refractory HTN
   - Worsening renal function (AKI on ACEi with heart failure or progressive CKD)
   - Recurrent flash pulmonary oedema

Rhabdomyolysis

Definition: skeletal muscle fibre and myocyte cell membrane breakdown due to medical or traumatic injury, leading to the release of intracellular contents, including potassium, myoglobin, creatine kinase (CK) and urates, into the circulation.

Buzzwords:
- **Risk factors:** trauma (e.g., crush injury, burns), recreational drugs or toxins (e.g., ecstasy, cocaine, amphetamine, alcohol), medications (e.g., statins, erythromycin, steroids), myositis, exertional (e.g., strenuous exercise), infection (e.g., influenza, EBV, HIV, *S. pyogenes*, *S. aureus*)
- **Presentation:** elderly patient with a history of a fall and long lie; younger patient presenting after trauma (e.g., long bone fracture) and immobilisation; swollen, painful muscles; paraesthesia; confusion; dehydration; tea-coloured urine; arrhythmias

Investigations:
- **Electrocardiogram (ECG):** evidence of hyperkalaemia (see Cardiology and ECGs in an Hour)
- **Urine dipstick:** haematuria with no RBCs on microscopy
- **Venous blood gas (VBG):** metabolic acidosis with a high anion gap
- ***Blood*:** ↑ CK (5× upper limit normal), ↑ K$^+$, ↑ urea and creatinine, ↑ phosphate, ↓ calcium, ↑ APTT and PT (severe)
- Further tests to determine the underlying cause (e.g., muscle biopsy if a genetic aetiology, toxicology screen if illicit drug use is suspected)

Differentials: inflammatory myositis, infectious myositis, compartment syndrome, diabetic ketoacidosis (DKA), deep vein thrombosis (DVT), renal colic

Management:

1. Urgent treatment for hyperkalaemia if present
2. Fluid resuscitation
3. Urinary alkalinisation with bicarbonate (limited clinical evidence)
4. RRT (if anuric or unresponsive to rehydration therapy)

Polycystic Kidney Disease

Definition: an inherited group of disorders characterised by multiple renal cysts (see Figs 20.7 & 20.8) and multiple extra-renal manifestations. There are two types: autosomal-dominant (most common) and autosomal recessive.

- **Autosomal dominant:** PKD1 (most common, chromosome 16 abnormality) and PKD2 (chromosome 4 abnormality)
- **Autosomal recessive:** chromosome 6 abnormality, occurs commonly in infancy, severe renal impairment with a poor prognosis

This section focuses on autosomal-dominant PKD.

Buzzwords:
- **Risk factors:** family history of PKD, family history of a cerebrovascular event
- **Presentation:** flank pain, haematuria, LUTS, hypertension, palpable kidneys, subarachnoid haemorrhage, incidental finding of a low GFR

Investigations:
- **Urine dipstick, urinalysis and MC&S:** proteinuria, haematuria, coliforms are the most common pathogen
- **Blood:** ↑ FBC, ↑ urea and creatinine
- **US:** see Table 20.8
- ***Next generation sequencing*:** infants and children with very early–onset progressive disease and progressive disease with a negative family history

Differentials: Wilms' tumour, simple cyst, tuberous sclerosis, von Hippel-Lindau

Management:

1. **Supportive:** increase water intake to 3–4 L/day, avoid contact sports, lifestyle advice
2. **Antihypertensive therapy:** ACEi or ARB
3. **Antibiotics** (if suspected UTI or infected renal cysts)
4. **Analgesia:** may require cyst decompression if very large
5. **Urgent neurosurgical referral** +/− intervention (if suspected SAH)
6. CKD management and RRT (dialysis or transplant) if required

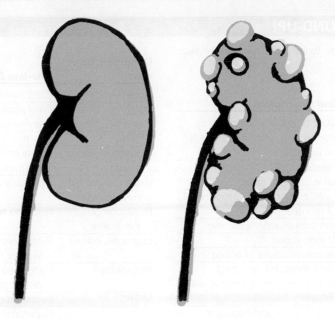

Normal kidney   Polycystic kidney disease

Fig 20.7 Normal kidney and Polycystic Kidney Disease. (Illustrated by Hollie Blaber.)

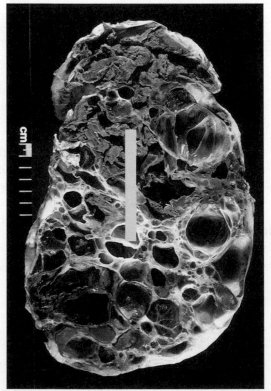

Fig 20.8 Pathology Specimen of a Polycystic Kidney. (With permission from Uthman, E., Houston, TX, USA, CC BY 2.0.)

TABLE 20.8	**Ultrasound Diagnostic Criteria**
If Positive Family History	**Without Family History**
2× unilateral or bilateral renal cysts and <30 years of age	Bilateral renal enlargement and cyst **or** Multiple bilateral renal cysts and hepatic cysts **and**
2× cysts in each kidney and 30–59 years of age	
4× cysts in each kidney and >60 years of age	No manifestations of alternative cystic disease

CHEMICAL PATHOLOGY

BLOOD GASES

Basic Principles

Definitions:

- **pH:** refers to the amount of hydrogen ions in the blood. A normal pH is between 7.35 and 7.45
- **PaO_2 (partial pressure of oxygen):** refers to the amount of oxygen dissolved in the blood. The reference range is between 11–13 kPa
- **$PaCO_2$ (partial pressure of carbon dioxide):** refers to the amount of carbon dioxide dissolved in the blood. The reference range is between 4.7–6.0 kPa. Carbon dioxide is excreted via the lungs

THE ONE-LINE ROUND-UP!

Here are some key words to help you remember each condition/concept

Condition/Concept	One-line Description
UTIs	<65 years of age = urine dip, everyone else, urine culture, >10⁵ cfu = antibiotics
AKI	STOP (sepsis, toxins, optimise volume, prevent harm)
CKD	eGFR <60 and/or ACR >3 mg/mmol for 3 months
RRT	Filtration acute, dialysis chronic
Acute RRT	AEIOU indications
Renal transplant	CMV is classic cause of failure
MCD	Child with relapsing-remitting nephrotic syndrome, treated with steroids
FSGS	Scarred glomeruli and podocyte damage
MN	Underlying condition or new medication started and nephrotic syndrome
Thin basement membrane disease	Benign asymptomatic haematuria
IgA nephropathy	Adult post URTI or GI infection and gross haematuria

Condition/Concept	One-line Description
Alport syndrome	Can't see, can't pee, can't hear a bee
PSGN	Child post-pharyngitis with cola-coloured urine
RPGN	Haematuria and crescents on biopsy
Diabetic kidney disease	Poorly controlled diabetes and proteinuria
Hypertensive kidney disease	Diagnosis of exclusion
Hepatorenal syndrome	HAS and terlipressin
Lupus nephritis	Proteinuria, ANA and dsDNA positive with wire-loop lesions on biopsy
Amyloidosis	Congo red stain and apple-green birefringence
MGRS	Renal deposition of immunoglobulin
RTA	Hyperchloraemic metabolic acidosis requiring bicarbonate
Interstitial nephritis	Nonoliguric AKI
Renovascular disease	Fibromuscular dysplasia, string of beads appearance
Rhabdomyolysis	Crush injury with ↑ CK
PKD	Flank pain, haematuria, LUTS

- **HCO₃ (bicarbonate):** refers to the amount of bicarbonate in the blood. The reference range is between 22–26 mmol/L. Bicarbonate is excreted and reabsorbed via the kidneys
- **Lactate:** under normal conditions, lactate levels are <2 mmol/L. Higher lactate levels may be caused by:
  - Poor oxygenation or poor tissue perfusion (e.g., sepsis, heart failure, shock, pulmonary oedema, anaemia)
  - Increased oxygen demand or metabolism (e.g., liver/kidney failure, AIDS, leukaemia)
  Acid-base disturbance:
- A **low blood pH (<7.35)** indicates that the blood is more acidic (**acidaemia**). Acidosis may occur due to acid (CO_2) retention (e.g., lung disease) or due to a base (HCO_3) loss (e.g., kidney disease)
- A **high blood pH (>7.45)** indicates that the blood is more alkaline (**alkalaemia**). Alkalosis occurs due to

base (HCO_3) retention (e.g., kidney disease) or due to acid (CO_2) loss (e.g., lung disease)
- Both the respiratory and renal systems work together to maintain the acid-base balance (see Fig. 20.9). When one system fails, the other may **compensate** in order to maintain the pH within the normal range

Blood Gas Analysis

1. Know the normal ranges:
   - **pH:** 7.35–7.45
   - **PaO₂:** 11.0–13.0 kPa
   - **PaCO₂:** 4.7–6.0 kPa
   - **HCO₃:** 22–26 mmol/L
   - **Base excess (BE):** -2 to +2 mmol/L
   - **Lactate:** <2 mmol/L
2. Determine if there is respiratory failure and the type of respiratory failure (see Table 20.9)
3. Determine if there is an acid-base disturbance (see Table 20.10)

4. Determine the cause of the acid-base imbalance:
- **Metabolic acidosis:** calculate the anion gap to determine the cause:
  - **Anion gap** = $([Na^+] + [K^+]) - ([Cl^-] + [HCO_3^-])$ mmol/L
  - Reference range is 10–20 mEq/L (10–20 mmol/L).
  - A normal anion gap indicates **bicarbonate loss** (e.g., diarrhoea) or reduced acid secretion by the kidneys (e.g., renal disease)

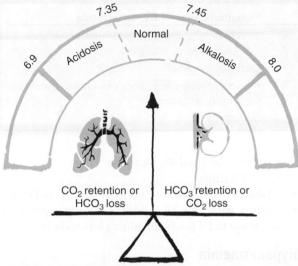

Fig 20.9 Acid-Base Disturbances. (Illustrated by Hollie Blaber.)

- An increased anion gap indicates the **presence of other anions** (e.g., lactate, ketones, toxins)
- **Metabolic alkalosis:** look at the clinical picture to determine the cause. Main causes:
  - Acid loss (e.g., vomiting, diuretics)
  - Acid shift into the cells (hypokalaemia leads to H^+ moving into the cells and K^+ moving out)
  - Bicarbonate administration (e.g., IV fluids)
- **Respiratory acidosis:** main causes are those that lead to type 2 respiratory failure (see Table 20.9).
- **Respiratory alkalosis:** causes include conditions that lead to hyperventilation (e.g., anxiety, infection, asthma, thyrotoxicosis)

5. Determine if there is compensation

The body tries to compensate for any pH changes by increasing or decreasing the respiratory rate (which affects the CO_2 levels) or by increasing or decreasing the secretion of bicarbonate via the kidneys. Compensation by the lungs can occur rapidly. However, compensation by the kidneys is a much slower process.

To determine if there is compensation, check the direction of the **$PaCO_2$ and HCO_3^-**.
- If levels of CO_2 and HCO_3^- are going in the **same direction** (i.e., both are either increased or decreased), it means there is compensation. If the pH is normal, it means there is full compensation.

TABLE 20.9	**Type 1 Respiratory Failure vs Type 2 Respiratory Failure**	
	Type 1 Respiratory Failure	**Type 2 Respiratory Failure**
Arterial blood gas	• Low PaO_2 • Normal or low $PaCO_2$	• Low PaO_2 • High $PaCO_2$
Causes	Any disorder that leads to failed **oxygenation** (oxygen is not getting into the circulation): • Pulmonary oedema • Pneumonia • Pulmonary embolism	Any disorder that leads to failed **ventilation** (oxygen is not getting in and carbon dioxide is not getting out): • Chronic obstructive pulmonary disease • Obstructive sleep apnoea • Chest wall deformities • CNS disorders (e.g., stroke) • Neuromuscular junction disorders (e.g., Guillain-Barre, myasthenia gravis) • Medication (e.g., benzodiazepines, opioids)
Presentation	Hyperventilation, dyspnoea, agitation, tachycardia, cyanosis	May be tachypnoeic or have shallow breathing depending on cause, confusion/drowsiness is a late sign
Management	Treat the underlying cause Oxygen supplementation +/– CPAP	Treat the underlying cause +/– BiPAP

TABLE 20.10   **Acid-Base Disturbances**

	Metabolic Acidosis	Respiratory Acidosis	Metabolic Alkalosis	Respiratory Alkalosis
pH [7.35–7.45]	Low	Low	High	High
PaCO$_2$ [4.7–6.0 kPa]	Normal	High	Normal	Low
HCO$_3^-$ [22–26 mmol/L]	Low	Normal	High	Normal
Base excess [–2 to +2]	Low	Normal	High	Normal

TABLE 20.11   **Hypernatraemia**

Fluid Status and Presentation	Urine Osmolality	Potential Cause of Hypernatremia
Hypovolemic (dry mucous membrane, tachycardia, poor urine output)	High (concentrated urine)	Severe dehydration (e.g., poor oral intake, diarrhoea, vomiting, diuretics)
	Low (dilute urine)	Diabetes insipidus
Euvolemic	Normal urine	Mild dehydration (e.g., poor oral intake, diarrhoea, vomiting, diuretics)
Hypervolemic (peripheral oedema)	Low (dilute urine)	Sodium gain (e.g., excess IV fluids)

- If both levels go in **opposite directions**, then it means there is coexisting metabolic and respiratory acidosis

SODIUM

Hypernatraemia

Definition: a high sodium concentration (>146 mmol/L). The normal reference range is 133–146 mmol/L. Causes of hypernatraemia can be divided by the fluid status (i.e., hypovolaemic, euvolaemic and hypervolaemic). Fluid status can be determined by examining the patient. Urine osmolality can be used to distinguish between potential causes (see Table 20.11).
Buzzwords:
- **Risk factors:** water loss, diabetes insipidus, sodium gain
- **Presentation:** fatigue, weakness, confusion, seizures
Investigations:
- **Blood:** U&E (hypernatraemia), serum osmolality (high osmolality = more particles in the serum)
- **Urine osmolality:** may be normal, low (= dilute urine) or high (= concentrated urine)
Management: treat the underlying cause:
- **Dehydration:** replace with IV fluids. Ideally avoid 0.9% NaCl or Hartmann's as they contain a high sodium concentration. You may use any of the following:

- 0.18% NaCl and 4% Dextrose
- 5% Dextrose
- **Diabetes insipidus:** see Endocrinology in an Hour
- **Sodium gain:** stop IV fluids if clinically appropriate or change to IV fluids containing less sodium

Hyponatraemia

Definition: the normal sodium reference range is 133–146 mmol/L. Hyponatraemia is defined as a low serum sodium (<133 mmol/L).
Buzzwords:
- **Risk factors:** increasing age, hospitalisation, diuretics, selective serotonin reuptake inhibitors (SSRIs), antipsychotics (e.g., haloperidol and phenothiazines), carbamazepine, underlying medical conditions (e.g., heart failure, kidney disease, liver disease, endocrine disorder)
- **Presentation:** depends on speed of onset of hyponatraemia
  - **Acute hyponatraemia:** likely symptomatic. Symptoms may include nausea, vomiting, lethargy, muscle cramps, weakness, confusion, seizures, reduced Glasgow Coma Scale score
  - **Chronic and gradual-onset hyponatraemia:** may be asymptomatic/have few symptoms even if a severe hyponatraemia
Investigations:
- **Blood:**
  - U&E to confirm hyponatraemia

TABLE 20.12 Hyponatraemia

Fluid Status	Urine Osmolality	Urine Sodium	Cause of Hyponatraemia
Hypovolaemic	High (≥100 mOsm/kg)	High (>30 mmol/L)	Occurs when there is fluid and sodium loss due to renal causes: • Primary adrenal insufficiency • Renal/cerebral salt wasting
	High (≥100 mOsm/kg)	Low (<30 mmol/L)	Occurs when there is fluid and sodium loss due to extrarenal causes: • Diarrhoea, vomiting • 'Third spacing'
Euvolemic	High (≥100 mOsm/kg)	High (> 30 mmol/L)	Occurs when there is normal sodium in the body but increased fluid, which dilutes the sodium: • Syndrome of inappropriate secretion of antidiuretic hormone • Secondary adrenal insufficiency • Hypothyroidism
	High (≥100 mOsm/kg)	Low (<30 mmol/L)	Primary polydipsia
Hypervolemic	High (≥100 mOsm/kg)	Low (<30 mmol/L)	Occurs when there is increased fluid and sodium retention, but more fluid than sodium: • Heart failure • Liver cirrhosis • Nephrotic syndrome

- Blood tests to rule out other causes: thyroid function tests (TFTs), cortisol level, liver function tests (LFTs), nT-proBNP
- Determine if there is **true** hyponatraemia by measuring the serum osmolality:
  - Low plasma osmolality (<275 mOsmol/kg) = true hyponatraemia
  - Normal plasma osmolality (275–295 mOsmol/kg). In the presence of hyponatraemia, this may indicate pseudohyponatremia, which is caused by high levels of serum lipids or proteins
  - High plasma osmolality (>295 mOsmol/kg). May be caused by hyperglycaemia
3. Determine the cause of true hyponatraemia by measuring *three* things: *fluid status, urine osmolality, and urine sodium* (see Table 20.12)

Management: Avoid rapid correction to prevent osmotic demyelination syndrome.
- **Mild:** monitor
- **Moderate/severe:** treatment depends on the fluid status and severity of the presentation:
  - Hypovolaemic hyponatraemia: IV fluids (hypertonic saline may be used under specialist supervision)
  - Euvolemic hyponatraemia: treat the underlying cause if possible

- Hypervolemic hyponatraemia: fluid restriction

POTASSIUM

Hyperkalaemia

Definition: a high serum potassium (>5.5 mmol/L).
Causes:
- **Renal:** AKI, drugs, CKD, renal tubular acidosis (Type IV)
- **Tissue breakdown:** rhabdomyolysis, tumour lysis, haemolysis
- **Endocrine:** DKA, Addison's, metabolic acidosis
- **Diet** (rare)
- **Pseudo-hyperkalaemia:** raised potassium due to lysis of RBCs (most commonly due to a prolonged transit time to the lab)

Investigations:
- **Blood:** ABG/VBG/U&E show K >5.5mmol/L
- **ECG:** Progressive changes (see Fig. 20.10 & 20.11)
  - PR prolongation
  - Flattened or absent P waves
  - Tall, tented T waves
  - Wide QRS (>0.12 s)
  - Ventricular tachycardia
  - Bradycardia
  - 'Sine wave' appearance

TABLE 20.13   **Management of Hyperkalaemia**

Hyperkalaemia	Management

Mild (5.5–5.9 mmol/L)	1. Treat cause
	2. Remove potassium from the body (if necessary):
	  • Calcium resonium 15–30 g or
	  • Sodium polystyrene sulfonate 15–30 g

Moderate (6.0–6.4 mmol/L)	1. Electrocardiography and cardiac monitoring
	2. Shift potassium into the cells with glucose/insulin: 10 units of short-acting insulin and 25 g glucose IV over 15–30 min
	3. Remove potassium from the body:
	  • Calcium resonium 15–30 g or
	  • Sodium polystyrene sulfonate 15–30 g

Severe (≥6.5 mmol/L) with ECG changes	1. Seek expert help, set up cardiac monitoring and do an ECG
	2. Shift potassium into the cells with glucose/insulin:
	  • 10 units of short-acting insulin AND
	  • 50 mL of 50% glucose IV over 15 min or 125 mL of 20% glucose IV over 15 min
	3. Shift potassium into the cells with salbutamol 10–20 mg NEB
	4. Remove potassium from body: consider dialysis if refractory to treatment

Severe (≥6.5 mmol/L) Without ECG Changes	1. Seek expert help, set up cardiac monitoring and do an ECG
	2. Cardioprotection with:
	  • 10 mL of 10% calcium chloride IV over 2–5 min OR
	  • 30 mL of 10% calcium gluconate IV over 2–5 min
	3. Shift potassium into cells with glucose/insulin: 10 units of short-acting insulin and 25 g glucose IV over 15–30 min
	4. Shift potassium into the cells with salbutamol 10–20 mg NEB
	5. Remove potassium from body: consider dialysis if refractory to treatment

• Cardiac arrest (e.g., pulseless electrical activity (PEA), ventricular fibrillation (VF)/pVT, asystole)

Management of hyperkalaemia in a non-cardiac arrest situation: see Table 20.13

Management of hyperkalaemia in the context of cardiac arrest:

1. **Cardioprotection** with:
   • 10 mL of 10% calcium chloride IV by rapid injection or
   • 30 mL of 10% calcium gluconate IV by rapid injection
2. **Shift potassium into the cells with glucose/insulin:** 10 units of short-acting insulin and 25 g glucose IV over 15–30 min
3. Sodium bicarbonate 50 mmol IV by rapid injection
4. Remove potassium from the body. Consider dialysis
5. Consider a mechanical chest compression device if prolonged CPR is needed

Hypokalaemia

Definition: a low serum potassium (<3.5 mmol/L). Causes include:

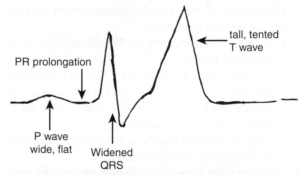

Fig 20.10 Electrocardiographic Changes in Hyperkalaemia. (Illustrated by Hollie Blaber.)

• **Decreased intake:** poor diet, malabsorption
• **Increased loss:** GI (e.g., diarrhoea), renal (e.g., renal tubular disorders, nephrogenic diabetes insipidus, dialysis)
• **Endocrine:** Cushing's, hyperaldosteronism
• **Drugs:** diuretics, laxatives, steroids, some antibiotics
• Magnesium loss
Buzzwords:

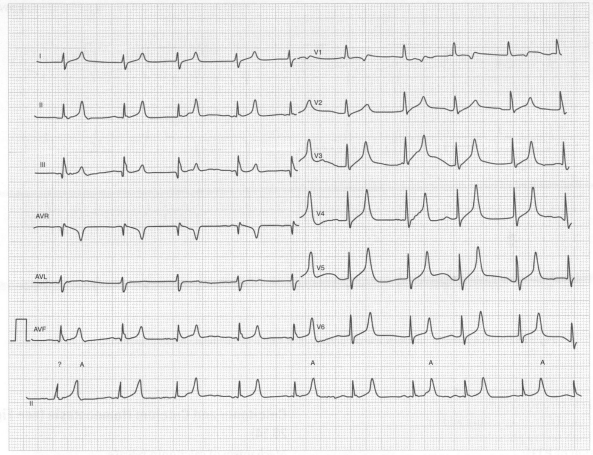

Fig 20.11 Hyperkalaemia on Electrocardiography. (With permission from Dr. Michael-Joseph F. Agbayani and Dr. Eddieson Gonzales, Manila, Philippines.)

- **Presentation:**
  - **Mild** (3.0–3.5 mmol/L): asymptomatic
  - **Moderate** (2.5–3.0 mmol/L): fatigue, weakness, muscle pain, constipation
  - **Severe** (<2.5 mmol/L): ascending paralysis, palpitations, ileus, respiratory failure, tetany, rhabdomyolysis

Investigations:
- **Blood:** U&E (hypokalaemia, hypomagnesemia)
- **ECG** (see Fig 20.12): U waves, T wave flattening, ST depression, arrhythmias, cardiac arrest

Management of hypokalaemia in a noncardiac arrest situation:
- **Mild**
  1. Oral potassium supplement
  2. Treat underlying cause
  3. Monitor potassium levels every few days
- **Severe**
  1. Seek expert advice

2. Cardiac monitoring
3. IV potassium chloride (maximum rate 20 mmol/h) – NEVER GIVE A BOLUS!
4. Treat underlying cause
5. Monitor potassium levels every 3 hours
- **Management of hypokalaemia in the context of cardiac arrest:**
  1. IV potassium 2 mmol/min for 10 min followed by 10 mmol over 5–10 min (senior input required!)
  2. Treat underlying cause
  3. Monitor potassium levels post-cardiac arrest

CALCIUM

Parathyroid Hormone (PTH) and Calcium Homeostasis (see Fig 20.13)

Mechanism of PTH release:

PTH is released by the chief cells of the four **parathyroid glands** in response to:

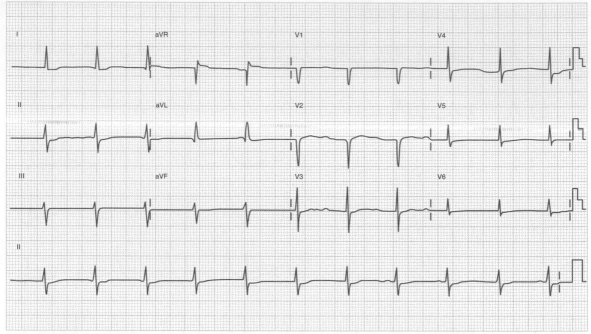

Fig 20.12 Hypokalaemia on Electrocardiography (K = 1.6). (With permission from Hammond, K., Wilson, M., Sanche, S., Wilson, T.W. (2009). Cocktail paralysis. *The American Journal of Medicine*. Elsevier.)

- Low serum calcium
- Low serum magnesium and/or
- High serum phosphate

Action of PTH:

PTH acts at three main sites:

- **Kidneys:** PTH **increases calcium reabsorption and decreases phosphate reabsorption** from the kidneys. It also stimulates the **formation of active Vitamin D** (Calcitriol and Ercalcitriol). Normal levels of active vitamin D are needed for PTH to exert its action at other sites (including the bones and small bowel)
- **Bones:** PTH stimulates osteoclast number and activity, leading to bone absorption and calcium release into the blood
- **Small bowel:** PTH stimulates calcium absorption from the gut.

Net effect of PTH: Serum calcium levels increase, and serum phosphate levels decrease.

When the serum calcium level is high, PTH release is suppressed (via **negative feedback**), thereby helping to reduce the serum calcium level.

Calcitonin and Calcium Homeostasis (see Fig 20.14)

Mechanism of calcitonin release:

Calcitonin is released by the parafollicular cells (C-cells) of the **thyroid gland** in response to:

- High serum calcium
- High serum magnesium and/or
- Low serum phosphate

Role of calcitonin:

Calcitonin has the opposite effect of PTH:

- **Kidneys:** calcitonin decreases calcium reabsorption
- **Bone:** calcitonin increases calcium deposition
- **Small bowel:** calcitonin decreases dietary uptake of calcium

Hyper and Hypocalcaemia

Definition:

- **Hypercalcaemia:** an adjusted (a.k.a., corrected) serum calcium concentration of ≥2.6 mmol/L on two separate occasions. The lab should provide you with the adjusted serum calcium level.

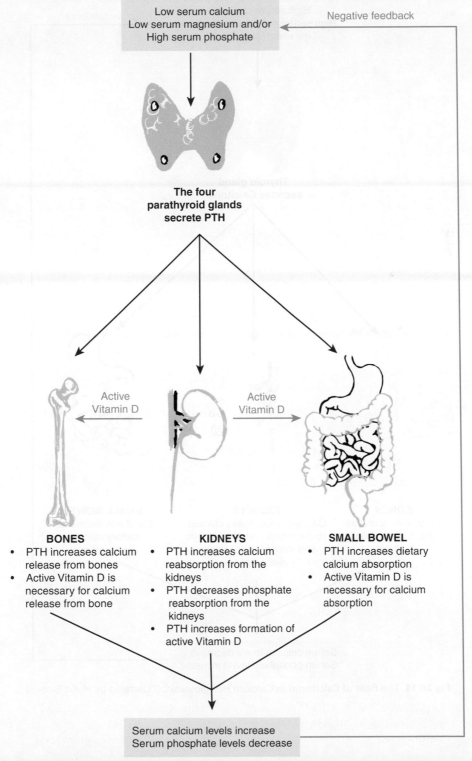

Fig 20.13 The Role of Parathyroid Hormone in Calcium Homeostasis. (Illustrated by Hollie Blaber)

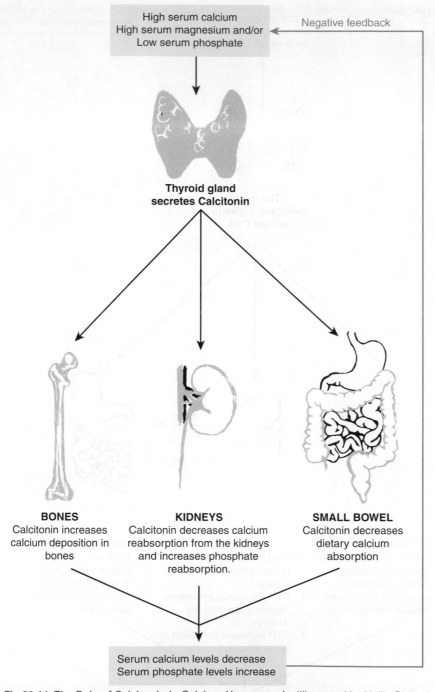

High serum calcium
High serum magnesium and/or
Low serum phosphate

Negative feedback

**Thyroid gland
secretes Calcitonin**

BONES
Calcitonin increases
calcium deposition in
bones

KIDNEYS
Calcitonin decreases calcium
reabsorption from the kidneys
and increases phosphate
reabsorption.

SMALL BOWEL
Calcitonin decreases
dietary calcium
absorption

Serum calcium levels decrease
Serum phosphate levels increase

Fig 20.14 The Role of Calcitonin in Calcium Homeostasis. (Illustrated by Hollie Blaber.)

TABLE 20.14 Hypercalcaemia vs Hypocalcaemia

Hypercalcaemia	Hypocalcaemia
Mnemonic: malignancy + RED GIF • **Malignancy** • **R**enal failure – AKI/CKD • **E**ndocrine – primary hyperparathyroidism, thyrotoxicosis, Addison's, phaechromocytoma • **D**rugs – thiazide diuretics, lithium, vitamin D, vitamin A, milk-alkali syndrome • **G**ranulomatous disease – TB, sarcoidosis • **I**mmobility • **F**amilial hypocalciuric hypercalcaemia	• Primary hypoparathyroidism • Pseudohypoparathyroidism • Secondary hyperparathyroidism (due to vitamin D deficiency of CKD) • Drugs: calcium-channel blockers, calcium chelators, bisphosphonates, calcitonin, drugs affecting vitamin D (e.g., phenytoin) • Rarer causes but important to know: rhabdomyolysis, tumour lysis syndrome

- **Adjusted serum calcium** = measured total calcium + [0.8 × (4 - serum albumin)]
- **Hypocalcaemia:** an adjusted serum calcium concentration of <2.1 mmol/L on two separate occasions
- See Table 20.14 for causes of hyper- and hypocalcaemia

Do not confuse the 'ionized' calcium (i.e., calcium that is not bound to albumin), total calcium and adjusted calcium values:

- The reference range for **ionized calcium** is 1.1–1.3 mmol/L. This value is measured by blood gas machines.
- The reference range for **total calcium** is 2.2–2.6 mmol/L. However, this value depends on the albumin level and needs to be adjusted (adjusted calcium). Total calcium values are measured by taking a blood sample (U&E).
- The reference range for **adjusted serum calcium** is 2.2–2.6 mmol/L. Corrected calcium values are calculated from the albumin and calcium levels.

Buzzwords:
- **Hypercalcaemia presentation:**
  - **Bone**: pain, deformities, osteoporosis, fragility fractures, pathological fractures in the context of a malignancy
  - **Renal:** including renal stones, nephrogenic diabetes insipidus, renal impairment
  - **Gastrointestinal:** abdominal pain, constipation, nausea, vomiting
  - **Psychiatric and neurological**: depression, lethargy, seizures
  - **Cardiac**: arrhythmias, ECG changes (see Investigations), hypotension
- **Hypocalcaemia presentation**: muscle cramps, muscle pain, twitching, Trousseau's sign (carpopedal

spasm caused by the BP cuff), Chvostek's sign (facial contraction caused by tapping the facial nerve)

Investigations:
- **ECG (see Fig 20.15):**
  - **Hypercalcemia:** short QT interval, prolonged QRS, flat T waves, AV block, cardiac arrest
  - **Hypocalcaemia**: QT prolongation, T wave inversion, sinus bradycardia, heart block, cardiac arrest
- **Blood:** U&E, bone profile, phosphate, magnesium, vitamin D, PTH (see Table 20.15)
- Further investigations may be required based on the suspected pathology.

Management:
- **Hypercalcemia:** Consult local guidelines and treat the underlying cause if possible, give fluids, specialist referral. Consider:
  - IV pamidronate 30–90 mg
  - IV furosemide 1 mg/kg
  - IV hydrocortisone 200–300 mg (in malignancy)
- **Hypocalcaemia:** Consult local guidelines and treat underlying cause if possible. If associated with hypomagnesaemia, replace magnesium first. If Vitamin D is low, replace. In mild hypocalcaemia cases, give PO calcium supplementation (e.g. Adcal D3). In severe cases, give 10-20ml 10% Calcium Gluconate in 50-100 mL of 5% Glucose IV over 5 to 10 minutes with ECG monitoring. Repeat if necessary, with senior input. In exceptional cases a continuous calcium infusion may be required. If infusion is required, dilute 100mL of 10% calcium gluconate (10 x 10ml ampoules) in 1L of 0.9% NaCl or 5% Glucose and infuse at a rate of 50-100 ml/hour. Note: Calcium chloride injections are available but are more irritant.

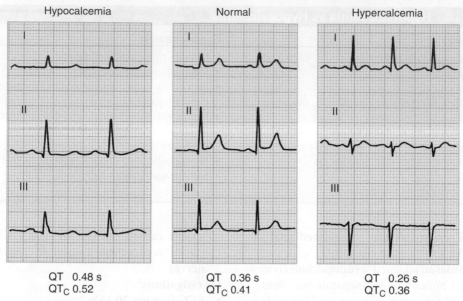

Fig 20.15 Hypocalcaemia vs Hypercalcaemia on ECG. With permission from Goldberger A.L. et al. (2013). Drug effects, electrolyte abnormalities, and metabolic factors (Fig. 10.7). In A. L. Goldberger et al. (Eds.), *Clinical electrocardiography: A simplified approach* (8th ed.) (pp. 92–100). Philadelphia, PA: Elsevier.)

TABLE 20.15   Blood Test Results in Calcium Disorders and Other Disorders

Pathology	PTH	Calcium	Phosphate	ALP
Hypercalcaemia of malignancy (may include metastatic disease)	Low	High	Low (or normal)	Varies depending on cause
Primary hyperparathyroidism – caused by a parathyroid adenoma (80%), MEN1/2A (20%) or carcinoma (<0.5%)	High	High	Low	High
Secondary hyperparathyroidism – caused by prolonged hypocalcaemia (CKD, chronic vitamin D deficiency)	High	Low (or normal)	High	High
Tertiary hyperparathyroidism – caused by parathyroid hyperplasia	High	High	High	High
Primary hypoparathyroidism – caused by parathyroid gland damage (e.g., autoantibodies, surgery, trauma) or a genetic disorder (e.g., DiGeorge)	Low	Low	High	Normal
Secondary hypoparathyroidism – caused by high calcium levels leading to reduced production of PTH	Low	High	High	Normal
Pseudohypoparathyroidism, in which target organs fail to respond to PTH	High	Low	Low	Normal
Osteomalacia	High	Low	Low	High
Paget's disease	Normal	Normal	Normal	High
Osteoporosis	Normal	Normal	Normal	Normal

MAGNESIUM

Hypermagnesaemia

Definition: The reference range for magnesium is 0.85–1.10 mmol/L. Hypermagnesemia is defined as a serum magnesium of >1.1 mmol/L. It is less common than hypomagnesaemia.

Causes:
- Reduced excretion due to kidney failure
- Increased intake (e.g., Mg-containing laxatives, 1V replacement)
- Occasionally – parenteral nutrition, lithium therapy, Addison's

Buzzwords:
- **Presentation:** asymptomatic, flushing, confusion, weakness, respiratory depression, atrioventricular (AV) block, cardiac arrest (at levels >6.0)

Investigations:
- **Blood:** U&E (usually hypocalcaemia coexists), magnesium (high)
- **ECG:** PR prolongation, QT prolongation, AV block

Management:
- Treat the underlying cause: stop Mg-containing medications (e.g., laxatives)
- If normal renal function, the body will remove the Mg itself. This can be enhanced with IV saline/furosemide
- Consider treatment when Mg is >1.75 mmol/L with 10% calcium chloride 5–10 mL IV
- Consider dialysis if CKD

Hypomagnesaemia

Definition: the reference range for magnesium is 0.85–1.10 mmol/L. Hypomagnesemia is defined as a serum magnesium of <0.6 mmol/L.

Causes:
- Malnutrition disorders (e.g., coeliac disease) and diarrhoea
- Surgical removal of the small intestines (magnesium is normally absorbed from the small intestine)
- Drugs: PPI, antibiotics, diuretics, IV fluids, chemotherapy agents, immunosuppressants

- Renal damage (e.g., ATN), inherited renal disorders (e.g., Gitelman's syndrome) and polyuria

Buzzwords:
- **Presentation:** normally asymptomatic until <0.5 mmol/L. If symptomatic:
  - **Neuromuscular symptoms:** weakness, tremor, paraesthesia, drowsiness, seizures, coma
  - **Cardiovascular symptoms:** arrythmias
  - **Other electrolytes:** likely low K^+ and Ca^{2+} as well

Investigations:
- **Blood:** magnesium (low), U&E and bone profile (hypomagnesemia usually coexists with low potassium and low calcium. Note: you cannot correct those abnormalities without also correcting the magnesium)
- **ECG:** flat p wave, PR prolongation, widened QRS, ST depression, T wave inversion, ventricular arrhythmias, torsade de pointes
- Tests to determine the cause are only done if the diagnosis is unclear from the history:
  - **24-h urinary magnesium excretion:** daily magnesium excretion >2 mEq (1 mmol or 24 mg) indicates renal losses
  - **Fractional excretion of magnesium (FEMg – see formula):** magnesium excretion of >3% indicates renal loss

Fractional excretion of magnesium formula:

$$FEMg = [(\text{Urinary Mg} \times \text{Plasma Creatinine})/(\text{Plasma Mg} \times \text{Urinary Creatinine} \times 0.7)] \times 100$$

Management:
- Treat the underlying cause
- If asymptomatic, no need for further treatment
- Oral therapy: various magnesium salts available for mild symptoms
- If severe or symptomatic, treat:
  - IV replacement: 5 g magnesium sulphate (10 mL; 20 mmol) in 1000 mL of 0.9% saline over 4–8 hours
  - Arrhythmia/torsades de pointes: 2 g 50% magnesium sulphate (4 mL; 8 mmol) IV over 10 min
  - Seizure: 2 g 50% magnesium sulphate (4 mL; 8 mmol) IV over 10 min

THE ONE-LINE ROUND-UP!

Here are some key words to help you remember each condition/concept.

Condition/Concept	One-line Description
T1RF	Failed oxygenation
T2RF	Failed ventilation
Anion gap	Anion gap = $([Na^+] + [K^+]) - ([Cl^-] + [HCO_3^-])$ mmol/L
Hypernatraemia	Usually dehydration
Hyponatraemia	Assess fluid status, get urine osmol/Na levels
Hyperkalaemia	Calcium, insulin/dextrose, salbutamol

Condition/Concept	One-line Description
Hypokalaemia	Malnutrition, U waves, check Mg
PTH	Raises calcium, reduces phosphate
Hypercalcaemia	Check PTH, check malignancy, give fluids
Hypocalcaemia	Trousseau's sign
Hypermagnesaemia	Renal failure, iatrogenic
Hypomagnesaemia	Check K, weakness, tremors, arrhythmias

READING LIST: RENAL MEDICINE IN AN HOUR

INFECTIONS
Urinary Tract Infection
NICE. (2018). *CKS: Urinary tract infection (lower) – men.* https://cks.nice.org.uk/topics/urinary-tract-infection-lower-men/. Accessed April 2021.

NICE. (2020). *CKS: Urinary tract infection (lower) - women.* https://cks.nice.org.uk/topics/urinary-tract-infection-lower-women/. Accessed April 2021.

NICE. (2018). *NG109: Urinary tract infection (lower): Antimicrobial prescribing.* https://www.nice.org.uk/guidance/ng109. Accessed April 2021.

Pyelonephritis
BMJ Best Practice. (2020). *Acute pyelonephritis.* https://bestpractice.bmj.com/topics/en-gb/3000111. Accessed April 2021.

NICE. (2018). *NG111: Pyelonephritis (acute): Antimicrobial prescribing.* https://www.nice.org.uk/guidance/ng111. Accessed April 2021.

KIDNEY INJURIES
Acute Kidney Injury (AKI)
BMJ Best Practice. (2020). *Acute kidney injury.* https://bestpractice.bmj.com/topics/en-gb/3000117. Accessed April 2021.

NICE. (2019). *NG148: Acute kidney injury: Prevention, detection and management.* https://www.nice.org.uk/guidance/ng148. Accessed April 2021.

NICE. (2018). *CKS: Acute kidney injury.* https://cks.nice.org.uk/topics/acute-kidney-injury/. Accessed April 2021.

NHS England. (2020). *Recommended minimum requirements of a care bundle for patients with AKI in hospital.* https://www.thinkkidneys.nhs.uk/aki/wp-content/uploads/sites/2/2020/03/AKI-care-bundle-2020.pdf. Accessed April 2021.

Chronic Kidney Disease
NICE. (2015). *CG182: Chronic kidney disease in adults: Assessment and management.* https://www.nice.org.uk/guidance/cg182. Accessed April 2021.

NICE. (2020). *CKS: Chronic kidney disease.* https://cks.nice.org.uk/topics/chronic-kidney-disease/. Accessed April 2021.

NICE. (2019). *TA599: Sodium zirconium cyclosilicate for treating hyperkalaemia.* https://www.nice.org.uk/guidance/ta599. Accessed April 2021.

Kidney Disease Improving Global Outcomes. (2012). *Clinical Practice Guideline for the evaluation and management of chronic kidney disease.* https://kdigo.org/guidelines/ckd-evaluation-and-management/.

Life in the Fast Lane. (2020). *Renal replacement therapy indications.* https://litfl.com/renal-replacement-therapy-indications/. Accessed April 2021.

Renal Replacement Therapy (RRT)
Gemmell, L., Docking, R., & Black, E. (2017). Renal replacement therapy in critical care. *BJA Education, 17*, 88–93.

Rayner, H., Imai, E., & Kher, V. (2019). Approach to renal replacement therapy. In J. Feehally, J. Floege, M. Tonelli, & R. J. Johnson (Eds.), *Comprehensive clinical nephrology* (6th ed.) (pp. 1036–1049). Elsevier.

Al-Shaikh, B., & Stacey, S. (2019). *Essentials of equipment in anaesthesia, critical care and perioperative medicine.* Elsevier.

NICE. (2018). *CKS: Acute kidney injury.* https://cks.nice.org.uk/topics/acute-kidney-injury/ [Accessed April 2021].

HEE e-LFH. (2020). *Anaesthesia e-LA, core training, Renal Replacement Therapy.* http://portal.e-lfh.org.uk. Accessed April 2021.

Renal Transplant
Mulley, W., & Kanellis, J. (2019). Evaluation and preoperative management of kidney transplant recipient and donor.

In J. Feehally, J. Floege, M. Tonelli, & R. J. Johnson (Eds.), *Comprehensive clinical nephrology* (6th ed.) (pp. 1163–1173). Elsevier.

Womer, K. (2019). Immunologic principles in kidney transplantation. In J. Feehally, J. Floege, M. Tonelli, & R. J. Johnson (Eds.), *Comprehensive clinical nephrology* (6th ed.) (pp. 1141–1153). Elsevier.

Cooper, J., Stites, E., & Wiseman, A. (2019). Prophylaxis and treatment of kidney transplant rejection. In J. Feehally, J. Floege, M. Tonelli, & R. J. Johnson (Eds.), *Comprehensive clinical nephrology* (6th ed.) (pp. 1163–1173). Elsevier.

Alquadan, K., Womer, K., & Casey, M. (2019). Immunosuppressive medications in kidney transplantation. In J. Feehally, J. Floege, M. Tonelli, & R. J. Johnson (Eds.), *Comprehensive clinical nephrology* (6th ed.) (pp. 1154–1162). Elsevier.

BNF. (2021). *Ciclosporin*. https://bnf.nice.org.uk/drug/ciclosporin.html. [Accessed April 2021].

BNF. (2021). *Tacrolimus*. https://bnf.nice.org.uk/drug/tacrolimus.html. [Accessed April 2021].

BNF. (2021). *Mycophenolate mofetil*. https://bnf.nice.org.uk/drug/mycophenolate-mofetil.html [Accessed April 2021].

Lenihan, C., & Tan, J. (2020). Clinical management of the adult kidney transplant recipient. In *Brenner and Rector's the kidney* (11th ed.) (pp. 2244–2287). Elsevier.

GLOMERULAR DISEASE

With Nephrotic Syndrome

Kidney Disease Improving Global Outcomes. (2012). *KDIGO Clinical Practice Guideline for Glomerulonephritis*. https://kdigo.org/wp-content/uploads/2017/02/KDIGO-2012-GN-Guideline-English.pdf. Accessed April 2021.

BMJ Best Practice. (2018). *Assessment of nephrotic syndrome*. https://bestpractice.bmj.com/topics/en-gb/356. Accessed April 2021.

BMJ Best Practice. (2019). *Membranous nephropathy*. https://bestpractice.bmj.com/topics/en-gb/941. Accessed April 2021.

BMJ Best Practice. (2020). *Minimal change disease*. https://bestpractice.bmj.com/topics/en-gb/940. Accessed April 2021.

With Haematuria

Kidney Disease Improving Global Outcomes. (2012). *KDIGO Clinical Practice Guideline for Glomerulonephritis*. https://kdigo.org/wp-content/uploads/2017/02/KDIGO-2012-GN-Guideline-English.pdf. Accessed April 2021.

National Kidney Foundation. (2017). *Thin basement membrane disease*. https://www.kidney.org/atoz/content/thin-basement-membrane-disease. Accessed April 2021.

BMJ Best Practice. (2020). *Alport's syndrome*. https://bestpractice.bmj.com/topics/en-gb/860. Accessed April 2021.

With Acute Kidney Injury

Kidney Disease Improving Global Outcomes. (2012). *KDIGO Clinical Practice Guideline for Glomerulonephritis*. https://kdigo.org/wp-content/uploads/2017/02/KDIGO-2012-GN-Guideline-English.pdf. Accessed April 2021.

BMJ Best Practice. (2018). *IgA nephropathy*. https://bestpractice.bmj.com/topics/en-gb/480. Accessed April 2021.

Rawla, P., Pafala, S. A., & Ludhwani, D. (2020). *Poststreptococcal glomerulonephritis*. StatPearls. https://www.ncbi.nlm.nih.gov/books/NBK538255/. Accessed April 2021.

Naik, R. H., & Shawar, S. H. (2020). *Rapidly progressive glomerulonephritis*. StatPearls. https://www.ncbi.nlm.nih.gov/books/NBK557430/. Accessed April 2021.

RENAL MANIFESTATIONS OF SYSTEMIC DISEASE

Diabetic Kidney Disease (DKD)

Wilkinson, I., Raine, T., Wiles, K., Goodhart, A., Hall, C., & O'Neill, H. (2017). *Oxford handbook of clinical medicine* (10th ed.). Oxford University Press.

Patient info. (2016). *Diabetic nephropathy*. https://patient.info/doctor/diabetic-nephropathy. Accessed April 2021.

Zac-Varghese, S., & Winocour, P. (2018). Managing diabetic kidney disease. *British Medical Bulletin, 125,* 55–66.

Kidney Disease Improving Global Outcomes. (2020). *Clinical Practice Guideline for Diabetes Management in Chronic Kidney Disease*. https://academic.oup.com/bmb/article/125/1/55/4677302. Accessed April 2021.

Hypertensive Kidney Disease

MSD Manual. (2021). *Hypertensive arteriolar nephrosclerosis*. https://www.msdmanuals.com/en-gb/home/kidney-and-urinary-tract-disorders/blood-vessel-disorders-of-the-kidneys/hypertensive-arteriolar-nephrosclerosis. Accessed April 2021.

Castillo-Rodriguez, E., Fernandez-Fernandez, B., Alegre-Bellassai, R., Kanbay, M., & Ortiz, A. (2019). The chaos of hypertension guidelines for chronic kidney disease patients. *Clinical Kidney Journal, 12,* 771–777. https://academic.oup.com/ckj/article/12/6/771/5575922. Accessed April 2021.

Hepatorenal Syndrome (HRS)

The European Association for the Study of the Liver. (2018). EASL Clinical Practice Guidelines for the management of patients with decompensated cirrhosis. *Journal of Hepatology, 69,* 406–460. https://easl.eu/wp-content/uploads/2018/10/decompensated-cirrhosis-English-report.pdf. Accessed April 2021.

Simonetto, D. A., Gines, P., & Kamath, P. S. (2020). Hepatorenal syndrome: pathophysiology, diagnosis and management. *British Medical Journal, 370,* 2687. https://www.bmj.com/content/370/bmj.m2687. Accessed April 2021.

BMJ Best Practice. (2019). *Hepatorenal syndrome*. https://bestpractice.bmj.com/topics/en-gb/402. Accessed April 2021.

Lupus Nephritis

Wilkinson, I., Raine, T., Wiles, K., Goodhart, A., Hall, C., & O'Neill, H. (2017). *Oxford handbook of clinical medicine* (10th ed.). Oxford University Press.

Kidney Disease Improving Global Outcomes. (2012). *KDIGO Clinical Practice Guideline for Glomerulonephritis*. https://kdigo.org/wp-content/uploads/2017/02/KDIGO-2012-GN-Guideline-English.pdf. Accessed April 2021.

Amyloidosis

Wilkinson, I., Raine, T., Wiles, K., Goodhart, A., Hall, C., & O'Neill, H. (2017). *Oxford handbook of clinical medicine* (10th ed.). Oxford University Press.

BMJ Best Practice. (2020). *Amyloidosis*. https://bestpractice.bmj.com/topics/en-gb/444 [Accessed April 2021].

Monoclonal Gammopathy Of Renal Significance (MGRS)

Leung, N., Bridoux, F., Batuman, V., et al. (2019). The evaluation of monoclonal gammopathy of renal significance: A consensus report of the International Kidney and Monoclonal Gammopathy Research Group. *Nature Reviews*, *15*, 45–59. https://www.nature.com/articles/s41581-018-0077-4. Accessed April 2021.

RENAL TUBULAR DISORDERS
Renal Tubular Acidosis (RTA)

BMJ Best Practice. (2020). *Renal tubular acidosis*. https://bestpractice.bmj.com/topics/en-gb/239. Accessed April 2021.

Patient Info. (2016). *Renal tubular disease*. https://patient.info/doctor/renal-tubular-disease. Accessed April 2021.

Interstitial Nephritis

BMJ Best Practice. (2020). *Acute interstitial nephritis*. https://bestpractice.bmj.com/topics/en-gb/938. Accessed April 2021.

Patient info. (2015). *Interstitial nephritides and nephrotoxins*. https://patient.info/doctor/interstitial-nephritides-and-nephrotoxins. Accessed April 2021.

Wilkinson, I., Raine, T., Wiles, K., Goodhart, A., Hall, C., & O'Neill, H. (2017). *Oxford handbook of clinical medicine* (10th ed.). Oxford University Press.

Renal Artery Stenosis

BMJ Best Practice. (2020). *Renal artery stenosis*. https://bestpractice.bmj.com/topics/en-gb/435. Accessed April 2021.

Patient info. (2016). *Renovascular disease*. https://patient.info/doctor/renovascular-disease. Accessed April 2021.

Badila, E., & Tintea, E. (2014). How to manage renovascular hypertension. *E-Journal of Cardiology Practice*, *13*. https://www.escardio.org/Journals/E-Journal-of-Cardiology-Practice/Volume-13/How-to-manage-renovascular-hypertension. Accessed April 2021.

Rhabdomyolysis

BMJ Best Practice. (2020). *Rhabdomyolysis*. https://bestpractice.bmj.com/topics/en-gb/167. Accessed April 2021.

Patient Info. (2015). *Rhabdomyolysis*. https://patient.info/doctor/rhabdomyolysis-and-other-causes-of-myoglobinuria. Accessed April 2021.

Williams, J., & Thorpe, C. (2013). Rhabdomyolysis. *Continuing Education in Anaesthesia Critical Care & Pain*, *14*, 163–166. https://academic.oup.com/bjaed/article/14/4/163/293634. Accessed April 2021.

Polycystic Kidney Disease (PKD)

BMJ Best Practice. (2020). *Polycystic kidney disease*. https://bestpractice.bmj.com/topics/en-gb/481.

Patient info. (2015). *Autosomal recessive polycystic kidney disease*. https://patient.info/doctor/autosomal-recessive-polycystic-kidney-disease. Accessed April 2021.

Wilkinson, I., Raine, T., Wiles, K., Goodhart, A., Hall, C., & O'Neill, H. (2017). *Oxford handbook of clinical medicine* (10th ed.). Oxford University Press.

Gimpel, C., Bergmann, C., Bockenhauer, D., et al. (2019). International consensus statement on the diagnosis and management of autosomal dominant polycystic kidney disease in children and young people. *Nature Reviews Nephrology*, *15*, 713–726. https://www.nature.com/articles/s41581-019-0155-2. Accessed April 2021.

READING LIST: CHEMICAL PATHOLOGY IN AN HOUR
Basic Principles

Lab Tests Online. (2019). *Blood Gases*. http://www.labtestsonline.org.uk. Accessed Feb 2021.

Blood Gas Analysis

Resuscitation Council. (2018). *Advanced Life Support Guidelines*. http://www.resus.org.uk. Accessed June 2020.

Medscape. (2015). *Anion gap*. https://emedicine.medscape.com/article/2087291-overview Accessed July 2020.

MDCALC. https://www.mdcalc.com/anion-gap#evidence. Accessed July 2020.

Lab Tests Online. (2019). *Blood gases*. http://www.labtestsonline.org.uk. Accessed Feb 2021.

Hypernatraemia

Patient info. (2016). *Hypernatremia*. https://patient.info/doctor/hypernatraemia Accessed June 2020

BMJ Best Practice. (2019). *Hypernatraemia*. https://bestpractice.bmj.com/topics/en-gb/1215 Accessed Feb 2021

Hyponatraemia

NICE. (2015). *CKS: Hyponatremia*. https://cks.nice.org.uk/topics/hyponatraemia/ Accessed June 2020.

Patient info. (2016). *Hyponatremia*. https://patient.info/doctor/hyponatraemia-pro Accessed June 2020.

Hyperkalaemia

Resuscitation Council. (2018). *Advanced Life Support Guidelines*. http://www.resus.org.uk. Accessed June 2020.

Hypokalaemia

Resuscitation Council. (2018). *Advanced Life Support Guidelines*. http://www.resus.org.uk. Accessed June 2020.

Patient info. (2017). *Hypokalaemia*. https://patient.info/doctor/hypokalaemia. Accessed June 2020.

Parathyroid Hormone (PTH) and Calcium Homeostasis

Patient info. (2017). *Hyperparathyroidism*. https://patient.info/doctor/hypoparathyroidism-pro. Accessed June 2020.

Calcitonin And Calcium Homeostasis

Patient info. (2017). *Hyperparathyroidism*. https://patient.info/doctor/hyperparathyroidism-pro Accessed June 2020.

Hypercalcaemia

NICE. (2019). *CKS: Hypercalcemia*. https://cks.nice.org.uk/topics/hypercalcaemia/ Accessed June 2020.

Resuscitation Council. (2018). *Advanced Life Support Guidelines*. http://www.resus.org.uk. Accessed June 2020.

Hypocalcaemia

Patient info. (2015). *Hypocalcaemia*. https://patient.info/doctor/hypocalcaemia. Accessed June 2020.

Resuscitation Council. (2018). *Advanced Life Support Guidelines*. http://www.resus.org.uk. Accessed June 2020.

Patient info. (2014). *Hypoparathyroidism*. https://patient.info/doctor/hypoparathyroidism-pro. Accessed June 2020.

Medscape. (2018). *Hypoparathyroidism*. https://emedicine.medscape.com/article/122207-overview. Accessed June 2020.

Hypermagnesaemia/Hypomagnesaemia

Resuscitation Council. (2018). *Advanced Life Support Guidelines*. http://www.resus.org.uk. Accessed June 2020.

Patient info. (2014). *Magnesium disorders*. https://patient.info/doctor/magnesium-disorders. Accessed June 2020.

NICE. (2013). *Evidence summary [ESUOM4]: Preventing recurrent hypomagnesaemia: oral magnesium glycerophosphate*. https://www.nice.org.uk/advice/esuom4/chapter/Key-points-from-the-evidence Accessed June 2020.

Medscape. (2018). *How is FE of magnesium used in the diagnosis of hypomagnesemia?*. https://www.medscape.com/answers/2038394-36012/how-is-fe-of-magnesium-used-in-the-diagnosis-of-hypomagnesemia Accessed June 2020.

21

Respiratory Medicine in an Hour

Gregory Oxenham, Phil Wild, Berenice Aguirrezabala Armbruster and Peter Goodrem

OUTLINE

EMERGENCIES

The following emergencies are covered in Emergency Medicine in an Hour:

- Anaphylaxis
- Pneumothorax
- Pulmonary embolism

PHYSIOLOGY

Key Concepts and Equations

- **VENTILATION (V):** the movement of air into and out of the lungs during a single breathing cycle
- **MINUTE VENTILATION (MV):** the total volume of air exhaled from the lungs in 1 min
  - *MV = respiratory rate (RR) × tidal volume (Vt)*
- **ALVEOLAR VENTILATION:** the total volume of air that reaches the alveoli and contributes to gas exchange
  - *Alveolar ventilation (Va) = RR × [Vt – Dead Space Volume (Vd)]*
  - *Va = RR × (Vt – Vd)*
- **ANATOMICAL DEAD SPACE:** the volume of the airways not contributing to gas exchange (i.e., the bronchi/trachea). With a tidal volume of 500 mL, the anatomical dead space is ~150 mL.
- **PHYSIOLOGICAL DEAD SPACE:** in healthy individuals, this is almost identical to the anatomical

dead space. The *physiological* dead space represents the volume of lung that does not eliminate CO_2. The size of the physiological dead space is important because, if the physiological dead space increases (for instance, with pneumonia in which gas exchange is impaired), the patient must increase their MV to maintain adequate gas exchange.

- **PERFUSION (Q):** the volume of blood (in litres) flowing through the pulmonary circulation each minute. The pulmonary circulation is at a lower pressure than the systemic circulation because the pressure required to move blood to and away from the alveoli is less than what is required to pump blood to the whole body. Perfusion within the lungs is mostly gravity dependent, so blood flow to the apices is low when compared to the bases whilst in an upright position. This difference is reduced in the supine position.
- **HYPOXIC PULMONARY VASOCONTRICTION:** a physiological response to alveolar hypoxia. When the PAO_2 decreases, the pulmonary arterioles supplying that area of the lungs *vasoconstrict* and limit blood flow to hypoxic alveoli. In adults, this is important because hypoxic pulmonary vasoconstriction *limits blood flow to poorly ventilated areas of the lung* (see Fig 21.1). In the foetus, the hypoxic alveolar environment leads to a high pulmonary

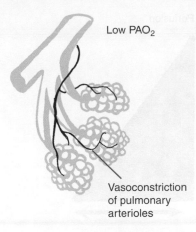

Low PAO₂

Vasoconstriction
of pulmonary
arterioles

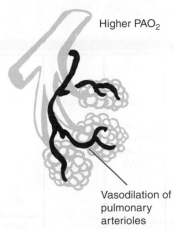

Higher PAO₂

Vasodilation of
pulmonary
arterioles

Fig 21.1 Hypoxic Pulmonary Vasoconstriction. (Illustrated by Hollie Blaber.)

vascular resistance, and most of the cardiac output is diverted from the lungs (see Paediatrics in an Hour).

V/Q Ratio

Ventilation and perfusion are separate dynamic *processes* that must be balanced to achieve adequate gas exchange. A normal value is approximately 1.

- **Example:** if ventilation through part of the lung is 4 L/min and the perfusion is 5 L/min, the V/Q ratio is 4/5 or 0.8. By decreasing ventilation, the V/Q ratio will decrease. By decreasing perfusion, the V/Q ratio will increase.

Extreme V/Q ratios:

- An area with ventilation but no perfusion (V/Q ratio of infinity) is *dead space. An example of this is a pulmonary embolism.*
- An area with perfusion but no ventilation (V/Q ratio of 0) is described as a *shunt. An example of this is a pneumonia.*

The distribution of inhaled gases and pulmonary blood flow is not uniform throughout the lungs. *Both ventilation and perfusion are greater at the lung bases than the apices.* The drop in perfusion from the base to the apex is *far greater* than the drop in ventilation when comparing the base and apex. Accordingly, the V/Q ratio is different between the base and the apex of normal lungs (see Fig 21.2).

V/Q Mismatch

V/Q mismatches are the most common explanation for hypoxaemia. Other causes are diffusion limitations, hypoventilation and low inspiratory oxygen pressure. These causes must also be considered in all cases, as they may coexist.

- An abnormal V/Q ratio can be either above or below the normal range (0.8–1.0)
- A V/Q mismatch reduces both the uptake of O_2 and the output of CO_2
- Hypoxaemia is seen more commonly than hypercapnia. An increase in ventilation will clear CO_2 quicker than it will increase the PaO_2
- The blood from areas of V/Q mismatch will have a reduced PaO_2, resulting in hypoxaemia when mixed with blood from areas with a normal V/Q ratio
- The degree of V/Q mismatch can be measured using the *alveolar-arterial PO_2 difference.* A good rule of thumb is that if the PaO_2 is $<(FiO_2 - 10)$, there is V/Q mismatch
- A-a gradient = $PAO_2 - PaO_2$ (this means (Alveolar – arterial))

RESPIRATORY INVESTIGATIONS

Lung Volumes and Spirometry

Definitions: (see Figs 21.3 and 21.4 and Table 21.1)

- **Tidal volume (Vt):** the volume of air in one normal breath
- **Forced vital capacity (FVC):** the volume of air measured after one maximal inspiration followed by one maximal expiration

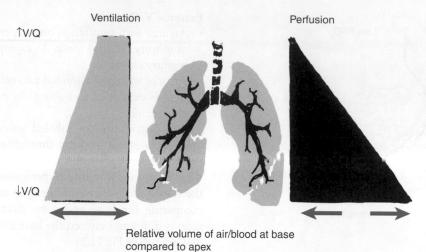

Ventilation

↑V/Q

↓V/Q

Perfusion

Relative volume of air/blood at base
compared to apex

Fig 21.2 V/Q Variation in a Normal Lung. (Illustrated by Hollie Blaber.)

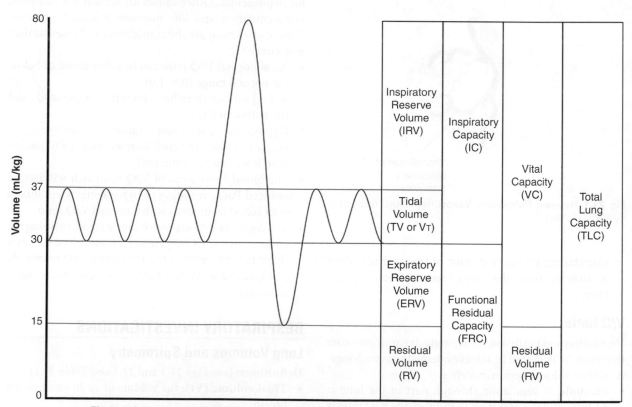

Fig 21.3 Lung Volumes. (With permission from *Kapwatt at English Wikipedia, CC BY-SA 3.0.*)

TABLE 21.1   Spirometry Patterns

Spirometry pattern	FEV1	FVC	FEV1:FVC	Causes
Obstructive	Reduced	Normal or reduced	<70%	Asthma, chronic obstructive pulmonary disease, bronchiectasis, alpha-1 antitrypsin deficiency, cystic fibrosis
Restrictive	Normal or reduced	Reduced	Normal or increased	Fibrosis, neuromuscular conditions, obesity

FEV1, Forced expiratory volume in 1 sec; FVC, forced vital capacity.

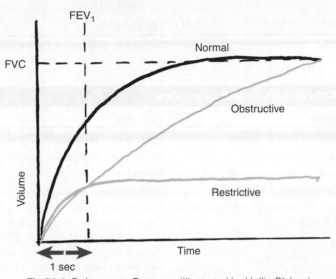

Fig 21.4 Spirometry Patterns. (Illustrated by Hollie Blaber.)

- **Forced expiratory volume in 1 sec (FEV1):** the volume of air measured after 1 sec of forced expiration from a maximal inspiration
- **Residual volume (RV):** the volume remaining in the lungs after a maximal expiration
- **Functional residual capacity (FRC):** the volume remaining in the lungs after a normal expiration

Peak Expiratory Flow Rate (PEFR)

- Measures the peak rate of airflow as the patient blows into the tube
- Best predicted values are derived from the age, height and sex
- Helps assess the severity of any airflow limitations
- Peak flow diaries are recommended for patients and are more useful than a single measurement

OBSTRUCTIVE DISORDERS

Asthma

Definition: a chronic inflammatory condition of the airways, which are hyperresponsive and easily constrict in response to a wide range of stimuli/triggers. Characterised by a reversible airway obstruction

Buzzwords:
- **Risk factors:** atopy (or family history of atopy)
- **Common triggers:** animals, mould, cold weather, respiratory tract infections, occupational allergens (classically bakers), drugs (e.g., nonsteroidal antiinflammatory drugs (NSAIDs), beta blockers), stress and emotions
- **Presentation:** shortness of breath (SOB), wheezing, cough (commonly at night), diurnal variation/PEFR variation

TABLE 21.2 Asthma Guidelines for Adults >17 years of Age

	Indication	As required:	Regular: NICE Guidelines for Adults >17 years of age	Regular: BTS Guidelines for Adults >17 years of age
STEP 1	Symptoms 3 times per week Night-time symptoms Severe asthma attack in last 2 years	SABA	Low dose ICS	Low dose ICS
STEP 2	Uncontrolled asthma with step 1	SABA	Low dose ICS + LTRA	Low dose ICS + LABA
STEP 3	Uncontrolled asthma with step 2	SABA	Low dose ICS + LABA +/- LTRA	Medium dose ICS + LABA or LTRA
STEP 4	Uncontrolled asthma with step 3	SPECIALIST REFERRAL		

ICS, Inhaled corticosteroid; LABA, long-acting beta 2 agonist; LTRA, leukotriene-receptor antagonist; SABA, short-acting beta 2 agonist.

TABLE 21.3 Drug Abbreviations and Examples

Abbreviation	Definition	Example
SABA	Short-acting beta 2 agonist	Salbutamol, Terbutaline
ICS	Inhaled corticosteroid	Beclomethasone, Budesonide, Fluticasone
LTRA	Leukotriene-receptor antagonist	Montelukast
LABA	Long-acting beta 2 agonist	Salmeterol, Formoterol
ICS + LABA	Inhaled corticosteroid and long-acting beta 2 agonist	May be prescribed as separate inhalers or as a MART meter (a single inhaler device combining both drugs). There are a number of MART meters that you should be aware of (all contain formoterol): **Symbicort and DuoResp** = Formoterol (LABA) + Budesonide (ICS) **Fostair** = Formoterol (LABA) + Beclomethasone (ICS)

Investigations:
- **Symptom diary:** to identify triggers
- **PEFR:** diurnal variation, reduced values with increasing symptoms
- **Spirometry with bronchodilator reversibility:** obstructive picture with resolution after bronchodilator administration
- **Fractional exhaled nitric oxide (FeNO):** FeNO >40 parts per billion
- **Challenge testing:** induction of bronchospasm with subsequent reversibility

Differentials: COPD, allergic bronchopulmonary aspergillosis (ABPA), heart failure, cystic fibrosis (CF), foreign body aspiration

Management:
1. If occupational asthma (symptoms commonly worse at work), patient should be referred to a specialist

2. Symptoms should guide management as per guidelines (see Tables 21.2 & 21.3)

Two guidelines are available: NICE and BTS.

Acute Asthma

Definition: an acute worsening of usual asthma symptoms, specifically SOB and wheezing.

Buzzwords:
- **Risk factors (for severity of the attack):** previous ITU admission, previous intubation, history of brittle asthma/poor treatment response, escalating short-acting beta 2 agonist (SABA) use, respiratory infection
- **Presentation:** see Table 21.4

Investigations: clinical assessment is most important
- **PEFR:** see Table 21.4
- **Arterial blood gas (ABG):** see Table 21.4

TABLE 21.4 Asthma Severity Indicators

NB: if the patient possesses any life-threatening features, they should be treated as such

	Moderate	Severe	Life-threatening	Near-fatal
Peak expiratory flow rate	50%–75% of best or predicted	33%–50% of best or predicted	<33% of best or predicted	
Respiratory rate (breaths/min)	<25	>25		
Heart rate (beats/min)	<110	>110		
Blood gas			Normal $PaCO_2$ PaO_2 <8 kPa SaO_2 <92%	High $PaCO_2$
Other	Normal speech	Can't complete sentences	**C**yanosis **H**ypotension **E**xhaustion **S**ilent chest **T**achycardia Reduced Glasgow Coma Scale score	Requiring mechanical ventilation with raised inflation pressures

- **Chest x-ray (CXR):** often normal but may show consolidation if concurrent infection. Important to rule out a pneumothorax (PTX).
- **Bloods:** normal or ↑ WCC, ↑ CRP, ↑ neutrophils if bacterial infection

Differentials: COPD exacerbation, pneumonia, foreign body aspiration, congestive heart failure, anaphylaxis, PTX

Management:

Acute management

1. Oxygen: 15 L/min via non-rebreather (for all patients including those with COPD. Once stable, must titrate in COPD patients)
2. Salbutamol 5mg nebuliser (driven with oxygen), can be continuous ('back-to-back')
3. Prednisolone 40 mg PO (IV hydrocortisone if the PO route is not appropriate)
4. Ipratropium bromide 500micrograms nebuliser (driven with oxygen), 4–6 hourly
5. IV magnesium sulphate
6. Escalate: ITU referral if evidence of impending respiratory failure/respiratory or cardiac arrest (see Anaesthetics and Critical Care in an Hour)

Post-acute management:

1. Once stable, wean nebuliser use and aim to switch to inhalers

2. Serial PEFR monitoring. Readings should be moving toward baselines before discharging (at least 75% of predicted or previous best)
3. Assess for triggers (e.g., lower respiratory tract infection (LRTI), antigens)
4. Inhaler review to check inhaler technique and optimize management
5. Monitor for hypokalaemia if large amounts of salbutamol have been given

Discharge plan:

1. Asthma action plan in place (for all patients!)
2. Continue prednisolone for a minimum of 5 days (up to 14 days maximum)
3. Review with a general practitioner at 2 days post-discharge is recommended

Bronchiectasis

Definition: a chronic inflammatory lung disease characterised by dilated and thick-walled bronchi

Buzzwords:

- **Risk factors:** previous severe or recurrent infections (e.g., tuberculosis (TB) or childhood pneumonia), impaired mucous clearance (e.g., primary ciliary dyskinesia, CF, obstruction (e.g., distal to an obstructing mass))
- **Presentation:** a productive cough classically with large sputum volumes, SOB, coarse crackles (incl.

squawks, pops), recurrent infective episodes with a tendency towards chronic colonising bacteria (*Pseudomonas, Haemophilus*), clubbing

Investigations:

- **Sputum sample:** if there is purulent sputum/recurrent infections, to guide antibiotic choices
- **High-resolution CT:** tram-track sign, signet-ring sign, dilated peripheral bronchi
- **CFTR/chloride sweat test:** >30 mmol/L in CF (consider in patients without an obvious aetiology)
- **QuantiFERON:** positive if the patient has latent TB

Differentials: pneumonia, chronic bronchitis, TB, CF

Management:

1. Conservative: smoking cessation, flu vaccine, airway clearance via pulmonary physiotherapy
2. Mucolytics can help with expectoration (especially for thick and sticky sputum)
3. Sputum MC&S (yearly and during exacerbations) are essential for targeting antibiotic therapy
4. Consider prophylactic antibiotics
5. Lung transplantation

Chronic Obstructive Pulmonary Disease

Definition: airway inflammation related to smoking and smoke exposure (90% cases), harmful substances (e.g., fumes) or an alpha-1 antitrypsin deficiency. Persistent respiratory symptoms and airflow obstruction that is usually progressive and not reversible. A combination of two pathologies: chronic bronchitis and emphysema.

Buzzwords:

- **Risk factors:** cigarette smoke exposure (primary or secondary), occupational exposure to hazardous aerosols, family history of COPD in those under 40 years of age (alpha-1 antitrypsin)
- **Presentation:** chronic productive cough, wheezing, SOB (rest or exertional), hyperinflation, cyanosis, features of right heart failure (*cor pulmonale*)

Investigations:

- **Spirometry+bronchodilator test:** post-bronchodilator FEV1/FVC of <0.7 confirms a persistent airflow obstruction. Low FEV1 correlates with the severity
- **CXR:** coarse bronchovascular markings, hyperinflation with flattened hemidiaphragms, may see cardiomegaly/bullae. Important to screen for lung cancer
- **Alpha-antitrypsin levels:** if family history or early onset, the ZZ genotype associated with the most severe phenotype

Differentials: asthma, congestive cardiac failure (CCF), bronchiectasis

Management:

Long-term management: see Fig 21.5

Long-term oxygen therapy (LTOT) for COPD:

- Indications:
  - Persistent hypoxia of <7.3 kPA when breathing room air
  - *Or* a resting PaO_2 of <8.0 kPA *if* signs of peripheral oedema, evidence of polycythaemia or pulmonary hypertension
- An ABG must be taken on air and on the proposed oxygen prescription to ensure the patient does not retain CO_2
- Patient must not smoke due to fire hazard

Osteoporosis prophylaxis and capillary blood glucose (CBG) monitoring: for those who require repeated courses of steroids

Acute Exacerbation of COPD (Infective vs Non-infective)

Definition: a sustained deterioration of an individual's baseline symptoms, acute in onset and beyond day-to-day variation. Viral triggers are far more common than bacterial ones. Other triggers include smoking/allergens. **Common infective organisms** include *H. influenza, Rhinovirus, Streptococcus pneumoniae*.

Buzzwords:

- **Risk factors:** as for COPD *PLUS* the winter months, continued smoking, more severe COPD, on LTOT, previous intubation/ventilation or non-invasive ventilation (NIV)
- **Presentation:** SOB, wheezing, productive cough with increased sputum production or a change in colour, fever (if an infective origin), drowsy (if type 2 respiratory failure (T2RF))

Investigations:

- **ABG:** type 1 respiratory failure (T1RF) ($\downarrow pO_2$) or T2RF ($\downarrow pO_2$, $\uparrow pCO_2$, $\downarrow pH$)
- **Bloods:** $\uparrow$ WCC, $\uparrow$ CRP, $\uparrow$ neutrophils
- **CXR:** hyperinflation +/- consolidation
- **Sputum sample** (if purulent sputum): specific organism identified
- **Blood cultures** (if pyrexia): specific organism identified
- **Theophylline levels** (if the patient is on theophylline): 10–20 mg/L at 4–6 h post-dose

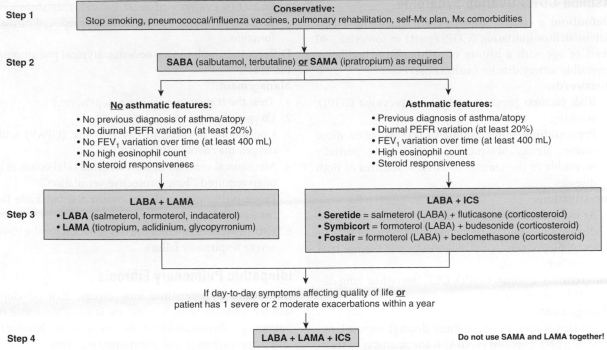

Fig 21.5 Long-term Management of Chronic Obstructive Pulmonary Disease Adapted from the 2019 NICE Guidelines. (Illustrated by Berenice Aguirrezabala Armbruster.) *FEV1*, Forced expiratory volume in 1 sec; *ICS*, inhaled corticosteroid; *LABA*, long-acting beta 2 agonist; *LAMA*, long-acting muscarinic antagonists; *PEFR*, peak expiratory flow rate; *SABA*, short-acting beta 2 agonist, *SAMA*, short-acting muscarinic antagonists.

Differentials: CCF, acute coronary syndrome (ACS), pneumonia, pulmonary embolism (PE), PTX

Management:

Hospital management:

1. Nebulised bronchodilator therapy
   a. Salbutamol 5 mg
   b. Ipratropium 500 micrograms
2. Oxygen therapy
   a. Target an SpO_2 of 88%–92% via Venturi mask (controlled flow) due to the risk of T2RF and perform an urgent ABG
   b. If the pCO_2 is >6, continue to target 88%–92%. If the pCO_2 is <6, target >94% unless the patient has previously had episodes of T2RF requiring NIV/invasive ventilation
   c. Once oxygen therapy has been established, perform another ABG after 2 hours, paying particular attention to any rises in the pCO_2
3. Oral steroids
   a. Prednisolone 30 mg OD for 5 days
4. Antibiotic therapy: consider if there is purulent sputum, consolidation on CXR or elevations in inflammatory markers (follow local guidelines)
   a. Oral first line: amoxicillin 500 mg TDS for 5 days or doxycycline or clarithromycin
   b. Oral second line (if no improvement in 2–3 days): co-amoxiclav, levofloxacin, co-trimoxazole
   c. IV first line: follow local guidelines
   d. IV second line: check with microbiology
5. IV aminophylline
   a. If poor response to bronchodilators
   b. Monitor levels and perform an electrocardiogram (ECG) at 24 h after administration
6. NIV if persistent hypercapnia despite optimal medical treatment
7. Consider intubation and mechanical ventilation if there is a poor response or the patient is not able to tolerate NIV (and patient is deemed eligible by an intensivist)

Asthma-COPD Overlap Syndrome

Definition: a clinical syndrome encompassing a persistent airflow limitation (COPD part) in someone >40 years of age with a history of asthma/bronchodilator-reversible airway disease (asthma part)

Buzzwords:

- **Risk factors:** previous asthma or previous COPD, smoking
- **Presentation:** as for asthma/COPD but often more severe, airway obstruction that is only partially reversible in the context of asthma, features of both diseases

Investigations:

- **As for asthma/COPD:** results show elements of both disease (e.g., partial bronchodilator reversibility) or inconclusive results for diagnosing one disease over the other

Differentials: asthma, COPD, CCF, interstitial lung disease (ILD), bronchiectasis

Management:

- Inhaled steroid (using asthma dosing) with a long-acting beta 2 agonist (LABA) is the mainstay of treatment

Prognosis: more frequent exacerbations, worse quality of life, higher mortality and more rapid decline in lung function than either asthma/COPD alone

RESTRICTIVE DISORDERS

Acute Respiratory Distress Syndrome

Definition: an acute inflammatory lung disease caused by a trigger and characterised by:

- Onset within 7 days of the triggering event
- Bilateral opacities in the lungs on CXR/CT
- Respiratory failure with an associated decrease in the PaO_2/FiO_2 ratio (used in grading acute respiratory distress syndrome (ARDS))

Buzzwords:

- **Risk factors:** trauma, sepsis, pancreatitis, aspiration, influenza, chemotherapy, coronavirus disease 2019 (COVID-19) – many potential causes
- **Presentation:** severe hypoxia, decreased lung compliance, recent significant physical insult

Investigations:

- **ABG:** decreased PaO_2/FiO_2 ratio, usually T1RF
- **CXR:** bilateral opacities
- **CT chest:** diffuse coalescent opacities, gravity dependent, quickly evolving

- **ECHO** (if evidence of heart failure): may show evidence of pulmonary hypertension or reduced cardiac function

Differentials: pulmonary oedema, atypical pneumonia, PE, ILD

Management:

1. Treat the trigger (e.g., trauma, sepsis, etc.)
2. Oxygen therapy
3. Continuous positive airway pressure (CPAP) with oxygen may avoid intubation
4. Mechanical ventilation with targeted tidal volumes is often required ('lung-protective ventilation')
5. Prone positioning and neuromuscular blockade for the first 48 h
6. Extra-corporeal membrane oxygenation for the most severe respiratory failure

Idiopathic Pulmonary Fibrosis

Definition: an interstitial lung disease that develops without known cause. It is the most common cause of pulmonary fibrosis and leads to a progressive deterioration in gas exchange and pulmonary function.

Buzzwords:

- **Risk factors:** idiopathic
- **Presentation:** chronic cough, SOB, clubbing, fine end-inspiratory crepitations, cyanosis, right heart failure

Investigations:

- **Spirometry:** restrictive pattern, reduced lung volumes
- **High-resolution CT:** honeycombing, minimal ground glass, septal thickening, traction bronchiectasis

Differentials: secondary ILD from toxins (e.g., asbestos), drugs (e.g., nitrofurantoin, amiodarone) and connective tissue diseases (e.g., sarcoidosis, rheumatoid arthritis), CCF, COPD, lung cancer

Management:

- **Supportive:** home oxygen therapy, pulmonary rehabilitation, smoking cessation
- **Antifibrotics:** pirfenidone or nintedinib if the FVC is 50%–80% of predicted without deterioration by >10% in 12 months
- **Lung transplantation** (single or double lung)

Pulmonary Sarcoidosis

Definition: a multisystem granulomatous disorder of unknown aetiology that typically presents in younger adults. The majority of patients have lung involvement, although other organs (e.g., heart, liver, skin, kidneys, central nervous system) may also be involved.

Buzzwords:

- **Risk factors:** younger age, black heritage
- **Presentation:**
  - Acute presentation: cough, dyspnoea, fatigue, fever, arthralgia, weight loss, erythema nodosum (EN)
  - Löfgren syndrome consists of EN, bilateral hilar adenopathy, arthralgia and fevers
  - Chronic presentation: insidious onset usually presenting with features of pulmonary fibrosis
  - Other extrapulmonary features: ocular (e.g., uveitis), rash, palpitations, confusion

Investigations:

- **CXR:** bilateral hilar adenopathy (acute presentation), reticular opacities (upper zones > lower zones) and fibrosis (chronic presentation). CXR is also requested to exclude TB.
- **Bloods:** angiotensin-converting enzyme (ACE) is elevated in 75% (though not sensitive nor specific), hypercalcaemia, raised ESR
- **High-resolution CT:** hilar and mediastinal lymphadenopathy, ground glass, irregular thickening of the broncho-vascular bundles, mid/upper lobe predominance
- **Biopsy:** evidence of a non-caseating granuloma is usually required for diagnosis (unless Löfgren's)
- **Spirometry:** required to stage lung involvement. Spirometry is commonly normal, although patients can have mild obstructive or restrictive patterns). A significant restrictive defect is in keeping with pulmonary fibrosis

Differentials: TB, lung cancer, ILD

Management:

1. Observation and regular follow-ups: mild acute presentations usually remit spontaneously
2. Glucocorticoids if the symptoms are intolerable, hypercalcaemia, progressive lung disease or extrapulmonary involvement
3. Immunosuppression (steroid sparing) if there is deteriorating lung function, worsening radiographic changes or resistance to steroid treatment

OCCUPATIONAL LUNG DISEASE

Asbestos-related Pleuropulmonary Disease

Definition: an inflammatory lung disease caused by asbestos inhalation. This includes:

- **Asbestosis:** progressive, diffuse pulmonary fibrosis caused by asbestos inhalation
- **Pleural disease:** plaques and benign asbestos effusion
- **Malignancies:** non-small cell/small cell lung cancers (NSCLC/SCLC) and malignant pleural mesothelioma – *see end of chapter*

Buzzwords:

- **Risk factors:** occupational exposure (e.g., shipbuilding, mining, insulation fitting), living with an exposed person (e.g., washing their clothes)
- **Presentation:**
  - **Asbestosis:** progressive dyspnoea, chronic cough, fine end-inspiratory crepitations, clubbing
  - **Pleural disease:** pleural plaques are usually asymptomatic, possibly signs of a unilateral effusion
  - **Malignancy:** weight loss, haemoptysis, chest pain, back pain, effusion

Investigations:

- **Spirometry:** restrictive – reduced lung volumes, normal FEV1:FVC
- **CXR:** pleural plaques (classic), effusion. If a bulky ipsilateral hilum, round lung lesions and a unilateral effusion, consider malignancy
- **High-resolution CT:** pleural plaques, effusion, fibrosis and honeycombing
- **Pleural aspirate** (if effusion): exudative, typically blood-stained – only ~25% have a malignant cytology

Differentials: ILD, lung cancer, COPD, acute interstitial pneumonia, silicosis

Management:

Asbestosis:

- Smoking cessation and pneumococcal/flu vaccination
- Monitor for progressive respiratory failure
- LTOT for those with resting hypoxaemia

Pleural plaques:

- As for asbestosis
- Plaques have no malignant potential and should be considered benign. However, all effusions should be investigated for malignancy. If proven to be benign, no treatment +/- effusion drainage for symptomatic relief

Malignancy: see end of chapter

Hypersensitivity Pneumonitis (Extrinsic Allergic Alveolitis)

Definition: an immune-related lung disease triggered by allergens and resulting in inflammatory and fibrotic lung changes. Bird-fancier's lung and farmer's lung are both types of hypersensitivity pneumonitis (HP)

- **Acute**: within 4–6 hours, inflammatory, often reversible
- **Sub-acute**: onset of days to short weeks, often reversible
- **Chronic**: >6 weeks and usually months/years of insidious symptoms, fibrotic phenotype, less reversible

Buzzwords:

- **Risk factors**: birdkeepers, farmers, exposure to bioaerosols
- **Presentation:**
  - **Acute**: cough, fever, dyspnoea, tightness, fine crackles, gets better when the allergen is avoided
  - **Chronic**: insidious cough, progressive dyspnoea, fatigue, weight loss, clubbing, diffuse crackles

Investigations: a detailed exposure history is important!

- **CXR**: normal during the acute phase, fibrosis during chronic phase
- **High-resolution CT**: normal in the acute phase; honeycombing, ground glass, septal thickening, nodules in the chronic phase
- **Spirometry**: restrictive
- **Bronchoscopy and bronchoalveolar lavage (BAL)**: lymphocytes in hypersensitivity pneumonitis

Differentials: other ILDs, asthma, pneumonia, asbestosis, silicosis

Management:

1. Avoid trigger
2. Glucocorticoids if acute/sub-acute
3. Trial glucocorticoids +/- immunosuppression if chronic (limited efficacy)

INFECTION

Acute Bronchitis

Definition: a self-limiting LRTI that involves inflammation of the bronchi

Buzzwords:

- **Risk factors**: viral (90%) or atypical bacterial exposure, smoking, exposure to pollution
- **Presentation**: cough (usually worse at night or with exercise, may be productive), mild constitutional symptoms (e.g., sore throat, headache, mild fever, mild shortness of breath)
  - **Compared to pneumonia**: less systemically unwell, no focal signs of pneumonia on a chest exam, no new hypoxia

Investigations: typically a clinical diagnosis

- **CXR**: if performed, does not show a pneumonia

Differentials: asthma, pneumonia, postnasal drip, COVID-19, pulmonary oedema, reflux oesophagitis, lung cancer

Management:

1. Smoking cessation advice
2. Simple analgesia
3. Antibiotics if systemically unwell or at a higher risk of complications (e.g., >80 years of age, CCF, immunosuppression) – consider investigating with blood tests/CXR, blood cultures
4. Consider antibiotics if the patient is at higher risk of complications:
   - First line: 5-day course of oral doxycycline
   - First line in pregnancy: 5-day course of oral amoxicillin

Community-acquired Pneumonia

Definition: a community-acquired infection in which the alveoli become filled with microorganisms, fluid and inflammatory cells. Most common pathogens include *S. pneumonia*, *H. influenzae* and respiratory viruses (which account for one third of cases). '**Atypical**' pneumonia encompasses pneumonias that do not respond to first-line treatment and commonly present with a dry cough, flu-like symptoms, deranged LFT/U&Es and bilateral pneumonia. Typical examples are respiratory viruses, *Legionella* and *Mycoplasma*. **Severity** of a community-acquired pneumonia (CAP) is determined by calculating the CURB-65 (or the CRB-65 in the community, since there is often limited access to blood tests for urea) (see Table 21.5):

- 0–1: low risk (<3% risk of death)
- 2: moderate risk (3%–15%)
- 3–5: high risk (>15%)

Buzzwords:

- **Risk factors**: increasing age, COPD, smoking, immunosuppression, CF, bronchiectasis, diabetes, winter months
- **Presentation**: productive cough, dyspnoea, pleuritic pain, fever, reduced breath sounds, crepitations, bronchial breath sounds
  - *Legionella*: hyponatraemia, air-conditioning exposure
  - *Mycoplasma*: erythema multiforme, encephalitis, uveitis, haemolytic anaemia

Investigations: if diagnosed clinically and managed in community, no tests are indicated

TABLE 21.5	**CURB65 Score**	
C	Confusion	1 point
U	Urea >7 mmol/L	1 point
R	Respiratory rate ≥ 30 breaths/min	1 point
B	Blood pressure ≤60 mmHg dia-stolic or <90 mmHg systolic	1 point
65	Age ≥ 65 years	1 point

- **Bloods:** ↑ WCC/CRP, +/- ↑ lactate
- **CXR:** consolidation. **Repeat in 6/52** to look for an underlying pathology that may have triggered the pneumonia (especially in those >50 years of age or a smoker)
- **Blood cultures:** +/- organism
- **COVID-19/flu swab:** if clinical concern (although routine at time of writing)
- *Legionella*/**pneumococcal urinary antigens/respiratory virus screen**

Differentials: acute bronchitis, COVID-19, PE, lung cancer, collapse

Management: many cases of acute cough resolve spontaneously and do not require antibiotics

CURB-65 (or CRB-65) of 0–1 point: treat in the **community**
- PO first line: Amoxicillin
- Alternatively, Doxycycline, clarithromycin or erythromycin (in pregnancy) if penicillin allergic

CURB-65 (or CRB-65) of 2 points: treat as an **inpatient**
- PO first line: Amoxicillin (if atypical then amoxicillin AND clarithromycin or erythromycin)
- Alternatively, Clarithromycin or doxycycline if penicillin allergic

CURB-65 (or CRB-65) of 3 or more points: treat as an inpatient and consider **escalation to ITU** if appropriate
- PO first line: Co-amoxiclav AND clarithromycin or erythromycin
- Consult local guidelines if penicillin allergic

Consider hospital referral if:
- Symptoms not improving on oral antibiotics or unable to take oral antibiotics
- Previous antibiotic resistance
- Young adults/children
- Older, frailer or significant comorbidities

Hospital-acquired Pneumonia

Definition: as for CAP, but evidence that the infection began at least 48 h after being in the hospital or following a recent discharge from the hospital

Buzzwords:
- **Risk factors:** hospital stay, immunosuppressed, previous recurrent infections, critical care and invasively ventilated
- **Presentation:** as for CAP, escalating hospital 'early warning score'

Investigations:
- As for CAP
- Consider a high-resolution CT in the critically unwell: may show acute interstitial pneumonia, organising pneumonia, aspiration, lung abscess, empyema – these are more common following a hospital stay with a respiratory infection

Differentials: as for CAP, but with different causative pathogens, including *Staphylococcus aureus* and methicillin-resistant *Staphylococcus aureus* (MRSA)

Management: follow local guidance on antibiotics, usually broad spectrum

Common regimens:
- Non-severe symptoms/signs
  - Co-amoxiclav PO
  - *Penicillin allergy:* doxycycline PO *or* co-trimoxazole PO *or* cefalexin PO
- Severe symptoms/signs or sepsis
  - Tazocin IV (tazobactam and piperacillin)
  - Ceftazidime IV
- If MRSA likely:
  - Vancomycin IV *or* teicoplanin IV – in addition to primary IV antibiotics

Empyema

Definition: a collection of pus in the pleural space, most commonly developing after an episode of pneumonia.

Buzzwords:
- **Risk factors:** recent pneumonia, diabetes, immunosuppression, bronchiectasis, chest surgery, TB
- **Presentation:** recurrent 'swinging' fevers in someone treated for pneumonia, night sweats, cough, dyspnoea, weight loss, pleuritic pain, reduced expansion/breath sounds

Investigations:
- **Bloods:** ↑ WCC/CRP +/- lactate
- **CXR:** complex effusion +/- pleural thickening
- **Thoracic ultrasound and pleural fluid aspirate:** a multi-loculated effusion requires aspiration as a minimum to send a MC&S for isolation of an organism. Fluid is exudative/turbid. If the fluid pH is <7.2, then a full drainage with a chest drain is indicated.

Differentials: parapneumonic effusion, sepsis, PE, lung abscess

Management:

1. Prolonged course of antibiotics (minimum 2 weeks and up to 6 weeks)
2. Chest drain insertion
3. Referral to thoracic surgery for consideration of video-assisted thoracic surgery if no improvement or ongoing clinical decline

Lung Abscess

Definition: a cavitating area of suppurative lung infection with the localised formation of a fibrous wall. Most commonly caused by anaerobes, *S. aureus* and Gram-negative rods (*Klebsiella*).

Buzzwords:

- **Risk factors:** necrotising pneumonia (e.g., *S. aureus*), septic emboli (e.g., tricuspid endocarditis, intravenous drug use), necrotising tumours, aspiration, vasculitis
- **Presentation:** swinging fever, foul-tasting purulent sputum, cough, pleuritic pain, haemoptysis, tachypnoea, clubbing, may develop empyema

Investigations:

- **Bloods:** ↑ WCC/CRP
- **CXR:** walled cavity +/- fluid level, may show consolidation/empyema. Multiple foci in cases of septic emboli
- **Chest CT:** may show a microemboli or an obstructing bronchial mass as the cause. Can guide aspiration.
- **Bronchoscopy:** may show an obstruction, can collect pus sample for antibiotic guidance

Differentials: empyema, pneumonia, lung cancer, TB

Management:

1. Most cases (80%–90%) are managed with IV antibiotics for 2–3 weeks followed by PO for 4–8 weeks
2. Pulmonary physiotherapy
3. If this approach fails to work, may require bronchoscopic/CT-guided drainage or a surgical excision. Surgical excisions are associated with high morbidity (e.g., provoking empyema, pneumatocele)

COVID-19

Given the rapidly changing nature of the pandemic, information within this section may soon be out of date.

Definition: a disease caused by severe acute respiratory syndrome coronavirus 2 (SARS-CoV-2) that primarily spread by respiratory droplets. Symptom onset is 5–6 days after exposure on average but can take up to 14 days.

Buzzwords:

- **Risk factors:** contact with confirmed cases
- **Severity factors:** male, increasing age, obesity (BMI >30 kg/m²), type 2 diabetes mellitus, hypertension, ethnic origin (Bangladeshi, Chinese, Indian, Pakistani, Other Asian, Caribbean, Other Black ethnicity)
- **Presentation:** variable, from asymptomatic to multiorgan failure with severe pneumonia and ARDS-like features
  - Any or all of the following **symptoms**: fever, dry cough, dyspnoea, malaise, headache, muscle aches, diarrhoea, vomiting, loss of smell/taste and rashes (especially in younger people)
  - Hypercoagulable state

Investigations:

- **Bloods:** ↓ lymphocytes, raised acute-phase reactants (e.g., CRP, ferritin), **typically a normal** WCC unless a superimposed bacterial infection
- **ABG:** T1RF (or normal in mild cases)
- **CXR:** bilateral diffuse infiltrates (hazy opacifications). Often normal in early /asymptomatic cases
- **SARS CoV-2 PCR:** naso/pharyngeal swab
- **CTPA:** to investigate for a PE, a crucial differential – shows features in keeping with CXR. The D-dimer is *not* a reliable marker because it is usually elevated in unwell COVID-19 patients. Consider in a patient with acute deterioration and a rising RR or FiO₂

Differentials: influenza, upper respiratory tract infection (URTI), CAP, PE

Management:

Mild illness: stay at home and isolate, fluids, antipyretics (e.g., paracetamol)

Requiring hospital admission:

1. Oxygen if hypoxaemia
2. CPAP if persistent hypoxaemia despite escalating oxygen delivery
3. NIV in T2RF
4. Dexamethasone 6 mg PO OD 10/7 if hypoxic/in respiratory distress/ARDS/septic. Monitor CBG
5. Remdesivir in hospitalised patients with comorbidities for 5/7
6. Tocilizumab for ventilated patients without a superimposed bacterial infection
7. Antibacterials as per CURB-65 if concerns of a superimposed bacterial pneumonia

8. Critical care management if requiring organ support (respiratory, renal or cardiovascular)

MALIGNANCY

Malignant Pleural Mesothelioma

Definition: a rare malignancy of mesothelial cells, most commonly found in the pleura. Gradual onset and poor prognosis, with most presenting at an advanced stage.

Buzzwords:
- **Risk factors:** asbestos exposure
- **Presentation:** 25–40-year latency period post-exposure, chest pain, dyspnoea, weight loss, fatigue, unilateral pleural effusion

Investigations:
- **CXR:** plaques, volume loss, unilateral effusion
- **Pleural aspirate:** exudate, may be bloody. Send cytology (only 25% have positive cytology)
- **High-resolution CT:** pleural thickening, extension of the tumour, reduced volume hemithorax
- **Pleural biopsy (if the cytology is negative and diagnosis remains uncertain):** histological confirmation
- **MRI:** assess for soft-tissue spread
- **PET-CT:** search for distant metastases (although unlikely to change management)

Differentials: lung cancer, benign pleuropulmonary disease

Management:
- First line is usually chemotherapy (adjuvant or neo-adjuvant)
- Surgery has limited benefits in treatment. Partial pleurectomy for debulking/palliation
- Pleurodesis (surgical or medical) is as effective as a pleurectomy for managing effusions but should strongly consider indwelling pleural catheter (permanent chest drain)
- Palliative radiotherapy to reduce pain
- Advise about compensation schemes if related to an occupational exposure

Prognosis:
- Stage and grade have the greatest influence
- Poor prognostic features: poor performance status, age >75 years of age, elevated lactate dehydrogenase (LDH) and haematologic abnormalities

Lung Cancer

Definition: second most common type of cancer in the United Kingdom. The most important distinction histologically is between SCLC and NSCLC, which are staged using the TNM system (8th edition). Metastases are common at presentation, with common sites including the liver, bone, adrenals and brain.

- **SCLC** (15%–20%): arise from endocrine cells, are responsible for most paraneoplastic syndromes. More likely to be extensive at presentation
- **NSCLC** (75%–80%): includes squamous, adenocarcinoma and large cell lung cancer

Buzzwords:
- **Risk factors:** cigarette smoke exposure (implicated in 90% of lung cancer), asbestos exposure, some occupational exposures (e.g., coal dust and diesel fumes)
- **Presentation:** cough, dyspnoea, haemoptysis, weight loss, pain, effusion, clubbing
- **Complications:** metastases, lung collapse distal to the obstructing tumour, superior vena cava obstruction (SVCO), hoarseness (if recurrent laryngeal compression), Horner's syndrome, phrenic nerve palsy, effusion

Investigations:
- **Bloods:** ↑ platelets, anaemia, ↑ calcium with metastasis/paraneoplastic effects
- **CXR:** peripheral nodule (spiculation more indicative of cancer), hilar enlargement, consolidation (non-resolving), collapse, effusion, bony metastasis
- **Pleural aspirate (if effusion):** exudate, may be bloody. Send for microbiology and cytology.
- **CT TAP (thorax, abdomen, pelvis):** if suspicious of cancer or for staging in established cancer
- ***CT-guided/bronchoscopic biopsy*:** confirms the diagnosis/guides treatment based on histology
  - **Biopsy*:** breast, colon, prostate and renal cancer commonly spread to the lung, **assess if these are the primary**
- **Bronchoscopy + endobronchial USS:** to assess spread, can guide surgical appropriateness
- **PET-CT/radionucleotide bone scan:** to identify metastasis

> **URGENT CHEST X-RAY (WITHIN 2/52) INDICATIONS**
>
> - *Age >40 years and two of the following* (or just one with a history of smoking): cough, fatigue, shortness of breath, chest pain, weight loss, appetite loss
> - Or any of the following: persistent or recurrent chest infection, clubbing, supraventricular lymphadenopathy or persistent cervical lymphadenopathy, chest signs consistent with lung cancer, thrombocytosis

Differentials: CAP, TB, metastasis from other primary malignancy

Management:

1. **2-week-wait (2WW) referral for:** CXR that suggests lung cancer *or* age >40 years with unexplained haemoptysis
2. Smoking cessation advice
3. Multidisciplinary team (MDT) consensus on management and treatment
4. Chemotherapy – different regimens for NSCLC and SCLC. First line for SCLC
5. Monoclonal antibodies and tyrosine kinase inhibitors – depending on tumour genetics
6. Lobectomy/pneumonectomy/radical radiotherapy may be curative – perform spirometry prior to this.
   a. Surgery is more likely to be successful for NSCLC in early-stage disease

Palliative treatment:

- SVCO – see Palliative Care and Oncology in an Hour
- Endobronchial obstruction: surgical debulking/laser, radiotherapy, stenting
- Brain metastases: dexamethasone +/- radiotherapy
- Bone metastases: radiotherapy for pain
- Pleural effusion: drainage of a symptomatic effusion +/- pleurodesis

Prognosis: 5-year survival is less than 10%. Much improved rates of survival seen in those with localised cancer that is surgically resected.

Pulmonary Vascular Disease and Pulmonary Hypertension

Definition: a disease of the pulmonary circulation that affects the pressure within the pulmonary artery. A mean pulmonary artery pressure (PAP) of ≥25 mmHg at rest is considered pulmonary hypertension. Most symptoms of pulmonary hypertension are caused by right heart failure (*cor pulmonale*). There are **five types (simplified):**

1. **Pulmonary arterial hypertension:** idiopathic or associated with connective tissue disease
2. **Pulmonary hypertension due to left heart disease:** left ventricular systolic/diastolic dysfunction, mitral stenosis
3. **Pulmonary hypertension due to lung disease:** COPD, ILD, sleep apnoea
4. **Pulmonary hypertension due to a chronic arterial obstruction:** chronic PE, congenital pulmonary artery stenosis

5. **Multifactorial pulmonary hypertension:** haemolytic anaemia, sarcoidosis, chronic kidney disease

Buzzwords:

- **Risk factors:** idiopathic pulmonary arterial hypertension is more common in young women
- **Presentation:** SOB, syncope, ascites, peripheral oedema, raised JVP, clubbing, loud P2 and splitting of S2

Investigations:

- **CXR:** enlarged pulmonary arteries/right atrium – may show underlying ILD/sarcoid
- **ECG:** right ventricular hypertrophy – right axis deviation, right ventricular strain pattern (ST depression and T-wave inversion in V1-3 and inferior leads), P pulmonale
- **ECHO:** large right chambers, distended septum, elevated PA pressure and assess for tricuspid regurgitation
- **Cardiac catheterisation (right heart catheter with pulmonary capillary wedge pressures):** essential for a definite diagnosis – mean PAP of ≥25 mmHg at rest. Patient inhales nitric oxide while the heart is catheterised to determine if the vasculature is reactive (i.e., the pulmonary vessels relax and the PAP falls) or if the obstruction is fixed – guides treatment
- **CT (PA):** if concerned that PE/ILD is the underlying cause

Differentials: CCF, aortic stenosis, liver/renal failure

Management:

1. Treat underlying cause
2. Strongly advise patients to avoid pregnancy (12%–17% maternal death rate)
3. For those with *reactive* pulmonary vasculature following cardiac catheterisation (see earlier): high-dose calcium-channel blockers (e.g., diltiazem)
4. For those without *reactive* pulmonary vasculature following cardiac catheterisation (see above):
   - Phosphodiesterase inhibitors (e.g., sildenafil)
   - Endothelin-receptor antagonists (e.g., bosentan)
   - Prostanoids (continuous IV infusion)
   - Diuretics if oedema/RHF
5. LTOT if hypoxic
6. Consider for transplant referral (lung or heart/lung)

THE ONE-LINE ROUND-UP!

Here are some key words to help you remember each condition/concept.

Condition/Concept	One-line Description
Asthma	Wheeze, diurnal variation and night-time cough
Acute asthma	Severity assessment
Bronchiectasis	Large volume of sputum in someone with previous or recurrent infections
COPD	Breathless smoker with recurring wheeze/chest infections
Acute exacerbation of COPD	Worsening SOB above natural variation
Asthma-COPD overlap syndrome	Features of both asthma and COPD
ARDS	Hypoxia with bilateral infiltrates following a major injury/illness
Idiopathic pulmonary fibrosis	Fine inspiratory crackles and clubbing
Pulmonary sarcoidosis	Bilateral hilar lymphadenopathy
Asbestosis	Progressive fibrosis

Condition/Concept	One-line Description
Asbestos pleural disease	Benign effusions, plaques and reduced lung volumes
Hypersensitivity pneumonitis	Farmers and bird-fanciers!
Acute bronchitis	Mildly ill with a cough
CAP	Chest signs, CURB-65 and consolidation on CXR
Hospital-acquired pneumonia	Pneumonia >48 h after admission
Empyema	Swinging fevers after pneumonia treatment
Lung abscess	Septic emboli, needs drainage
COVID-19	Bilateral hazy opacification
Malignant pleural mesothelioma	Asbestos, bloody unilateral effusion, weight loss
Lung cancer	Smoker with cough, haemoptysis and weight loss
Pulmonary hypertension	Young woman with right heart failure

READING LIST: RESPIRATORY MEDICINE IN AN HOUR

PHYSIOLOGY

West, J., & Luks, A. (2016). *West's respiratory physiology: The essentials* (10th ed.). Wolters Kluwer.

OBSTRUCTIVE DISORDERS
Asthma (Including Acute Asthma)

NICE. (2020). *CKS: Asthma.* [https://cks.nice.org.uk/topics/asthma/- Accessed March 2022].

British Thoracic Society. (2019). *BTS/SIGN guideline for the management of asthma 2019.* [https://www.brit-thoracic.org.uk/quality-improvement/guidelines/asthma/- Accessed March 2022].

BNF. (2022). *Treatment summary: Acute asthma.* [https://bnf.nice.org.uk/treatment-summary/asthma-acute.html- Accessed March 2022].

Bronchiectasis

NICE. (2021). *CKS: Bronchiectasis.* [https://cks.nice.org.uk/topics/bronchiectasis/- Accessed March 2022].

COPD (Including COPD Exacerbations)

NICE. (2018). *NG114: Chronic obstructive pulmonary disease (acute exacerbation): Antimicrobial prescribing.* [https://www.nice.org.uk/guidance/ng114 Accessed March 2022].

NICE. (2019). *NG115: Chronic obstructive pulmonary disease in over 16s: Diagnosis and management.* [https://www.nice.org.uk/guidance/ng115-Accessed March 2022].

Patient Info. (2019). *Acute exacerbations of COPD.* [https://patient.info/doctor/acute-exacerbations-of-copd#:~:text=An%20exacerbation%20of%20COPD%20causes,Increased%20dyspnoea. -Accessed March 2022].

NICE. (2019). *CKS: Chronic obstructive pulmonary disease.* [https://cks.nice.org.uk/topics/chronic-obstructive-pulmonary-disease/- Accessed March 2022].

Asthma-COPD Overlap Syndrome

BMJ. (2017). Clinical Review: Asthma-COPD overlap syndrome: Pathogenesis, clinical features, and therapeutic targets. *British Medical Journal*, 358, j3772.

Halpin, D. (2016). *Clinical features should be used to assess asthma–COPD overlap.* Guidelines in Practice. https://www.guidelinesinpractice.co.uk/respiratory/clinical-features-should-be-used-to-assess-asthma-copd-overlap/352787.article.

RESTRICTIVE DISORDERS
ARDS

Faculty of Intensive Care Medicine. (2018). *Guidelines on the management of acute respiratory distress syndrome.* [https://www.ficm.ac.uk/sites/ficm/files/documents/2021-10/Guidelines_on_the_Management_of_Acute_Respiratory_Distress_Syndrome.pdf- Accessed March 2022].

Pulmonary Fibrosis

NICE guidelines. (2017). *CG163: Idiopathic pulmonary fibrosis in adults: Diagnosis and management.* [https://www.nice.org.uk/guidance/cg163- Accessed March 2022].

NICE. TA504: Pirfenidone for treating idiopathic pulmonary fibrosis. [https://www.nice.org.uk/guidance/ta504 Accessed March 2022].

Pulmonary Sarcoidosis

King, T. (2020). *Treatment of pulmonary sarcoidosis. Initial therapy with glucocorticoids.* UpToDate. https://www.uptodate.com. [Accessed 8 August 2020].

King, T. (2019). *Clinical manifestations and diagnosis of pulmonary sarcoidosis.* UpToDate. http://www.uptodate.com. [Accessed 9 August 2020].

OCCUPATIONAL LUNG DISEASE
Asbestos Related Pleuropulmonary Disease

King, T. (2020). *Asbestos related pleuropulmonary disease.* UpToDate. http://www.uptodate.com. Accessed 9 August 2020.

Hypersensitivity Pneumonitis (a.k.a. Extrinsic Allergic Alveolitis)

King, T. (2019). *Hypersensitivity pneumonitis (extrinsic allergic alveolitis): Clinical manifestations and diagnosis.* UpToDate. http://www.uptodate.com. [Accessed 11 August 2020].

King, T. (2019). *Hypersensitivity pneumonitis (extrinsic allergic alveolitis): Treatment, prognosis, and prevention.* UpToDate. http://www.uptodate.com. [Accessed 11 August 2020].

INFECTION
Acute Bronchitis

NICE. (2020). *CKS: Chest infections – adult.* [https://cks.nice.org.uk/topics/chest-infections-adult/- Accessed March 2022].

NHS. (2020). *Bronchitis.* http://nhs.uk/conditions/bronchitis. [Accessed 29 November 2020].

Community-acquired Pneumonia

NICE. (2020). *CKS: Chest infections – adult.* [https://cks.nice.org.uk/topics/chest-infections-adult/- Accessed March 2022].

NICE. (2019). *CKS: Pneumonia (community-acquired): Antimicrobial prescribing.* [https://www.nice.org.uk/guidance/ng138- Accessed March 2022].

BNF. Respiratory system infections, antibacterial therapy. [https://bnf.nice.org.uk/treatment-summary/respiratory-system-infections-antibacterial-therapy.html- Accessed March 2022].

Hospital-acquired Pneumonia

NICE. (2019). *NG139: Pneumonia (hospital-acquired): Antimicrobial prescribing.* [https://www.nice.org.uk/guidance/ng139- Accessed March 2022].

NICE. (2020). *NG173: COVID-19 rapid guideline: Antibiotics for pneumonia in adults in hospital.* [https://www.nice.org.uk/guidance/ng173- Accessed March 2022].

Empyema

NHS. (2018). *Conditions: Empyema.* http://www.nhs.uk/conditions/empyema. [Accessed 13 August 2020].

Wilkinson, I. (2017). Complications of pneumonia. In *Oxford handbook of clinical medicine* (10th ed.) (p. 170). Oxford University Press.

Lung Abscess

Knott, L. (2019). *Lung abscess. Patient info.* http://www.patient.info [Accessed 14 August 2020].

Wilkinson, I. (2017). Complications of pneumonia. In *Oxford handbook of clinical medicine* (10th ed.) (p. 170). Oxford University Press.

COVID-19

NICE. (2020). *CKS: Coronavirus (COVID-19).* [https://cks.nice.org.uk/topics/coronavirus-covid-19/management/- Accessed March 2022].

NICE. (2020). *NG173: COVID-19 rapid guideline: Antibiotics for pneumonia in adults in hospital.* [https://www.nice.org.uk/guidance/ng173- Accessed March 2022].

Bell, D., & Knipe, H. (2020). *COVID-19: Summary. Radiopaedia.* https://radiopaedia.org/. [Accessed 17 August 2020].

WHO. Coronavirus disease (COVID-19). [https://www.who.int/emergencies/diseases/novel-coronavirus-2019. Accessed March 2022].

MALIGNANCY
Malignant Pleural Mesothelioma

Woolhouse, I., Bishop, L., Darlison, L., et al. (2018). British Thoracic Society Guideline for the investigation and management of malignant pleural mesothelioma. *Thorax, 73,* i1–i30.

Pass, H., et al. (2020). *Initial management of pleural mesothelioma.* UpToDate. http://www.uptodate.com. [Accessed 8 August 2020].

Lung Cancer

Wilkinson, I. (2017). Lung tumours. In *Oxford handbook of clinical medicine* (10th ed.) (pp. 175–176). Oxford University Press.

NICE. (2021). *CKS: Lung and pleural cancers: Recognition and referral.* [https://cks.nice.org.uk/topics/lung-pleural-cancers-recognition-referral/- Accessed March 2022].

NICE. (2019). *NG122: Lung cancer: Diagnosis and management.* [https://www.nice.org.uk/guidance/ng122- Accessed March 2022].

Pulmonary Vascular Disease

NICE. (2019). *NG115: Managing pulmonary hypertension and cor pulmonale.* [https://www.nice.org.uk/guidance/ng115/evidence/a-managing-pulmonary-hypertension-and-cor-pulmonale-pdf-6602768750- Accessed March 2022].

European Society of Cardiology. (2015). Guidelines for the diagnosis and treatment of pulmonary hypertension. *European Heart Journal, 37,* 67–119.

22

Rheumatology in an Hour

Dolcie Paxton, Berenice Aguirrezabala Armbruster and Emma Clark

INFLAMMATORY ARTHRITIS WITH PREDOMINANTLY PERIPHERAL JOINT INVOLVEMENT

Rheumatoid Arthritis

Definition: a chronic autoimmune disease characterised by inflammation of the synovial joints leading to chronic erosive arthritis and other extra-articular features. Rheumatoid arthritis (RA) increases cardiovascular risk (uncontrolled RA accelerates atherosclerosis), fracture risk (uncontrolled RA promotes bone resorption) and depression (impact of the long-term condition and change in life roles). It is the most common inflammatory arthritis.

Buzzwords:
- **Risk factors:** 30–50 years of age, female, family history, smoking
- **Presentation:**
  - **Articular:** symmetrical polyarthritis, small joints, distal interphalangeal joints (DIPs) spared, stiffness >1 h
  - **Features of long-standing uncontrolled disease (Articular):** Boutonnière deformity, Swann neck, Z-thumb, ulnar deviation, subluxation (see Figs 22.1 and 22.2)

- **Features of long-standing uncontrolled disease (Extra-articular):** Mnemonic **CRAPP-E-SOFAS** – **C**arpel tunnel, **R**aynaud's, **A**naemia, **P**ulmonary fibrosis, **P**ericarditis, **E**ye (scleritis or episcleritis), **S**jögren's syndrome, **O**steoporosis, **F**elty's syndrome (RA, splenomegaly, neutropenia), **A**tlantoaxial subluxation, **S**kin vasculitis (Fig 22.3)

Investigations:
- **Blood:** ↑ C-reactive protein (CRP)/erythrocyte sedimentation rate (ESR), ↓ haemoglobin (Hb), ↑/↔ platelets
- **Antibody testing:** anti-cyclic citrullinated peptide (anti-CCP) present in 80% and highly specific, rheumatoid factor (RhF) present in 60%, antinuclear antibody (ANA) present in 30%
- **X-ray: SPEL** – **S**oft tissue swelling, **P**eri-articular osteoporosis, **E**rosions, **L**oss of joint space (symmetrical)
- **Ultrasound:** synovitis, effusion, hypervascularity, early erosions
- **Monitoring:** Disease Activity Score (DAS)-28. High is >5.1, moderate is 3.2–5.1, low is <3.2, remission is <2.6
- **Screening before disease-modifying antirheumatic drug (DMARD) use:** the following tests should be negative to proceed with DMARD use:

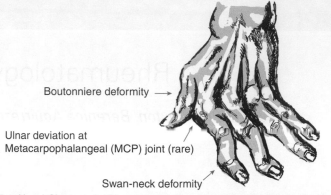

Boutonniere deformity →

Ulnar deviation at
Metacarpophalangeal (MCP) joint (rare)

Swan-neck deformity

Fig 22.1 Hand Changes in Rheumatoid Arthritis. (Illustrated by Hollie Blaber.)

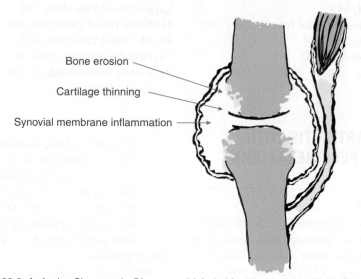

Bone erosion

Cartilage thinning

Synovial membrane inflammation

Fig 22.2 Articular Changes in Rheumatoid Arthritis. (Illustrated by Hollie Blaber.)

- **Infectious diseases:** hepatitis B and human immunodeficiency virus (HIV) serology, varicella-zoster antibody
- **Tuberculosis (TB) testing:** QuantiFERON, T-spot, Mantoux test
- **Chest X-ray (CXR):** TB, malignancy, pulmonary fibrosis
- **Blood:** full blood count (FBC), urea and electrolytes (U&Es), liver function tests (LFTs)

Differentials: psoriatic arthritis, systemic lupus erythematosus (SLE), polyarticular gout, osteoarthritis (OA). A similar presentation in a child <16 years may be suggestive of juvenile idiopathic arthritis.

Management:
1. Analgesia: nonsteroidal anti-inflammatory drugs (NSAIDs) are common first-line agents
2. Steroids (e.g., prednisolone) for acute flares
3. Conventional DMARDs to maintain remission (monotherapy first, can add additional DMARDs if unresponsive):
    - Methotrexate (+ folic acid)
    - Sulfasalazine (safe in pregnancy)
    - Hydroxychloroquine (safe in pregnancy)
    - Leflunomide
4. Biologic DMARDs if unresponsive to two trials of conventional DMARDs. Some examples:

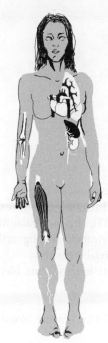

Eyes: Episcleritis, Scleritis, Keratoconjunctivitis sicca

Respiratory: Rheumatoid nodules, Interstitial Fibrosis, Pleuritis, Caplan syndrome

Cardiovascular:
- **Heart:** Valvular lesions, Pericarditis, Myocarditis
- **Peripheral:** Oedema, Vasculitis, Raynaud's phenomenon

Musculoskeletal: Tenosynovitis, Myositis, Carpal Tunnel Syndrome, Rheumatoid nodules

Neurology: Peripheral neuropathy

Other: Amyloidosis, Felty syndrome, Siögren syndrome, Lymphadenopathy

Fig 22.3 Extraarticular Changes in Rheumatoid Arthritis. (Illustrated by Hollie Blaber.)

- Anti-tumour necrosis factor (anti-TNF) agents: etanercept, infliximab, adalimumab
- Anti-CD20: rituximab
- Anti-interleukin (IL)-6: tocilizumab
5. Management of cardiovascular risk, fracture risk and depression
6. Physiotherapy and occupational therapy to aid self-management

Psoriatic Arthritis

Definition: a progressive inflammatory arthritis involving the joints and connective tissue that affects about 5%–25% of patients with psoriasis. The most common form of psoriatic arthritis (PsA) mimics rheumatoid arthritis, with symmetrical small joint involvement and without axial involvement. For this reason, it is presented here despite its common classification within the *seronegative spondyloarthropathies*.

Buzzwords:
- **Risk factors:** psoriasis, HLA-B27
- **Patterns of presentation:** DR SAM
  - **D**istal arthritis of DIP joints
  - **R**heumatoid-like symmetrical polyarthritis (**most common**)
  - **S**pondylitic pattern with sacroiliitis

  - **A**symmetrical oligoarthritis (often affects the knee)
  - **M**utilans (arthritis mutilans): not a presentation pattern but can be the result of longstanding rheumatoid-like psoriatic arthritis
- **Other musculoskeletal (MSK) features:** dactylitis (swelling of an entire digit due to inflammation of the flexor tendon sheaths)
- **Non-MSK features:** psoriatic plaques, nail changes (e.g., pitting, subungual hyperkeratosis, onycholysis)

Investigations:
- **Blood:** ↑ CRP/ESR
- **X-ray:** DIP erosion, 'pencil-in-cup' deformity in late stages (Fig 22.4)
- **Antibody testing:** normal as 'seronegative'
- **To monitor:** FBC, U&E, LFTs may be deranged as a treatment complication

Differentials: RA, gout, erosive OA, reactive arthritis

Management:
1. Analgesia: NSAIDs are common first-line agents.
2. Steroids (e.g., prednisolone) for acute flares
3. Conventional DMARDs to maintain remission:
   a. Methotrexate (+ folic acid)
   b. Sulfasalazine (safe in pregnancy)
   c. Leflunomide

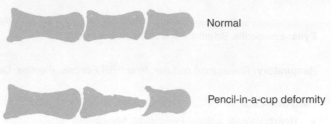

Fig 22.4 Pencil-in-cup Deformity. (Illustrated by Hollie Blaber.)

3. Biologic DMARDs if unresponsive to two conventional DMARDs or there is axial disease alone: anti-TNF agents (e.g., etanercept, infliximab, adalimumab), ustekinumab (cytokine modulator)
4. Management of cardiovascular risk, fracture risk and depression
5. Physiotherapy and occupational therapy to aid self-management

INFLAMMATORY ARTHRITIS WITH AXIAL INVOLVEMENT

The following three conditions (as well as psoriatic arthritis) are part of a family of **seronegative spondyloarthropathies.** They are all associated with **HLA-B27** and share similar clinical, radiographical and laboratory features, including:
- Axial arthritis and sacroiliitis
- Asymmetrical large-joint oligoarthritis or monoarthritis
- Enthesitis (inflammation at the sites where tendons/ligaments attach to bone)
- Dactylitis (inflammation of an entire digit)
- Extra-articular: uveitis, psoriaform rashes, oral ulcers, aortic regurgitation, inflammatory bowel disease (IBD)

HLA-B27 is rarely tested for in clinical practice.

Reactive Arthritis

Definition: an inflammatory arthritis that manifests several days to weeks after exposure to certain bacterial infections

Buzzwords:
- **Causes:** 1–4 weeks after an enteric infection (e.g., *Campylobacter*, *Salmonella*, *Shigella*, *Yersinia*), a venereal infection (e.g., *Chlamydia*) or a streptococcal sore throat

- **Presentation:**
  - **Can't see:** iritis, uveitis, conjunctivitis
  - **Can't pee:** urinary tract infection (UTI), sexually transmitted infection (STI), circinate balanitis
  - **Can't bend my knee:** asymmetrical oligoarthritis (particularly the knee), axial arthritis
  - **Can't stand on my feet:** keratoderma blennorrhagica

Investigations:
- **Blood:** ↑ CRP/ESR, FBC (↓ Hb, ↑ white blood cells (WBC) and ↑ platelets)
- **Antibody testing:** normal as 'seronegative'
- **Joint aspiration:** negative for crystals and bacteria
- **Serology for possible infectious causes:** *Campylobacter*, *Streptococcus*, *Salmonella*, *Shigella*, *Yersinia* or *Chlamydia*, but often unhelpful as the *infection has usually cleared by the time the arthritis presents.*
- **Slit-lamp examination if evidence of uveitis:** presence of white cells in the anterior chamber, hazy aqueous humour with flare, hypopyon may be present
- **Monitoring:** FBC, U&E, LFTs may be deranged as a treatment complication, x-ray may demonstrate sacroiliitis and enthesitis in the chronic phase

Differentials: other seronegative spondyloarthropathies, septic arthritis, RA, post-viral arthritis

Management:
1. Physiotherapy
2. NSAIDs, corticosteroids (intra-articular or systemic)
3. Treatment of the underlying infection *in the unlikely case that an infection is still present* (see note above) will clear the underlying cause but will not shorten the duration of joint disease
4. Relapse/chronic disease may require conventional DMARDs (e.g., methotrexate, sulfasalazine). Biological DMARDs can be helpful for axial disease

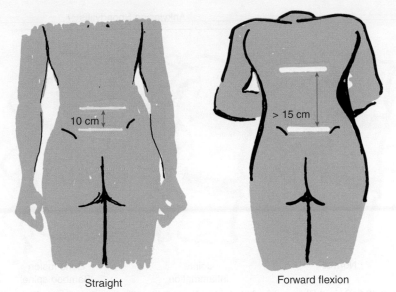

10 cm

> 15 cm

Straight

Forward flexion

Fig 22.5 Schober's Test. Normal if forward flexion is >15 cm. (Illustrated by Hollie Blaber.)

Enteropathic Arthritis

Definition: a spondylarthritis associated with a range of gastrointestinal pathologies, including IBD. Joint involvement may present before, simultaneously or after the diagnosis of IBD.

Buzzwords:
- **Risk factors:** IBD, Whipple's disease, coeliac disease, intestinal bypass surgery, HLA-B27
- **Presentation:** asymmetrical large joint oligoarthritis, sacroiliitis, abdominal pain, changes in bowel habits, gastrointestinal bleeding, erythema nodosum, pyoderma gangrenosum, uveitis

Investigations:
- **Blood:** ↑ CRP/ESR, FBC (↑ WBC, ↑ platelets, ↓ Hb)
- **Antibody testing:** normal as 'seronegative'
- **X-ray:** soft tissue swelling, peri-articular osteopenia, occasionally erosions
- **Sigmoidoscopy/colonoscopy:** to identify a gastrointestinal cause if indicated by the symptoms (see Gastroenterology in an Hour)
- **Monitoring:** FBC, U&E, LFTs may be deranged as a treatment complication

Differentials: RA, other seronegative spondyloarthropathies

Management:
1. Treat IBD (see Gastroenterology in an Hour): control of the underlying gastrointestinal disease may improve the arthritis
2. Steroids (prednisolone) for acute flares
3. Conventional DMARDs to maintain remission:
   a. Methotrexate (+ folic acid)
   b. Sulfasalazine (safe in pregnancy)
   c. Hydroxychloroquine (safe in pregnancy)
4. Biologic DMARDs if unresponsive to conventional DMARDs
5. Physiotherapy and occupational therapy to aid self-management

Ankylosing Spondylitis

Definition: a chronic progressive inflammatory arthropathy primarily involving the axial skeleton

Buzzwords:
- **Risk factors:** male, age 20–30 years, family history
- **Presentation:**
  - **Spinal:** morning back pain relieved by exercise, spinal stiffness, reduced Schober's test (Fig 22.5), alternating buttock pain, reduced chest expansion, increased thoracic kyphosis (question-mark posture), occasionally peripheral large-joint mono/oligoarthritis

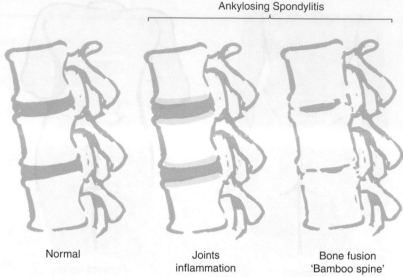

Ankylosing Spondylitis

| Normal | Joints inflammation | Bone fusion 'Bamboo spine' |

Fig 22.6 Spinal Changes in Ankylosing Spondylitis. (Illustrated by Hollie Blaber.)

- **Extraspinal:** **A**nterior uveitis, **A**utoimmune bowel disease, **A**pical lung fibrosis, **A**ortic regurgitation, **A**myloidosis, **A**chilles' tendonitis, **A**trioventricular node block (*Remember this as all A's!*)

Investigations:

- **Blood:** ↑ CRP/ESR
- **Spinal x-ray:** sacroiliitis, syndesmophytes, squaring of the vertebrae, bamboo spine in late disease (Fig 22.6)
- **Magnetic resonance imaging (MRI):** sacroiliac joint inflammation, enthesitis, inflammatory changes (e.g., bone marrow oedema)
- **Monitoring:** x-ray/MRI often used to check for radiographic disease progression, a Bath Ankylosing Spondylitis Disease Activity Index (BASDAI) score of >4 indicates active disease

Differentials: other seronegative spondyloarthropathies

Management:

1. Exercise and physiotherapy to maintain posture and mobility
2. NSAIDs
3. Steroid injections can provide short-term relief
4. Anti-TNF agents if NSAIDs fail to control disease
5. DMARDs may be considered for peripheral joint disease
6. Self-management (e.g., through the National Ankylosing Spondylitis Society (NASS) weekly community exercise classes)

CONNECTIVE TISSUE DISORDERS

Systemic Lupus Erythematous

Definition: a chronic multisystem autoimmune disease with a relapsing-remitting course. SLE is thought to be caused by inflammatory processes triggered by the formation of immune complexes involving autoantibodies and complement consumption.

Buzzwords:

- **Risk factors:** family history, ultraviolet (UV) light exposure, medications (e.g., isoniazid, hydralazine), female, child-bearing age, African Caribbean and South Asian descent
- **Presentation:** photosensitive (often malar) rash, malaise, alopecia, oral ulcers, new-onset Raynaud's, symmetrical polyarthritis, renal impairment, haemolytic anaemia, seizures, psychosis, serositis (e.g., pleuritis, pericarditis)

Investigations:

- **Blood:** FBC (↓ Hb, ↓ WBC, ↓ platelets), U&E (reduced renal function), coagulation screen (↑ activated partial thromboplastin time [APTT]), ↑ CRP/ESR
- **Urinalysis:** red cells, red blood cell casts, proteinuria in lupus nephritis
- **Immune markers:** anti-double-stranded DNA (anti-dsDNA) and anti-Smith are specific, ANA positive (95% sensitive, less specific), anti-histone antibody in drug-induced lupus, low C3 and C4 (complement)

- **Monitoring:** FBC, U&E, LFTs may be deranged as a treatment complication, low C3/C4 in active disease, raised anti-dsDNA in active disease

Differentials: variable and depending on the presentation

Management:
1. **Lifestyle:** avoid sun exposure, smoking cessation, manage cardiovascular risk factors
2. **Skin, musculoskeletal and systemic symptoms:** **hydroxychloroquine** is first line
3. **Maintenance** therapy with **azathioprine** or **methotrexate**
4. **Organ-threatening or resistant disease:** remission-induction therapy with **cyclophosphamide or mycophenolate mofetil (MMF)** and steroids. Further options include belimumab (a B-cell activating factor inhibitor) and rituximab.

Sjögren's Syndrome

Definition: a systemic autoimmune disease characterised by lymphocytic infiltration of the exocrine glands, especially the salivary and lacrimal glands. Sjögren's syndrome can occur alone (primary) or with another autoimmune disease (secondary).

Buzzwords:
- **Risk factors:** female, SLE, RA, systemic sclerosis
- **Presentation:** dry eyes, dry mouth (salivary stones, eating difficulties, candidiasis), parotid enlargement, cough, dyspareunia, arthralgia, fatigue, interstitial lung disease, polyneuropathy, renal tubular acidosis, Raynaud's, vasculitis, myositis

Investigations:
- **Blood:** FBC (↓ platelets, ↓ Hb), ↑ ESR, ↑ gamma globulins
- **Schirmer's test:** positive test. A filter paper is placed in the lower conjunctival sac. The test is positive if less than 5 mm of the paper is wetted after 5 min
- **Serology:** anti-Ro/anti-La positive, RhF positive, ANA positive
- **Biopsy of salivary gland:** mononuclear cell infiltrates (B cells, T cells and dendritic cells) in perivascular and periductal areas, focus score of >1

Differentials: SLE, RA, systemic sclerosis

Management:
1. Lifestyle: good oral hygiene, good fluid intake
2. Moisture replacement: artificial tears, saliva substitute mouth rinse
3. Muscarinic agonists: pilocarpine

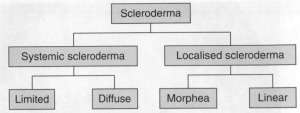

Fig 22.7 Scleroderma Classification. (With permission from © 2022 National Scleroderma Foundation.)

4. Hydroxychloroquine for arthralgia
5. Steroids and immunomodulators for resistant, systemic involvement

Scleroderma

Definition: a multisystem **autoimmune disease** affecting the skin and internal organs characterised by increased fibroblast activity, resulting in **vascular damage and fibrosis**. Fibrosis occurs in the skin, gastrointestinal tract, heart, lungs and other organs. Vascular manifestations include pulmonary arterial HTN, renal disease, Raynaud's and ischaemia of the extremities.

Classification of scleroderma (Fig 22. 7):
- **Systemic scleroderma:** can be further subdivided by the degree of skin involvement
  - **Limited systemic sclerosis** (a.k.a., CREST syndrome): skin fibrosis restricted to the extremities (i.e., the hands, distal arms, distal legs), face and neck.
    CREST features may be present (**C**alcinosis, **R**aynaud phenomenon, o**E**sophageal dysfunction, **S**clerodactyly, **T**elangiectasia)
  - **Diffuse systemic scleroderma:** Widespread skin fibrosis (including the chest, abdomen, upper arms and legs). Internal organ involvement is more common in this subtype
- **Localised scleroderma:** can be further subdivided according to skin involvement:
  - **Morphoea localised scleroderma:** the skin fibrosis is waxy and oval shaped
  - **Linear localised scleroderma:** the skin fibrosis is linear

Buzzwords:
- **Risk factors:** peak onset at 40 years of age, female, family history, radiation therapy, infectious agents (e.g., Cytomegalovirus, Parvovirus B19, Epstein-Barr virus, Hepatitis B virus), chemical exposure

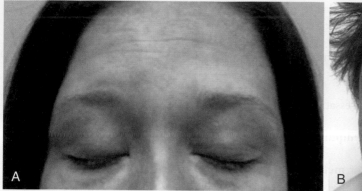 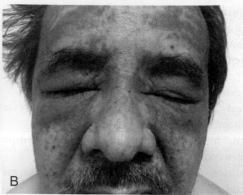

Fig 22.8 Heliotrope Rash in (A) Lighter Skin and (B) Darker Skin. Panel A: With permission from DeWane, M.E., Waldman, R., Lu, J. (2020). Dermatomyositis: Clinical features and pathogenesis. *Journal of the American Academy of Dermatology*; Panel B: With permission from Filho, F.B., Brito, D.P., Queiroz, R.M., Mello, D.F.R.E., Valentin, M.V.N. (2019). Man with erythematous rash and muscle weakness. *Annals of Emergency Medicine*. Elsevier.

- **Presentation:** depends on the subtype (see the classification above)

Investigations:
- **Blood:** FBC (↓ Hb, ↑ platelets), ↑ ESR, ↑ creatinine
- **Urinalysis:** proteinuria
- **Antibody testing:** anti-centromere (limited) positive, anti-Scl-70 (diffuse) positive, anti-RNA-III positive, ANA positive (in 30%)
- **Monitoring:** due to the multisystem nature of this disease and the severe complications that can develop, the monitoring protocol is extensive and based on the symptoms and autoantibodies present. Monitoring can include lung function tests, computed tomography (CT) imaging of the chest, electrocardiography (ECG), echocardiography, oesophageal manometry and endoscopy.

Differentials: SLE, polymyositis or dermatomyositis, mixed connective tissue disease

Management: difficult to treat, complications are managed individually
- **Skin thickening:** cyclophosphamide, methotrexate
- **Raynaud's:** nifedipine or losartan. Intravenous (IV) iloprost in severe cases
- **Calcinosis:** bisphosphonates, consider surgical removal
- **Gastrointestinal symptoms:** proton-pump inhibitors (PPIs), prokinetic agents
- **Scleroderma renal crisis:** angiotensin-converting enzyme inhibitors (ACEi), renal replacement therapy
- **Interstitial lung disease:** cyclophosphamide

- **Pulmonary HTN:** phosphodiesterase type 5 (PDE-5) inhibitors, endothelin-receptor antagonists (e.g., bosentan, ambrisentan)

Polymyositis and Dermatomyositis

Definition: an autoimmune disorder characterised by inflammation of muscle, causing symmetrical, proximal muscle weakness. May be idiopathic, associated with a connective tissue disease or a paraneoplastic phenomenon (e.g., lung, pancreas, ovaries, bowel). Dermatomyositis is a variant of the disease in which *skin manifestations are prominent* (e.g., purple (heliotrope) rash on the cheeks and eyelids).

Buzzwords:
- **Risk factors:** female, other autoimmune diseases (e.g., myasthenia gravis, Hashimoto's thyroiditis), malignancy (dermatomyositis)
- **Presentation:**
  - **Polymyositis:** symmetrical, proximal muscle weakness; dysphagia; dysphonia; respiratory weakness; Raynaud's
  - **Dermatomyositis:** as above, *plus skin signs* such as a heliotrope rash (Fig 22.8A,B), shawl sign (macular rash over the back and shoulders), nail-fold erythema, Gottron papules (Fig 22.9A,B)

Investigations
- **Blood:** ↑ lactate dehydrogenase (LDH), ↑ creatinine kinase (CK), ↑ aspartate aminotransferase (AST)/alanine aminotransferase (ALT)

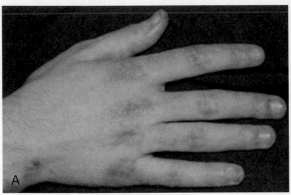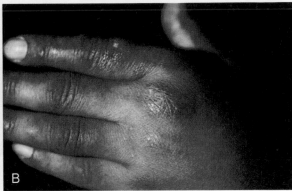

Fig 22.9 Gottron Papules in (A) Lighter Skin and (B) Darker Skin. (Panel A: Courtesy Julie V. Schaffer, MD; Panel B: With permission from Krachmer, J.H., Palay, D.A. Immunologic disorders of the cornea. In *Cornea atlas*. Elsevier.)

- **Antibody testing:** anti-Mi-2 positive (specific for dermatomyositis), ANA positive, anti-Jo-1 positive, anti-signal recognition particle (SRP) positive
- **MRI muscle:** evidence of myositis
- **Muscle biopsy:** endomysial inflammatory infiltrate (I-cells) surrounding and invading non-necrotic muscle fibres
- **Screen for malignancy:** tumour markers, CXR, mammography, pelvic/abdominal ultrasound scan (USS), CT scan
- **Monitoring:** FBC, U&E, LFTs – results depending on the drug treatment used

Differentials: muscular dystrophy, polymyalgia rheumatica, carcinomatous myopathy, rhabdomyolysis

Management:
1. Physical activity to maintain muscular strength
2. Immunosuppression
   a. High-dose oral steroids are first line
   b. Methotrexate, tacrolimus, MMF or azathioprine can be considered
   c. IV immunoglobulins (IVIG) if refractory

INHERITED COLLAGEN DISORDERS

Marfan Syndrome

Definition: a systemic disorder of **connective tissue** inherited as an **autosomal-dominant** trait and caused by mutations in the **FBN1 gene** (encodes fibrillin 1, helps maintain the structure of connective tissue)

Buzzwords:
- **Risk factors:** genetics

- **Presentation:**
  - **MSK:** tall stature, long arms and fingers (arachnodactyly), arm span-to-height ratio of >1.05, Steinberg's thumb and Walker-Murdoch sign (Fig 22.10), hypermobility, arthralgias, scoliosis, pectus carinatum/excavatum
  - **Non-MSK:** high arched palate, aortic root dilation (valve regurgitation, aortic dissection/rupture), mitral valve prolapse and regurgitation, upwards lens subluxation, myopia, glaucoma, retinal detachment, dural ectasia, pneumothorax, skin striae

Investigations: Marfan syndrome is usually diagnosed clinically. The following investigations are used to assess for complications:
- **Echocardiogram (annually):** progressive aortic root dilation, valve disease
- **CT aorta:** aortic root dilation or ascending aortic dissection, valve disease
- **Slit-lamp examination:** visualisation of subluxed/dislocated lens, elevated intraocular pressure
- **MRI spine** (if back pain/neurological symptoms): evidence of dural ectasia

Differentials: Ehlers-Danlos syndrome, homocystinuria

Management: preventing death from aortic disease is the focus of treatment. Pregnant females are at particular risk.
1. **Lifestyle:** avoid intense exercise and contact sports
2. **Prophylactic beta blockers** are used to lower the risk of aortic rupture and to slow aortic root dilatation
3. **Surgical:** aortic root replacement

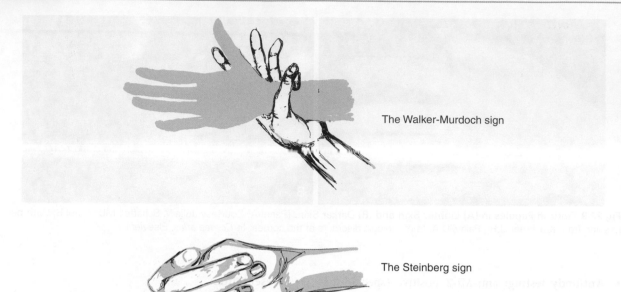

The Walker-Murdoch sign

The Steinberg sign

Fig 22.10 Walker-Murdoch Sign (positive if the thumb and fifth finger overlap) and Steinberg Sign (positive if the thumb tip extends from the palm of hand). (Illustrated by Hollie Blaber.)

Ehlers-Danlos Syndrome

Definition: a group of rare inherited connective tissue disorders with **multiple subtypes** (13 subtypes) caused by mutations in the genes involved in collagen synthesis and structure. Ehlers-Danlos syndrome (EDS) is most commonly inherited with an autosomal-dominant pattern. EDS of the hypermobility type is common but has no known genetic associations and is closely linked to fibromyalgia.

Buzzwords:

- **Risk factors:** female
- **Presentation:** hyperextensible skin, joint hypermobility (dislocation, subluxation, arthralgia), tissue fragility (mucosal bleeding, vessel/organ rupture), cardiac involvement (e.g., valve prolapse, aortic root dilation), pneumothorax, uterine and anal prolapse

Investigations: EDS is usually diagnosed **clinically**. The following investigations are used to assess for complications:

- **Echocardiogram:** aortic dilation, mitral valve prolapse

Differentials: fibromyalgia, Marfan syndrome, chronic fatigue syndrome

Management: treatment and management are focused on patient education, physiotherapy and preventing serious complications

METABOLIC BONE DISEASE

Osteoporosis

Definition: a progressive bone disease characterised by a low bone mineral density (BMD) and microarchitectural deterioration of bone tissue. This condition leads to an increased risk of fragility fractures.

Buzzwords:

- **Risk factors:** increasing age, post-menopausal, glucocorticoids, low body mass index (BMI), diabetes mellitus (DM), hyperthyroidism, chronic kidney disease (CKD), coeliac disease, chronic pancreatitis, IBD, female, family history, Cushing's, inflammatory arthritis, previous fragility fracture, smoking, alcohol, myeloma, selective serotonin reuptake inhibitors (SSRIs), anti-epileptics, aromatase inhibitors
- **Presentation:** fragility fractures involving the vertebrae, proximal femur, distal radius, humerus

Investigations:

- **Blood:** normal calcium, normal alkaline phosphatase (ALP), normal phosphate, normal parathyroid hormone (PTH)
- **Dual-energy x-ray absorptiometry (DEXA) scan to calculate the T-score and Z-score**

- **T-score:** the number of standard deviations from the mean bone density of a 30-year-old adult (<−2.5 is osteoporosis; −1.5 to −2.5 is osteopenia)
- **Z-score:** the number of standard deviations from the mean bone density of an age/gender-matched control (a Z-score of <2 indicates a low BMD)

Differentials: osteomalacia, multiple myeloma, metastatic bone malignancy

Management: the main aim of treatment is to reduce the risk of fractures

1. **Lifestyle factors:** smoking cessation, maintaining a healthy BMI, reducing alcohol intake, fall prevention, weight-bearing exercise
2. **FRAX tool:** assessment of the fracture risk is a key to planning future management
3. **Physiotherapy:** to reduce the risk of further falls
4. **Supplementation:** calcium and vitamin D supplementation
5. **Bisphosphonates** (e.g., alendronic acid is first line). NB. patients must take one tablet a week on the same day. Patients should take the tablet with water, sit up, and have nothing to eat or drink for 30 min.
6. If oral bisphosphonates are not tolerated, consider referral to a specialist for further treatment options (e.g., denosumab (subcutaneous injection every 6 months), zoledronate (IV injection once a year)).

Paget's Disease (Osteitis Deformans)

Definition: increasingly rare. A localised disorder of bone characterised by uncontrolled bone turnover (excessive osteoclastic resorption and increased osteoblastic activity). This condition results in expanded, weakened bone with sclerotic and lytic areas. It most commonly affects the pelvis, skull, femur, sacrum, tibia and radius

Buzzwords:
- **Risk factors:** family history, male, >55 years of age
- **Presentation:** asymptomatic in 70%, bone pain, pathological fractures, asymmetrical bone involvement
- **Complications:** deafness, radiculopathy, high-output cardiac failure, osteosarcoma, OA, spinal cord compression, head enlargement, saber tibia

Investigations:
- **Blood:** ↑ ALP, normal phosphate, normal calcium
- **X-ray:** localised sclerosis, coarse and irregular trabecular patterning, bone expansion, thickened calvarium, **'blade of grass'** lesions (Fig 22.11) in

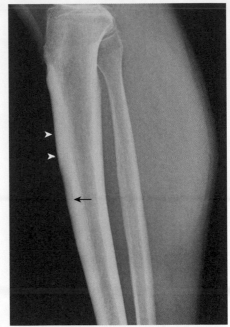

Fig 22.11 Thickening of the Anterior Tibia *(arrowheads)* with a 'Blade of Grass' Appearance Distally *(arrow)*. (With permission from Carlsen, D., Hassan, T.S., Lewi, J.E. (2015). The physical therapist's leg pain: Paget's disease. *The American Journal of Medicine.* Elsevier.)

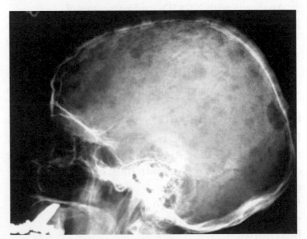

Fig 22.12 'Cotton Wool' Skull Pattern (With permission from Mettler, F.E. (2019). Head and soft tissues of face and neck. In *Essentials of radiology.* Elsevier.)

diseased long bones, **'cotton wool'** pattern in the skull (Fig 22.12)
- **Bone scintigraphy:** will show active bone lesions and therefore can demonstrate the extent of disease – can guide which areas to x-ray

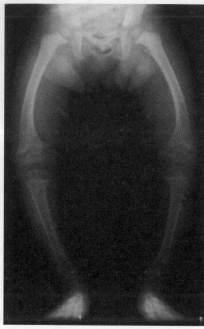

Fig 22.13 Rickets Radiograph. (With permission from Mrich. English Wikipedia., CC BY-SA 1.0.)

Differentials: osteomalacia
Management:
1. Analgesia with NSAIDs and paracetamol
2. Zoledronic acid IV 5 mg – a single dose induces remission in most patients (per oral (PO) risedronate is second line)
3. Surgical interventions as indicated: arthroplasty, fixation of fractures, realignment osteotomies if there is significant deformity amendable to surgical correction

Osteomalacia/Rickets

Definition: a metabolic bone disease characterised by incomplete mineralization of the underlying mature organic bone matrix (osteoid), most often due to a vitamin D deficiency.
- **Rickets:** seen in children
- **Osteomalacia:** after epiphysis fusion

Buzzwords:
- **Risk factors:** vitamin D deficiency (malabsorption, lack of sunlight, diet), renal failure, drug induced (e.g., anticonvulsants), liver disease, family history (e.g., inherited vitamin D resistance)
- **Presentation**
  - **Rickets:** knock-kneed/bow-legged (Fig 22.13), bone pain, craniotabes, osteochondral swelling, Harrison's sulcus

- **Osteomalacia:** bone pain and tenderness, proximal myopathy, fractures

Investigations:
- **Blood:** ↑ PTH, ↑ ALP, ↓ calcium, ↓ phosphate, ↓ vitamin D
- **X-ray:** loss of cortical bones, Looser's zones (pseudofractures), cupped metaphysis in rickets
- **Monitoring:** measure calcium weekly initially. Should see improved plasma levels with treatment

Differentials: Paget's disease, osteoporosis
Management: calcium and vitamin D supplements

MYALGIAS

Fibromylagia

Definition: a syndrome characterised by chronic, widespread MSK pain with tender points at specific anatomical sites. The cause remains unknown.

Buzzwords:
- **Risk factors:** most common in middle-aged women
- **Presentation:** widespread pain for >3 months, fatigue, sleep disturbance, headaches, cognitive impairment ('fibro fog')

Investigations: this is a **clinical diagnosis** based on symptoms and an examination of tender points (9 pairs in total – see Fig 22.14), although assessments should be conducted for organic disease. **Monitoring** is performed by clinical assessments alone.

Differentials: polymyalgia rheumatica (PMR), RA, hypothyroidism, vitamin D deficiency, vasculitis
Management: nonpharmacological treatment is key:
- Patient education
- Cognitive behavioural therapy
- Graduated exercise program involving aerobic exercise and strength training
- Analgesia is no longer recommended
- Antidepressants have a role in improving pain and function.

Polymyalgia Rheumatica

Definition: an inflammatory condition of unknown cause most commonly affecting the older population. PMR shares the same demographic characteristics as giant cell arteritis (GCA), and they frequently occur together.

Buzzwords:
- **Risk factors:** >50 years of age

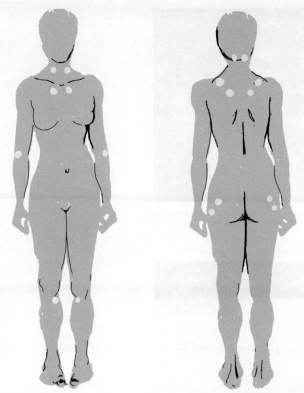

Fig 22.14 Fibromyalgia Tender Points. (Illustrated by Hollie Blaber.)

- **Presentation:** bilateral shoulder and/or pelvic girdle pain, worse with movement, stiffness, insidious onset (<2 weeks), low-grade fever, fatigue, anorexia, weight loss, depression, **normal muscle strength**

Investigations: often diagnosed **clinically** by a rapid response to steroid therapy

- **Blood:** thyroid function tests (TFTs), creatine kinase (CK), FBC, U&E all normal in PMR, ESR is typically >40, ↑ ALP in 30%

Differentials: GCA, polymyositis, recent-onset RA, hypothyroidism

Management:

1. Trial of PO prednisolone 15 mg/day for 1 week then assess for improvement. A clinical response is expected in 1 week, with normalisation of inflammatory markers in 4 weeks
2. Taper steroids according to the clinical response
3. Consider DMARDs for recurrent relapses

CRYSTAL ARTHROPATHIES

Gout

Definition: a type of arthropathy characterised by hyperuricaemia and the deposition of urate crystals leading to an acute inflammatory arthritis and, if untreated, chronic joint disease

Buzzwords:

- **Risk factors:** male, high purine diet (e.g., red meat, shellfish), diuretics, HTN, myeloproliferative disease, psoriasis, CKD, alcohol, tacrolimus, ACEi
- **Presentation:** severe acute pain, swelling, erythema, maximum inflammation/pain develops <24 h, can't bear touch or pressure to affected joint, mono- or oligo-arthritis, tophi, first metatarsophalangeal (MTP) joint in most cases

Investigations:

- **Blood:** ↑ WBC and CRP, serum urate may be normal in the acute phase
- **Joint aspiration:** negative birefringent needle-shaped monosodium urate crystals (*mnemonic 'gout negative needles'*)
- **X-ray:** useful only in chronic gout. Para-articular erosions with **'overhanging edges'** of bone are characteristic of gout (Fig 22.15)
- **Monitoring:** serum urate. Usually measured 4–6 weeks after an acute attack to confirm hyperuricaemia (urate levels > 380 micromol/L). NB: normal levels do not exclude a diagnosis of gout. Should decrease with allopurinol/febuxostat treatment

Differentials: septic arthritis, reactive arthritis, haemarthrosis, pseudogout

Management:

- **Acute:**
  - Colchicine and/or NSAIDs are first-line agents with PPIs (choice depends on renal function and comorbidities)
  - Corticosteroids are second line
- **Long term**
  - Lifestyle factors and modification
  - Consider urate-lowering therapy (e.g., **allopurinol** or **febuxostat**) for long-term prevention following confirmation of the diagnosis, particularly if: >2 attacks in 12 months, presence of tophi, chronic gouty arthritis, renal impairment, history of urolithiasis, use of a diuretic or cytotoxic drug. Wait 2 weeks following the first attack before starting. Co-prescribe colchicine or a low-dose NSAID to prevent an acute

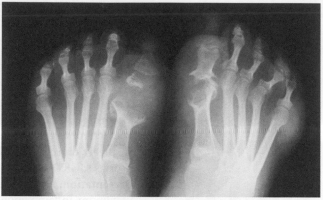

Fig 22.15 X-ray of Chronic Tophaceous Gout. (Photograph courtesy Dr Jorge Jaimes.)

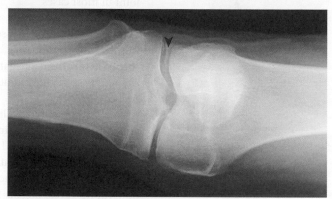

Fig 22.16 Chondrocalcinosis of Menisci *(arrowhead).* (With permission from Klatt, E.C. (2020). Bones, joints, and soft tissues. In *Robbins and Cotran Atlas of Pathology.* Elsevier.)

attack of gout whilst initiating therapy. NB: do not stop during an acute attack. Titrate the dose of allopurinol against the serum urate.

Pseudogout

Definition: an inflammation in the joints caused by the deposition of calcium pyrophosphate crystals in intra-articular and periarticular tissues

Buzzwords:

- **Risk factors:** OA, hyperparathyroidism, steroids, hypothyroidism, haemochromatosis, Wilson's disease, acromegaly, dialysis. Can be provoked by illness/surgery
- **Presentation:** acute mono- or oligo-arthropathy, most commonly affects the knee

Investigations:

- **Blood:** ↑ WBC and CRP

- **Joint aspiration:** positively birefringent, rhomboid-shaped crystals under polarised light microscopy *(mnemonic 'pseudogout positive rhomboid')*
- **X-ray:** chondrocalcinosis (Fig 22.16) and other soft tissue calcium deposition

Differentials: septic arthritis, reactive arthritis, gout, OA

Management: treatment is largely symptomatic

1. NSAIDs, colchicine, steroids in the acute phase
2. Chronic disease can be managed with anti-inflammatories or methotrexate in resistant disease

LARGE-VESSEL VASCULITIS

Giant Cell Arteritis

Definition: an immune-mediated vasculitis charac-terised by granulomatous inflammation in the walls of medium and large-sized arteries. Primarily affects the carotid artery and its extracranial branches. GCA can cause sudden and potentially irreversible vision loss in the elderly (usually due to anterior ischaemic optic neuropathy); therefore, it is considered a rheumatological emergency.

Buzzwords:

- **Risk factors:** >50 years of age, PMR, female
- **Presentation:** fever, malaise, fatigue, headache, temporal artery and scalp tenderness, jaw claudication, prominent temporal arteries plus or minus pulsation, amaurosis fugax, diplopia, sudden vision loss

Investigations:

- **Blood:** ↑ ESR, ↑ platelets, ↑ ALP, normocytic anaemia
- **Fundoscopy:** pale swollen optic disc with haemorrhages – anterior ischaemic optic neuropathy. **Consult ophthalmology if any suspicion of this condition**
- **Temporal artery biopsy:** granulomatous inflammation, multinucleated giant cells. False negatives can occur due to skip lesions.
- **Temporal artery ultrasound:** may show wall thickening (halo sign), stenosis or occlusion
- **Monitoring:** CRP/ESR should decrease if steroids are started and symptoms improve

Differentials: PMR, migraine, Takayasu's arteritis (<50 years of age)

Management:

1. Steroids: 40–60 mg of prednisolone. May require IV pulse methylprednisolone therapy if visual symptoms are present. Taper steroids gradually, guided by symptoms and the ESR
2. PPIs and consider bone health and bisphosphonates with high-dose steroid use
3. Tocilizumab if unresponsive to steroids

Takayasu's Arteritis

Definition: a rare granulomatous vasculitis of the aorta, its main branches and the pulmonary arteries. Systemic symptoms are common in the early phase of disease; however, as the disease progresses, the consequences of vascular inflammation become apparent, with arterial stenosis, thrombosis and aneurysms.

Buzzwords:

- **Risk factors:** female, <40 years of age, more common in children, Asian ethnicity

- **Presentation:** dependent on which vessels are affected – limb claudication with exertion, chest pain, weight loss, fatigue, vascular bruits, unequal blood pressures, absent pulses, hypertension (due to renal artery stenosis)

Investigations:

- **Blood:** ↑ WBC and CRP, normocytic anaemia, U&E derangement with renal artery involvement
- **CT angiography:** segmental narrowing or occlusion, occasionally dilation of affected vessels
- **Fluorodeoxyglucose-positron emission tomography (FDG-PET):** more sensitive test, increased uptake highlights inflammation in vascular walls
- **Monitoring:** monitor inflammatory markers and radiological progression with relevant imaging dependent on the disease site

Differentials: other causes of a large-vessel vasculitis (e.g., syphilis, tuberculosis, SLE, RA, Behçet's disease)

Management:

1. Steroids are first line. Azathioprine, methotrexate, cyclophosphamide are also commonly used in steroid-resistant cases
2. Biological drugs (e.g., anti-TNF inhibitors like rituximab) appear to be effective
3. Aspirin for prevention of ischaemic events if there are no contraindications
4. Management of HTN
5. Surgery: long-segment stenosis with excessive fibrosis or occlusion requires bypass

MEDIUM-VESSEL VASCULITIS

Polyarteritis Nodosa

Definition: a necrotizing vasculitis of medium-sized arteries causing aneurysms, bleeds and thrombosis

Buzzwords:

- **Risk factors:** hepatitis B/C, HIV, middle-aged males, family history
- **Presentation:** fever, arthralgia, weight loss, livedo reticularis, palpable purpura, sensorimotor polyneuropathy, haematuria and proteinuria due to renal impairment, HTN, abdominal pain from visceral vasculitis

Investigations:

- **Blood:** ↑ WBC and neutrophils, ↑ eosinophils (in 30%), ↓ Hb, ↑ ESR, ↑ creatinine/urea, ↓ complement
- **Serology:** anti-neutrophil cytoplasm antibodies (ANCA) negative– (if ANCA positive, test strongly indicates an alternative diagnosis)

- **Urinalysis:** possible proteinuria, casts, haematuria
- **Hepatitis and HIV serology:** positive cases associated with polyarteritis nodosa (PAN), especially hepatitis B
- **Angiography:** microaneurysms in the small- and medium-sized arteries of the kidneys and abdominal viscera
- **Tissue biopsy:** a focal and segmental transmural necrotising inflammation of medium-sized vessels
- **Monitoring:** monitor inflammatory markers

Differentials: diseases with vasculitic features (e.g., RA, SLE), other vasculitides

Management:
1. Prednisolone is first line
2. Add a DMARD if needed (e.g., azathioprine or cyclophosphamide)
3. Treatment of active hepatitis or HIV if indicated

SMALL-VESSEL VASCULITIS

Granulomatosis with Polyangiitis (Formerly Wegener's Granulomatosis)

Definition: an autoimmune condition associated with a necrotizing granulomatous vasculitis usually involving the upper and lower respiratory tract and kidneys

Buzzwords:
- **Risk factors:** male, 40–50 years of age
- **Presentation:** nasal crusting and epistaxis, sinusitis, ear discharge or tympanic membrane perforation, saddle-shaped nose, haemoptysis, rapidly progressive glomerulonephritis, cANCA positive

Investigations:
- **Blood:** ↓ Hb, ↑ platelets, ↑ ESR, ↑ creatinine/urea, ↓ complement
- **Serology:** cANCA positive in >90%. Some express pANCA
- **Urinalysis:** proteinuria, red cell casts, haematuria if renal involvement
- **Chest X-ray:** bilateral nodules. Infiltrates seen in pulmonary haemorrhage
- **Renal biopsy:** epithelial crescents in Bowman's capsule
- **Tissue biopsy:** granulomatous inflammation

Differentials: diseases with vasculitic features (e.g., RA, SLE), eosinophilic granulomatosis with polyangiitis (EGPA), anti-glomerular basement membrane (anti-GBM) disease

Management:
1. **Induce remission** with corticosteroids and DMARDs. Cyclophosphamide for severe disease
2. **Maintenance of remission** with ongoing DMARD/steroid therapy

3. **Plasma exchange in patients with severe renal disease** and in patients presenting with pulmonary haemorrhage

Eosinophilic Granulomatosis with Polyangiitis (Formerly Churg-Strauss Syndrome)

Definition: a systemic autoimmune vasculitis associated with late-onset asthma, eosinophilia and rapidly progressive glomerulonephritis

Buzzwords:
- **Risk factors:** asthma, allergic rhinitis, sinusitis
- **Presentation:** sinusitis, allergic rhinitis, **asthma**, pulmonary infiltrates, **eosinophilia,** haematuria, mononeuritis multiplex. Can present as a glomerulonephritis with renal failure/HTN

Investigations:
- **Blood:** ↑ eosinophils, ↑ ESR, ↓ Hb
- **Serology:** positive pANCA in 30%–40%
- **Urinalysis:** proteinuria, red cell casts, microscopic haematuria in renal involvement
- **Chest X-ray:** transient infiltrates, effusion
- **Biopsy (lung or kidney commonly):** small necrotising granulomas. Necrotising vasculitis involving the small arteries and venules

Differentials: granulomatosis with polyangiitis (GPA), PAN, haematological malignancy

Management:
1. **Induce remission:** high-dose corticosteroids
2. **Severe disease:** cyclophosphamide
3. Biologics (e.g., rituximab) if refractory
4. Monitor for complications in other organ systems

Henoch-Schönlein Purpura

Definition: the most common cause of vasculitis in childhood. Henoch-Schönlein purpura (HSP) is characterised by the classic tetrad of **rash, abdominal pain, arthritis and glomerulonephritis**. It is usually seen in children following an infection and, in most cases, resolves with symptomatic treatment. 90% of cases occur in those <10 years of age.

Buzzwords:
- **Risk factors:** male, age 3–15 years, prior upper respiratory tract infection
- **Presentation:** palpable purpuric rash over the buttocks and extensor surfaces of arms and legs (Fig 22.17A, B); **mildly unwell,** abdominal pain, diarrhoea, polyarthritis, haematuria, renal failure

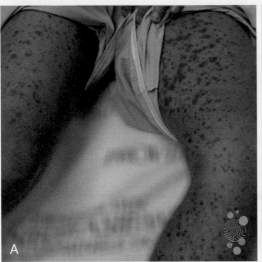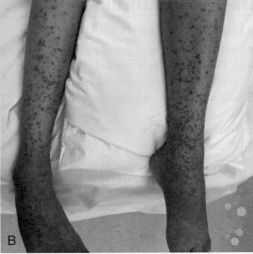

Fig 22.17 Henoch-Schönlein Purpura in (A) Darker Skin and (B) Lighter Skin. (Panels A and B with permission from *SKIN DEEP*.)

Investigations:
- **Blood:** ↑ WBC and CRP, ↑ platelets, ↑ eosinophils, ↑ creatinine/urea, ↑ immunoglobulin A (IgA)
- **Urinalysis:** proteinuria, haematuria (20%–40%)
- **Skin biopsy:** leucocytoclastic vasculitis with IgA deposition
- **Monitoring:** monitor inflammatory markers, renal function, blood pressure and urinalysis

Differentials: intussusception, meningococcal septicaemia, other causes of glomerulonephritis, connective tissue disease

Management:
1. Supportive
2. Treatment of the nephropathy is generally supportive. Can use steroids and immunosuppressants in exceptional cases. <1% progress to end-stage renal failure

VARIABLE VESSEL VASCULITIS

Behçet's Disease

Definition: a complex multisystem disorder with a presumed autoimmune-mediated inflammation of the arteries and veins. It commonly involves the skin, mucosa, joints, eyes, nervous system and gastrointestinal system.

Buzzwords:
- **Risk factors:** eastern Mediterranean (e.g., Turkey) origin, male, young adults, family history
- **Presentation:** skin pathergy (hypersensitivity), oral ulcers, genital ulcers, eye involvement (e.g.,

anterior uveitis, retinal vasculitis), thrombophlebitis and deep vein thrombosis, arthralgia, neurological involvement (e.g., aseptic meningitis, memory impairment), abdominal pain, colitis, erythema nodosum

Investigations: this diagnosis is mostly a **clinical** one
- **Blood:** ↑ WBC and CRP, ↓ Hb
- **Pathergy test:** positive in 60%. This test involves making multiple punctures with a sterile needle into the forearm and observing the reaction over 24–48 h. The test is positive if any of the following are present: papules, pustules or ulcers at the sites of puncture.
- **Antiphospholipid antibodies:** positive in 25%
- **Monitoring:** monitor inflammatory markers, renal function, blood pressure and urinalysis

Differentials: varied given the huge variation in presentation. Includes other systemic inflammatory disorders (e.g., Takayasu's, EGPA), sarcoidosis, herpes infection, seronegative spondyloarthropathies

Management:
1. Topical corticosteroids for oral/genital ulcers. Colchicine can be used to treat frequent attacks of aphthous ulceration or arthritis
2. DMARDs for severe cases and for those with major organ involvement/major vessel disease
3. Central nervous system involvement requires the most intensive treatment with steroids and immunosuppression

PAEDIATRIC RHEUMATOLOGY

Juvenile Idiopathic Arthritis (JIA)

Definition: Most common type of arthritis affecting children < 16 years old. There are different types of JIA including oligoarthritis, polyarthritis, systemic, psoriatic arthritis, enthesitis-related and undifferentiated. Aetiology remains unknown.

Buzzwords:

- **Risk factors:** combination of environmental and genetic factors
- **Presentation:** Joint swelling, stiffness, pain and inflammation. Other body parts may be affected. If lower limb joints are affected patient may present with a limp. Patients may also present with fatigue, fever, rash and/or anterior uveitis.

Investigations: clinical diagnosis. Musculoskeletal examination includes pGALS (paediatric Gait, Arms, Legs, Spine) and pREMS (paediatric Regional Examination of the Musculoskeletal System). Bloods and imaging may be used to exclude other differentials.

Differential: trauma, Legg-Calve-Perthes, Developmental hip dysplasia, Slipped upper femoral epiphysis, malignancy

Management: Management is conducted by a multidisciplinary team (MDT)

- Refer to paediatric rheumatology team
- 1st line: NSAIDs and intra-articular Corticosteroids
- If refractory to 1st line therapy consider DMARDs (e.g. Methotrexate)
- Consider Biological agents if inadequate response to other therapies

ANTIBODY TABLE

See Table 22.1 for a summary of the antibodies present in different rheumatological conditions.

TABLE 22.1   Antibodies

Disease	Antibodies
Seronegative spondyloarthropathies	RhF negative
Rheumatoid arthritis	RhF positive ~80% Anti-CCP (~96% specific) – also prognostic ANA positive ~30%
Systemic lupus erythematous	ANA positive in >95% Anti-dsDNA ~60% sensitive, highly specific Anti-Smith Anti-histone (drug induced) Anti-Ro/La ~15%
Sjögren's disease	RhF positive ~100% ANA positive ~70% Anti-Ro Anti-La
Systemic sclerosis	ANA positive ~90% Anti-centromere antibody (limited sclerosis) Anti-SCL-70 (diffuse sclerosis) Anti-topoisomerase I Anti-RNA polymerase III
Antiphospholipid syndrome	Lupus anticoagulant Anti-beta-2 glycoprotein antibodies
Polymyositis, dermatomyositis	Anti-Jo-1 Anti-Mi-2 (highly specific)
Mixed connective tissue disease	Anti u1-snRNP

ANA, Antinuclear antibody; CCP, cyclic citrullinated peptide; dsDNA, double-stranded DNA; RhF, rheumatoid factor.
Lab Tests Online UK. https://labtestsonline.org.uk/. Accessed March 2021; Clunie, G., Wilkinson, N., Nikiphorou, E. & Jadon, D. (2018). *Oxford handbook of rheumatology*, (4th ed.). Oxford University Press; Patient info. (2016). *Plasma autoantibodies disease associations*. https://patient.info/doctor. Accessed March 2021; GP Online. *Interpreting rheumatology tests*. https://gponline.com. Accessed March 2021.

THE ONE-LINE ROUND-UP!

Here are some key words to help you remember each condition/concept.

Condition/Concept	One-line Description
Rheumatoid arthritis	Symmetrical polyarthropathy
Psoriatic arthritis	DRSAM
Ankylosing spondylitis	Syndesmophytes
Reactive arthritis	Arthritis, UTI and eye problems
Enteropathic arthritis	Arthritis and IBD
Systemic lupus erythematous	Malar rash and anti-dsDNA
Sjögren's syndrome	Dry mucous membranes
Scleroderma	CREST
Polymyositis	Symmetrical proximal muscle weakness
Dermatomyositis	Heliotrope rash
Marfan syndrome	Tall, large arm span
Ehlers-Danlos syndrome	Hypermobility
Osteoporosis	Elderly with hip/wrist/vertebrae/humeral fractures
Paget's disease	Rapid bone turnover
Osteomalacia/rickets	Soft bones secondary to a vitamin D deficiency
Fibromyalgia	18 pain points
Polymyalgia rheumatica	Shoulder and pelvic girdle pain
Gout	Podagra, negatively birefringent
Pseudogout	Chondrocalcinosis
Giant cell arteritis	Headache and jaw claudication
Takayasu arteritis	Loss of pulses
Polyarteritis nodosa	Sensorimotor polyneuropathy, livedo reticularis, abdominal pain
Granulomatosis with polyangiitis	Saddle nose deformity, upper respiratory tract symptoms
Eosinophilic granulomatosis with polyangiitis	Poorly controlled asthma, allergic rhinitis, limb weakness
Henoch-Schönlein purpura	Purpuric rash and well
Behçet's	Mediterranean, mouth/genital lesions and eye problems
JIA	Joint pain, swelling, stiffness in <16 years old

READING LIST: RHEUMATOLOGY IN AN HOUR

INFLAMMATORY ARTHRITIS

Rheumatoid Arthritis

NICE. (2020). *CKS: Rheumatoid arthritis.* https://cks.nice.org.uk/topics/rheumatoid-arthritis/. [Accessed August 2020].

Smolen, J. S., Landewé, R., Bijlsma, J., et al. (2017). EULAR recommendations for the management of rheumatoid arthritis with synthetic and biological disease-modifying antirheumatic drugs: 2016 update. *Annals of the Rheumatic Diseases, 76,* 960–977.

Clunie, G., Wilkinson, N., Nikiphorou, E., & Jadon, D. (2018). *Oxford handbook of rheumatology* (4th ed.). Oxford University Press.

Psoriatic Arthritis

Coates, L. C., Tillett, W., Chandler, D., et al. (2013). The 2012 BSR and BHPR guideline for the treatment of psoriatic arthritis with biologics. *Rheumatology (Oxford), 52,* 1754–1757.

Gossec, L., Smolen, J. S., Ramiro, S., et al. (2016). European League Against Rheumatism (EULAR) recommendations for the management of psoriatic arthritis with pharmacological therapies: 2015 update. *Annals of the Rheumatic Diseases, 75,* 499–510.

Patient info. (2016). *Psoriatic arthritis.* https://patient.info/doctor/psoriatic-arthritis-pro. [Accessed February 2021].

Reactive Arthritis

Patient info. (2015). *Reactive arthritis.* https://patient.info/doctor/reactive-arthritis-pro. [Accessed August 2020].

BMJ Best Practice. (2021). *Reactive arthritis*. https://bestprac-tice.bmj.com/topics/en-gb/597 [Accessed March 2021].

Enteropathic Arthritis
Clunie, G., Wilkinson, N., Nikiphorou, E., & Jadon, D. (2018). *Oxford handbook of rheumatology* (4th ed.). Oxford University Press.
Patient info. (2015). *Enteropathic arthropathies*. https://pa-tient.info/doctor/enteropathic-arthropathies [Accessed August 2020].

Ankylosing Spondylitis
NICE. (2019). *CKS: Ankylosing spondylitis*. https://cks.nice.org.uk/topics/ankylosing-spondylitis/ [Accessed August 2020].
Hamilton, L., Barkham, N., Bhalla, A., et al. (2017). BSR and BHPR guideline for the treatment of axial spondyloar-thritis (including ankylosing spondylitis) with biologics. *Rheumatology (Oxford), 56*, 313–316.
BMJ Best Practice. (2021). *Ankylosing spondylitis*. https://bestpractice.bmj.com/topics/en-gb/366 [Accessed March 2021].

CONNECTIVE TISSUE DISORDERS
Systemic Lupus Erythematous
Patient info. (2020). *Systemic lupus erythematous*. https://patient.info/doctor/systemic-lupus-erythematosus-pro. [Accessed February 2021].
Gordon, C., Amissah-Arthur, M. B., Gayed, M., et al. (2018). The British Society for Rheumatology guideline for the management of systemic lupus erythematosus in adults. *Rheumatology (Oxford), 57*, e1–e45.

Sjögren's Syndrome
BMJ Best Practice. (2019). *Sjogren's syndrome*. https://bestprac-tice.bmj.com/topics/en-gb/175 [Accessed August 2020].
Price, E. J., Rauz, S., Tappuni, A. R., et al. (2017). The British Society for Rheumatology guideline for the management of adults with primary Sjögren's Syndrome. *Rheumatology (Oxford), 56*, 1828.

Scleroderma
Clunie, G., Wilkinson, N., Nikiphorou, E., & Jadon, D. (2018). *Oxford handbook of rheumatology* (4th ed.). Oxford University Press.
Patient info. (2016). *Systemic sclerosis*. https://bestpractice.bmj.com/topics/en-gb/175 [Accessed August 2020].
Denton, C. P., Hughes, M., Gak, N., et al. (2016). BSR and BHPR guideline for the treatment of systemic sclerosis. *Rheumatology (Oxford), 55*, 1906–1910.

Polymyositis and Dermatomyositis
Clunie, G., Wilkinson, N., Nikiphorou, E., & Jadon, D. (2018). *Oxford handbook of rheumatology* (4th ed.). Oxford University Press.

Patient info. (2016). *Myositis – polymyositis and dermatomy-ositis*. https://patient.info/doctor/myositis-polymyosi-tis-and-dermatomyositis [Accessed August 2020].

INHERITED COLLAGEN DISORDERS
Marfan Syndrome
Patient info. (2016). *Marfan's syndrome*. https://patient.info/doctor/marfans-syndrome-pro [Accessed August 2020].
BMJ Best Practice. (2018). *Marfan syndrome*. https://best-practice.bmj.com/topics/en-gb/514 [Accessed July 2020].

Ehlers Danlos Syndrome
Patient info. (2017). *Ehlers-Danlos syndrome*. https://patient.info/doctor/ehlers-danlos-syndromes [Accessed August 2020].
The Royal College of General Practitioners. *The Ehlers Danlos toolbox*. https://www.rcgp.org.uk/clinical-and-research/resources/toolkits/ehlers-danlos-syndromes-toolkit.aspx. [Accessed August 2020].

METABOLIC BONE DISEASE
Osteoporosis
NICE. (2021). *CKS: Osteoporosis - prevention of fragility frac-tures*. https://cks.nice.org.uk/topics/osteoporosis-preven-tion-of-fragility-fractures/ [Accessed March 2022].
National Osteoporosis Guideline Group. (2017). *NOGG 2017: Clinical guideline for the prevention and treatment of osteoporosis*.

Paget's Disease
Patient info. (2017). *Paget's disease of bone*. https://patient.info/doctor/pagets-disease-of-bone-pro [Accessed March 2021].
Singer, F. R., Bone, H. G., 3rd., Hosking, D. J., Lyles, K. W., Murad, M. H., Reid, I. R., Siris, E. S., & Endocrine Soci-ety.. (2014). Paget's disease of bone: an endocrine society clinical practice guideline. *The Journal Of Clinical Endocri-nology & Metabolism, 99*, 4408–4422.

Osteomalacia/Rickets
Patient info. (2015). *Vitamin D deficiency including osteomala-cia and rickets*. https://patient.info/doctor/vitamin-d-defi-ciency-including-osteomalacia-and-rickets-pro [Accessed March 2021].
BMJ Best Practice. (2021). *Osteomalacia*. https://bestpractice.bmj.com/topics/en-gb/517 [Accessed February 2021].

MYALGIAS
Fibromyalgia
Macfarlane, G. J., Kronisch, C., Dean, L. E., et al. (2017). EULAR revised recommendations for the management of fibromyalgia. *Annals of the Rheumatic Diseases, 76*, 318.
Patient info. (2014). *Fibromyalgia*. https://patient.info/doctor/fibromyalgia-pro [Accessed August 2020].

Polymyalgia Rheumatica

NICE. (2019). *CKS: Polymyalgia Rheumatica.* https://cks.nice. org.uk/topics/polymyalgia-rheumatica/ [Accessed August 2020].

Dasgupta, B., Borg, F. A., Hassan, N., et al. (2010). BSR and BHPR guidelines for the management of polymyalgia rheumatica. *Rheumatology (Oxford), 49,* 186–190.

CRYSTAL ARTHROPATHIES

Gout

NICE. (2018). *CKS: Gout.* https://cks.nice.org.uk/topics/gout/ [Accessed August 2020].

Hui, M., Carr, A., Cameron, S., et al. (2017). The British Society for Rheumatology guideline for the management of gout. *Rheumatology (Oxford), 56,* e1–e20.

Pseudogout

Patient info. (2015). *Calcium pyrophosphate deposition – including pseudogout.* https://patient.info/doctor/calcium-pyrophosphate-deposition-including-pseudogout-pro [Accessed August 2020].

BMJ Best Practice. (2019). *Calcium pyrophosphate deposition.* https://bestpractice.bmj.com/topics/en-gb/370 [Accessed March 2021].

LARGE-VESSEL VASCULITIS

Giant Cell Arteritis

NICE. (2020). *CKS: Giant cell arteritis.* https://cks.nice.org. uk/topics/giant-cell-arteritis/ [Accessed August 2020].

Mackie, S. L., Dejaco, C., Appenzeller, S., et al. (2020). British Society for Rheumatology guideline on diagnosis and treatment of giant cell arteritis. *Rheumatology (Oxford), 59,* e1–e23.

Takayasu Arteritis

BMJ Best Practice. (2018). *Takayasu's arteritis.* https://bestpractice.bmj.com/topics/en-gb/1064 [Accessed March 2021].

Patient info. (2015). *Takayasu's arteritis.* https://patient.info/ doctor/takayasus-arteritis. [Accessed March 2021].

MEDIUM-VESSEL VASCULITIS

Polyarteritis Nodosa

Patient info. (2015). *Polyarteritis nodosa.* https://patient.info/ doctor/polyarteritis-nodosa-pro [Accessed August 2020].

BMJ Best Practice. (2021). *Polyarteritis nodosa.* https://bestpractice.bmj.com/topics/en-gb/351 [Accessed March 2021].

SMALL-VESSEL VASCULITIS

Granulomatosis with Polyangiitis (Formerly Wegener's Granulomatosis)

Clunie, G., Wilkinson, N., Nikiphorou, E., & Jadon, D. (2018). *Oxford handbook of rheumatology* (4th ed.). Oxford University Press.

Patient info. (2015). *Granulomatosis with polyangiitis.* https:// patient.info/doctor/granulomatosis-with-polyangiitis-wegeners-granulomatosis-pro [Accessed August 2020].

Eosinophilic Granulomatosis with Polyangiitis (Formerly Churg-Strauss Syndrome)

Clunie, G., Wilkinson, N., Nikiphorou, E., & Jadon, D. (2018). *Oxford handbook of rheumatology* (4th ed.). Oxford University Press.

Patient info. (2016). *Churg-Strauss syndrome.* https://patient. info/doctor/churg-strauss-syndrome-pro [Accessed August 2020].

Henoch Schoenlein Purpura

Clunie, G., Wilkinson, N., Nikiphorou, E., & Jadon, D. (2018). *Oxford handbook of rheumatology* (4th ed.). Oxford University Press.

Patient info. (2019). *Henoch-Schonlein purpura.* https:// patient.info/doctor/henoch-schonlein-purpura-pro [Accessed August 2020].

VARIABLE-VESSEL VASCULITIS

Behcet's Disease

Patient info. (2016). *Behcet's disease.* https://patient.info/doctor/behcets-disease-pro. [Accessed March 2021].

Hatemi, G., Christensen, R., Bang, D., et al. (2018). Update of the EULAR recommendations for the management of Behçet's syndrome. *Annals of the Rheumatic Diseases, 77,* 808.

PAEDIATRICS RHEUMATOLOGY

Juvenile idiopathic arthritis

Ruperto, N. & Angelo R. Principles of management of juvenile idiopathic arthritis. *Oxford textbook of rheumatology.* Oxford, UK: Oxford University Press. Oxford Medicine Online. https://oxfordmedicine.com/view/10.1093/ med/9780199642489.001.0001/med-9780199642489-chapter-96. [Accessed Apr 2022].

SC(NHS)FT. (2015). 346. *Medical guidelines for paediatric medicine.*13.1 Juvenile Idiopathic Arthritis www.sheffield-childrens.nhs.uk. [Accessed March 2022].

Arthritis Foundation: Juvenile idiopathic arthritis (JIA) [https://www.arthritis.org/diseases/juvenile-idiopathic-arthritis. [Accessed March 2022].

23

Trauma and Orthopaedics in an Hour

Berenice Aguirrezabala Armbruster, Nagarjun Konda, Dolcie Paxton, Yvonne Chang, Michael Whitehouse, Karanjit Mangat and James Li

ANATOMY

Bones (see Figs 23.1 and 23.2)

Carpal bones mnemonic:
- **Proximal Row: S**he **L**ooks **T**oo **P**retty (Scaphoid, Lunate, Triquetrum, Pisiform)
- **Distal Row: T**ry **T**o **C**atch **H**er (Trapezium, Trapezoid, Capitate, Hamate). The trapezium is at the base of the thumb for the starting point.

Tarsal bones mnemonic: **T**iger **C**ubs **N**eed **MILC**
- **T**alus
- **C**alcaneus
- **N**avicular
- **M**edial, **I**ntermediate, **L**ateral **C**uneiforms

Brachial Plexus (see Fig 23.3)

Definition: the brachial plexus is a network of nerves arising from the spinal roots C5–T1. The brachial plexus innervates the upper limb. Terminal branches consist of the following nerves and branches:
- **Musculocutaneous (C5–C7):** see Table 23.1
- **Axillary (C5–C6):** see Table 23.2

- **Median nerve (C6–T1):** see Table 23.3
  - **Forearm:** muscular branches, anterior interosseous branch, palmar cutaneous nerve
  - **Hand:** recurrent branch, palmar digital branch
- **Radial nerve (C5–T1):** see Table 23.4
  - **Arm:** muscular branches
  - **Forearm and hand:** posterior interosseous branch, superficial branch
- **Ulnar nerve (C8–T1):** see Table 23.5
  - **Forearm:** motor branches, palmar cutaneous branch, dorsal cutaneous branch
  - **Hand:** superficial branch and deep branch

Buzzwords:
- **Risk factors for brachial plexus injury:**
  - **Neonates:** large birthweight, shoulder dystocia, multiparity, assisted delivery
  - **Adults:** trauma, clavicle surgery
- **Presentation:** depends on where the injury occurs
  - **Upper root injury (Erb's palsy, C5–C6 injury):** occurs due to a forceful widening of the angle between the shoulder and head. The following movements are lost/reduced: shoulder abduction, elbow flexion. Sign: 'waiter's tip'

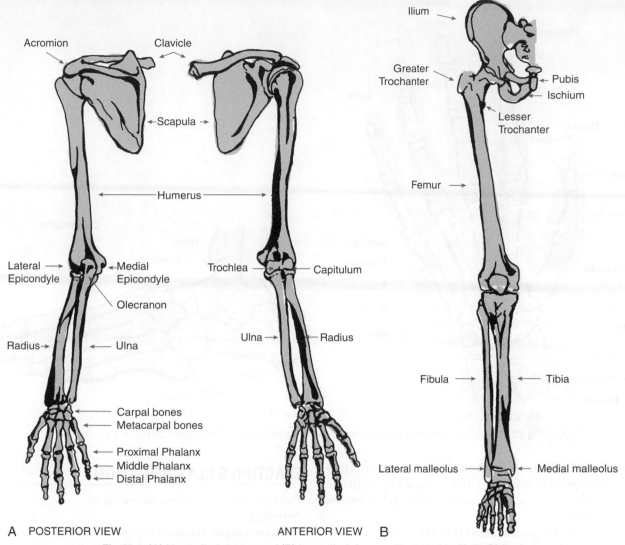

Fig 23.1 (A) Upper limb bones and (B) lower limb bones. (Illustrated by Hollie Blaber.)

- **Lower root injury (Klumpke's palsy, C8–T1 injury):** occurs due to forceful shoulder abduction. Shoulder and elbow movements are maintained, but wrist and hand movements are lost/reduced. Sign: 'claw hand'
- **Terminal branch injury:** see Tables 23.1–23.5
NB: All intrinsic muscles of the hand are innervated by the ulnar nerve except the LOAF muscles, which are innervated by the median nerve. LOAF muscles:
- **L**umbricals (lateral two)
- **O**pponens pollicis
- **A**bductor pollicis brevis

- **F**lexor pollicis brevis
The radial nerve has no intrinsic innervation to the hand. The radial nerve and posterior interosseous branch innervate ALL extensors of the upper limb, wrist and hand.

Lumbar and Sacral Plexus (see Fig 23.4)
Definition:
- **Lumbar plexus:** a network of nerves arising from the spinal roots L1–L4. Terminal branches include:
  - **Femoral nerve (L2–L4):** See Table 23.6
  - **Obturator nerve (L2–L4):** See Table 23.7

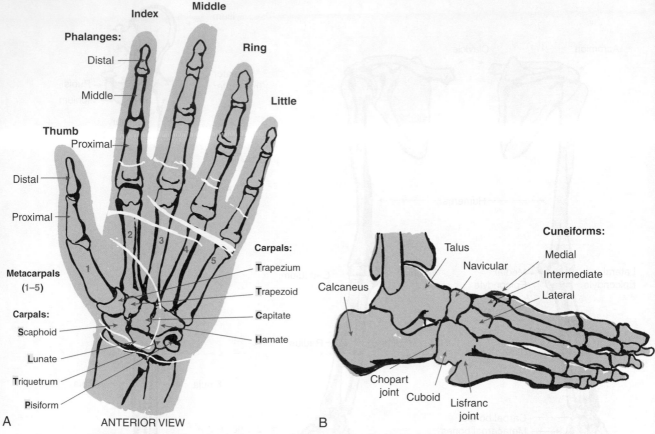

Fig 23.2 (A) Hand and wrist bones and (B) foot and ankle bones. (Illustrated Dr Hollie Blaber.)

- **Sacral plexus:** a network of nerves arising from the spinal roots L4–S4 (L4 is shared by both the lumbar and sacral plexuses). Terminal branches include:
  - **Superior gluteal nerve (L4–S1)**
  - **Inferior gluteal nerve (L5–S2)**
  - **Sciatic nerve (L4–S3):** See Table 23.8. The sciatic nerve then divides into the:
    - Tibial nerve (L4–S3)
    - Common peroneal (fibular) nerve (L4–S2)
  - **Pudendal nerve (S2–S4).** The pudendal nerve then divides into the:
    - Peroneal nerve
    - Dorsal nerve of the penis (or clitoris)

Buzzwords:
- **Risk factors:** trauma, degenerative changes
- **Presentation:** depends on the location of the injury. Nerve function may be lost or decreased (see Table 23.6, 23.7 and 23.8)

FRACTURES CLASSIFICATION

Fractures may be classified according to:

Aetiology
- **Stress/fatigue fracture:** repetitive, normal force in normal bone
- **Traumatic fracture:** abnormal force in normal bone
- **Pathological fracture:** normal force in abnormal bone

Severity: markers of severity include open vs. closed, fracture-dislocation

Localization:
- **Bone:** describes the bone involved. Each bone is given a number: Humerus (1), Radius/Ulna (2), Femur (3), Tibia/Fibula (4)
- **Location:** describes where in the bone the fracture lies. Each bone is divided into segments and a number is given: Proximal segment (1), middle-diaphyseal segment (2), distal segment (3)

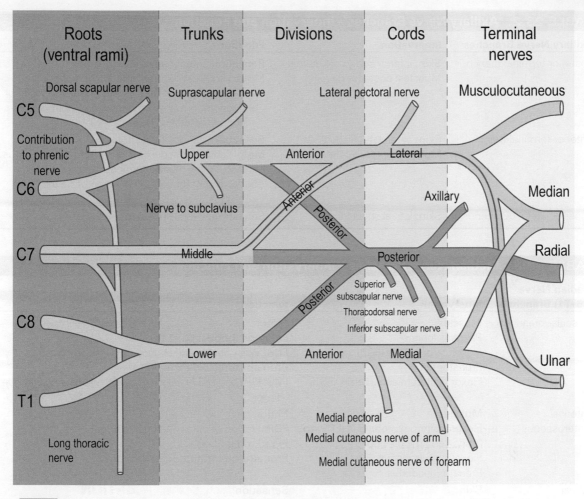

Fig 23.3 Brachial Plexus. (Adapted with permission from Drake, R.L., Vogl, A.W., Mitchell, A. (Eds.), *Gray's Anatomy for Students* (2nd ed). Elsevier, Churchill Livingstone. Copyright 2010.)

TABLE 23.1	Musculocutaneous Nerve Branches – Innervation and Function	
Musculocutaneous Nerve Branches	**Innervation**	**Function**
Muscular branches	**Muscles ('BBC' mnemonic):** Brachialis Biceps brachii Coracobrachialis	**Motor:** **Brachialis:** Foreram flexor at elbow joint **Biceps brachii:** Forearm flexor at elbow joint. Accessory arm flexor at glenohumeral joint (GHJ) **Coracobrachialis:** Arm flexor at GHJ.
Lateral cutaneous	**Skin:** lateral side of forearm	**Sensation:** lateral side of forearm

TABLE 23.2 Axillary Nerve Branches – Innervation and Function

Axillary Nerve Branches	Innervation	Function
Posterior terminal branch	**Skin:** inferior surface of deltoid **Muscles:** posterior deltoid, teres minor	**Sensation:** inferior surface of deltoid **Motor:** shoulder external rotation and abduction 15°–180° (supraspinatus is the primary muscle for abduction from 0°–15° but also contributes to the action of the deltoid from 15°–90°)
Anterior terminal branch	**Skin:** anterolateral shoulder **Muscles:** anterior deltoid	**Sensation:** anterolateral shoulder **Motor:** shoulder abduction 15°–180° (supraspinatus is the primary muscle for abduction from 0°–15° but also contributes to the action of deltoid from 15°–90°)
Superior lateral cutaneous	**Skin:** lateral shoulder	**Sensation:** lateral shoulder

TABLE 23.3 Median Nerve Branches – Innervation and Function

Median Nerve (C6–T1) Branches	Innervation	Function
Muscular branches	**Muscles:** Palmaris longus Flexor carpi radialis (FCR) Pronator teres Flexor digitorum superficialis (FDS)	**Motor:** **Palmaris longus:** Wrist flexor. **FCR:** Wrist flexion and abduction. **Pronator teres:** Forearm pronation. **FDS:** PIPJ and MCPJ flexion of index, middle, ring and little finger
Anterior interosseous	**Muscles:** Flexor digitorum profundus (FDP) to index and middle finger Flexor pollicis longus (FPL) Pronator quadratus	**Motor:** **FDP:** Flexion of index and middle finger. **FPL:** Thumb flexor **Pronator quadratus:** Forearm pronation
Palmar	**Skin:** Palmar surface of the lateral three and a half digits Dorsal surface of the lateral three and a half fingertips	**Sensation:** Palmar surface of the lateral three and a half digits Dorsal surface of the lateral three and a half fingertips **Autonomous area of innervation:** tip of index finger
Recurrent	**Muscles:** thenar muscles ('pollicis' – abductor pollicis brevis, flexor pollicis brevis, opponens pollicis)	**Motor:** thumb abduction, flexion and opposition

MCPJ, Metacarpophalangeal joint; PIPJ, proximal interphalangeal joint.

Morphology:
- **Type:** describes the fracture pattern. For diaphyseal fractures, the morphology can be simple, wedge or multifragmentary. For proximal or distal segment fractures, the morphology may be extra-articular, partial articular or complete articular. A letter is given for the type (see Fig 23.5).

- **Group:** describes the fracture pattern in more detail. A number is given:
  - **For extra-articular:** avulsion (1), simple (2), wedge or multifragmentary (3)
  - **For partial articular:** simple (1), split and/or depressed (2), fragmentary (3)
  - **For complete articular:** simple (1), multifragmentary (2)

TABLE 23.4   **Radial Nerve Branches – Innervation and Function**

Radial Nerve (C5–T1) Branches	Innervation	Function
Muscular	Muscles: Brachioradialis Extensor carpi radialis longus (ECRL) Anconeus	Motor: Brachioradialis: Accessory elbow flexor. ECRL: Wrist extension and abduction. Anconeus: Ulna abduction in pronation. Accessory elbow extensor.
Posterior interosseous	Muscles: Extensor digitorum (ED) Extensor digiti minimi (EDM) Extensor carpi ulnaris (ECU) Extensor carpi radialis brevis (ECRB)	Motor: ED: extension of index, middle, ring and little finger EDM: extension of little finger ECU: wrist extension and abduction ECRB: wrist extension and abduction
Superficial	Skin: Dorsolateral surface of the hand Dorsal surface of lateral three and a half fingers except the tips	Sensation: Dorsolateral surface of the hand Dorsal surface of lateral three and a half fingers except the tips **Autonomous area of innervation:** first web space

TABLE 23.5   **Ulnar Nerve Branches – Innervation and Function**

Ulnar Nerve (C8–T1) Branches	Innervation	Function
Motor	Muscles: Flexor carpi ulnaris (FCU) Medial (or ulnar) side of the flexor digitorum profundus (FDP)	Motor: **FCU:** Wrist flexion and adduction **Medial side of FDP:** Ring and little finger DIPJ flexion
Palmar	Skin: hypothenar eminence	Sensation: hypothenar eminence
Dorsal	Skin: Dorsal medial surface of the hand Dorsal surface of little finger and half of ring finger	Sensation: Dorsal medial surface of the hand Dorsal surface of little and half of ring finger
Superficial	Skin: Palmar surface of little finger and half of ring finger Muscle: Palmaris brevis	Sensation: Little finger and half of ring finger Autonomous area of innervation: tip of little finger Motor: Improves grip
Deep	Muscles ('HIMA' mnemonic): Hypothenar muscles ('digiti minimi') Interossei muscles Medial two lumbricals (3rd and 4th) Adductor pollicis	Motor: Hypothenar muscles: little finger opposition, flexion and abduction Palmar interossei: adduction of thumb, index, ring and little finger ('PAD') Dorsal interossei: abduction of index, middle and ring finger ('DAB') Adductor pollicis: thumb adduction

DIPJ, Distal interphalangeal joint.

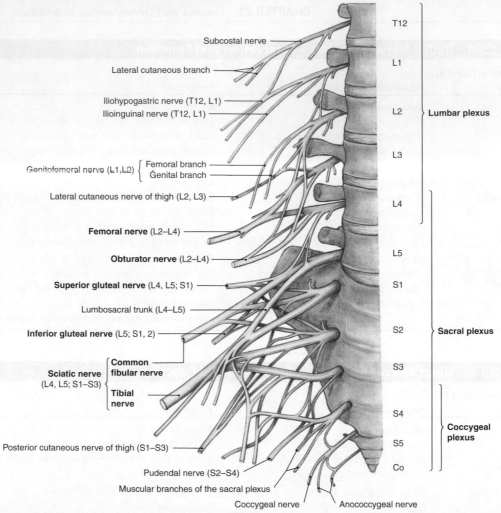

Fig 23.4 Lumbar and Sacral Plexuses. (With permission from Paulsen, Waschke. *Sobotta Atlas of Human Anatomy*, 16th ed. (2018). © Elsevier GmbH, Urban & Fischer, Munich.)

TABLE 23.6 Femoral Nerve Branches – Innervation and Function

Femoral Nerve (L2–L4) Branches	Innervation	Function
Muscular	**Muscles:** all anterior compartment muscles of the thigh and one medial compartment muscle. (Mnemonic: Queen Songs Improve Party Playlists) • Quadriceps femoris (vastus lateralis, vastus intermedius, vastus medialis, rectus femoris) • Sartorius • Iliacus • Psoas • Pectineus (medial compartment muscle)	**Motor:** Hip flexion, knee extension. Pectineus assists in hip adduction
Cutaneous: medial cutaneous, intermediate cutaneous, saphenous nerve	**Skin:** medial and anterior aspects of the thigh	**Sensation:** over the medial and anterior aspects of the thigh
Articular	**Joint:** hip and knee joint	**Joint:** innervation of synovial fluid, ligaments, fibrous capsule

TABLE 23.7 Obturator Nerve Branches – Innervation and Function

Obturator Nerve (L2–L4) Branches	Innervation	Function
Muscular branches	**Muscles:** all medial compartment muscles except for the pectineus (mnemonic: **All Good Orthopods**) • Adductor longus, brevis, magnus • Gracilis • Obturator externus	**Motor:** Hip adduction, internal and external rotation
Cutaneous branches	**Skin:** medial aspect of the thigh	**Sensation:** medial aspect of the thigh
Articular branches	**Joint:** hip and knee joint	**Joint:** innervation of synovial fluid, ligaments, fibrous capsule

TABLE 23.8 Sciatic Nerve Branches – Innervation and Function

Sciatic Nerve (L4–S3) Branches	Innervation	Function
Main trunk muscular branches	**Muscles:** all muscles of the posterior compartment of the thigh (the hamstrings): • Biceps femoris • Semitendinosus • Semimembranosus	**Motor:** Knee flexion, Hip extension
Tibial nerve has the following branches: Muscular Cutaneous (sural nerve) Articular	**Muscles:** all muscles in the superficial posterior compartment of the leg (mnemonic: **GPS**) • Gastrocnemius • Plantaris • Soleus All muscles in the deep posterior compartment of the leg (mnemonic: **Pongy Feet From Trainers**) • Popliteus • Flexor hallucis longus • Flexor digitorum longus • Tibialis posterior **Skin:** lateral side of the leg, foot and 5th toe **Joint:** knee joint	**Motor:** Knee flexion, plantar flexion **Sensation:** lateral side of the leg, foot and 5th toe **Joint:** innervation of synovial fluid, ligaments, fibrous capsule
Common peroneal (fibular) nerve divides into: • Deep peroneal (motor + cutaneous), • Superficial peroneal (motor + cutaneous)	DEEP PERONEAL **Muscle:** all muscles in the anterior compartment of the leg (mnemonic: **FEET**) • Fibularis tertius (peroneus) • Extensor hallucis longus • Extensor digitorum longus • Tibialis anterior **Skin:** web between 1st and 2nd toe SUPERFICIAL PERONEAL **Muscle:** all muscles in the lateral compartment of the leg: fibularis longus and fibularis brevis **Skin:** lateral aspect of leg and dorsum of foot (except web between 1st and 2nd toe)	DEEP PERONEAL: **Motor:** Foot dorsiflexion, eversion and inversion **Sensation:** web between 1st and 2nd toe SUPERFICIAL PERONEAL **Motor:** Foot plantar flexion and eversion **Sensation:** lateral aspect of leg and dorsum of foot (except web between 1st and 2nd toe)

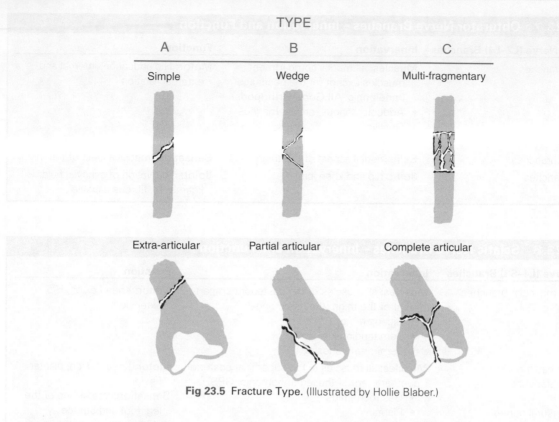

TYPE

A	B	C
Simple	Wedge	Multi-fragmentary

Extra-articular	Partial articular	Complete articular

Fig 23.5 Fracture Type. (Illustrated by Hollie Blaber.)

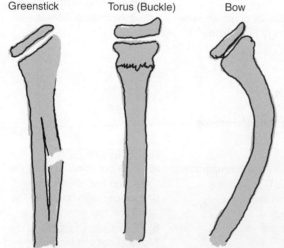

Greenstick   Torus (Buckle)   Bow

Fig 23.6 Paediatric Fractures. (Illustrated by Hollie Blaber.)

- **Subgroup:** used only for complete articular fractures. It describes the metaphyseal fracture pattern. A number is given for the subgroup: Simple articular with a simple metaphyseal pattern (1), Simple articular with a multifragmentary metaphyseal pattern (2),

Multifragmentary articular with a multifragmentary metaphyseal (3).

- **Paediatric fractures:** greenstick, torus (buckle), bow (plastic deformation), growth plate (see Fig 23.6 & Fig 23.7)

Displacement: if a fracture has moved from its anatomical position, it is called a displacement. The movement of the **distal** fragment is described in relation to the **proximal** fragment, i.e., assuming the proximal fragment has remained in the normal position (see Figure 23.8). The following terminology is used to describe **displaced** fractures (mnemonic STAR):

- **S**hortening/lengthening
- **T**ranslation (posterior/anterior/lateral/medial shift) of the distal fragment respective to the proximal fragment. The amount of translation is expressed as a percentage of the width of the bone at the level of the fracture.
- **A**ngulation (varus/valgus in the coronal plane, lateral/medial in the sagittal plane). The angle is measured as the deviation from the long axis of the proximal fragment.

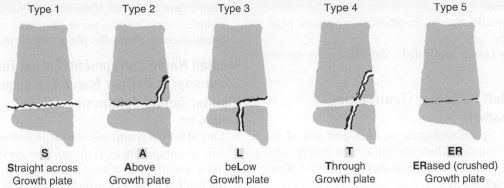

Fig 23.7 Salter-Harris Classification of Growth Plate Fractures. Type 2 is the most common. (Illustrated by Hollie Blaber.)

Type 1	Type 2	Type 3	Type 4	Type 5
S	**A**	**L**	**T**	**ER**
Straight across Growth plate	**A**bove Growth plate	be**L**ow Growth plate	**T**hrough Growth plate	**ER**ased (crushed) Growth plate

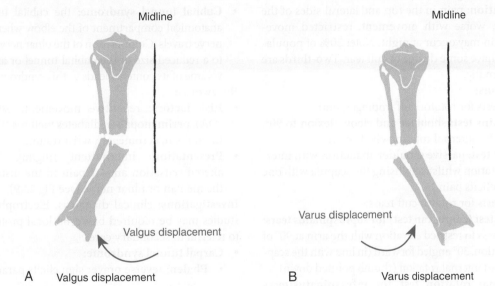

Fig 23.8 (A) **Valgus** and (B) **varus displacements.** The midline represents the anatomical position of the proximal fragment. The distal fragment is used to describe the displacement. (Illustrated by Hollie Blaber.)

- Rotation. The degree of rotation can be difficult to assess on radiographs and is best appreciated clinically.

UPPER LIMB ELECTIVE

Epicondylitis

Definition:
- **Medial epicondylitis (golfer's elbow):** caused by common **flexor** tendon overuse. The origin of the common flexor tendon lies on the medial epicondyle of the humerus.
- **Lateral epicondylitis (tennis elbow):** caused by common **extensor** tendon overuse. The origin of the common extensor tendon lies on the lateral epicondyle of the humerus.

Buzzwords:

- **Causes:**
  - **Golfer's elbow:** repetitive strain on wrist flexion and, to a lesser extent, finger flexion (e.g., striking the floor in golf)
  - **Tennis elbow:** repetitive strain on wrist extension and, to a lesser extent, finger extension (e.g., tennis backhand stroke)
- **Presentation:**
  - **Golfer's elbow:** tender medial epicondyle; painful, resisted wrist flexion, finger flexion and forearm pronation
  - **Tennis elbow:** tender lateral epicondyle; painful, resisted wrist and middle finger extension

Investigations: clinical diagnosis

Differentials: bursitis, gout, pseudogout, ulnar neuritis (medial side), radio-capitellar osteoarthritis (lateral side)

Management:

- **Conservative:** activity modification, analgesia, physiotherapy
- **Surgery (rarely indicated):** debridement ± tendon repair

Rotator Cuff Pathology (Tear/Strain/Tendinopathy)

Definition: an inflammation or tearing of any of the rotator cuff muscles. There are four rotator cuff muscles (mnemonic 'SITS'): **S**upraspinatus, **I**nfraspinatus, **T**eres minor, **S**ubscapularis.

Buzzwords:

- **Risk factors:** age, history of trauma
- **Presentation:** pain in the top and lateral sides of the shoulder, worse with movement, restricted movement, pain may occur at night. Note: 20% of population will have some degree of cuff tear. Two-thirds are asymptomatic.

Investigations:

- Special tests for rotator cuff impingement:
  - **Hawkins test:** shoulder and elbow flexion to 90°, shoulder internal rotation elicits pain
  - **Neers test:** passive shoulder abduction with internal rotation whilst stabilising the scapula with one hand elicits pain
- Special tests for rotator cuff tears:
  - **Jobe's test (empty can test) for supraspinatus tears:** weakness to resisted elevation with the arm at 90° of abduction, 30° angled forward (in line with the scapula) and internal rotation (thumb pointed down)
  - **External rotation test for infraspinatus/teres minor tears:** weakness to external rotation with the elbow at 90° and adducted
  - **Lift-off test for a subscapularis tear:** weakness/inability of the patient to lift the hand off the back when placed on the lower lumbar spine with the palm facing out. Alternatively, the **belly press test** is useful for older patients with more restricted/stiffer joints and those with recent injuries, as they find this test more tolerable. In this test, the palms are placed on the belly and the elbows are pushed forward while the patient attempts to resist the examiner pushing the elbows back.
- **Ultrasound or MRI:** to assess the rotator cuff

Management:

- Analgesia, corticosteroid injections and physiotherapy
- Consider surgery if the pain is persistent despite conservative treatment. Options include an arthroscopic or open rotator cuff repair. If the tear is irreparable, options include suprascapular nerve ablation, arthroscopic debridement or even arthroplasty (reverse prosthesis)

Median Nerve Entrapment (Carpal Tunnel Syndrome) and Ulnar Nerve Entrapment (Cubital Tunnel Syndrome)

Definition:

- **Carpal tunnel syndrome:** the carpal tunnel is an anatomical compartment of the wrist where the median nerve and the flexor tendons run. Compression of the median nerve either due to a reduced size of the carpal tunnel or an increased volume of its contents leads to this syndrome.
- **Cubital tunnel syndrome:** the cubital tunnel is an anatomical compartment of the elbow where the ulnar nerve travels. Compression of the ulnar nerve either due to a reduced size of the cubital tunnel or an increased volume of its contents leads to this syndrome.

Buzzwords:

- **Risk factors:** repetitive movement, osteoarthritis (OA), perimenopause, diabetes mellitus (DM), hypothyroidism, acromegaly, wrist trauma
- **Presentation:** intermittent tingling, numbness, altered sensation and/or pain in the distribution of the median or ulnar nerve (see Fig 23.9)

Investigations: clinical diagnosis. Electrophysiological studies may be required based on local protocols prior to referral to secondary care.

- **Carpal tunnel syndrome:**
  - **Phalen:** reverse prayer sign elicits paraesthesias

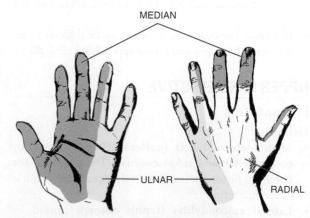

Fig 23.9 Sensory Supply by the Median Nerve (*grey*), Ulnar Nerve (*yellow*) and Radial Nerve (*uncoloured*). (Illustrated by Hollie Blaber.)

- **Tinel:** tapping on the median nerve elicits paraesthesia
- **Durkan's test:** pressure over the proximal edge of the carpal ligament elicits symptoms
- **Hand elevation test:** both hands are elevated above the head, which elicits paraesthesia in <2 min
- **Cubital tunnel syndrome:**
  - Ulnar nerve may be irritable on palpation
  - Rule out an ulnar nerve subluxation (out of the groove)
  - Note: A positive Tinel's test is often seen

Management:
- Lifestyle modifications (e.g., avoiding repetitive movements) and physiotherapy
- Wrist splints at night for carpal tunnel syndrome
- Corticosteroid injection for carpal tunnel syndrome (may provide relief for up to 18 months, although often less)
- Surgical decompression may be considered for patients with persistent or severe symptoms

UPPER LIMB TRAUMA

Distal Radial Fractures

Definition:

Extra-articular distal radial fractures:
- **Colles':** extra-articular distal radial fracture with dorsal displacement (see Fig 23.10) (mnemonic 'Collie **D**og = **C**olles' **D**orsal displacement')
- **Smith's:** extra-articular distal radial fracture with volar displacement (see Fig 23.10)

Intra-articular distal radial fractures:
- **Barton's:** intra-articular distal radial fracture with dorsal displacement (mnemonic '**B**ad **D**og = **B**arton's **D**orsal displacement)

- **Volar Barton's:** intra-articular distal radial fracture with volar displacement

Buzzwords:
- **Risk factors:** osteoporosis risk factors (e.g., steroid use, age, female, early menopause), trauma
- **Presentation:** pain, deformity, redness ± neurovascular compromise

Investigations:
- **X-ray** two views (AP and lateral) (see Radiology in an Hour)
- **CT:** if the fracture is complex and/or it is required for surgical planning
- **MRI:** can be useful if the diagnosis is equivocal, may reveal significant soft tissue injuries or other fractures (e.g., scaphoid)

Management:

Closed fractures:
- **Dorsal displacement (Colles' fracture) without significant deformity/neurovascular compromise:**
  - Closed manipulation under regional anaesthesia with a plaster cast with 3-point moulding in neutral flexion for 4 weeks
  - Fracture clinic within 72 h
  - Early mobilisation as pain allows once the plaster is removed
- **Dorsal displacement (Colles' fracture) with significant deformity/neurovascular compromise:**
  - Age <65 years: if possible, a closed manipulation and K wires. If not possible to achieve a satisfactory reduction, then an open reduction and internal fixation
  - Age >65 years: non-operative treatment may be suitable unless there is significant deformity or neurological compromise

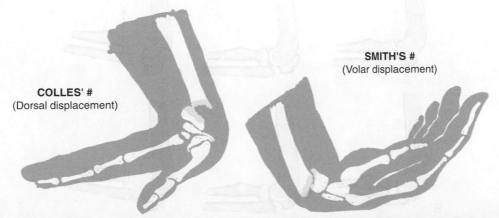

COLLES' #
(Dorsal displacement)

SMITH'S #
(Volar displacement)

Fig 23.10 Mechanism of Injury in a Colles' Fracture and Smith's Fracture. (Illustrated by Hollie Blaber.)

- **Volar displacement (Smith's fracture) regardless of deformity/neurovascular compromise:** these fractures are unstable and require an open reduction and plate fixation within 1 week
- **Intra-articular fractures (Barton's and reverse Barton):** an open reduction and plate fixation is recommended within 72 h

Open fractures:

- Initial surgical exploration and debridement
- Fixation if skin closure is achievable
- Complex wounds may need plastic surgery input

Scaphoid Fractures

Definition: a fracture of the scaphoid bone that occurs due to a fall on an outstretched hand (FOOSH). These fractures have a high risk of avascular necrosis (AVN) due to the retrograde radial blood supply by the **dorsal carpal branch of the radial artery.** Scaphoid fracture classification:

- Scaphoid waist fractures (most common)
- Scaphoid proximal pole fractures
- Distal scaphoid fractures

Buzzwords:

- **Risk factors:** young male
- **Presentation:** there is a strong possibility of a scaphoid fracture if ≥2 of the following examination findings are present: anatomical snuffbox tenderness,

tenderness when axially loading the thumb and/or scaphoid tubercle tenderness

Investigations:

- Consider an **MRI** for first-line imaging if a scaphoid fracture is suspected
- **X-ray scaphoid series** (AP, lateral, two obliques) and wrist X-ray (see Radiology in an Hour)

Differentials: sprain, radial fracture, De Quervain's tenosynovitis, scapholunate ligament tear

Management:

- **Minimally displaced fracture:** scaphoid cast until clinical/radiographic union (typically 8 weeks)
- **Displaced fracture:** if a waist or scaphoid fracture is displaced by more than 2 mm, fixation is recommended

Olecranon Bursitis

Definition:

- **Bursitis:** inflammation of the bursa. Note: Bursitis may occur anywhere in the body that bursae are located. Common sites include olecranon, trochanteric, various knee bursae and the adventitious bursae overlying the hallux valgus
- **Infective bursitis:** inflammation and infection of the bursa
- **Septic bursitis:** bursa inflammation, infection and associated septicaemia

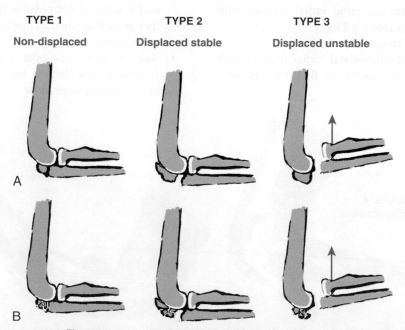

Fig 23.11 Mayo Classification of Olecranon Fractures.

TYPE 1 — Non-displaced   TYPE 2 — Displaced stable   TYPE 3 — Displaced unstable

Buzzwords:

- **Risk factors:** mechanical stress on bursa, rheumatoid arthritis (RA), penetrating injuries, infection of a nearby joint
- **Presentation:**
  - Bursitis: pain, tenderness, erythema and warmth around affected bursa. Limited movement
  - Infective bursitis: as above ± fever
  - Septic bursitis: bursitis presentation + septicaemia signs/symptoms (e.g., fever, hypotension)

Investigations:

- **Bursa aspiration** (always check with senior colleagues first) for microscopy, cultures and sensivities (MC&S)
- **Blood cultures:** *Staphylococcus aureus* is the most common microorganism identified.
- **Blood:** there may be ↑ WCC, ↑ CRP/ESR
- **Ultrasound (US) or MRI:** consider for assessment of the soft tissues and to identify a foreign body if in doubt

Differentials: cellulitis, gout, pseudogout

Management:

- **Inflammatory bursitis:** analgesia
- **Infective bursitis:** analgesia + antibiotics (NICE Guidelines: Initially Flucloxacillin. If penicillin allergic then Clarithromycin. Once cultures are back, treat based on sensitivities) ± surgical debridement
- **Septic bursitis:** sepsis protocol + analgesia + antibiotics (NICE Guidelines: Initially Flucloxacillin. If penicillin allergic then Clarithromycin. Once cultures are back, treat based on sensitivities) ± surgical debridement

Olecranon Fractures

Definition: a fracture of the olecranon, usually as a result of direct trauma. Fractures are classified according to the Mayo classification system (see Fig 23.11):

- **Type 1** (non-displaced), **Type 2** (displaced and stable, ulno-humeral joint preserved), **Type 3** (displaced and unstable, ulnar-humeral joint disrupted)
- **Type A** (transverse), **Type B** (comminuted)

Buzzwords:

- **Risk factors:** FOOSH, twisting injury, direct trauma
- **Presentation:** posterior elbow pain and swelling ± ulnar nerve injury

Investigations: X-ray (AP and lateral)

Differentials: olecranon bursitis, gout, pseudogout, septic arthritis

Management:

- **Nondisplaced fracture:** mobilise as pain allows and repeat X-rays to monitor for displacement

- **Displaced fracture:** tension-band construct (using wires or sutures) or plate fixation.
- Consider nonoperative management regardless of the fracture configuration in a low-demand, comorbid elderly patient, as there is a high risk of complications with ORIF in this group.

Shoulder Dislocation

Definition: an **anterior dislocation** (more common) occurs as a result of forced abduction and external rotation. A **posterior dislocation** (less common, may occur in seizures/electrocution) occurs as a result of forced adduction and internal rotation.

Buzzwords:

- **Risk factors:** hypermobility syndrome, female, trauma
- **Presentation:** shoulder pain/deformity, reduced range of motion

Investigations: X-ray – AP, axillary, scapula Y view (see Radiology in an Hour)

- **Anterior glenohumeral joint (GHJ) dislocation:** humeral head lies medial and inferior to the glenoid
- **Posterior GHJ dislocation:** 'light bulb sign' on the AP view

Differentials: fracture, subluxation

Management: reduction under sedation – several methods exist (beyond the scope of this book). Indications for surgery include an inability to reduce, a symptomatic rotator cuff tear, fracture dislocation and recurrent instability (or a high risk of). For further information, see the BESS guidelines on traumatic shoulder instability.

Proximal Humeral Fracture

Definition: the proximal humerus includes the anatomical neck (old epiphyseal plate), surgical neck, greater tuberosity (insertion point of three rotator cuff muscles – supraspinatus, infraspinatus, teres minor) and the lesser tuberosity (insertion of one rotator cuff muscle – subscapularis) of the humerus. Common fracture in the elderly population who have osteoporotic bone.

Buzzwords:

- **Risk factors:** elderly, osteoporosis
- **Presentation:** pain, reduced range of motion ± axillary nerve damage

Investigations:

- **X-ray:** True AP (**Grashey view**), scapular Y, axillary lateral

- **CT** for surgical planning
- **Neer classification:** number of parts involved (greater tuberosity, lesser tuberosity, articular surface, shaft)

Management:
- **Conservative management:** the majority of proximal humerus fractures can be managed conservatively using a collar and cuff. Appropriate if:
  - Minimal displacement
  - Poor surgical candidate
- **Surgery** is considered if there is significant displacement, head-splitting fractures, fracture dislocations:
  - Closed reduction and percutaneous pinning (CRPP)
  - Open reduction and internal fixation (ORIF)
  - Intramedullary nailing
  - Hemiarthroplasty
  - Reverse total shoulder

Clavicle Fracture

Definition: usually results from trauma/fall on the shoulder. Classification based on the position (medial, middle and lateral third) and degree of displacement
Buzzwords:
- **Risk factors:** children, contact sports
- **Presentation:** pain, swelling around the clavicle, reduced range of motion ± neurovascular compromise. May have a concurrent pneumothorax
Investigations:
- **X-ray:** AP and cephalic view tilt, check for pneumothoraces
Management:
- Conservative management in a sling for the majority of fractures
- Surgical indications: open fracture, impending skin breakdown or necrosis, symptomatic non-union, neurovascular compromise
- Consider surgery if severely displaced and shortened

LOWER LIMB ELECTIVE

Knee Ligament Injuries

Definition: injury to any of the four ligaments involved in knee stability:
- **Anterior cruciate ligament (ACL) injury:** occurs due to a **twisting** motion. There may be an associated medial collateral ligament (MCL) injury and meniscal tear
- **Posterior cruciate ligament (PCL) injury:** occurs when the knee is flexed and the tibia is forced **posteriorly**

- **Medial collateral ligament (MCL) injury:** occurs due to direct trauma to the **lateral** aspect of the knee (**valgus stress**)
- **Lateral collateral ligament (LCL) injury:** occurs due to direct trauma to the **medial** aspect of the knee (**varus stress**)
Buzzwords:
- **Risk factors:** sports, road traffic accidents
- **Presentation:**
  - **ACL:** hemarthrosis, pain, reduced range of motion (ROM), sensation of a 'pop'
  - **PCL:** 'knee gives way', unable to bear weight
  - **MCL:** localised tenderness
  - **LCL:** diagnosis may be missed, as instability may be less common
Investigations:
- Special test for ACL injuries:
  - **Anterior drawer test:** knee flexion to 90° and pulling the proximal tibia anteriorly shows an increased laxity of the ACL injury without a firm endpoint when translating the tibia anteriorly
  - **Lachman test:** a variant of the anterior drawer test, but the knee is flexed to 15° instead of 90° and the femur is fixed with the examiner's other hand
- Special test for PCL injuries:
  - **Posterior drawer test:** knee flexion to 90° and pushing the proximal tibia posteriorly shows increased laxity
- Special test for MCL injury:
  - **Valgus stress test:** knee valgus stress shows increased laxity with a MCL injury. Test is done with the knee in slight flexion
- Special test for LCL injury:
  - **Varus stress test:** knee varus stress shows increased laxity with an LCL injury. Test is done with the knee in slight flexion
- **MRI:** to confirm the diagnosis
Differentials: other ligamentous ruptures, fracture, meniscal tear
Management:
- **ACL:** These injuries have no ability to repair on their own. If there are persistent symptoms of instability, a surgical repair or reconstruction is required.
- **PCL:** These injuries may be able to heal on their own.
- **MCL:** These injuries typically heal well on their own over 6–8 weeks. No surgical intervention is needed, although physiotherapy and a brace may be offered for symptomatic relief.

- **LCL:** These injuries may not heal on their own and are usually treated with a surgical repair, fixation or graft augmentation if symptomatically unstable. These injuries usually happen in combination with other injuries requiring fixation.

Meniscal Tear

Definition: commonly occurs as a result of a traumatic tear in the young who have a normal meniscus or a degenerative tear in the elderly. There may be an associated ACL and/or MCL injury, which is much more likely to occur with a traumatic tear. Classification is based on the location, size and pattern.

Buzzwords:
- **Risk factors:** young, sports, elderly (degenerative changes)
- **Presentation:** knee pain, joint effusion, locked knee (unable to fully extend), 'click' sensation

Investigations:
- **Clinical diagnosis:** a combination of history and examination showing pain in the affected compartment, joint line tenderness and mechanical symptoms. Positive meniscal provocation tests, such as Thessaly and McMurray's
- **X-ray:** to rule out a fracture
- **MRI:** to confirm a meniscal tear

Management:
- Conservative treatment for degenerative tears: physiotherapy ± knee injection for symptomatic relief
- Surgical options for traumatic tears, preservation of the meniscus is preferred in this group:
  - Partial menisccectomy
  - Meniscal repair
  - Meniscal transplant

LOWER LIMB TRAUMA

Hip Fracture

Definition: fractures of the proximal femur anywhere from the femoral head up to 5 cm below the lesser trochanter. Hip fractures are classified according to the fracture location in relation to the hip joint capsule (see Fig 23.12).
- **Intracapsular:** includes subcapital, transcervical and basicervical
- **Extracapsular:** includes trochanteric and subtrochanteric

Intracapsular fractures are at risk of inducing AVN of the femoral head due to the retrograde blood supply to the femoral head.

- Majority of the blood supply is from the lateral and medial circumflex arteries (branches of the femoral artery)
- Small contribution from the ligamentum teres artery and intramedullary supply

Intracapsular neck of femur (NOF) fractures can also be classified according to the fracture pattern using the Garden classification system (see Fig 23.13):
- **Garden 1:** Incomplete NOF fracture, minimal displacement or valgus impacted
- **Garden 2:** Complete NOF fracture **without** displacement
- **Garden 3:** Complete NOF fracture with **partial** displacement
- **Garden 4:** Complete NOF fracture with **full** displacement

Buzzwords:
- **Risk factors:** osteoporosis, malignancy
- **Presentation:** shortened and externally rotated leg, pain in groin/thigh that may radiate to the knee

Investigations:
- **Blood:** routine preoperative blood tests (e.g., FBC, U&E, G&S) and postoperative blood tests (e.g., FBC, U&E)
- **X-ray (pelvis AP and lateral hip):** Shenton's line may be disrupted on the AP film, fracture may be confirmed on the lateral film

Management:
1. Analgesia whilst waiting for surgery, including a fascia iliaca block
2. Surgery with an aim of the patient being able to fully bear weight (without restriction) in the immediate postoperative period (see Table 23.9)
3. Postsurgery:
   - Early mobilisation and physiotherapy
   - Orthogeriatric assessment if elderly to assess risk factors and manage accordingly
   - Venous thromboembolism (VTE) prophylaxis for 28 days post-NOF fracture

Standards for the management of NOF fractures are dictated by national guidelines and are outlined in the Best Practice Tariff (BPT) for Fragility Hip Fractures

Ankle Fractures

Definition:
- Weber classification for fibula fractures depending on the position in relation to the syndesmosis (see Fig 23.14):
  - **Weber A** (fibular fracture below the tibiofibular syndesmosis): likely *stable*

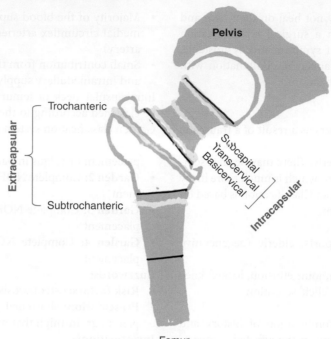

Fig 23.12 Hip Fractures. (Illustrated by Hollie Blaber.)

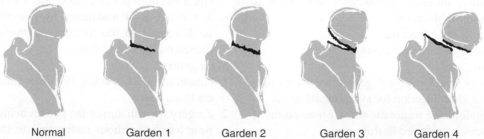

Fig 23.13 Garden Classification System for Hip Fractures. (Illustrated by Hollie Blaber.)

TABLE 23.9	**Hip Fracture Management Options**	
Hip Fractures	**Fracture Pattern**	**Management**
Nondisplaced intracapsular	Subcapital Transcervical Basicervical	Low risk of AVN; therefore, consider fixation of the femoral head and monitoring Counsel patients that a further operation may be needed if AVN develops or non-union occurs For elderly/high-risk patients, replacement rather than fixation may be most appropriate Note that a basicervical fracture tends to be treated more like a trochanteric fracture
Displaced intracapsular	Subcapital Transcervical Basicervical	High risk of AVN NICE guidelines: • **Offer a total hip replacement if** able to walk independently with no more than one stick AND No cognitive impairment AND Medically fit for anaesthesia and the procedure • **Otherwise offer hemiarthroplasty** • Consider fixation in very young patients
Extracapsular	Trochanteric	Dynamic hip screw or intramedullary if reverse oblique pattern
	Subtrochanteric	Intramedullary nail

AVN, Avascular necrosis.

- **Weber B** (fibular fracture at the level of the tibiofibular syndesmosis): may or may not be stable. Requires assessment of the ankle mortise for congruency
- **Weber C** (fibular fracture above the tibiofibular syndesmosis): likely *unstable*
- Ankle fractures can also be classified according to malleolar fracture involvement:
  - Unimalleolar
  - Bimalleolar: medial and lateral malleolar fractures
  - Trimalleolar: medial, lateral and posterior malleolar fractures

Buzzwords:
- **Risk factors:** high-energy sports, osteoporosis, smoking
- **Presentation:** pain, bruising, swelling, ankle deformity, may be unable to weight bear

Investigations: the examination will guide which imaging to request:
- **Ankle X-ray:** to include AP, lateral and **mortise** views (the mortise view allows for an assessment of talar shift, see Fig 23.15). Note: be aware that if the patient is not fully weightbearing (due to pain/reluctant to do so), the mortise view may look normal even in the presence of instability
- **Whole-leg X-ray:** to rule out a Maisonneuve injury (suspect if there is proximal fibular tenderness or a talar shift on the mortise view with no distal fibular fracture)
- Consider CT imaging for surgical planning if there is a complex fracture pattern or you are unsure if the syndesmosis has been disrupted

Differentials: deltoid ligament tear

Management:
- Reduction and splinting
- **Stable fractures (Weber A, Weber B without a talar shift):**
  - Analgesia, splinting, weight bearing as tolerated
  - Consider a repeat weight-bearing X-ray to assess stability
  - Thromboprophylaxis as per local protocols
  - Follow up in 6 weeks
- **Unstable fractures (Weber C, Weber B with a talar shift):**
  - Open reduction internal fixation (ORIF)
  - Postsurgery: analgesia, weight bearing as tolerated, thromboprophylaxis, 6-week follow-up
  - >60 years of age: a closed reduction and ankle casting is equivalent to internal fixation for unstable malleolar fractures

Osteomyelitis

Definition: an infection of the bone or bone marrow arising from direct/contiguous spread (e.g., cellulitis, abscess, trauma, surgery) or haematogenous spread. This condition results in inflammatory destruction of the bone and necrosis (sequestrum). A large sequestrum that remains in situ acts as a focus for ongoing infection. The most common pathogen is *S. aureus*. Other pathogens include *Escherichia coli*, *Pseudomonas* and *Streptococcus*.

Buzzwords:
- **Risk factors:** vascular disease, trauma, diabetic feet, intravenous drug use (IVDU), sickle cell disease, immunosuppression, chronic skin infections, prosthesis, chronic joint disease
- **Presentation:** pain, tenderness, erythema, warmth, reduced ROM, effusion in neighbouring joints, signs of systemic infection

Investigations:
- **Blood:** ↑ WCC and CRP
- **X-ray:** changes take 10–14 days or longer to appear. They may include haziness, decreased bone density, subperiosteal reaction, sequestrum and involucrum

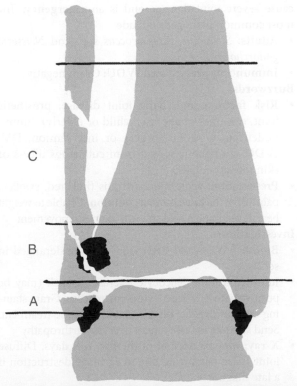

Fig 23.14 Weber Fractures. (Illustrated by Hollie Blaber.)

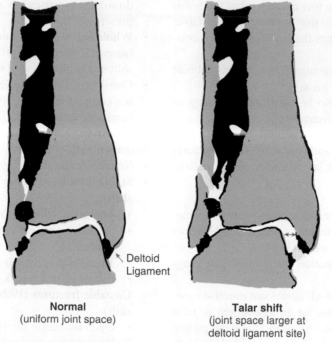

Normal
(uniform joint space)

Talar shift
(joint space larger at
deltoid ligament site)

↖ Deltoid
Ligament

Fig 23.15 Normal Ankle Joint vs a Talar Shift. (Illustrated by Hollie Blaber.)

- **MRI (more sensitive than X-ray):** may show signs of infection in the medullary canal or surrounding soft tissues, bone destruction
- **Blood cultures:** sensitivities will guide therapy
- **Bone biopsy and culture (intra-operative):** sensitivities will guide therapy

Differentials: gout, septic arthritis

Management:

1. IV antibiotics for 4–6 weeks in most cases. Chronic infection may require long-term (>3 months) treatment, usually oral. Follow local microbiology guidelines. BNF recommendations for patients without diabetes or a prosthesis include:
   - IV flucloxacillin (consider adding fusidic acid or rifampicin for first 2 weeks)
   - **If penicillin allergic:** IV clindamycin (consider adding fusidic acid or rifampicin for first 2 weeks)
   - **If *S. aureus* is suspected:** IV vancomycin or teicoplanin (consider adding fusidic acid or rifampicin for first 2 weeks)
2. Debridement to drain pus and remove sequestra if severe

Septic Arthritis

Definition: an infection of one or more joints caused by pathogenic inoculation of microorganisms into the joint, either directly or by haematogenous spread. It can cause severe joint damage and is an **emergency.** The most common pathogens include:

- **Adults:** *S. aureus*, *Streptococcus* spp. and *Neisseria gonorrhoea*
- **Immunosuppressed and IVDU:** Gram negative

Buzzwords:

- **Risk factors:** underlying joint disease, prosthetic joint, extremes of age (e.g., child or elderly), immunodeficiency, recent surgery or intervention, DM, IVDU, contiguous spread from cutaneous ulcers or skin infection, CKD
- **Presentation:** acute monoarthritis (hot, red, swollen, painful) of the **knee is most common.** Unable to weight bear, fever, joint is held still with pain on movement

Investigations:

- **Blood:** ↑ WCC and CRP, U&E may be deranged in sepsis
- **Joint aspiration:** leucocyte esterase dipstick (may be positive with ≥ 2+ leucocytes), microscopy, Gram staining and cultures for diagnosis and to guide treatment. Send samples for assessment of crystal arthropathy
- **X-ray:** may be normal in the first few days. Diffuse joint space narrowing due to cartilage destruction if a late diagnosis

- **Blood cultures:** if an organism is found, sensitivities will guide antibiotic therapy

Differentials: crystal arthropathy, reactive arthritis, trauma, flare-up of OA

Management:

1. **Antibiotics for 4–6 weeks** (initially IV for 2 weeks) according to local microbiology guidelines. Follow local guidelines. BNF recommendations for patients without DM or a prosthesis include:
   - IV flucloxacillin *or*
   - **If penicillin allergic:** IV clindamycin
   - **If *S. aureus* suspected:** IV vancomycin or teicoplanin
   - **If Gram negative or gonococcal suspected:** IV cefotaxime or ceftriaxone
   - Seek expert advice if the patient has diabetes or a prosthesis
2. **Surgical management:** drainage of the joint if severe or an open washout in theatre
3. **Monitor for complications:** osteomyelitis, arthritis

OPEN FRACTURES

Definition: fracture with an overlying break in the skin. Open fractures have a significantly increased risk of infection and subsequent complications. May be an orthopaedic emergency requiring an urgent intervention

Buzzwords:

- **Risk factors:** road traffic accidents, high-energy injuries
- **Presentation:** may present with multiple injuries, requiring the Advanced Trauma Life Support (ATLS) approach

Gustillo-Anderson Classification (determined post-debridement):

- Type I: wound <1 cm, minimal contamination or soft tissue damage
- Type II: wound 1–10 cm, moderate soft tissue damage
- Type IIIA: wound >10 cm, contamination, extensive soft tissue injury
- Type IIIB: significant periosteal stripping requiring soft tissue coverage (local or free flap)
- Type IIIC: open fracture with a vascular injury requiring repair

Investigations:

- **Blood:** blood cultures, FBC, U&E, CRP
- **Trauma CT:** head to toe (in the polytrauma patient)
- **CT angiography:** of the affected limb if there is vascular compromise and for planning a soft tissue reconstruction

Management: (Guidelines: BOAST Open Fractures)

- ATLS approach for identifying other life- or limb-threatening injuries
- IV antibiotics within 1 h (pre-hospital if needed) and tetanus vaccine
- Examination and documentation of the neurovascular status
- Remove gross contamination and cover with saline-soaked gauze
- Reduction and splinting with a post-reduction examination of the neurovascular status
- If vascular compromise, emergency vascular referral – revascularisation of the limb should occur within 4 h
- Photography of the injury
- Referral to major trauma centre (MTC) as per BOAST guidelines
- Initial washout and debridement with joint plastic surgery and orthopaedics involvement
- Definitive fixation only when concurrent skin coverage is achievable at the same time

OSTEOARTHRITIS

Definition: Osteoarthritis is a chronic disorder characterised by a progressive loss of cartilage at the synovial joints and degeneration of the underlying bone.

Buzzwords:

- **Risk factors:** family history, aging, female, obesity, previous joint injury, hypermobility, occupation involving manual labour, haemochromatosis, acromegaly, hyperparathyroidism, crystal deposition disease
- **Presentation:** long history of reduced ROM, joint stiffness <30 min, pain exacerbated by movement and relieved by rest, crepitus, bony swelling or deformity
  - **Hand (see Fig 23.16):** Heberden's nodes (distal interphalangeal joint (DIPJ)), Bouchard's nodes ((proximal interphalangeal joint (PIPJ)), joint line tenderness, thumb carpometacarpal (CMC) squaring
  - **Hip:** pain/tenderness on internal rotation, Trendelenburg's sign (see Fig 23.17)
  - **Knee:** pain/tenderness usually on medial side

Investigations:

- **X-ray:** mnemonic LOSS – **L**oss of joint space, **O**steophytes, **S**ubchondral cysts, **S**ubarticular sclerosis.

Differentials: bursitis, tendonitis, muscular pain

Management:

- Physiotherapy
- Analgesia

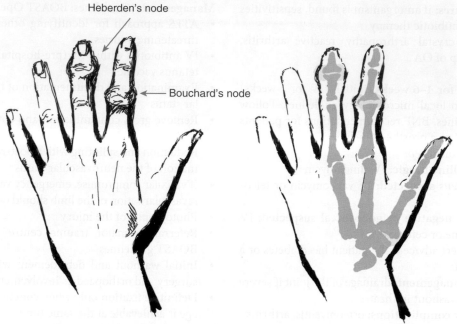

Fig 23.16 Heberden's Nodes and Bouchard's Nodes. (Illustrated by Hollie Blaber.)

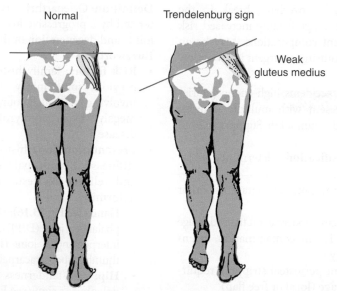

Fig 23.17 Trendelenburg Sign (to test for abductor muscle weakness). The patient stands on one leg and the anterior superior iliac spine (ASIS) of both hips are identified. Normally, the patient can maintain both ASIS aligned due to strong abductor muscles. However, abductor muscle weakness of the standing leg will cause the unsupported side to drop or the patient to tilt excessively in an attempt to achieve balance. This finding indicates a positive Trendelenburg's test. Abductor muscle weakness has multiple causes including osteoarthritis and a previous hip surgery. (Illustrated by Hollie Blaber.)

- Referral to an orthopaedic surgeon if symptoms are refractory to medical management and there is a significant impact on the person's quality of life
- Elective joint replacement may be considered

SPINE

Scoliosis

Definition:
- **Functional scoliosis:** apparent scoliosis due to an extraspinal cause (e.g., leg-length discrepancy)
- **Structural scoliosis:** lateral angulation of the spine in the coronal plane with a Cobb's angle of >10°
- **Types:** idiopathic (80%), congenital, neuromuscular (e.g., cerebral palsy, poliomyelitis), metabolic (e.g., Hunter's syndrome)
- **Types by age:** infantile (age <3 years), juvenile (age 3–10 years), adolescent (age 10 years until skeletal maturity), adult (skeletally mature)

Buzzwords:
- **Risk factors:** trauma, malignancy, male (infantile scoliosis), female (juvenile and adolescent scoliosis)
- **Presentation:** asymptomatic in mild disease (curvatures of 10°–20°), symptomatic with pain/disability for larger curvatures. Adam's forward-bend test is positive (scoliosis is more prominent on flexion)

Investigations:
- **X-ray:** AP and lateral view to determine the Cobb angle. Lateral bending views for surgical planning
- **CT:** to assess the vertebra in detail for surgical planning
- **MRI:** to assess the soft tissue in detail for surgical planning and to assess neurological compromise

Differentials: functional scoliosis

Management: management depends on the severity, neurological compromise and quality of life. Options include:
- **Conservative:** observation, analgesia, orthoses, physiotherapy
- **Surgical:** thoracoplasty, instrumental fusion

BONE AND CARTILAGE TUMOURS

See Tables 23.10–23.13 and Fig 23.18 for a summary of bone and cartilage tumours. See Radiology in an Hour for radiographs of these conditions.

PAEDIATRIC TRAUMA AND ORTHOPAEDICS

Developmental Dysplasia of the Hip

Definition: an array of conditions ranging from hip subluxation and acetabular immaturity to hip dislocation.

TABLE 23.10	Benign Bone Tumours		
Benign Bone Tumours	**Osteoid Osteoma**	**Osteoblastoma**	**Giant Cell Tumours (Osteoclastoma)**
Risk factors	Age 5–25 years, male	Age 10–30 years, male	Age 20–40 years, female
Presentation	Pain at night, worse with exercise, better with NSAIDs	No pain at night, pain cannot be relieved by NSAIDs	Joint pain, reduced range of movement
Location and size	Diaphysis of long bones <1.5-cm diameter	Metaphysis of long bones and spine >1.5-cm diameter	Epiphysis of long bones May grow into the joint
X-ray appearance	Central nidus (radiolucent/black area) surrounded by a sclerotic (dense white) area	Central nidus (radiolucent/black area) surrounded by a sclerotic (dense white) area	'Soap bubble' appearance
Management	NSAIDs	Surgical excision	Surgical excision and regular follow-up
Prognosis	Usually self-resolving	Slow growing Malignant transformation is rare	Fast-growing tumour. Malignant transformation in 10% cases to osteosarcomas
Differentials	Growing pains, fracture, bone infarction, soft tissue injury, other tumours		

NSAIDs, Nonsteroidal antiinflammatory drugs.

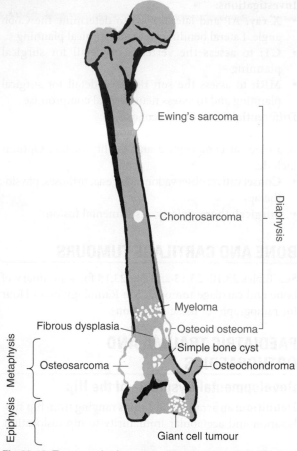

Fig 23.18 Tumours by Location. (Illustrated by Hollie Blaber.)

Labels on figure:
- Ewing's sarcoma
- Chondrosarcoma
- Diaphysis
- Myeloma
- Fibrous dysplasia
- Osteoid osteoma
- Simple bone cyst
- Osteosarcoma
- Osteochondroma
- Giant cell tumour
- Metaphysis
- Epiphysis

Developmental dysplasia of the hip (DDH) affects 1%–3% of newborns with screening occurring at the 6–8-week newborn physical examination performed by general practitioners.

Buzzwords:
- **Risk factors:** sibling with DDH, breech presentation, oligohydramnios, neuromuscular disorders
- **Presentation:** examination may show asymmetry: asymmetrical gluteal or thigh skin folds, reduced range of motion (ROM), limb-length discrepancy. Older children may present with a painless limp

Investigations:
- **Screening:** Barlow's test (screen for a dislocatable hip) and Ortolani's test (screen for a dislocated hip). See Fig 23.19
- **US:** subluxation or dislocation. Only to confirm an abnormal hip examination due to the high false-positive rate. Useful in infants <6 months of age
- **Pelvic X-ray:** useful for infants >6 months of age once the femoral head ossification centre has developed (see Radiology in an Hour)

Differentials: Legg-Calve-Perthes disease

Management:
- **Conservative:** dynamic flexion-abduction orthosis (Pavlik harness)
- **Surgical:** if no response to the harness or diagnosed after 6 months of age, a closed reduction with adductor or psoas tenotomy

Benign Cartilage Tumours	Enchondroma	Osteochondroma	Chondroblastoma
TABLE 23.11	**Benign Cartilage Tumours**		
Risk factors	Age 20–50 years	Adolescence	Age 10–19 years, male
Presentation	Asymptomatic (most common) or pain, pathological fracture, deformity, swelling	Painless lump (most common). Can be painful if surrounded structures are compressed	Pain, swelling, effusion
Location	Small bones Epiphysis of long bones	Metaphysis of long bones	Epiphysis of long bones
X-ray	'Pop-corn' appearance	'Mushroom' appearance	Small lytic lesion surrounded by a thin sclerotic area
Management	Observation if asymptomatic Consider surgery if symptomatic	Observation if asymptomatic. Consider surgery if symptomatic	Surgical excision
Prognosis	Risk of malignant transformation into chondrosarcoma is 1% for a single lesion. If multiple lesions, then the risk varies from 30%–100%	Malignant transformation is rare	
Differentials	Growing pains, fracture, bone infarction, soft tissue injury, other tumours		

TABLE 23.12 Malignant Bone Tumours

Malignant Bone Tumours	Ewing's Sarcoma	Osteosarcoma
Risk factor	Age 10–20 years, male, Caucasian	Children and adolescents, male, genetic link with Li-Fraumeni syndrome and retinoblastoma
Presentation	Pain and local mass effect	Pain and local mass effect
Location	Spine, long bones and shoulder	Metaphysis of long bones
X-ray	'Onion skin' appearance	'Sun burst' appearance with formation of a 'Codman triangle'
Management	Chemotherapy and surgical excision ± radiotherapy. Follow-up required	Chemotherapy and surgical excision
Prognosis	5-year survival is 60%. It can recur after surgical excision and can metastasise to other sites	5-year survival is 60%–80%. It may metastasise to other sites in 10%–20% cases
Differentials	Growing pains, fracture, bone infarction, soft tissue injury, other tumours	

TABLE 23.13 Malignant Cartilage Tumour

Malignant Cartilage Tumour	Chondrosarcoma
Risk factors	Age 30–60 years
Presentation	Pain and local mass effect
Location	Spine, pelvis, shoulder and/or jaw
X-ray	'Moth eaten' appearance. Tumour size of >4 cm
Management	Surgical excision ± radiotherapy. Chemotherapy is usually not effective except for de-differentiated chondrosarcoma (a subtype of chondrosarcoma)
Prognosis	Grade I: 5-year survival is 83%. Grade II–III: 5-year survival is 53%
Differentials	Growing pains, fracture, bone infarction, soft tissue injury, other tumours

Legg-Calve-Perthe Disease

Definition: avascular necrosis of the proximal femoral epiphysis resulting in abnormal growth of the epiphysis. Usually seen in children 3–10 years of age

Buzzwords:

- **Risk factors:** male, caucasian, skeletal dysplasias, hypercoagulable states
- **Presentation:** onset over weeks with no history of trauma. Flexion deformity of the hip, painless limp. Late presentation involves limitations in all hip movements and an antalgic gait

Investigations:

- **Blood:** FBC (normal, ↑ ESR)
- **Bilateral hip X-rays (AP and frog lateral views):** femoral head collapse, widening of the joint space (see Radiology in an Hour)
- **MRI:** femoral head collapse and fragmentation

Differentials: septic arthritis, sickle cell disease, juvenile idiopathic arthritis, transient synovitis of the hip

Management:

- **Conservative:** physiotherapy, restriction of weight-bearing, NSAIDs
- **Surgical:** proximal femoral osteotomy

Slipped Upper Femoral Epiphysis

Definition: instability and anterosuperior displacement of the proximal femoral growth plate (epiphysis). A slipped upper femoral epiphysis (SUFE) is the most common hip disorder of adolescents, mainly affecting those 11–13 years of age.

Buzzwords:

- **Risk factors:** obesity, hypothyroidism, hypopituitarism, growth hormone deficiency, vitamin D deficiency
- **Presentation:** pain in the hip or groin or referred pain to the knee. Pain is worse with running and jumping, limp may be present

Investigations: bilateral hip X-rays (AP and frog lateral views) shows epiphyseal line widening or femoral head displacement (see Fig 23.20 and Radiology in an Hour)

BARLOW'S TEST

Hip flexion + adduction + light posterior pressure

Positive test = femoral head dislocates

ORTOLANI'S TEST

Hip flexion + abduction + light anterior pressure

Positive test = femoral head reduces into acetabulum

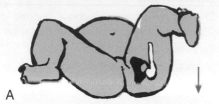 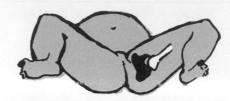

Fig 23.19 (A) Barlow and (B) Ortolani Tests. (Illustrated by Hollie Blaber.)

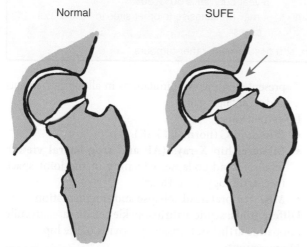

Fig 23.20 Slipped Femoral Epiphysis. (Illustrated by Hollie Blaber.)

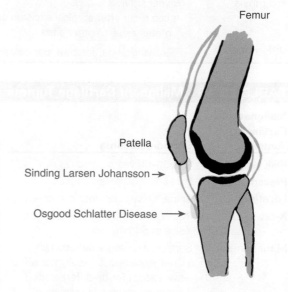

Fig 23.21 Osgood-Schlatter Disease vs Sinding-Larsen-Johansson Disease. (Illustrated by Hollie Blaber.)

Differentials: Perthes' disease, osteomyelitis, hip fracture, septic arthritis

Management: surgery – in situ screw fixation (minimally invasive) ± prophylactic fixation of contralateral hip

Osgood-Schlatter Disease

Definition: traction apophysitis of the tibial tuberosity due to overuse, causing anterior knee pain (see Fig 23.21). Osgood-Schlatter disease (OSD) commonly occurs during the adolescent growth spurt.

Buzzwords:

- **Risk factors:** OSD in the contralateral knee, male, adolescents, sporting activities
- **Presentation:** swelling, pain, erythema and localised tenderness over the tibial tuberosity on palpation

Investigations: knee X-ray may be normal. Enlarged tibial tuberosity, irregularity of the apophysis (see Radiology in an Hour)

Differentials: Sinding-Larsen-Johansson disease (SLJD), fracture, malignancy, osteomyelitis

Management:

- **Conservative:** rest from sport or a reduction in duration/intensity, ice, physiotherapy, analgesia
- **Surgery:** for persistent disease – osteoplasty of tibial tuberosity, rarely required

Osteochondritis Dissecans

Definition: a disease affecting subchondral bone, commonly the knee in children and adolescents with open growth plates. The exact cause is not known but it may be due to inflammation, ischaemia, a genetic predisposition or repetitive trauma.

Buzzwords:

- **Risk factors:** male, trauma, repetitive loading, weight-bearing exercises, family history
- **Presentation:** joint pain that is worse with activity, joint locking. Common sites include the anteromedial aspect of the knee, ankle and lateral aspect of the elbow

Investigations:

- **X-rays:** intra-articular loose body, osteochondral lesion
- **CT:** to identify the site and size of loose body

Differentials: meniscal tear, septic arthritis, osteochondral fracture, OSD, SLJD, osteoarthritis

Management:

- **Conservative:** analgesia, physiotherapy, load reduction
- **Surgery:** arthroscopic subchondral drilling/debridement/excision

Congenital Talipes Equinovarus

Definition: also known as clubfoot, it is characterised by an altered foot morphology in a newborn (see Fig 23.22). Common birth defect affecting 1 in 1000 newborns.

Buzzwords:

- **Risk factors:** family history, male, neuromuscular diseases
- **Presentation:** the hindfoot is in varus, with an adducted forefoot, and the ankle in equinus and cannot be dorsiflexed. The sole of the foot points medially.

Investigations: Usually a clinical diagnosis, AP X-rays can be useful to determine the severity

Differentials: metatarsus adductus

Management:

- **Conservative:** manipulation and casting using the Ponseti method. Maintenance is with a nightly brace for 3 years
- **Surgery:** for a fixed deformity involving an Achilles tenotomy

Radial Head Subluxation (Pulled Elbow)

Definition: also known as nursemaid's elbow, it is caused by a subluxation of the radial head from the encircling annular ligament (see Fig 23.23) and affects children less than 6 years of age.

Buzzwords:

- **Risk factors:** age <6 years, female
- **Presentation:** a sudden history of pain from axial pulling of the arm. The elbow is flexed and pronated, often held against the abdomen with tenderness around the radial head

Investigations:

- **X-rays** if a fracture is suspected or a reduction is unsuccessful

Differentials: Monteggia fracture, congenital dislocation of radial head, non-accidental injury (NAI)

Management: conservative – manipulation either with a pronation or supination method, parent education to prevent reoccurrence, screen for NAI

Osteogenesis Imperfecta

Definition: also known as brittle bone syndrome, it is classified into seven types ranging from osteoporotic bones to multiple fractures and affecting the teeth and sclera.

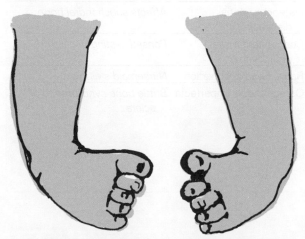

Fig 23.22 Congenital Talipes Equinovarus. (Illustrated by Hollie Blaber.)

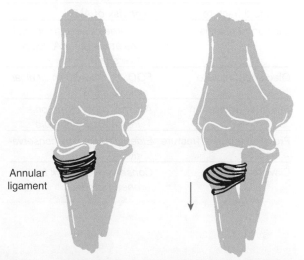

Annular ligament

Fig 23.23 Radial Head Subluxation. (Illustrated by Hollie Blaber.)

Buzzwords:
- **Risk factors:** mutations in type 1 collagen genes
- **Presentation:** childhood fractures, blue sclera, impaired dentition, joint hypermobility, short stature, heart valve deformities

Investigations:
- **US:** prenatally – limb deformity, abnormal skull shape

- **X-rays:** multiple fractures, osteoporotic bones
- **Genetic testing:** mutations in collagen genes

Differentials: achondrogenesis, NAI

Management:
- **Conservative:** physiotherapy and bracing
- **Medical:** bisphosphonates
- **Surgery:** intramedullary rod placement

THE ONE-LINE ROUND-UP!

Here are some key words to help you remember each condition/concept.

Condition/Concept	One-line Description
Epicondylitis	**Medial (golfer's elbow):** flexor tendon overuse. **Lateral (tennis elbow):** extensor tendon overuse
Rotator cuff pathology	**Rotator cuff impingement:** Hawkins test, Neers test. **Rotator cuff tears:** Jobe's test (supraspinatus), external rotation (infraspinatus/ teres minor), lift-off test (subscapularis)
Median and ulnar nerve entrapment	Carpal tunnel = median. cubital = ulnar. Numbness/ tingling/pain in nerve distribution
Distal radial fracture	FOOSH, Colles' = dorsal. Smith's = volar. Barton's = intra-articular
Scaphoid fracture	High risk of AVN
Olecranon bursitis	Tenderness/warmth/erythema at bursa – RA, repetitive strain
Olecranon fracture	FOOSH, elbow pain ±/ ulnar nerve signs
Shoulder dislocation	Anterior most common. Posterior = 'lightbulb'
Proximal humeral fracture	Elderly fall, mostly conservative Mx
Clavicle fracture	Conservative, check for pneumothorax

Condition/Concept	One-line Description
Osteoarthritis	Degenerative, LOSS on x-ray
Knee ligament injuries	ACL/PCL – drawer test, MCL/ LCL – valgus/varus stress test
Meniscal tear	Pain, locking, clicking – after trauma
Neck of femur fracture	Intracapsular vs extracapsular
Ankle fractures	Unstable = Weber C and Weber B with a talar shift
Osteomyelitis	Diabetic feet, vascular disease – long-term Abx
Septic arthritis	Emergency, acute, knee most common
Open fractures	Fracture with skin break
Scoliosis	Cobb's angle >10 degrees
DDH	Barlow & Ortolani Tests
Perthe's disease	3–10 years of age
SUFE	11–13 years of age, obesity
OSD	Apophysitis of tibial tuberosity
Osteochondritis dissecans	Affects subchondral bone
Congenital talipes equinovarus	Ponseti casting
Radial head subluxation	Nursemaid's elbow
Osteogenesis imperfecta	Brittle bone syndrome, blue sclera

READING LIST: TRAUMA AND ORTHOPAEDICS IN AN HOUR

Anatomy

Duckworth, A., Porter, D., & Ralston, S. (2016). *Churchill's pocketbook of orthopaedics, trauma and rheumatology* (2nd ed.). Elsevier.

Bowden, G., McNally, M., Thomas, S., & Gibson, A. (2010). *Oxford handbook of orthopaedics and trauma*. Oxford University Press.

Richard Drake, R., Wayne Vogl, A., & Mitchell, A. (2015). *Gray's anatomy for students* (3rd ed.). Elsevier.

Ellis, H., & Mahadevan, V. (2013). *Clinical anatomy: Applied anatomy for students and junior doctors*. Wiley-Blackwell.

Ortho info. (2015). *Brachial plexus injuries*. https://orthoinfo.aaos.org/en/diseases--conditions/brachial-plexus-injuries. [Accessed March 2021].

Patient info. (2015). *Brachial plexus assessment and common injuries*. https://patient.info/doctor/brachial-plexus-assessment-and-common-injuries. [Accessed March 2021].

Refai, N. A., & Tadi, P. (2021). *Anatomy, bony pelvis and lower limb, thigh femoral nerve*. StatPearls. StatPearls Publishing. https://www.ncbi.nlm.nih.gov/books/NBK556065/.

Lam, J. H., & Bordoni, B. (2021). *Anatomy, shoulder and upper limb, arm abductor muscles*. StatPearls. StatPearls Publishing. https://www.ncbi.nlm.nih.gov/books/NBK537148/.

Fracture Classification

AO Surgery reference. *Simple fracture, Oblique*. https://surgeryreference.aofoundation.org/orthopedic-trauma/adult-trauma/tibial-shaft/simple-fracture-oblique/definition. [Accessed April 2021].

AO Surgery reference. *23-M/2.1 Metaphyseal, torus/buckle fractures, both bones*. https://surgeryreference.aofoundation.org/orthopedic-trauma/pediatric-trauma/distal-forearm/23-m-21/definition?searchurl=%2fSearchResults. [Accessed April 2021].

Meinberg, E. G., Agel, J., Roberts, C. S., Karam, M. D., & Kellam, J. F. (2018). Fracture and dislocation classification compendium – 2018. *Journal of Orthopaedic Trauma, 32,* S1–S10. https://doi.org/10.1097/BOT.0000000000001063

UPPER LIMB ELECTIVE
Epicondylitis

Duckworth, A., Porter, D., & Ralston, S. (2016). *Churchill's pocketbook of orthopaedics, trauma and rheumatology* (2nd ed.). Elsevier.

BMJ Best Practice. (2020). *Epicondylitis*. https://bestpractice.bmj.com/topics/en-gb/978. [Accessed Dec 2020].

NICE. (2017). *CKS: Tennis elbow*. https://cks.nice.org.uk/topics/tennis-elbow/. [Accessed Dec 2020].

Rotator Cuff Pathology

Tokish, J. M., Decker, M. J., Ellis, H. B., Torry, M. R., & Hawkins, R. J. (2003). The belly-press test for the physical examination of the subscapularis muscle: Electromyographic validation and comparison to the lift-off test. *Journal of Shoulder and Elbow Surgery, 12,* 427–430. https://doi.org/10.1016/s1058-2746(03)00047-8

Royal College of Surgeons of England (RCS), British Orthopaedic Association (BOA). (2014). *Commissioning guide: Subacromial shoulder pain*.

NICE. (2017). *CKS: Shoulder pain*. https://cks.nice.org.uk/topics/shoulder-pain/. [Accessed April 2021].

Median Nerve Entrapment And Ulnar Nerve Entrapment

NICE. (2020). *CKS: Carpal tunnel syndrome*. https://cks.nice.org.uk/topics/carpal-tunnel-syndrome/. [Accessed April 2021].

BOA. (2019). *Carpal-Tunnel_Syndrome-Guide-Final*. https://www.boa.ac.uk/resources/carpal-tunnel-syndrome-guide-final--pdf.html. [Accessed April 2021].

Guysandstthomas.nhs. *Cubital tunnel syndrome*. https://www.guysandstthomas.nhs.uk/resources/patient-information/therapies/hand-therapy/cubital%20tunnel%20syndrome.pdf.

Amirfeyz, R., Gozzard, C., & Leslie, I. J. (2005). Hand elevation test for assessment of carpal tunnel syndrome. *The Journal of Hand Surgery (European Volume), 30,* 361–364.

Mason, W., Ryan, D., Khan, A., et al. (2017). Injection versus Decompression for Carpal Tunnel Syndrome-Pilot trial (INDICATE-P)-protocol for a randomised feasibility study. *Pilot Feasibility Studies, 3,* 20. https://doi.org/10.1186/s40814-017-0134-y.

UPPER LIMB TRAUMA
Distal Radial Fractures

BOA. (2017). *The management of distal radial fractures*. https://www.boa.ac.uk/resources/boast-16-pdf.html. [Accessed Nov 2020].

Scaphoid Fractures

Clementson, M., Björkman, A., & Thomsen, N. O. (2020). Acute scaphoid fractures: guidelines for diagnosis and treatment. *EFORT Open Review, 5,* 96–103. https://doi.org/10.1302/2058-5241.5.190025

Duckworth, A., Porter, D., & Ralston, S. (2016). *Churchill's pocketbook of orthopaedics, trauma and rheumatology* (2nd ed.). Elsevier.

Bowden, G., McNally, M., Thomas, S., & Gibson, A. (2010). *Oxford handbook of orthopaedics and trauma*. Oxford University Press.

NICE. (2016). *NG38: Fractures (non-complex): Assessment and management.* https://www.nice.org.uk/guidance/ng38/chapter/Recommendations.

Dias, J. J., Brealey, S. D., Fairhurst, C., et al. (2020). Surgery versus cast immobilisation for adults with a bicortical fracture of the scaphoid waist (SWIFFT): A pragmatic, multicentre, open-label, randomised superiority trial. *Lancet, 396,* 390–401. https://doi.org/10.1016/S0140-6736(20)30931-4

Olecranon Bursitis

Torok, E., Moran, E., & Cooke, F. (2016). *Oxford handbook of infectious diseases and microbiology* (2nd ed.). Oxford University Press, 775–776.

BMJ Best Practice. *Bursitis.* https://bestpractice.bmj.com/topics/en-gb/523. [Accessed November 2020].

Olecranon Fractures

Duckworth, A., Porter, D., & Ralston, S. (2016). *Churchill's pocketbook of orthopaedics, trauma and rheumatology* (2nd ed.). Elsevier.

Bowden, G., McNally, M., Thomas, S., & Gibson, A. (2010). *Oxford handbook of orthopaedics and trauma.* Oxford University Press.

Nazifi, O., Gunaratne, R., D'Souza, H., & Tay, A. (2021). The use of high strength sutures and anchors in olecranon fractures: A systematic review. *Geriatr Orthop Surg Rehabil, 12,* 2151459321996626. https://doi.org/10.1177/2151459321996626.

Chen, M. J., Campbell, S. T., Finlay, A. K., Duckworth, A. D., Bishop, J. A., & Gardner, M. J. (2021). Surgical and nonoperative management of olecranon fractures in the elderly: A systematic review and meta-analysis. *Journal of Orthopaedic Trauma, 35,* 10–16. https://doi.org/10.1097/BOT.0000000000001865

Shoulder Dislocation

Duckworth, A., Porter, D., & Ralston, S. (2016). *Churchill's pocketbook of orthopaedics, trauma and rheumatology* (2nd ed.). Elsevier.

Bowden, G., McNally, M., Thomas, S., & Gibson, A. (2010). *Oxford handbook of orthopaedics and trauma.* Oxford University Press.

Proximal Humeral Fracture

Pencle, F. J., & Varacallo, M. (2021). *Proximal humerus fracture.* StatPearls. StatPearls Publishing. https://www.ncbi.nlm.nih.gov/books/NBK470346/.

Jo, M. J., & Gardner, M. J. (2012). Proximal humerus fractures. *Current Reviews in Musculoskeletal Medicine, 5,* 192–198. https://doi.org/10.1007/s12178-012-9130-2

Clavicle Fracture

Patient info. (2014). *Clavicle fractures.* https://patient.info/doctor/clavicle-fracture. [Accessed April 2021].

LOWER LIMB ELECTIVE
Knee Ligament Injuries

Willmott, H. (2015). *Trauma and orthopaedics at a glance.* Wiley-Blackwell.

Duckworth, A., Porter, D., & Ralston, S. (2016). *Churchill's pocketbook of orthopaedics, trauma and rheumatology* (2nd ed.). Elsevier.

Bowden, G., McNally, M., Thomas, S., & Gibson, A. (2010). *Oxford handbook of orthopaedics and trauma.* Oxford University Press.

White, T. O., Mackenzie, S. P., Gray, A. J., & McRae, R. (2016) *McRae's orthopaedic trauma and emergency fracture management.*

Meniscal Tear

Willmott, H. (2015). *Trauma and orthopaedics at a glance.* Wiley-Blackwell.

Duckworth, A., Porter, D., & Ralston, S. (2016). *Churchill's pocketbook of orthopaedics, trauma and rheumatology* (2nd ed.). Elsevier.

Bowden, G., McNally, M., Thomas, S., & Gibson, A. (2010). *Oxford handbook of orthopaedics and trauma.* Oxford University Press.

LOWER LIMB TRAUMA
Hip Fractures

NICE. (2011). *Hip fracture management Clinical guideline [CG124].* https://www.nice.org.uk/guidance/cg124. [Accessed Dec 2020].

Willmott, H. (2015). *Trauma and orthopaedics at a glance.* Wiley-Blackwell.

Duckworth, A., Porter, D., & Ralston, S. (2016). *Churchill's pocketbook of orthopaedics, trauma and rheumatology* (2nd ed.). Elsevier.

Bowden, G., McNally, M., Thomas, S., & Gibson, A. (2010). *Oxford handbook of orthopaedics and trauma.* Oxford University Press.

Ankle Fractures

BOAST. (2016). *The management of ankle fractures.* https://www.boa.ac.uk/resources/boast-12-pdf.html. [Accessed Feb 2021].

AITKEN. (2019). *Crash course rheumatology and orthopaedics.* Elsevier.

Mayo Clinic. *Broken ankle.* https://www.mayoclinic.org/diseases-conditions/broken-ankle/symptoms-causes/syc-20450025. [Accessed Feb 2021].

Patient info. (2016). *Ankle fractures.* http://www.patient.info/doctor. [Accessed Feb 2021].

Keene, D. J., Lamb, S. E., Mistry, D., Tutton, E., Lall, R., Handley, R., Willett, K., & Ankle Injury Management (AIM) Trial Collaborators. (2018). Three-Year follow-up of a trial of close contact casting vs surgery for initial treatment of unstable ankle fractures in older adults. *Journal of the American Medical Association, 319,* 1274–1276. https://doi.org/10.1001/jama.2018.0811

Osteomyelitis

Clunie, G., Wilkinson, N., Nikiphorou, E., & Jadon, D. (2018). *Oxford handbook of rheumatology* (4th ed.). Oxford University Press.

Patient info. (2016). *Osteomyelitis.* https://patient.info/doctor/osteomyelitis-pro. [Accessed 24 August 2020].

BMJ Best Practice.. (2018). *Osteomyelitis.* https://bestpractice.bmj.com/topics/en-gb/3000178. [Accessed July 2020].

Septic Arthritis

Clunie, G., Wilkinson, N., Nikiphorou, E., & Jadon, D. (2018). *Oxford handbook of rheumatology* (4th ed.). Oxford University Press.

Patient info. (2016). *Septic arthritis.* https://patient.info/doctor/septic-arthritis-pro. [Accessed 24 August 2020].

Knapper, T., Murphy, R. J., Rocos, B., Fagg, J., Murray, N., & Whitehouse, M. R. (2021). Utility of bedside leucocyte esterase testing to rule out septic arthritis. *Emergency Medicine Journal, 38,* 707–710. https://doi.org/10.1136/emermed-2020-209842.

Open Fractures

BOAST. (2020). *Management of arterial injuries Associated with Extremity Fracture and Disclocations.* https://www.boa.ac.uk/resources/boast-6-pdf.html. [Accessed Feb 2021].

BOAST. (2017). *Open fractures.* https://www.boa.ac.uk/resources/boast-4-pdf.html. [Accessed April 2021].

Osteoarthritis

Nice. (2018). *CKS: Osteoarthritis.* https://cks.nice.org.uk/topics/osteoarthritis/. [Accessed April 2021].

Clunie, G., Wilkinson, N., Nikiphorou, E., & Jadon, D. (2018). *Oxford handbook of rheumatology* (4th ed.). Oxford University Press.

Scoliosis

Bowden, G., McNally, M., Thomas, S., & Gibson, A. (2010). *Oxford handbook of orthopaedics and trauma.* Oxford University Press.

Bone and Cartilage Tumours

Duckworth, A., Porter, D., & Ralston, S. (2016). *Churchill's pocketbook of orthopaedics, trauma and rheumatology* (2nd ed.). Elsevier.

Bowden, G., McNally, M., Thomas, S., & Gibson, A. (2010). *Oxford handbook of orthopaedics and trauma.* Oxford University Press.

LUQMANI. (2013). *Textbook of Orthopaedics, Trauma and Rheumatology* (2nd ed.). Elsevier.

Patient info. (2015). *Bone tumours.* https://patient.info/doctor/bone-tumours. [Accessed Feb 2021].

Orthoinfo. *Osteoid osteoma, osteoblastoma, giant cell tumour, chondrosarcoma.* http://www.orthoinfo.aaos.org. [Accessed Feb 2021].

Biondi, N. L., & Varacallo, M. (2020). *Enchondroma.* StatPearls. StatPearls Publishing. https://www.ncbi.nlm.nih.gov/books/NBK536938/.

Limaiem, F., Tafti, D., & Rawla, P. (2020). *Chondroblastoma.* StatPearls. StatPearls Publishing. https://www.ncbi.nlm.nih.gov/books/NBK536947/.

Bone Cancer Research Trust. http://www.bcrt.org.uk. [Accessed Feb 2021].

PAEDIATRIC TRAUMA AND ORTHOPAEDICS

Developmental Dysplasia of the Hip

BMJ Best Practice. (2020). *Developmental dysplasia of the hip.* https://bestpractice.bmj.com/topics/en-gb/742. [Accessed January 2021].

Patient info. (2015). *Developmental dysplasia of the hip.* https://patient.info/doctor/developmental-dysplasia-of-the-hip-pro. [Accessed January 2021].

Perthes' Disease

BMJ Best Practice. (2018). *Legg-Calvé-Perthes' disease.* https://bestpractice.bmj.com/topics/en-gb/751. [Accessed January 2021].

Patient info. (2020). *Perthes' disease.* https://patient.info/doctor/perthes-disease-pro. [Accessed January 2021].

Slipped Upper Femoral Epiphysis

BMJ Best Practice. (2018). *Slipped capital femoral epiphysis.* https://bestpractice.bmj.com/topics/en-gb/757. [Accessed January 2021].

Patient info. (2016). *Slipped capital femoral epiphysis.* https://patient.info/doctor/slipped-capital-femoral-epiphysis-pro. [Accessed January 2021].

Osgood-Schlatter Disease

NICE. (2020). *CKS: Osgood-Schlatter disease.* https://cks.nice.org.uk/topics/osgood-schlatter-disease/. [Accessed January 2021].

BMJ Best Practice. (2019). *Osgood-Schlatter's disease.* https://bestpractice.bmj.com/topics/en-gb/588. [Accessed January 2021].

Patient info. (2014). *Osgood-Schlatter disease.* https://patient.info/doctor/osgood-schlatter-disease-pro. [Accessed January 2021].

Osteochondritis Dissecans

BMJ Best Practice.. (2018). *Osteochondritis dissecans.* https://bestpractice.bmj.com/topics/en-gb/591. [Accessed January 2021].

Patient info. (2016). *Osteochondritis dissecans.* https://patient.info/doctor/osteochondritis-dissecans. [Accessed January 2021].

Congenital Talipes Equinovarus

BMJ Best Practice. (2020). *Equinovarus foot deformity*. https://bestpractice.bmj.com/topics/en-gb/745. [Accessed January 2021].

Patient info. (2017). *Talipes equinovarus*. https://patient. info/doctor/talipes-equinovarus. [Accessed January 2021].

Radial Head Subluxation

Patient info. (2014). *Radial head subluxation*. https://patient.info/ doctor/radial-head-subluxation. [Accessed January 2021].

Osteogenesis Imperfecta

Patient info. (2016). *Osteogenesis imperfecta*. https://patient.info/ doctor/osteogenesis-imperfecta. [Accessed January 2021].

24

Urology in an Hour

Mark Lam, Cherrie Ho and Marcus Drake

GENITOURINARY ANATOMY AND KEY PRINCIPLES

Anatomy Overview

Urology as a surgical specialty encompasses the management of medical and surgical diseases of the male and female urinary tracts (kidneys, ureters, bladder, urethra) and the male reproductive system (testes, epididymis, vas deferens, seminal vesicles, prostate and penis). The relevant genitourinary anatomy along with the common conditions affecting the respective organs are demonstrated in Figs 24.1–24.3.

Lower Urinary Tract Symptoms

Definition: a constellation of symptoms related to the quality and control of micturition. Lower urinary tract symptoms (LUTS) can be divided into:

- **Storage:** urgency, urinary frequency, nocturia, urinary incontinence
- **Voiding:** hesitancy, weak or intermittent stream, straining, terminal dribbling
- **Post-micturition:** post-micturition dribble, sensation of incomplete emptying

Investigations:

- **Urinalysis** (if a suspected urinary tract infection (UTI)): negative urine dip
- **Bladder diary and symptom score:** storage, voiding and post-micturition symptoms

- **Digital rectal examination (DRE) and prostate-specific antigen (PSA):** PSA levels within age-specific reference ranges, a benign-feeling prostate on a DRE
- **Flow rate and post-void residual volume:** abnormal flow (e.g., slow flow rate, high post-void residual volume)
- **Cystoscopy:** a lack of an underlying pathology (e.g., malignancy)
- **Imaging** (e.g., ultrasound (US), computed tomography (CT) or magnetic resonance imaging (MRI): a lack of an underlying pathology (e.g., malignancy, stones, strictures, etc.)

Differentials: UTI, urological malignancy

Management: detailed information is given in individual condition sections.

Urinary Retention

Definition: an inability to pass urine. Common causes include benign prostatic enlargement (BPE), urethral strictures, prostate and other pelvic malignancies, UTIs, neurological causes (e.g., diabetic autonomic neuropathy, multiple sclerosis (MS), cord compression, neurogenic bladder) and antimuscarinic drugs.

- **Acute** retention: **painful**, palpable or percussible bladder and **unable** to pass urine

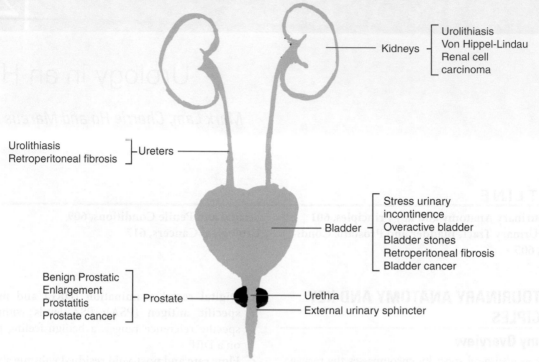

Kidneys — [Urolithiasis
Von Hippel-Lindau
Renal cell
carcinoma]

Urolithiasis
Retroperitoneal fibrosis } — Ureters

Bladder — [Stress urinary
incontinence
Overactive bladder
Bladder stones
Retroperitoneal fibrosis
Bladder cancer]

Benign Prostatic
Enlargement
Prostatitis
Prostate cancer } — Prostate

Urethra
External urinary sphincter

Fig 24.1 Urinary Tract Anatomy. (Illustrated by Hollie Blaber.)

- **Chronic** retention: **nonpainful**, palpable or percuss-ible bladder **after** passing some urine

Buzzwords:

- **Risk factors:** >50 years of age; male; previous reten-tion; pelvic or urological surgery; spinal or epidural anaesthesia; neurological or urological comorbidi-ties; anti-muscarinic, alpha agonist or opiate medica-tion use
- **Presentation:**
  - **Acute:** suprapubic pain, reduced urine output (U/O), inability to pass urine (micturate), BPE and neurological deficits (e.g., limb weakness, saddle anaesthesia) might be identified
  - **Chronic:** LUTS (storage, voiding and post-micturition)

Investigations:

- **Bladder scan:** abnormal if >200 mL (post void) or >500 mL (acute retention)
- **Blood** (suspected UTI): ↑/↔ WCC and CRP (only if UTI), ↑ creatinine, ↑ urea, ↓ eGFR (if chronic retention)
- **US renal tract:** ± hydronephrosis
- **MRI spine (if suspected spinal cord compression):** ± spinal cord compression

Differentials: UTI, appendicitis, abdominal aortic aneurysm (AAA), ovarian pathology (e.g., torsion, cyst), bowel obstruction

Management:

- If acute, recurrent acute or acute-on-chronic retention:
  - Admit to hospital
  - Immediate urethral catheterisation and measure the volume drained
  - Treat the underlying cause (e.g., if BPE, prescribe tamsulosin)
  - If >1000 mL, monitor for post-obstructive diure-sis and renal function
  - Trial without catheter (TWOC) at 24–48 h after insertion (if no renal impairment)
- If chronic:
  - Referral to urologist for consideration of a surgi-cal intervention
  - Either long-term, intermittent or no catheterisation with monitoring of renal function and urinary volumes

Urinary Incontinence

Definition: involuntary leakage of urine. The main types of urinary incontinence (UI) are:

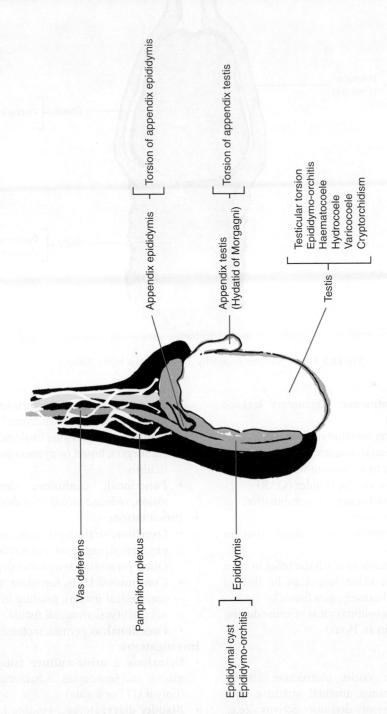

Torsion of appendix epididymis

Torsion of appendix testis

Appendix epididymis

Appendix testis
(Hydatid of Morgagni)

Testicular torsion
Epididymo-orchitis
Haematocoele
Hydrocoele
Varicocoele
Cryptorchidism

Testis

Vas deferens

Pampiniform plexus

Epididymal cyst
Epididymo-orchitis

Epididymis

Fig 24.2 Testicular Anatomy. (Illustrated by Hollie Blaber.)

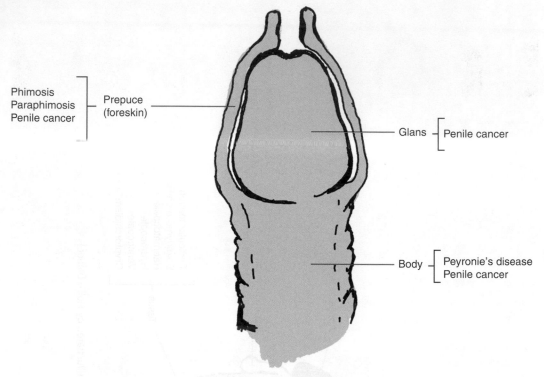

Phimosis
Paraphimosis
Penile cancer
— Prepuce
(foreskin)

Glans ⎤ Penile cancer

Body ⎤ Peyronie's disease
Penile cancer

Fig 24.3 Penile Surface Anatomy. (Illustrated by Hollie Blaber.)

- **Stress urinary incontinence:** involuntary leakage with effort or exertion
- **Urgency incontinence:** involuntary leakage accompanied by or immediately preceded by the sudden and compelling desire to urinate, of which the most common cause is an overactive bladder (OAB)
- **Mixed urinary incontinence:** a combination of stress and urgency symptoms
- **Overflow:** urinary retention and leakage from an overdistended bladder
- **Functional:** patient unable to reach the toilet in time
- **Continuous:** constant urine loss. Can be due to underlying anatomical cause (e.g., a fistula)
- **Nocturnal enuresis:** involuntary loss of urine during sleep (see Paediatrics in an Hour)

Buzzwords:
- **Risk factors:**
  - **Overflow:** bladder outlet obstruction (BOO) (e.g., BPE, malignancy, urethral stricture, urethral valves), loss of detrusor activity (e.g., angiotensin-converting enzyme inhibitors (ACEi),

antidepressants, antimuscarinics, antiparkinsonian drugs, cauda equina syndrome)
  - **Continuous:** previous urological or gynaecological surgery, bowel or gynaecological cancer, diverticulitis
  - **Functional:** confusion, dementia, impaired vision, reduced mobility or dexterity
- **Presentation:**
  - **Overflow:** straining to void, sensation of incomplete emptying, post-micturition dribble, LUTS. Other presenting symptoms depend on the cause
  - **Continuous:** UTIs, faeculent urine, pneumaturia (colovesical fistula), pooling of urine in the vaginal tract (vesicovaginal fistula)
  - **Functional:** as per risk factors

Investigations:
- **Urinalysis ± urine culture (suspected UTI):** ↑/↔ nitrites and leukocytes, ± bacteriuria $>10^5$ CFU/mL (only if UTI or fistula)
- **Bladder diary:** storage, voiding or post-micturition symptoms

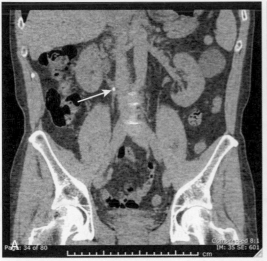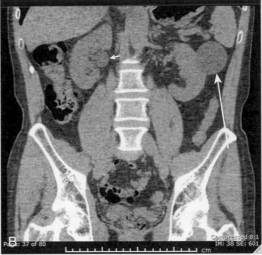

Fig 24.4 (A) A 4-mm calculus within the proximal right ureter *(arrow)* with (B) mild right hydronephrosis, a dilated renal pelvis *(small arrow)* and an incidental left renal cyst *(large arrow)*. (Image provided courtesy of Prof S. Gandhi, North Bristol NHS Trust.)

- **Bladder scan:** ± urinary retention
- **Urodynamic tests:** ± abnormality of detrusor contractility, bladder compliance, bladder sensation or capacity

Differentials: UTI, urogenital fistula, ectopic ureter, atrophic vaginitis, urethritis

Management:
1. **Conservative:**
   - Treat reversible causes (e.g., reduce caffeine intake, avoid excess fluid intake, weight loss, smoking cessation, etc.)
   - Absorbent containment products
   - Pelvic floor exercises
2. **Medical:** antimuscarinics and/or mirabegron
3. **If incontinence is untreatable + symptomatic:** bladder catheterisation as a last resort
4. Definitive management dependent on the type:
   - **Overflow UI:** Treat the underlying condition (e.g., if due to BOO, consider BOO surgery)
   - **Continuous UI (due to a fistula):** Resection of the fistula and repair of the bladder and involved viscera
   - **Functional UI:** Manage the underlying condition (e.g., if mobility related, consider aids or an occupational therapy assessment)

UPPER URINARY TRACT, BLADDER AND PROSTATIC CONDITIONS

Urolithiasis

Definition: the formation and presence of calculi or stones within the urinary tract (Fig. 24.4). The **types of stones** that are formed can be classified into infectious or noninfectious, or related to genetic defects or drugs:
- **Infectious:** struvite (commonly causes staghorn calculi), carbonate apatite, ammonium urate
- **Noninfectious stones:** calcium oxalate (most common type), calcium phosphate or mixed oxalate and phosphate, uric acid
- **Genetic:** cystine, xanthine, 2.8 dihydroxyadenine

Buzzwords:
- **Risk factors:** 40–60 years of age, urological anatomical abnormalities (e.g., horseshoe kidney, ureteric stricture), family history, hypertension (HTN), gout, red meat, myeloproliferative disease, hyperparathyroidism, low fluid intake, metabolic disorders, diuretics, UTI (*Proteus mirabilis*)
- **Presentation:** acute onset, waves of severe **flank pain radiating to the groin**, lasts minute to hours, unable to stay still, often associated with **nausea and vomiting,** may have dysuria, frequency and straining

Investigations:

- **Urinalysis ± urine culture:** haematuria, ↑/↔ nitrites and leukocytes (if UTI or infectious stone)
- **Blood:** ↑/↔ WCC and CRP (if UTI present), ↑ creatinine and urea (if hydronephrosis present; NB: emergency if single kidney)
- ***Non-contrast CT of the kidney, ureter and bladder (KUB) or US KUB (pregnant or child)*:** radiopacity in the renal tract, echogenic foci
- Abdominal US/CT may be done if a AAA is suspected
- **Stone analysis:** see definition section

Differentials: UTI, pyelonephritis, AAA

Management:

1. **Medical:** nonsteroidal anti-inflammatory drugs (NSAIDs), usually **PR diclofenac** and IV paracetamol. Consider opioids if both NSAIDs and paracetamol are contraindicated or not effective
2. **If signs of sepsis and/or anuria in obstructive uropathy:** urgent decompression with a percutaneous nephrostomy (not if a clotting abnormality) or ureteric stenting (not if unfit for general anaesthesia), urine and blood culture, IV antibiotics
3. Dependent on the size and location of the stone:
   - Asymptomatic renal stone <5 mm: watchful waiting
   - Renal stone <10 mm: shockwave lithotripsy (SWL) or consider a ureteroscopy (URS) if an SWL failed, is contraindicated or is unsuitable due to anatomy
   - Renal stone of 10–20 mm: URS or SWL (consider a percutaneous nephrolithotomy (PCNL) if both unsuccessful)
   - Renal stone >20 mm: PCNL
   - Distal ureteric stone <10 mm: medical expulsive therapy (alpha-blockers, e.g., tamsulosin), SWL or consider URS if an SWL failed, is contraindicated or is unsuitable due to anatomy
   - Ureteric stone 10–20 mm: URS (consider SWL or PCNL)
4. **Prevention:** increase fluid intake, reduce salt intake, restrict calcium intake, consider potassium citrate (>50% calcium oxalate stones) and thiazides (>50% calcium oxalate stones and hypercalciuria)

Stress Urinary Incontinence

Definition: involuntary leakage of urine with effort or exertion. Stress urinary incontinence (SUI) is caused by a failure of the urethral sphincter to remain closed with increased intra-abdominal pressures.

Buzzwords:

- **Risk factors:** older age, previous pregnancy, pelvic organ prolapse, obesity, UTIs, neurological disorders, constipation, family history, smoking and drugs, genitourinary surgery
- **Presentation:** older female, urine leakage when coughing, sneezing or exercise

Investigations:

- **Urinalysis + urine culture:** negative
- **Bladder diary:** storage, voiding or post-micturition symptoms
- **Bladder scan:** normal
- **Urodynamic tests:** urodynamic stress incontinence, normal detrusor contractility, bladder compliance, bladder sensation or capacity

Differentials: UTI, medication-induced urinary incontinence, OAB

Management:

1. Conservative:
   - Reduce caffeine intake, avoid excess fluid intake, weight loss, smoking cessation, etc.
   - Absorbent containment products (whilst waiting for treatment)
   - Six-month trial of supervised pelvic floor muscle training (PFMT)
2. If conservative management fails, referral to secondary care for:
   - **Medical:** offer duloxetine **only if** unsuitable for surgery and after counselling – **not first line**
   - **Surgical:** colposuspension, autologous rectus fascial sling, retropubic mid-urethral mesh sling (not currently used due to severe complications) and intramural urethral bulking agents (consider only if other surgical options are unsuitable)

Overactive Bladder

Definition: urinary urgency, typically accompanied by an increased voiding frequency and nocturia with or without urgency UI in the absence of a UTI or underlying pathology.

Buzzwords:

- **Risk factors:** increasing age, obesity
- **Causes:** idiopathic, neurological disorders (e.g., MS, stroke, spinal cord injury)
- **Presentation:** urgency, nocturia, increased frequency, urgency UI, abdominal discomfort

Investigations:

- **Urinalysis ± urine culture:** negative

- **Symptom score and bladder diary:** storage symptoms
- **Bladder scan** (if voiding symptoms or recurrent UTI): ± urinary retention
- **Urodynamic tests:** abnormality of detrusor contractility (detrusor overactivity), bladder sensation or capacity

Differentials: UTI, urolithiasis, SUI

Management:

1. **Conservative:** 6-week trial of bladder training (urgency UI and mixed UI)
2. **Medical:** antimuscarinic drugs (e.g., oxybutynin, solifenacin, tolterodine), beta-3 agonists (e.g., mirabegron)
3. **If above unsuccessful:**
   - Increase the dose, use an alternative drug (e.g., a beta-3 agonist if an antimuscarinic agent was tried) or a combination of these
   - If nocturia is the main feature of OAB and it is affecting the quality of life (QoL): consider desmopressin with careful monitoring of electrolytes (especially serum sodium)
4. If unresponsive to medical management, options include:
   - Botulinum A toxin (following local MDT review)
   - Percutaneous sacral or posterior tibial nerve stimulation
   - Augmentation cystoplasty
   - Urinary diversion

Bladder Stones

Definition: formation of calculi within the bladder

- **Primary:** in the absence of a urinary tract pathology
- **Secondary:** in the presence of a urinary tract pathology
- **Migratory:** passed from the upper urinary tract

Buzzwords:

- **Risk factors:** BOO (most common), neurogenic bladder dysfunction, catheters, bladder diverticula, passed ureteric calculi
- **Presentation:** urinary frequency, terminal haematuria, dysuria at the end of micturition, suprapubic pain worsened by exercise or movement. In children: pulling the penis, retention, enuresis and rectal prolapse (due to straining)

Investigations:

- **Urinalysis ± urine culture:** haematuria, ↑ nitrite and leukocyte (if infectious stone)
- **Blood:** ↑ WCC and CRP (infection), ↑ creatinine and urea (hydronephrosis)

- **X-ray KUB:** radio-opaque stones
- **Stone analysis:** see Urolithiasis section

Differentials: urolithiasis, UTI, bladder cancer, renal cancer

Management:

Surgical options include:

- Transurethral cystolitholapaxy (adults)
- Percutaneous transurethral cystolitholapaxy (children and adults with larger bladder stones)
- Open cystostomy (if the stone is too large for endoscopic management)

Benign Prostatic Enlargement

Definition: an increase in the size of the prostate gland in the absence of a malignancy (Fig. 24.5). BPE can lead to LUTS through two processes:

- An increase in benign prostatic tissue narrowing the urethral lumen (nodular hyperplasia)
- An increase in prostatic smooth muscle tone

Buzzwords:

- **Risk factors:** >50 years of age, family history
- **Presentation:** voiding symptoms (e.g., poor stream, hesitancy, intermittency, straining, incomplete emptying and post-micturition dribble), storage symptoms (e.g., increased frequency, urgency, nocturia), palpable bladder after voiding (if chronic retention), enlarged and smooth prostate

Investigations:

- **Urinalysis ± urine culture** (if suspected UTI or prostatitis): negative in uncomplicated BPE
- **PSA:** normal levels for age
- **International Prostate Symptoms Score:** mild, moderate or severe LUTS
- **Bladder scan:** >300 mL post-void residual volume if chronic retention
- **Transrectal USS:** >30 mL volume

Differentials: prostate cancer, prostatitis

Management:

1. **Conservative:** lifestyle advice and watchful waiting if manageable symptoms
2. **Medical:** alpha blockers (e.g., doxazosin, tamsulosin) or 5-alpha-reductase inhibitors (e.g., finasteride, dutasteride) for a large-volume prostate or a combination
3. **Surgical:** transurethral resection of prostate (TURP), UroLift, transurethral vaporisation of prostate, Holmium laser enucleation of prostate, open prostatectomy (if prostate is >80 g)

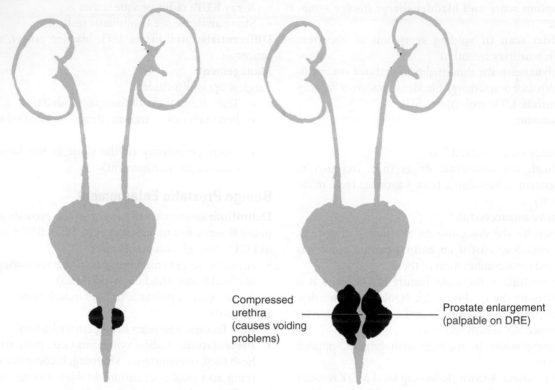

Compressed urethra (causes voiding problems)

Prostate enlargement (palpable on DRE)

Fig 24.5 Benign Prostatic Enlargement. *DRE,* Digital rectal examination. (Illustrated by Hollie Blaber.)

4. **Interventional radiology:** prostate artery embolization

Prostatitis

Definition: inflammation within the prostate
Buzzwords:

- **Risk factors:** UTI (*E. coli* most common), BPE, urethral instrumentation, trauma, sexually transmitted infections (STIs) (chlamydia or gonorrhoea), <50 years of age (acute), >50 years of age (chronic)
- **Presentation:**
  - **Acute:** dysuria, increased frequency, urgency, pain (perineal, penile, rectal), acute retention, voiding symptoms, lower back pain, tender and boggy prostate, fever
  - **Chronic:** perineal, suprapubic, scrotal or penis pain (at least 3 months), LUTS, erectile dysfunction, painful ejaculation, anxiety, depression

Investigations:

- **Urinalysis ± urine culture:** ↑/↔ nitrites and leukocytes and bacteriuria >10^5 CFU/mL
- **Blood:** ↑ WCC and CRP

- **Blood cultures (if febrile):** specific organism is identified
- **Urethral swabs ± STI screen (if suspected STI):** significant growth of organism
- **To monitor:** ↑ PSA in acute and chronic prostatitis with a return to normal after successful treatment

Differentials: UTI, BPE, prostate cancer
Management:
Acute:

1. **Referral to hospital if:** unable to take oral antibiotics, severe symptoms, signs of a serious underlying condition (e.g., sepsis, acute retention, abscess), immunocompromise, pre-existing urological condition (e.g., BPE, indwelling catheter)
2. **Oral antibiotic for 14 days according to local microbiology guidelines. BNF recommendations:**
   - **Oral first-line agent:** ciprofloxacin or ofloxacin (if either unsuitable, trimethoprim)
   - **Oral second-line agent (on specialist advice):** levofloxacin or co-trimoxazole
3. Intravenous antibiotics for severe cases. BNF recommendations:

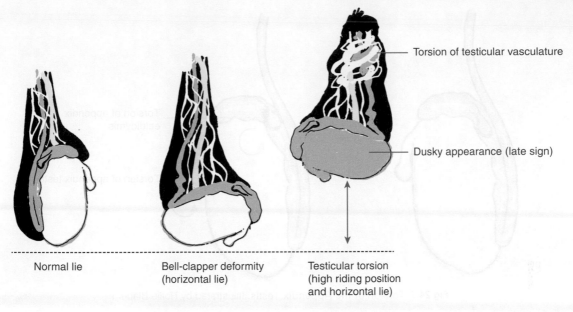

Torsion of testicular vasculature

Dusky appearance (late sign)

Normal lie

Bell-clapper deformity
(horizontal lie)

Testicular torsion
(high riding position
and horizontal lie)

Fig 24.6 Testicular Torsion. (Illustrated by Hollie Blaber.)

- **IV first-line agent:** amikacin, ceftriaxone, cefuroxime, ciprofloxacin, gentamicin or levofloxacin
- **IV second-line agent:** consult local microbiologist

Chronic:

1. Medical:
   - Paracetamol and ibuprofen. Do not offer opioids.
   - Alpha blocker for 4–6 weeks if significant LUTS
   - A single course of antibiotics if symptoms are present for <6 months. NICE recommendations: trimethoprim or doxycycline for 4–6 weeks
   - Stool softener if painful defecation
   - Targeted cognitive behavioural therapy, counselling or antidepressants if psychosocial symptoms
2. Referral to urologist if:
   - diagnostic uncertainty
   - severe symptoms
   - treatment failure
3. **Referral to chronic pain team** if no response to treatment (especially those suffering from chronic non-bacterial prostatitis)

SCROTAL AND PENILE CONDITIONS

Testicular Torsion

Definition: a urological emergency caused by twisting of the testicle on the spermatic cord, which can compromise the blood supply and lead to ischaemia of testicular

tissue (Fig. 24.6). Peak incidence occurs at 12–18 years of age but can occur in neonates and adults.

Buzzwords:

- **Risk factors:** bell-clapper deformity, testicular tumour, undescended testis, trauma, exercise
- **Presentation: sudden-onset scrotal pain**, on-and-off pain (intermittent torsion), suprapubic pain (children), **nausea and vomiting**, may come on during physical activity or after trauma, **high-riding testicle**, transverse lie, no pain relief with elevation of the scrotum (**negative Prehn's sign**), **absent cremasteric reflex**
- Be aware that torsion of the appendix testis (a.k.a., hydatid of Morgagni) may present similarly to testicular torsion (Fig. 24.7). However, in the former condition, the pain is less severe and insidious, and patients may present with the **blue dot sign.** Similarly, torsion of the appendix epididymis can be a rare presentation of an acute scrotum in children (Fig. 24.7)

Investigations:

- *Principally a **clinical diagnosis.** Investigations should not delay being taken to the theatre*
- **Urinalysis ± urine culture (to rule out UTI):** negative
- **Urethral swab ± STI screen (to rule out STI):** specific organism identified (see Epididymo-orchitis)

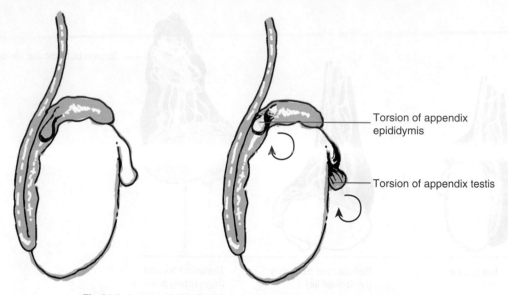

Torsion of appendix epididymis

Torsion of appendix testis

Fig 24.7 Torsion of the Appendix Testis. (Illustrated by Hollie Blaber.)

- **Doppler ultrasound (RARELY DONE; only consider if not planning an exploration):** absent blood flow to testis. The finding of absent testis blood flow on an ultrasound scan (USS) is an unacceptable error of practice; the patient should have been taken to theatre

Differentials: epididymo-orchitis, strangulated inguinal hernia, torsion of the appendix testis, torsion of the appendix epididymis

Management:
1. Analgesia and antiemetics preoperatively
2. Surgical exploration and detorsion. If torsion is confirmed: bilateral orchidopexy to prevent further torsion episodes (the bell-clapper abnormality predisposing to torsion can occur bilaterally). Orchidectomy may be required if a testis is nonviable

Epididymo-orchitis

Definition: a clinical syndrome consisting of pain, swelling and inflammation of the epididymis with or without inflammation of the testes.

Buzzwords:
- **Risk factors:** >19 years of age, STIs (chlamydia or gonorrhoea), UTIs (*E. coli* or *Enterococcus faecalis*), mumps, BOO, instrumentation of the urinary tract, urine reflux, immunocompromise (e.g., uncontrolled diabetes mellitus (DM) – examine carefully for **Fournier's gangrene**)

- **Presentation:** onset over **hours to days**, unilateral pain and tenderness (generally not as severe as torsion), diffuse swelling and erythema, usually **no** nausea and vomiting, relief of pain with elevation of the testes (**positive Prehn's sign**), urethral discharge, signs of UTI

Investigations:
- **Urethral swab or first-pass urine** (if suspected STI): specific organism identified
- **Urinalysis ± urine culture** (if suspected UTI): ↑/↔ nitrites and leukocytes and bacteriuria >10^5 CFU/mL
- **Blood:** ↑ WCC and CRP
- **Scrotal USS** (if suspected abscess): ± abscess visualised
- **IgM saliva sample** (if suspected mumps): ± IgM identified

Differentials: testicular torsion, infected hydrocele, strangulated inguinal hernia, testicular tumour

Management:
1. If likely secondary to a STI, treat according to local microbiology guidelines. NICE recommendations:
   - **First line:** treat empirically with ceftriaxone IM (or cefixime PO) and doxycycline PO (add azithromycin if gonorrhoea is likely)
   - **Second line:** ofloxacin PO or levofloxacin PO
   - Referral to genitourinary medicine
2. If likely secondary to an enteric organism (e.g., *E. coli*), treat according to local microbiology guidelines. NICE recommendations:

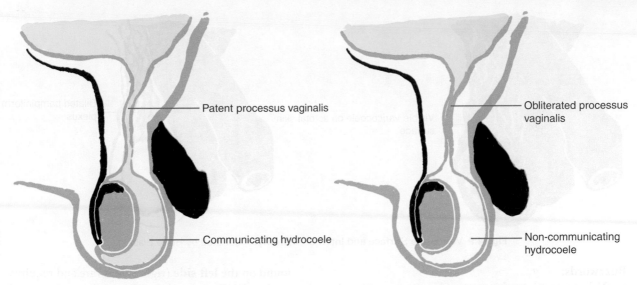

Fig 24.8 Communicating vs Non-communicating Hydrocoele. (Illustrated by Hollie Blaber.)

- **First line:** treat empirically with ofloxacin PO or levofloxacin PO (or co-amoxiclav if quinolones are contraindicated)
3. If idiopathic or viral (mumps): Analgesia, bed rest, scrotal elevation
4. If symptoms are severe and the patient is systemically unwell consider hospital admission

Hydrocoele

Definition: a collection of serous fluid between the layers of the tunica vaginalis. These can be congenital (secondary to a patent processus vaginalis (PPV)) or acquired. There are two types of hydrocoeles (Fig. 24.8):
- **Communicating hydrocoele:** a PPV allows peritoneal fluid to flow between the peritoneum and tunica vaginalis
- **Non-communicating (simple hydrocoele):** more fluid is being produced by the tunica vaginalis than is being absorbed

Buzzwords:
- **Risk factors:** premature infant, late descent of testis, increased intra-abdominal pressure, trauma, infection, torsion, varicocele operation, testicular tumour
- **Presentation:** infants (typically congenital) or adults (typically acquired), acute or chronic, painless and nontender, smooth swelling, **transilluminates,** can get above the swelling (cannot get above an inguinal hernia)

Investigations:
- Typically a **clinical diagnosis.** Further investigations may include:
- **US scrotum** (if suspected malignancy): presence or absence of a hydrocoele and causative factor (e.g., testicular tumour)

Differentials: epididymal cyst, inguinal hernia, testicular cancer, epididymo-orchitis

Management:
1. If uncertain of the underlying cause in primary care: referral to secondary care
2. Infant or toddler with hydrocele since birth:
   - Reassurance, likely to resolve by 2 years of age
   - If still present at 2 years of age, referral to a paediatric surgeon for ligation of the PPV
3. Adult with hydrocoele:
   - If simple noncommunicating with no underlying pathology: conservative management, reassurance and scrotal support
   - If unfit for surgery or patient declines surgery: conservative management
   - If large and symptomatic: exploratory surgery, Jaboulay (inversion of sac) or Lord's (plication of sac)

Epididymal Cyst

Definition: a benign cystic swelling of the epididymis. If the cyst contains spermatozoa, it may be referred to as a spermatocele.

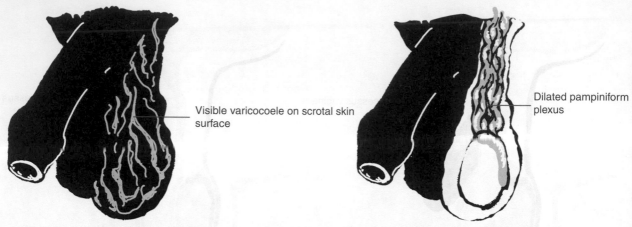

Visible varicocoele on scrotal skin surface

Dilated pampiniform plexus

Fig 24.9 Varicocele Surface and Internal Anatomy. (Illustrated by Hollie Blaber.)

Buzzwords:
- **Risk factors:** rarely cystic fibrosis, von Hippel-Lindau (vHL) syndrome, polycystic kidney disease (PCKD)
- **Presentation:** middle-aged male, chronic, painless, nontender, fluctuant, smooth, can be bilateral, testis separate from the lump, can get above the swelling, '**Chinese lantern**' appearance on transillumination

Investigations: typically a clinical diagnosis. No further investigations required unless there is diagnostic uncertainty.
- **US scrotum (if diagnostic uncertainty):** presence or absence of an epididymal cyst

Differentials: varicocele, hydrocoele
Management:
1. If diagnostic uncertainty in primary care: referral for a routine US of the scrotum
2. If symptomatic: routine referral to urology
   - Treatment is usually not necessary
   - If the patient has failed conservative management, consider a surgical removal (risk of recurrence and possible subsequent subfertility)

Varicocele

Definition: an abnormal dilatation of the internal spermatic veins and pampiniform venous plexus of the spermatic cord (Fig 24.9).
Buzzwords:
- **Risk factors:** family history
- **Presentation:** rare before puberty, may present with infertility, painless scrotal swelling more commonly

found on the **left side** (right side is rare and requires an US KUB), scrotal heaviness, '**bag of worms**' appearance, dilation of veins increases on standing. If associated with haematuria and abdominal pain, consider **Nutcracker syndrome** (compression of the left renal vein by the aorta and superior mesenteric artery)

Investigations: typically a clinical diagnosis. No further investigations are required unless there is a suspected underlying condition.
- **Doppler US scrotum** (diagnostic uncertainty or unable to examine the testicle): presence or absence of a varicocele
  - Semen analyses (in suspected infertility): ↓ sperm count
- **Serum follicle-stimulating hormone (FSH) and testosterone** (if suspected infertility): ↑ FSH and ↔ or ↓ testosterone
- **Imaging** (e.g., CT, MRI or USS (if suspected retroperitoneal mass)): presence or absence of a retroperitoneal mass

Differentials: epididymal cyst, hydrocoele
Management:
- If diagnostic uncertainty/symptomatic/right-sided varicocele suspicious of a renal malignancy in primary care: referral to urology
- Typically, no treatment is necessary
- **Medical and surgical:** embolization or surgical ligation if symptomatic, bilateral large varicocele, varicocele in a solitary testis or subfertility (although no evidence of significant benefit to pregnancy rates following a surgical intervention)

Cryptorchidism (Undescended Testes)

Definition: a testis that is absent from the scrotum due to an incomplete descent from the abdomen through the inguinal canal. It can be classified as a:

- **True undescended testis:** lies along the normal path of descent in the abdomen or inguinal region
- **Ectopic testis:** testis lies outside the normal path of descent (e.g., femoral region, perineum, superficial inguinal pouch)
- **Retractile testis:** testis has completed the descent into the scrotum but can be found in a suprascrotal position along the normal path of descent due to an overactive cremasteric reflex

Buzzwords:

- **Risk factors:** family history, low birth weight and small for gestational age, preterm, twins, congenital adrenal hyperplasia (CAH), Prader-Willi, disorders of sexual development, previous inguinal hernia surgery
- **Presentation:** baby or infant, testis palpable during a warm bath (retractile), lump in the groin or abdomen (ectopic), hypospadias, ambiguous genitalia, large contralateral testis (suggests testicular absence or atrophy)

Investigations: typically a clinical diagnosis. No further investigations are required unless there is an unclear diagnosis

- **US or MRI abdomen and pelvis** (if the testis is not palpable along the inguinal canal): presence or absence of a testis

Differentials: retractile testis, ectopic testis, CAH, testicular agenesis

Management:

- Referral to a specialist is indicated if:
  - Suspected disorder of sexual development and/or bilateral undescended testes at birth (within 24 h)
  - Suspected bilateral undescended testes at 6–8 weeks (2-week-wait (2WW) referral)
  - Unilateral undescended testis at birth: review at 6–8 weeks and 4–5 months; if still undescended, refer to be seen at 6 months
- If retractile: annual follow-up due to a risk of permanent ascent
- If palpable testis: inguinal orchidopexy; should be performed ideally at 12 months and by 18 months
- If nonpalpable: diagnostic laparoscopy or inguinal exploration followed by an orchidopexy or orchidectomy (especially in a postpubertal boy or older as **increased risk of malignancy**)

Phimosis

Definition: an inability to retract the foreskin. This condition can be a **physiological** adherence of the foreskin to the glans, which is normal in infancy, with many males having a partially or fully retractable foreskin by 10 years of age. **Pathological** phimosis can occur at any age but is more common in adulthood due to scarring of the foreskin.

Buzzwords:

- **Risk factors:** balanitis xerotica obliterans (white fibrous scarring of the prepuce), STIs (genital herpes, syphilis), eczema, psoriasis, lichen sclerosis, Zoon's balanitis, penile cancer
- **Presentation:** poor stream, ballooning of the foreskin on micturition, 'spraying' or poor stream on micturition, recurrent attacks of balanitis or UTIs, dyspareunia, swelling and redness of the prepuce, shortened frenulum, white ring around the preputial orifice

Investigations:

- Primarily a **clinical diagnosis.** No further investigations are indicated.

Differentials: N/A

Management:

- Management is dependent on the presentation:
  - **Non-retractile foreskin and child is <2 years of age:** watchful waiting, avoid forcible retraction, personal hygiene advice, usually resolves over time
  - **Mild scarring:** topical steroid (betamethasone)
  - **Evidence of infection:** antibiotics
  - **If conservative measures fail:** referral to urology for circumcision

Paraphimosis

Definition: the inability to pull a retracted prepuce (foreskin) forward over the glans (Fig. 24.10). This is a **urological emergency** and, if not resolved, can lead to ischaemia of the glans.

Buzzwords:

- **Risk factors:** chronic balanoposthitis, **iatrogenic** (e.g., nonreplaced foreskin post-urinary catheterisation), trauma (e.g., sexual intercourse, forcible retraction, piercings)
- **Presentation:** painful erection, irritability (infants), pain and swelling of the glans, a visible constricting band around the coronal sulcus, penile ischaemia (blue skin, firm glans)

Investigations: primarily a clinical diagnosis. No further investigations indicated

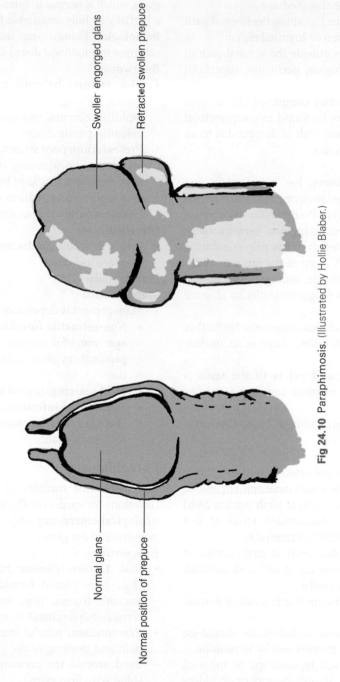

Fig 24.10 Paraphimosis. (Illustrated by Hollie Blaber.)

Swollen engorged glans

Retracted swollen prepuce

Normal glans

Normal position of prepuce

TABLE 24.1 Causes of Erectile Dysfunction

Vascular	Neurological	Hormonal	Anatomical	Drug Induced	Trauma	Psychogenic
Cardiovascular disease	Parkinson's disease	Hypogonadism	Peyronie's disease	Antihypertensives	Penile fracture	Generalised (e.g., disorders of sexual intimacy)
Atherosclerosis	Stroke	Hyperprolactinaemia	Micropenis and other penile anomalies	Beta blockers	Pelvic fractures	
Hypertension	Multiple sclerosis	Thyroid disease		Diuretics		
Diabetes		Cushing's disease		Antidepressants		Situational (e.g., performance-related issues)
Smoking	Tumours			Antipsychotics		
Surgery	Spinal cord disease			Hormonal agents		
Radiotherapy				Anticonvulsants		
Trauma	Neuropathies			Recreational drugs		

Differentials: N/A

Management:

1. **Acute:** manual pressure and reduction: compression of the foreskin and glans, and gradual reduction of the prepuce over the glans using the thumb and index fingers to apply counter pressure or applying upward pressure to the phallus. Application of **dextrose-soaked gauze** or ice packs

2. **Surgical** (if conservative measures are unsuccessful): dorsal slit reduction or circumcision

Erectile Dysfunction

Definition: the inability to attain and maintain an erection sufficient for satisfactory sexual performance. Erectile dysfunction (ED) can be classified as primary organic or primary psychogenic. See Table 24.1 for causes of erectile dysfunction.

Buzzwords:

- **Risk factors:** obesity, DM, cardiovascular disease, metabolic syndrome, HTN, smoking, lack of exercise, high alcohol consumption, previous pelvic surgery
- **Presentation:**
  - **Organic:** gradual onset of symptoms, lack of tumescence, normal libido, evidence of an underlying pathology (refer to Table 24.1)
  - **Psychogenic:** sudden onset of symptoms, decreased libido, good-quality spontaneous or self-stimulated erections, major life events, psychological issues (e.g., disorders of sexual intimacy, situational, anxiety, depression)

Investigations:

- International Index for Erectile Function (IIEF) or Sexual Health Inventory for Men: mild, moderate or severe ED

- **Fasting blood glucose** (if suspected DM): ≥7 mmol/L if DM is present
- **Lipid profile** (if suspected hypercholesterolaemia): ↑ cholesterol/LDL/triglycerides
- **Total testosterone** (if suspected hypogonadism): ↔ or ↓ levels

Differentials: medication related, depression, normal erectile function, spinal cord compression

Management:

1. Arrange referral to an appropriate specialty depending upon the findings and treat reversible causes
2. **Conservative:**
   - Lifestyle advice: weight loss, stop smoking, reduce alcohol consumption, exercise
   - Referral to psychosexual therapy
3. **Medical:**
   - PDE-5 inhibitors (e.g., sildenafil, tadalafil)
4. If PDE-5 inhibitors are unsuccessful, referral to urology/andrology clinic for alternative treatments:
   - Vacuum erection devices
   - Intracavernous injection
   - Intraurethral or topical alprostadil
   - Low-intensity shockwave therapy
   - Penile prosthesis

Priapism

Definition: a prolonged penile erection lasting more than 4 h in the absence of sexual stimulation and remaining despite an orgasm. This can be subclassified into:

- Ischaemic (most common and a urological emergency) – *the focus of this section*
- Non-ischaemic
- Stuttering

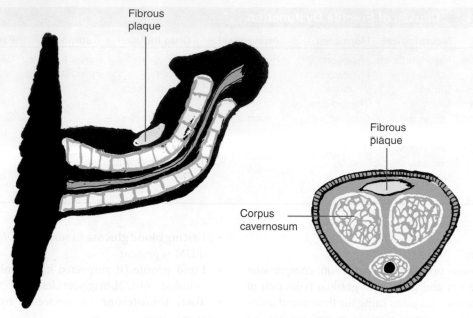

Fig 24.11 Peyronie's Disease. (Illustrated by Hollie Blaber.)

Buzzwords:
- **Risk factors:** family history, psychiatric conditions, drug abuse, genitourethral trauma
- **Causes:** haemoglobinopathies (e.g., sickle cell disease, thalassaemia, haematological malignancy), psychotropic medications (e.g., fluoxetine, risperidone, olanzapine), recreational drugs (e.g., cannabis, cocaine), malignancy, intracavernosal injections
- **Presentation:** painful erection, soft glans penis, evidence of a pelvic malignancy (e.g., palpable mass, lymphadenopathy)

Investigations:
- **Blood:** ↑ WCC (infection or blood dyscrasias), ↓ Hb and ↓ platelets (haemoglobinopathy)
- **Cavernosal blood gas:** pO_2 <30 mmHg, pCO_2 >60 mmHg, pH <7.25
- **Colour duplex US:** ± blood flow

Differentials: N/A

Management:
1. **Initial conservative measures:** local anaesthesia, intracorporeal or percutaneous access to the penile shaft and aspiration
2. **If step 1 is unsuccessful:** cavernosal irrigation with a 0.9% saline solution
3. **If step 2 is unsuccessful:** intracavernosal injection of phenylephrine

4. **If step 3 is unsuccessful:** surgical shunting or consider a primary penile implant (priapism present >48 h)

Peyronie's Disease

Definition: a penile connective tissue disorder characterised by fibrous plaque formation in the corpus cavernosum's tunica albuginea (Fig. 24.11). The inflammatory thickening leads to decreased elastic tissue and subsequent fibrosis and calcification, causing penile angulation or deformities.

Buzzwords:
- **Risk factors:** Dupuytren's contracture, DM, HTN, dyslipidaemia, smoking, alcohol excess, cardiomyopathy
- **Presentation:**
  - **Acute phase (up to 6 months):** penile pain during erections, changing penile deformity
  - **Stable phase (9–12 months):** pain disappears, palpable fibrous plaque at the site of angulation (stabilisation of the penile deformity), erectile dysfunction

Investigations: typically a clinical diagnosis. No further investigations are required

Differentials: normal anatomical curvature

Management:
1. Medical:
   - NSAIDs or extracorporeal shockwave treatment (pain during the acute phase)

- PDE-5 inhibitors (if ED or difficulty during sexual intercourse)
- Intralesional therapy (collagenase clostridium histolyticum or interferon)

2. Surgical: suturing, incision/excision and grafting or penile implants indicated for stable disease with a significant deformity preventing intercourse. Complications include penile shortening

UROLOGICAL CANCERS

Renal Cell Carcinoma

Definition: renal cell carcinoma is the most common solid lesion within the kidney and accounts for 90% of all kidney malignancies. There are three main types:

- **Clear cell:** most common and worse prognosis
- **Papillary**
- **Chromophobe:** least common and better prognosis

Other renal malignancies include transitional cell carcinoma, Wilms' tumour (see Paediatrics in an hour) and squamous cell carcinoma (SCC).

Buzzwords:

- **Risk factors:** smoking, obesity, HTN, family history, long-term dialysis, vHL, PCKD and horseshoe kidneys
- **Presentation:** asymptomatic, incidental finding. The classic triad of flank pain, visible haematuria and a palpable abdominal mass is rare. Constitutional symptoms (e.g., lethargy, weight loss), cervical lymphadenopathy, varicocele, bone pain, haemoptysis (cannonball metastases)

Investigations:

- **Urinalysis:** haematuria
- **Blood:** ↓ Hb, ↑ creatinine, ↑ calcium, ± metastasis markers (↑ PT, LFTs and LDH)
- **CT abdomen and pelvis:** renal mass ± metastasis
- **To monitor:** US abdomen and kidney and/or CT chest and abdomen (time schedule is risk-dependent)

Differentials: UTI, bladder cancer, urothelial cancer

Management: dependent on the stage (TNM staging) and following a discussion at a multidisciplinary team (MDT) meeting:

- **Localised tumour <7 cm in diameter (T1):** partial nephrectomy (open, laparoscopic or robot-assisted)
- **Localised tumour >7 cm in diameter (T2):** radical nephrectomy (open or laparoscopic)
- **Locally advanced (T3 and T4):** open radical nephrectomy

- **Metastatic disease:** tyrosine kinase inhibitors (e.g., sunitinib and pazopanib), immunotherapy agents (e.g., bevacizumab, nivolumab, ipilimumab), palliative nephrectomy for pain/bleeding, metastasectomy. Choice is determined by the level of risk

Prognosis:

- 80% of patients with RCC survive for 1 year
- 65% for 5 years
- 50% for 10 years or more
- A more favourable prognosis is based on the RCC type: chromophobe > papillary > clear cell
- For all RCC types, the prognosis worsens with the stage and grade

Bladder Cancer

Definition: cancer arising from the tissues of the bladder. Can be classified into **transitional cell carcinoma** (most common; can be papillary or non-papillary) or **non-transitional cell** (e.g., SCC, adenocarcinoma, sarcoma, small cell, metastases).

Buzzwords:

- **Risk factors:** male, increasing age, smoking, occupational exposures (e.g., industrial paint processing, dye, rubber and textiles), pelvis irradiation, cyclophosphamide, chronic inflammation (urolithiasis, indwelling catheters), schistosomiasis (specifically SCC), obesity, renal transplant
- **Presentation:** older male, painless gross (or microscopic) haematuria, dysuria (typical of carcinoma in situ (CIS) or an aggressive cancer), weight loss, unexplained and recurrent UTI

Investigations:

- **Urinalysis:** haematuria
- **US KUB** (non-muscle invasive): presence or absence of a bladder tumour ± obstruction
- **CT urography** (high-risk non-muscle invasive and all-muscle invasive): presence or absence of a suspected tumour
- **Flexible cystoscopy + biopsy:** presence or absence of a bladder malignancy
- **CT thorax, abdomen and pelvis** (TAP) (muscle invasive and metastatic bladder cancer): presence or absence of metastases
- **Monitoring:** flexible cystoscopy (initially at 3 months post-treatment); CT urography (recurrence); CT chest, abdomen and pelvis (metastatic recurrence); vitamin B12 (if use of bowel for ileal conduit)

Differentials: RCC, UTI, urothelial cancer

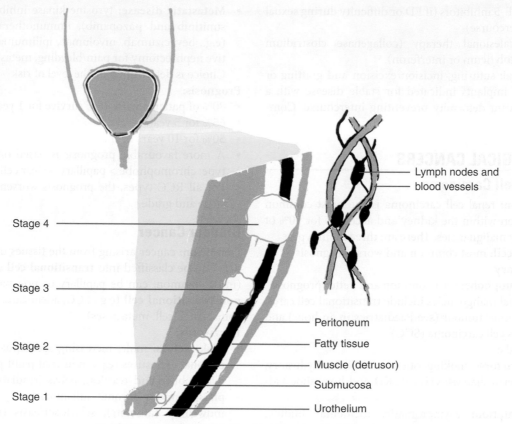

Lymph nodes and blood vessels

Stage 4

Stage 3

Peritoneum

Stage 2

Fatty tissue

Muscle (detrusor)

Submucosa

Stage 1

Urothelium

Fig 24.12 Bladder Cancer Staging. (Illustrated by Hollie Blaber.)

Management:

1. In primary care, non-urgent referral if:
   - ≥60 years of age and persistent unexplained UTI
2. In primary care, 2WW referral if:
   - ≥45 years of age + unexplained visible haematuria without UTI or persistent visible haematuria refractory to treatment of UTI
   - ≥60 years of age + unexplained nonvisible haematuria and dysuria or raised white cell count
3. **Secondary care treatment** is based on whether the tumour is non-muscle invasive (low, intermediate or high risk based on the tumour size and grading of cells) or muscle invasive and the presence or absence of metastases (Fig. 24.12):
   - **Non-muscle invasive, low risk:** TURBT + post-op single-dose intravesical mitomycin C
   - **Non-muscle invasive, intermediate risk:** TURBT + intravesical mitomycin C (at least six doses)

- **Non-muscle invasive, high risk:** TURBT then restaging TURBT (within 6 weeks) + intravesical BCG or radical cystectomy
- **Muscle invasive:** neoadjuvant chemotherapy and radical cystectomy or radical radiotherapy
- **If locally advanced/metastatic bladder cancer:** cisplatin-based chemotherapy regimen

3. Management of symptoms secondary to locally advanced/metastatic disease:
   - Bladder symptoms: palliative radiotherapy
   - Ureteric obstruction: nephrostomy or ureteric stenting
   - Bleeding: radiotherapy or embolisation
   - Pelvic pain: radiotherapy, nerve block or chemotherapy

Prognosis:

- Significantly worse prognostic factors for bladder cancer: higher grade, greater depth of invasion, presence of CIS

- Superficial tumour survival rate = 80%–90% at 5 years
- Metastatic bladder cancer survival rate = 10%–15% at 5 years

Prostate Cancer

Definition: a malignant tumour of the prostate, of which the most common type is adenocarcinoma (cancer of the glandular cells). Most are indolent and contained, whilst a minority can behave aggressively with local invasion or metastases

Buzzwords:
- **Risk factors:** older age, family history, Black ethnicity, high-fat diet, obesity
- **Presentation:** asymptomatic (localised cancer); LUTS; lower back pain; lethargy; weight loss; erectile dysfunction; bone pain (metastatic disease); hard, asymmetrical, craggy, nodular prostate

Investigations:
- **PSA level:** ≥3 ng/mL (if 50–69 years of age). NB: ↑ PSA may be seen in BPE, prostatitis, recent DRE, urinary tract instrumentation and recent ejaculation
- **Multiparametric MRI (if a clinically suspected T1 or T2 cancer):** presence or absence of a prostate mass
- **Transrectal ultrasound (TRUS)-guided needle biopsy:** presence of malignant cells
- **CT abdomen and pelvis (staging of a proven cancer if T or N will change the management):** presence or absence of metastases
- **Isotope bone scan** (intermediate- and high-risk disease): presence or absence of bony metastases
- **Monitoring:** PSA levels (6/52, every 6 months for 2 years, then yearly), isotope bone scan (watchful waiting + high risk of bone metastases)

Differentials: BPE, bladder cancer, chronic prostatitis

Gleason score, International Society of Urological Pathology (ISUP) grade and risk stratification:
- Grading uses the Gleason score (Fig. 24.13) from 1 (lowest) to 5 (highest)
- The grades of the two most common patterns are added together to give a score from 2 to 10. The first number is the predominant grade (e.g., 4+3=7 will be more aggressive than a score of 3+4=7)
- The ISUP group revised the Gleason score into simplified groups ranging from 1 to 5 (1 being least aggressive and 5 being most aggressive)
- These can be used alongside the PSA level and clinical staging to stratify patients from low to high risk to determine management. (see Table 24.2).

Management:
1. In primary care, referral on a 2WW pathway to urologist if:
   - Patient is between 50–69 years of age and the PSA level is ≥3.0 nanogram/mL
   - Prostate examination is suggestive of cancer
2. Dependent on the stage of cancer:
   - **Low-risk localised:** active surveillance (life expectancy >10 years, PSA levels every ~3–6 months, PR every ~6–12 months, prostate rebiopsy at 1 year), radical prostatectomy or radical radiotherapy (+ consider brachytherapy)
   - **Intermediate-risk localised:** radical prostatectomy or radical radiotherapy (+ consider brachytherapy) **with** androgen deprivation therapy (a luteinising hormone-releasing hormone (LHRH) agonist (e.g., goserelin) or gonadotropin-releasing hormone (GnRH) antagonist (e.g., degarelix)). Also consider active surveillance (patient chooses not to undergo surgery)
   - **High-risk localised** (if long-term control of disease is likely): radical prostatectomy + pelvic lymph node dissection or radical radiotherapy (+ brachytherapy) with androgen deprivation therapy
   - **Locally advanced:** radical prostatectomy + lymph node dissection, radical radiotherapy (+ brachytherapy) and hormonal therapy
   - **Metastatic:** hormonal therapy (or bilateral orchidectomy) and chemotherapy (docetaxel)
3. Manage complications of cancer and side effects of treatments:
   - **Tumour flare** (a temporary increase in testosterone levels due to LHRH agonists causing an increased size of vertebral metastases, which can endanger spinal cord function): medroxyprogesterone acetate or cyproterone acetate
   - **Osteoporosis:** bisphosphonates if the patient has osteoporosis (or denosumab if contraindicated)
   - **Gynaecomastia (due to bicalutamide):** prophylactic radiotherapy or tamoxifen if unsuccessful
   - **Erectile dysfunction:** PDE-5 inhibitor (e.g., sildenafil)

Prognosis:
- Prostate cancer is the second most common cause of death in males, with the overall survival depending upon the initial stage at diagnosis
- 5-year survival rate is 86%

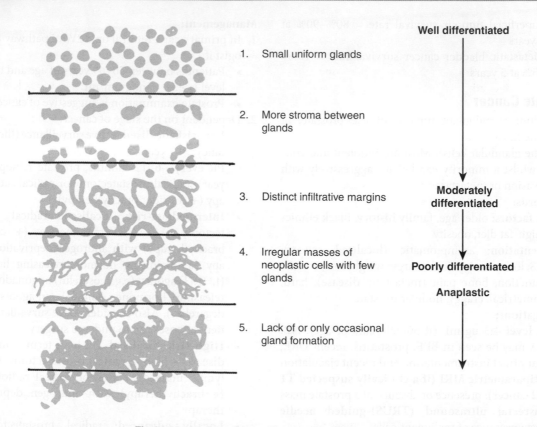

1. Small uniform glands — **Well differentiated**

2. More stroma between glands

3. Distinct infiltrative margins — **Moderately differentiated**

4. Irregular masses of neoplastic cells with few glands — **Poorly differentiated**

   Anaplastic

5. Lack of or only occasional gland formation

Fig 24.13 Gleason Score. (Illustrated by Hollie Blaber.)

TABLE 24.2 **Risk Stratification of Prostate Cancer**

Risk Category	PSA Level	Clinical Stage	Gleason Score	ISUP Grade Group
Low	<10 ng/mL	T1 to T2a	≤6	Grade Group 1
Intermediate Favourable	10–20 ng/mL	T2b	7 (3+4)	Grade Group 2
Intermediate Unfavourable			7 (4+3)	Grade Group 3
High	>20 ng/mL	≥T2c	8	Grade Group 4
			9 or 10	Grade Group 5

ISUP, International Society of Urological Pathology.

Testicular Cancer

Definition: the most common cancer in males between 20–40 years of age and accounting for 1% of all cancers. The primary testicular tumours can be categorised into:

- **Germ cell tumour** (most common)
  - Seminomas
  - Non-seminomatous (usually malignant): embryonal, teratoma, testicular choriocarcinoma, yolk sac, mixed germ cell

- **Non-germ cell tumour**
  - Leydig cell
  - Sertoli cell
  - Lymphoma (secondary testicular tumour) in older age group

Buzzwords:

- **Risk factors:** 25–35 years of age, White ethnicity, cryptorchidism, contralateral testicular cancer, family history, Klinefelter syndrome, Down syndrome, subfertility/infertility, infant hernia

- **Presentation:** chronic, typically a painless lump found after a trauma or infection, dragging sensation in the scrotum, secondary hydrocoele, haematospermia, dyspnoea (lung metastasis), abdominal mass (lymphadenopathy), gynaecomastia

Investigations:

- **Serum tumour markers:** ↑ AFP (non-seminomatous), ↑ β-hCG (choriocarcinoma and some pure seminomas), ↑ LDH (all germ cell tumours)
- **US doppler testis:** testicular mass
- **CT abdomen and pelvis:** evidence of extratesticular metastasis
- **MRI brain (if relevant symptoms or evidence of lung metastases):** presence or absence of brain metastases
- **Monitoring:** serum tumour markers, LH, FSH and testosterone, chest x-ray, CT abdomen and pelvis, CT chest and brain (for non-seminomatous germ cell tumours (NSGCTs) and seminomas >stage 1)

Differentials: hydrocoele, inguinal hernia, epididymal cyst

Management:

1. In primary care, 2WW pathway referral to urologist if:
   - Painless enlargement, or
   - Change in the shape or texture of a testis
2. In secondary care, initial treatment usually involves an inguinal radical orchidectomy, then further treatment is determined by the tumour type, staging and risk stratification
   - **NSGCT:** surveillance (low risk) or chemotherapy (high risk or metastases)
   - **Seminoma:** surveillance, adjuvant chemotherapy or radiotherapy (stage 1), radiotherapy or chemotherapy (stage II), chemotherapy (stage III or IV)
   - **Non-germ cell tumour:** chemotherapy (lymphoma)

Prognosis:

- 5-year survival of 95% for all testicular cancers

Penile Cancer

Definition: a disease in which malignant cells develop on the skin of the penis or within the penis. The most common penile malignancy is SCC. Commonly arises from the epithelium of the inner prepuce or glans.

Buzzwords:

- **Risk factors:** human papilloma virus, phimosis, chronic penile inflammation (balanoposthitis), psoralene and ultraviolet A phototherapy, smoking, multiple sexual partners, immunocompromise
- **Presentation:** lump, ulcer or erythematous lesion either on the glans or prepuce; painless, itching or burning sensation under the prepuce; discharge or bleeding from the lesion, inguinal lymphadenopathy

Investigations:

- **Penile biopsy:** histological evidence of a penile malignancy
- **Fine needle aspiration cytology (if inguinal nodes are palpable):** presence or absence of metastasis
- **CT/PET-CT chest, abdomen and pelvis (staging):** presence or absence or metastases
- **Monitoring:** CT (if suspected recurrence)

Differentials: balanitis, viral warts

Management:

1. In primary care, 2WW referral if penile mass or ulcerated lesion and an STI is excluded or treated
2. Combination of surgery, radiotherapy and chemotherapy
   - **Superficial non-invasive disease** (intraepithelial neoplasia): topical 5-FU, laser ablation or glans resurfacing
   - **Locally invasive but confined to the glans:** wide local excision ± reconstruction, glansectomy with split skin graft reconstruction
   - **Invasive and involving the penis:** partial amputation or total penectomy and formation of a perineal urethrostomy ± neoadjuvant radiotherapy or chemotherapy
   - **If palpable lymph nodes:** radical lymphadenectomy

Prognosis:

- 5-year survival rate is 74%
- Penile cancer and its treatment can significantly impact a patient's quality of life due to sexual dysfunction, voiding problems and cosmetic appearance

THE ONE-LINE ROUND-UP!

Here are some key words to help you remember each condition/concept.

Condition/Concept	One-line Description
LUTS	Storage, voiding, post-micturition
Urinary retention	>500 mL on bladder scan
Incontinence	Stress, urgency or both (mixed), overflow, functional, continuous
Urolithiasis	Loin-to-groin pain
Stress urinary incontinence	Pelvic floor training
Overactive bladder	Urgency, frequency and nocturia
Bladder stones	Dysuria at end of micturition
BPE	Poor flow, smooth prostate
Prostatitis	Tender, warm, boggy prostate
Testicular torsion	Sudden testicular pain
Epididymo-orchitis	Prehn's sign positive
Hydrocoele	Transilluminates
Epidymal cyst	Chinese lantern
Varicocele	'Bag of worms'
Cryptorchidism	High risk of malignancy
Phimosis	Tight foreskin
Paraphimosis	Iatrogenic post-catheterisation
Erectile dysfunction	PDE-5 inhibitor
Priapism	Sickle cell disease
Peyronie's disease	Dupuytren's contracture
Renal cell carcinoma	Flank pain, haematuria, abdominal mass
Bladder cancer	Painless haematuria
Prostate cancer	Craggy prostate
Testicular cancer	Painless testicular lump
Penile cancer	HPV infection

READING LIST: UROLOGY IN AN HOUR

Lower Urinary Tract Symptoms (LUTS)

NICE. (2019). *CKS: LUTS in men.* https://cks.nice.org.uk/topics/luts-in-men/. [Accessed April 2021].

European Association of Urology. (2021). *Management of non-neurogenic male LUTS.* https://uroweb.org/guideline/treatment-of-non-neurogenic-male-luts/. [Accessed April 2021].

NICE. (2015). *CG97: Lower urinary tract symptoms in men: management.* https://www.nice.org.uk/guidance/cg97. [Accessed April 2021].

Patient info. (2016). *Lower urinary tract symptoms in women.* https://patient.info/doctor/lower-urinary-tract-symptoms-in-women-pro. [Accessed April 2021].

Reynard, J., Brewster, S., Biers, S., & Neal, N. (2019). *Oxford handbook of urology* (4th ed.). Oxford University Press.

Urinary Retention

NICE. (2019). *CKS: LUTS in men.* https://cks.nice.org.uk/topics/luts-in-men/. [Accessed April 2021].

EAU Guidelines. (2021). *Management of non-neurogenic male LUTS.* https://uroweb.org/guideline/treatment-of-non-neurogenic-male-luts/. [Accessed April 2021].

NICE. (2015). *CG97: Lower urinary tract symptoms in men: management.* https://www.nice.org.uk/guidance/cg97. [Accessed April 2021].

Urinary Incontinence (UI)

NICE. (2019). *NG123: Urinary incontinence and pelvic organ prolapse in women: management.* https://www.nice.org.uk/guidance/ng123. [Accessed April 2021].

European Association of Urology. (2020). *Urinary incontinence.* https://uroweb.org/guideline/urinary-incontinence/. [Accessed April 2021].

NICE. (2019). *CKS: Incontinence- urinary, in women.* https://cks.nice.org.uk/topics/incontinence-urinary-in-women/. [Accessed April 2021].

Patient Info. (2019). *Urinary incontinence.* https://patient.info/doctor/urinary-incontinence-pro. [Accessed April 2021].

Urolithiasis

NICE. (2020). *CKS: Renal or ureteric colic – acute.* https://cks.nice.org.uk/topics/renal-or-ureteric-colic-acute/. [Accessed April 2021].

NICE. (2019). *NG118: Renal and ureteric stones: assessment and management.* https://www.nice.org.uk/guidance/ng118. [Accessed April 2021].

European Association of Urology. (2021). *Urolithiasis.* https://uroweb.org/guideline/urolithiasis/. [Accessed April 2021].

Stress Urinary Incontinence (SUI)

NICE. (2019). *NG123: Urinary incontinence and pelvic organ prolapse in women: management.* https://www.nice.org.uk/guidance/ng123. [Accessed April 2021].

European Association of Urology. (2020). *Urinary incontinence.* https://uroweb.org/guideline/urinary-incontinence/. [Accessed April 2021].

NICE. (2019). *CKS: Incontinence – urinary, in women.* https://cks.nice.org.uk/topics/incontinence-urinary-in-women/. [Accessed April 2021].

Patient info. (2019). *Urinary incontinence.* https://patient.info/doctor/urinary-incontinence-pro. [Accessed April 2021].

Overactive Bladder

NICE. (2019). *NG123: Urinary incontinence and pelvic organ prolapse in women: management.* https://www.nice.org.uk/guidance/ng123. [Accessed April 2021].

European Association of Urology. (2020). *Urinary incontinence.* https://uroweb.org/guideline/urinary-incontinence/. [Accessed April 2021].

Patient info. (2019). *Urinary incontinence.* https://patient.info/doctor/urinary-incontinence-pro. [Accessed April 2021].

Patient info. (2015). *Overactive bladder.* https://patient.info/doctor/overactive-bladder. [Accessed April 2021].

Bladder Stones

European Association of Urology. (2021). *Bladder stones.* https://uroweb.org/guideline/bladder-stones/. [Accessed April 2021].

Radiopaedia. (2021). *Urolithiasis.* https://radiopaedia.org/articles/urolithiasis?lang=gb. [Accessed April 2021].

Benign Prostatic Enlargement (BPE)

NICE. (2015). *CG97: Lower urinary tract symptoms in men: management.* https://www.nice.org.uk/guidance/cg97. [Accessed April 2021].

BMJ Best Practice. (2020). *Benign prostatic hyperplasia.* https://bestpractice.bmj.com/topics/en-gb/208. [Accessed April 2021].

Patient info. (2015). *Benign prostatic hyperplasia.* https://patient.info/doctor/benign-prostatic-hyperplasia. [Accessed April 2021].

Prostatitis

NICE. (2019). *CKS: Prostatitis – chronic.* https://cks.nice.org.uk/topics/prostatitis-chronic/. [Accessed April 2021].

NICE. (2019). *CKS: Prostatitis – acute.* https://cks.nice.org.uk/topics/prostatitis-acute/. [Accessed April 2021].

Testicular Torsion

BMJ Best Practice. (2020). *Testicular torsion.* https://bestpractice.bmj.com/topics/en-gb/506. [Accessed April 2021].

NICE. (2019). *CKS: Scrotal pain and swelling.* https://cks.nice.org.uk/topics/scrotal-pain-swelling/. [Accessed April 2021].

Epididymo-orchitis

NICE. (2019). *CKS: Scrotal pain and swelling.* https://cks.nice.org.uk/topics/scrotal-pain-swelling/. [Accessed April 2021].

Hydrocoele

BMJ Best Practice. (2020). *Hydrocele.* https://bestpractice.bmj.com/topics/en-gb/1104. [Accessed April 2021].

Patient info. (2016). *Hydrocele.* https://patient.info/doctor/hydrocele. [Accessed April 2021].

Epididymal Cyst

Patient info. (2014). *Epididymal cysts.* https://patient.info/doctor/epididymal-cysts. [Accessed April 2021].

NICE. (2019). *CKS: Scrotal pain and swelling.* https://cks.nice.org.uk/topics/scrotal-pain-swelling/. [Accessed April 2021].

Varicocele

NICE. (2019). *CKS: Scrotal pain and swelling.* https://cks.nice.org.uk/topics/scrotal-pain-swelling/. [Accessed April 2021].

Patient info. (2019). *Varicocele.* https://patient.info/doctor/varicocele-pro. [Accessed April 2021].

Cryptorchidism (Undescended Testes)

NICE. (2020). *CKS: Undescended testes.* https://cks.nice.org.uk/topics/undescended-testes/. [Accessed April 2021].

European Association of Urology. (2021). *Paediatric urology.* https://uroweb.org/guideline/paediatric-urology/. [Accessed April 2021].

Patient info. (2015). *Undescended and maldescended testes.* https://patient.info/doctor/undescended-and-maldescended-testes. [Accessed April 2021].

Phimosis

British Association of Urological Surgeons. (2020). *Tight foreskin (phimosis).* https://www.baus.org.uk/patients/conditions/13/tight_foreskin_phimosisv. [Accessed April 2021].

Patient info. (2018). *Phimosis and paraphimosis.* https://patient.info/mens-health/penis-problems/phimosis-and-paraphimosis. [Accessed April 2021].

Paraphimosis

Patient info. (2018). *Phimosis and paraphimosis.* https://patient.info/mens-health/penis-problems/phimosis-and-paraphimosis. [Accessed April 2021].

Bragg, B. N., Kong, E. L., & Leslie, S. W. (2020). *Paraphimosis.* StatPearls. https://www.ncbi.nlm.nih.gov/books/NBK459233/. [Accessed April 2021].

Erectile Dysfunction

NICE. (2019). *CKS: Erectile dysfunction.* https://cks.nice.org.uk/topics/erectile-dysfunction/. [Accessed April 2021].

Patient info. (2016). *Erectile dysfunction.* https://patient.info/doctor/erectile-dysfunction. [Accessed April 2021].

British Society for Sexual Medicine. (2018). *British Society for Sexual Medicine Guidelines on the management of erectile dysfunction in men - 2017.* http://www.bssm.org.uk/. [Accessed April 2021].

European Association of Urology. (2021). *Sexual and reproductive health.* https://uroweb.org/guideline/sexual-and-reproductive-health/. [Accessed April 2021].

Priapism

European Association of Urology. (2021). *Sexual and reproductive health.* https://uroweb.org/guideline/sexual-and-reproductive-health/. [Accessed April 2021].

Peyronie's Disease

European Association of Urology. (2021). *Sexual and reproductive health.* https://uroweb.org/guideline/sexual-and-reproductive-health/. [Accessed April 2021].

Patient info. (2015). *Peyronie's disease.* https://patient.info/doctor/peyronies-disease-pro. [Accessed April 2021].

Ibe, G., Parnham, A., & Pearce, I. (2020). Spotlight: Peyronie's disease management. *British Journal of Family Medicine.* https://www.bjfm.co.uk/spotlight-peyronie-s-disease-management. [Accessed April 2021].

Renal Cell Carcinoma

European Association of Urology. (2020). *Renal cell carcinoma.* https://uroweb.org/guideline/renal-cell-carcinoma/. [Accessed April 2021].

European Society for Medical Oncology. (2019). *Renal cell carcinoma: ESMO clinical practice guidelines.* https://www.esmo.org/guidelines/genitourinary-cancers/renal-cell-carcinoma. [Accessed April 2021].

Cancer Research UK. (2020). *Kidney cancer - survival.* https://www.cancerresearchuk.org/about-cancer/kidney-cancer/survival. [Accessed April 2021].

Bladder Cancer

NICE. (2015). *CKS: Urological cancers - recognition and referral.* https://cks.nice.org.uk/topics/urological-cancers-recognition-referral/. [Accessed April 2021].

NICE. (2015). *NG2: Bladder cancer: diagnosis and management.* https://www.nice.org.uk/guidance/ng2. [Accessed April 2021].

Patient info. (2015). *Bladder cancer.* https://patient.info/doctor/bladder-cancer-pro. [Accessed April 2021].

European Association of Urology. (2020). *Non-muscle-invasive bladder cancer.* https://uroweb.org/guideline/non-muscle-invasive-bladder-cancer/. [Accessed April 2021].

European Association of Urology. (2020). *Muscle-invasive and metastatic bladder cancer.* https://uroweb.org/guideline/bladder-cancer-muscle-invasive-and-metastatic/. [Accessed April 2021].

Prostate Cancer

NICE. (2017). *CKS: Prostate cancer.* https://cks.nice.org.uk/topics/prostate-cancer/. [Accessed April 2021].

Wilkinson, I. B., Raine, T., Wiles, K., Goodhart, A., Hall, C., & O'Neill, H. (2017). *Oxford handbook of clinical medicine* (10th ed.). Oxford University Press.

NICE. (2019). *NG131: Prostate cancer: diagnosis and management.* https://www.nice.org.uk/guidance/ng131. [Accessed April 2021].

Cancer Research UK. (2020). *Prostate cancer statistics.* https://www.cancerresearchuk.org/health-professional/cancer-statistics/statistics-by-cancer-type/prostate-cancer#heading-Two. [Accessed April 2021].

Testicular Cancer

European Association of Urology. (2021). *Testicular cancer.* https://uroweb.org/guideline/testicular-cancer/. [Accessed April 2021].

NICE. (2019). *CKS: Scrotal pain and swelling.* https://cks.nice.org.uk/topics/scrotal-pain-swelling/. [Accessed April 2021].

Teach Me Surgery. (2020). *Testicular cancer.* https://teachmesurgery.com/urology/genital-tract/testicular-cancer/. [Accessed April 2021].

Cancer Research UK. (2020). *Testicular cancer survival statistics.* https://www.cancerresearchuk.org/health-professional/cancer-statistics/statistics-by-cancer-type/testicular-cancer/survival. [Accessed April 2021].

Penile Cancer

European Association of Urology. (2018). *Penile cancer.* https://uroweb.org/guideline/penile-cancer/. [Accessed April 2021].

Teach Me Surgery. (2020). *Penile cancer.* https://teachmesurgery.com/urology/other/penile-cancer/. [Accessed April 2021].

Patient info. (2016). *Penile cancer.* https://patient.info/doctor/penile-cancer-pro. [Accessed April 2021].

Cancer Research UK. (2016). *Penile cancer survival statistics.* https://www.cancerresearchuk.org/health-professional/cancer-statistics/statistics-by-cancer-type/penile-cancer/survival. [Accessed April 2021].

Prescribing Appendix

HAEMATOLOGY

Anticoagulation

Unfractionated heparins: inhibit thrombin (IIa) and factor Xa

Low molecular weight heparins (LMWH): inhibit factor Xa and thrombin (IIa) to a lesser degree

Fondaparinux (a synthetic LMWH): inhibits factor Xa

Dabigatran, Argatroban, Bivalirudin: inhibit thrombin (IIa)

Rivaroxaban, Apixaban, Edoxaban: inhibit factor Xa

Warfarin: inhibits vitamin K dependent clotting factors (prothrombin (II), factor VII, factor IX, factor X)

Antiplatelet Therapy

See Table 1 for a summary of antiplatelet therapies and their uses.

TABLE 1 Antiplatelet Therapy

Drug	Mechanism of Action	Main Uses
Aspirin	Inhibits COX1, thus reducing thromboxane A2	Secondary prevention of cardiovascular disease Management of ACS, TIA, or acute ischaemic stroke
Clopidogrel	Irreversible inhibition of $P2Y_{12}$	Prevention of atherothrombotic events in ACS and percutaneous coronary intervention
Prasugrel	Irreversible inhibition of $P2Y_{12}$	Undergoing coronary angiography within 48 h of unstable angina or NSTEMI
Ticagrelor	Reversible inhibition of $P2Y_{12}$	Prevention of atherothrombotic events in patients with ACS
Tirofiban	GPIIb/IIIa antagonist	Prevention of myocardial infarction with angiography planned and chest pain within 12 h

Abbreviations used: acute coronary syndrome (ACS), transient ischaemic accident (TIA), non-ST elevation myocardial infarction (NSTEMI)

Transfusion Reactions

Monitor the patient's condition and vital signs before, during, and after blood transfusions to detect acute transfusion reactions. Always perform transfusions in areas that are appropriately staffed. See Table 2 for a summary of transfusion reactions and their management. For all acute transfusion reactions stop the transfusion and maintain IV access.

TABLE 2 Transfusion reactions

Reaction	Cause	Buzzwords	Management
Febrile non-haemolytic	Cytokines from transfused product	Rise in temperature by >1 deg, chills/rigours. Usually otherwise well	Consider paracetamol Most resolve in 2-3 h Monitor for acute haemolytic reaction
Mild allergic	Specific antigen from transfused product	Pruritis/urticaria/erythema, flushing. N+V	Monitor for anaphylaxis Antihistamine Consider restarting if symptoms settle
Anaphylactic	Specific antigen from transfused product	See Emergency Medicine in an Hour for features and management	
Acute (<24 h) haemolytic reactions	Patient antibodies to transfused RBCs or transfused antibodies to patient's RBCs. ABO incompatibility	Fever (earliest sign), dyspnoea, hypotension. Later: AKI, jaundice, possibly DIC Haemoglobinuria ↓haptoglobin, ↑bili rubin, ↑LDH Positive DAT	Identify if the correct product was given to the correct patient Inform blood bank Prevent further incompatible units from being given Urgent haematology review
Delayed (>24 h) haemolytic reactions	Patient antibodies to transfused RBCs – usually one that was in too low a concentration to be found on pre-transfusion testing	Usually milder than acute haemolytic reactions Unexpected ↓Hb with ↑bili, ↑LDH, positive DAT, new red cell antibody. Rarely, renal failure	Close follow up Identify antibody and find antigen-negative units for future transfusions. Monitor for the burden of haemolysis/renal failure
Bacterial contamination	Transfer of contaminated unit – most commonly platelets as they are stored at higher temperatures	Rapid onset of fever, chills, dyspnoea, hypotension, shock May progress to septic shock, DIC, renal failure. High mortality	As for sepsis – urgent IV Abx May require ICU care
Transfusion-associated lung injury (TRALI)	Antibodies in the transfused unit to HLA or granulocyte antigens	During or within hours of transfusion: onset of non-cardiogenic pulmonary oedema. Dyspnoea, hypoxia, tachycardia, hypotension	Supportive Oxygen +/- NIV +/- intubation Usually resolves in 48-96 h
Transfusion associated circulatory overload (TACO)	Circulatory overload due to increase in circulatory volume	During or shortly after transfusion. Acute respiratory distress, orthopnoea, hypertension, pulmonary oedema, peripheral oedema, raised jugular venous pressure (JVP), positive fluid balance. BNP may be elevated, consider an ECHO	Prevention is best. Identify high risk patients and ensure blood is given slowly. Diuretics may be given with the transfusion.
Graft-versus-host disease	Donor T-cells proliferate and recognise the host as foreign. Most common in patients with marked cellular immunodeficiencies	2-50 days after transfusion: rash, diarrhoea, liver failure, pancytopaenia. Mortality >90% - most die of infection	Prevention: irradiated blood to prevent leucocyte replication in at-risk patients

Abbreviations used: Acute Kidney injury (AKI), disseminated intravascular coagulation (DIC), lactate dehydrogenase (LDH), direct antiglobulin test (DAT), red blood cells (RBC), non-invasive ventilation (NIV)

ANAESTHETICS AND PERIOPERATIVE CARE

Anticoagulation for Venous thromboembolism (VTE) Prophylaxis

See Table 3.

General surgery: seven days LMWH or until enough mobility established

Cancer abdominal surgery: 28 days LMWH

Spinal surgery: 30 days LMWH

Elective hip replacement: 28 days LMWH + stockings **OR** ten days LMWH + Aspirin Low dose for a further 28 days

TABLE 3   Anticoagulation for VTE Prophylaxis

VTE Prophylaxis	Example	Indication
Unfractionated heparin	Heparin	Renally impaired, VTE prophylaxis
Low molecular weight heparin (LMWH)	Dalteparin Sodium Enoxaparin Sodium Tinzaparin Sodium	VTE Prophylaxis for all types of surgery (including T&O) VTE Treatment in DVT, PE, Pregnancy (stop at onset of labour)
Selective anti-Xa inhibitor	Fondaparinux	VTE Prophylaxis for all types of surgery (including T&O)

Abbreviations used: Venous thromboembolism (VTE), low molecular weight heparin (LMWH), deep vein thrombosis (DVT), pulmonary embolism (PE), trauma and orthopaedics (T&O)

Perioperative Medications: What to Stop and When See Table 4

TABLE 4   Perioperative Medication – What to Stop and When

CARDIOVASCULAR DRUGS	
Beta-blockers, Calcium Channel Blockers, Statins, Diuretics	Continue
ACE-inhibitors	Risk of profound hypotension – stop > two days before in those at risk of large haemorrhage (e.g., AAA repair) or having epidural anaesthesia
ANTICOAGULATION DRUGS	
Warfarin	**Elective surgery:** • Stop Warfarin five days prior to surgery and bridge with LMWH (i.e., start LMWH five days prior to surgery when you stop the Warfarin) • Stop LMWH on the day of surgery • Restart Warfarin and LMWH after the surgery and check daily for INR. Once INR is back to therapeutic range (usually 2-3), then stop LMWH **Emergency surgery which can be delayed 6-12 h** • Stop Warfarin, give Vitamin K (+/- dried prothrombin complex) • Check INR. When INR is < 1.5, then it is usually safe to proceed with surgery **Emergency surgery that cannot be delayed:** • Stop Warfarin, give Vitamin K AND dried prothrombin complex • Check INR. When INR is < 1.5, then it is usually safe to proceed with surgery
DOACs (apixaban, rivaroxaban, dabigatran etc)	• Dabigatran may be reversed in an emergency with idarucizumab • In an emergency, discuss with haematology • Stop >48 h before surgery and check clotting (though not a reliable indicator of residual effect)

Continued

TABLE 4   Perioperative Medication – What to Stop and When—cont'd

ANTIPLATELET DRUGS

Aspirin	Usually continued if 75 mg/day except in surgery involving: • Brain • Spinal canal • Prostate
Clopidogrel	Stopped five to seven days before

DIABETIC DRUGS

Insulin	Continue long-acting insulin. Examples of long-acting insulin (and brand) include: • Insulin glargine (Lantus, Toujeo, Basaglar) • Insulin detemir (Levemir) • Insulin degludec (Tresiba) Stop short/rapid-acting insulin and put the patient on a sliding scale. The sliding scale essentially replaces the short-acting insulin. Examples of short/rapid-acting insulin (and brand) include: • Lispro (Humalog) • Aspart (Novorapid)
Metformin	Continue

GYNAECOLOGY DRUGS

Combined oral contraceptive pill (COCP), HRT	Advised stop four weeks prior (alternative contraception required in case of COCP)

Abbreviations used: abdominal aortic aneurysm (AAA), low molecular weight heparin (LMWH), international normalised ratio (INR), combined oral contraceptive pill (COCP), hormone replacement therapy (HRT), Direct-acting oral anticoagulants (DOAC)

RENAL

Nephrotoxic Drugs

Acute changes in kidney function can lead to impaired clearance of patients regularly prescribed medications. The term 'nephrotoxic' should be used judiciously as few drugs have direct toxic effects on the kidneys. Many drugs can affect kidney function in those with existing renal impairment and intercurrent disease states (i.e., sepsis). The three main negative effects of drugs during acute kidney injury (AKI) are:

- Effects on renal, fluid, or electrolyte physiology
- Altered side effect profile in renal impairment
- Direct kidney damage

The most commonly encountered 'nephrotoxic' drugs are listed in Table 5. This list is not exhaustive, and consulting with the British National Formulary (BNF), your hospital pharmacist, and, if necessary, the renal team is essential.

With medicine management of patients with AKI, consider:

- Medication to be stopped
- Medication to be continued (no change to dosage or frequency)
- Medication to be altered (change to dosage +/- frequency +/- monitoring)
- Alternative medication
- Important information and advice given on discharge to patients, care providers, and health care professionals

TABLE 5 High-risk Medicines in AKI

Drug	Effects during AKI	Steps to take during AKI
NSAIDs/COX-II inhibitors	Reduced renal perfusion Interstitial nephritis	**Stopped/avoided**
Opioids (including Tramadol)	Accumulation of active metabolites	**Continued:** reduce dose and frequency
Benzodiazepines	Accumulation of active metabolites	**Continued:** reduce dose
Aminoglycosides (i.e., Gentamicin)	Ototoxicity Tubular cell damage	**Stopped/avoided**
Penicillins	Accumulation of active metabolites Interstitial nephritis (rare) and glomerulonephritis	**Continued:** reduce dose
Antivirals	Accumulation of active metabolites	**Continued:** reduce dose
ACEi/ARBs	Reduced GFR, especially when renal perfusion is compromised. Hyperkalaemia	**Stopped/avoided:** in haemodynamic instability, hypotension, or hyperkalaemia. **Continued in certain situations:** e.g., heart failure with adequate BP **Consider alternative medications** (e.g., CCBs, alpha-blockers, beta-blockers)
Antihypertensives (CCBs, alpha-blockers, beta-blockers, etc.)	Hypotension Reduce renal perfusion	**Continued (reduce dose) or stopped**
Thiazide and loop diuretics	Hypotension	**Stopped/avoided:** e.g., if hypotensive Loop diuretics>thiazides (thiazides can potentiate loop diuretic effects) **Continued:** high doses may be required in patients with fluid overload
Potassium-sparing diuretics i.e., spironolactone	Hyperkalaemia	**Stopped/avoided**
Metformin	Lactic acidosis	**Stopped/avoided:** if eGFR <30 mL/min
Contrast media	Tubular cell toxicity Contrast-induced nephropathy (uncertain significance)	Encourage oral hydration before and after IV contrast media administration Consider IV volume expansion with 0.9% NaCl or sodium bicarbonate if eGFR <30mL/min, renal transplant patients, large volume of contrast used or intra-arterial contrast use
Statins	Risk of rhabdomyolysis/cause AKI in the presence of rhabdomyolysis	**Stopped/avoided:** if AKI secondary to rhabdomyolysis. Otherwise, continue but monitor for side effects
Low molecular weight heparin	Accumulation of active metabolites	**Continued:** monitor anti-Xa levels and either reduce dose or consider alternative agent (unfractionated heparin)
Warfarin	Raised INR secondary to raised urea	**Continued or stopped:** monitor INR and either reduce dose or withhold depending on the indication for use
Direct oral anticoagulants	Accumulation of active metabolites	**Continued or stopped:** especially agents with high renal clearance (Dabigatran)

Abbreviations used: Non-steroidal anti-inflammatory drugs (NSAIDs), cytochrome c oxidase subunit 2 (COX-II), angiotensin-converting enzyme inhibitor (ACEi), angiotensin receptor blocker (ARB), glomerular filtration rate (GFR), blood pressure (BP), calcium channel blockers (CCB), acute kidney injury (AKI), international normalised ratio (INR)

CARDIOVASCULAR

Cardiovascular Drugs

See Table 6 for a summary of the contraindications and side effects of commonly used medications.

TABLE 6	Cardiovascular Drugs		
Drug	**Example**	**Contraindications**	**Side Effects**
ACE-inhibitors (-pril)	Enala**pril** Lisino**pril** Rami**pril**	• AKI/CKD • Bilateral renal artery stenosis • Hyperkalaemia • Pregnancy	Angioedema Dry cough Hyperkalaemia Hypotension Renal impairment
Beta-blocker (-olol)	**Non-selective (β1, β2):** Carvedilol, Propranolol **Selective (β1 only):** Atenolol, Bisoprolol, Metoprolol	• Asthma • Heart block • Raynaud • Simultaneous use of CCB with beta-blocker (risk of severe bradycardia and heart failure)	**Masked hypoglycaemia** **Masked tachycardia** (e.g., sepsis) Bronchospasm Bradycardia Erectile dysfunction Headache Hypotension Lethargy Sleep disturbances
Calcium channel blocker	**Rate limiting:** Diltiazem, Verapamil **Non-rate limiting:** Amlodipine, Nifedipine	**Rate limiting:** Heart failure, WPW syndrome, ventricular tachyarrhythmias **Non-rate limiting:** Unstable angina	**Rate limiting:** • Left ventricular depression • Constipation (Verapamil) **Non-rate limiting** • Headache (arterial dilation) • Flushing (arterial dilation) • Ankle swelling
Nitrates	Glyceryl Trinitrate (GTN) Isosorbide Mononitrate	• Hypersensitivity to nitrates • Hypotension (Systolic <100 mmHg) • Simultaneous use of Sildenafil with GTN (risk of serious hypotension)	• Dizziness • Headache • Flushing • Postural hypotension
Loop diuretics	Bumetanide Furosemide	• Anuria • Comatose states with liver cirrhosis • Renal failure • Severe hyponatraemia/hypokalaemia	**Decreases:** • **Hypocalcaemia (Loop diuretics only)** • Hypokalaemia • Hyponatraemia • Hypochloraemia **Increases:** • **Hypercalcaemia (Thiazide-like only)** • Hyperglycaemia • Hyperuraemia
Thiazide-like	Bendroflumethiazide Indapamide	• Addison's disease • Hypercalcaemia • Severe hyponatraemia/hypokalaemia	
Potassium-sparing diuretics	Amiloride Eplerenone Spironolactone	Hyperkalaemia	• Hyperkalaemia • Gynaecomastia (Spironolactone)

TABLE 6   Cardiovascular Drugs—cont'd

Drug	Example	Contraindications	Side Effects
Statin	Atorvastatin	• Active liver disease • Pregnancy • Breast-feeding	• Abnormal LFTs (most common) • Depression • Dizziness • GI disturbance • Headache • Muscle aches (myositis, myopathy, very rarely rhabdomyolysis) • Sleep disturbances • Thrombocytopenia

RHEUMATOLOGY

Conventional Disease-Modifying Antirheumatic Drugs (DMARDs) See Table 7

TABLE 7   Conventional DMARDs

Drug	Side Effects	Contraindications	Monitoring
Methotrexate	Mucositis, Pneumonitis, Liver toxicity, Myelosuppression	Avoid other anti-folate agents (trimethoprim, co-trimoxazole) Pregnancy	Baseline pregnancy test FBC LFTs U&E
Sulfasalazine	Gastrointestinal upset, Rash, Myelosuppression, Liver toxicity, Haemolysis, Lupus-like features, Reversible azoospermia	Glucose-6-phosphate dehydrogenase (G6PD) deficiency Porphyria Asthma	FBC LFTs U&E
Hydroxy-chloroquine	Gastrointestinal upset, Retinopathy, Photosensitive rash, Headaches, Tinnitus	COVID	FBC LFTs Vision
Leflunomide	Mucositis, rash, myelosuppression, hypertension, liver toxicity, terato-genicity	Pregnancy	Blood Pressure FBC LFTs U&E
Azathioprine	Photosensitivity reaction, myelosup-pression	Active infection	Thiopurine methyltransfer-ase (TPMT), FBC, LFTs prior to starting treatment FBC, LFT after starting

NB: conventional DMARDs safe in pregnancy: sulfasalazine, azathioprine, cyclosporin, hydroxychloroquine

Biological Disease-Modifying Antirheumatic Drugs (DMARDs) See Table 8

TABLE 8 Biological DMARDs			
Drug	**Side Effects**	**Contraindications**	**Monitoring**
Anti-TNF (e.g., Inflix-imab/ Etanercept)	Gastrointestinal upset, heart failure, hypersensitivity, fever, cytopenia	Previous or active tuberculosis, history of malignancy, demyelinating disease, severe heart failure	FBC only
Anti-CD20 (e.g., Rituximab)	Gastrointestinal upset, heart failure, hypersensitivity, fever, cytopenia	Previous or active tuberculosis, history of malignancy, demyelinating disease, severe heart failure	Immunoglobulin G at three months FBC

Other Drugs See Table 9

TABLE 9 Other Drugs Used in Rheumatology			
Drug	**Side Effects**	**Contraindications**	**Monitoring**
Allopurinol	Gastrointestinal upset, rash, kidney failure	Monitor liver and renal function	LFTs U&E
Alendronic acid	Oesophagitis, jaw necrosis, atypical hip fractures	Barret's oesophagus, renal impairment, poor dentition	N/A

GENERAL SURGERY

Surgical Site Infection

Definition: Local evidence of infection in a surgical site

Buzzwords:
- **Risk factors:** older patients, malnutrition, diabetes, colonisation with *S. Aureus*, traumatic/soiled wounds, smoking
- **Presentation:** at wound site - erythema, pain, swelling, pus. Delayed wound healing, wound dehiscence. More severe infections may present systemic features (fever, sepsis) and abscess formation deep in the wound.

Investigations:
- **Wound swab with culture/sensitivities:** identify organisms and appropriate treatment
- **Bloods:** often ↑ WCC and CRP
- Consider imaging (USS/CT/MRI) to identify collections

Differentials: normal post-incisional inflammation, necrotising fasciitis

Management:
- **Perioperative prevention:** - Decolonisation of *S. aureus* (mupirocin, chlorhexidine body wash), sterile technique, skin cleaning (commonly chlorhexidine). Prophylactic Abx (routine with the placement of prostheses; dirty/contaminated surgery such as bowel perforation; any surgery entering respiratory, GU or GI tracts; caesarean sections).
- **Postoperative prevention:** sterile dressing, advise against showering for 48 h, clean wound with sterile saline in first 48 h if required
- **Wound infection:** antibiotics to target most likely organism (based on local guidelines/culture results), consider opening wound/interventional radiology to drain pus/collections.

PALLIATIVE CARE AND ONCOLOGY

Nausea and Vomiting

Mechanism: Visceral, chemoreceptor trigger zone or vestibular stimulation by different triggers leads to the secretion of neurotransmitters which stimulate the medullary vomiting centre. This ultimately leads to nausea and vomiting.

Antiemetics See Table 11

To choose the best antiemetic, it is important to consider where it acts, its side effects, and warnings. See Fig. 1 and Table 10

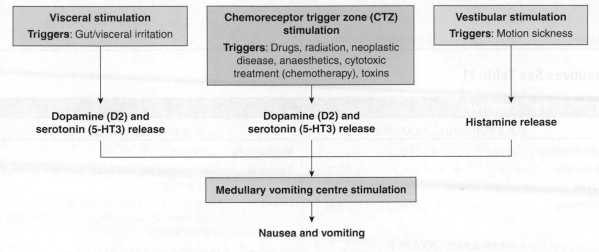

Fig. 1 Nausea and Vomiting Mechanism

TABLE 10 Antiemetics

DOPAMINE (D2) RECEPTOR ANTAGONIST		SEROTONIN (5-HT₃) RECEPTOR ANTAGONISTS	
Mechanism	Blocks dopamine receptors peripherally (visceral/GI tract) and/or centrally (CTZ).	**Mechanism**	Blocks serotonin receptors peripherally (visceral/GI tract) and/or centrally (CTZ).
Examples	Metoclopramide (central & peripheral) Domperidone (does not readily cross the blood-brain barrier) Haloperidol Phenothiazines such as prochlorperazine Chlorpromazine (central only)	**Examples**	Ondansetron
		Uses	N&V caused by peripheral (visceral/GI tract) and/or central (CTZ) stimulation.
Uses	N&V caused by peripheral (visceral/GI tract) and/or central (CTZ) stimulation.	**Side effects**	Severe constipation - avoid in post GI surgery or GI obstruction
Side effects	All are associated with sedation Metoclopramide is associated with oculogyric crisis in young patients (*especially in exams*), QT prolongation, and has a prokinetic effect	**Warning**	Avoid in children <12 or people <35kg Avoid in prolonged QT syndrome or use in conjunction with drugs at risk of causing prolonged QT syndrome (antipsychotics, SSRI, quinine)
Warning	Avoid all dopamine receptor antagonists (except Domperidone) in Parkinson's disease/Lewy body dementia		

Continued

TABLE 10 Antiemetics—cont'd

HISTAMINE (H₁) RECEPTOR ANTAGONISTS

Mechanism	Blocks H_1 receptors and ACh (muscarinic) receptors	**Side effects**	Drowsiness, confusion, dry mouth
Examples	Cyclizine Promethazine Cinnarizine	**Warnings**	Avoid in conditions susceptible to anticholinergic effects (e.g., Benign prostatic hyperplasia (BPH), acute angle closure glaucoma) and dementia/delirium
Uses	N&V triggered by vestibular stimulation.		

Laxatives See Table 11

TABLE 11 Laxatives

BULK FORMING LAXATIVES		SOFTENER LAXATIVE	
Mechanism	Increase the amount of stools	**Mechanism**	Softening of stools
Example	Ispaghula Husk, sterculia, methylcellulose	**Example**	Methylcellulose, docusate sodium, glycerol suppositories
Uses	Poor oral intake	**Usess**	Opioid-induced constipation, adhesions, palliative care. Normally prescribed with a stimulant
Warning	May exacerbate flatulence, bloating, and cramping	**Warning**	Poor efficacy when used alone
STIMULANT LAXATIVE		**OSMOTIC LAXATIVE**	
Mechanism	Increases motility	**Mechanism**	Increases and retains water in the large intestine
Example	Bisacodyl, senna, sodium picosulfate, glycerol suppositories Co-danthramer/co-danthrusate (only in palliative care)	**Example**	Lactulose, macrogol
Uses	Opioid-induced constipation, adhesions, palliative care. Normally prescribed with a softener	**Uses**	Opioid-induced constipation, adhesions, palliative care. Can be prescribed alone. Lactulose is for very mild constipation, macrogol is a stronger laxative
Warning	May cause abdominal cramps	**Warning**	Lactulose contains lactose (some people are intolerant)

WHO Analgesic Ladder

Originally for cancer pain - it can be used as a general guide (see Fig. 2):

- Non-opioid:paracetamol +/- NSAID
- Weak opioid:codeine, low dose tramadol
- Strong opioid:morphine, fentanyl, buprenorphine, methadone
- Adjuvant analgesics are drugs whose primary indication is not for pain (i.e., antidepressants, anticonvulsants, and antiarrhythmics)

Some advocate a fourth rung for acute severe pain not managed by the ladder. Here we see therapies such as nerve blocks, epidurals, PCA, and spinal stimulators

Commonly used analgesics are shown in Table 12.

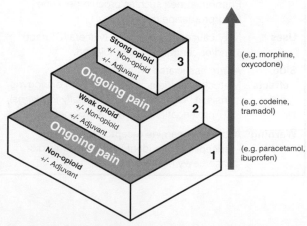

Fig. 2 WHO Analgesic Ladder Remember, combining non-opioids with opioids often reduces opioid requirements (and the SEs that come with them).

TABLE 12   Commonly used Analgesics

Name	Starting dose	Caution if...
NON-OPIOID		
Paracetamol	1 g PO QDS	Weight <50 Kg (give reduced dose)
Ibuprofen	400 mg PO TDS	Asthma, renal impairment, reflux disease, cardiac disease
WEAK OPIOID		
Codeine	15-60 mg PO QDS	Elderly, renal impairment, hepatic impairment
Tramadol	50-100 mg PO QDS	Elderly, renal impairment, hepatic impairment
STRONG OPIOID		
Morphine	2.5 mg-5 mg PO PRN	Renal/liver impairment, elderly, frail, previous reaction to opioids, already on other sedating medication
Oxycodone	1-2 mg PO PRN	EGFR <10 mL/min/1.73m^2
ADJUVANT		
Gabapentin	300 mg PO ON - titrate dose slowly to TDS	Elderly/reduced eGFR
Pregabalin	50-75 mg PO BD – titrate up as required	Elderly/reduced eGFR
Amitriptyline	10 mg PO ON – titrate as tolerated	Cardiac disease, risk of urinary retention, if on other antidepressants (serotonin toxicity)

PALLIATIVE CARE EXAMPLE CASE

Jane Doe has recently been diagnosed with metastatic breast cancer and is currently experiencing very mild pain that she says is relieved when she takes paracetamol.

1. Prescribe **REGULAR** Paracetamol 1g QDS PO

Jane Doe returns, stating she has quite good pain control, but she is experiencing some pain between doses. She has no other co-morbidities, good renal function, and no history of reflux.

2. Add **REGULAR** Naproxen 500 mg BD PO (caution in gastric, renal, and cardiac patients)

3. Consider prescribing PPI for gastric protection.

A month later, Jane Doe returns to the clinic and is experiencing worsening pain and is struggling to sleep. You prescribe some additional pain relief and ask her to return if the pain is still not controlled.

4. Prescribe **REGULAR** Codeine 60 mg QDS PO (this is in addition to the paracetamol and naproxen)

5. Prescribe **laxative** and **PRN antiemetic.**

A week later and Jane's pain is not well controlled. She has had little sleep and has stopped going to the shops and seeing friends because of the pain.

6. Switch Codeine to Morphine – Some calculations are required:
   - Calculate **current codeine dose** = 60 mg x4 = 240 mg codeine
   - 240 mg codeine = 24 mg morphine (see Palliative care and Oncology in an hour for more on conversions), but Jane is still in pain, so we need to increase the dose.
   - Start at 10 mg oral morphine (oramorph) 4 hourly
   - Calculate **daily morphine requirement** = 10 mg x 6 = **60 mg daily morphine requirement.**
   - Calculate **as required dose =** 1/6 of total daily morphine = 60 mg ÷ 6 = **10 mg oral morphine PRN**

Jane leaves the clinic with the following prescription:
- Paracetamol 1 g QDS PO
- Naproxen 500 mg BD PO
- Lansoprazole 15 mg OD PO

PALLIATIVE CARE EXAMPLE CASE—cont'd

- Docusate 120 mg OD PO
- Morphine sulphate 10 mg four-hourly PO
- Morphine sulphate 10 mg PO PRN (For breakthrough pain)

Jane returns to the clinic for a pain review. She says her pain is mostly well controlled, she is opening her bowels regularly, and she has experienced no other symptoms. She is regularly taking three PRN doses of her oramorph, and so you decide you must increase her morphine dose.

7. Increase oral morphine dose – Some more calculations
   - Calculate daily morphine requirements = regular morphine dose (60 mg) + PRN doses required (3 x 10 mg) = **90 mg daily morphine requirement.**
   - Give total requirement in six divided daily doses = 90 mg ÷ 6 = **15 mg oral morphine four-hourly**
   - Calculate new as required dose = 1/6 of total daily morphine requirements = 90 mg ÷ 6 = **15 mg oral morphine PRN**

Jane feels her pain is now well controlled, but she is still tired as she is waking up regularly to take her medications. You decide to switch her to a slow-release form of morphine, so she has to take it only twice a day.

8. Switch stable morphine dose to slow-release opiate (e.g., zomorph) - A couple more calculations
   - Calculate the daily **stable** morphine requirement = 6 x 15 mg = **90 mg daily oral morphine requirement**

- Give total requirement in two divided daily doses = 90 mg ÷ 2 = **45 mg oral morphine (modified release) BD**
- Calculate as required dose = 1/6 of total daily morphine requirements = 90 mg ÷ 6 = **15 mg oral morphine PRN**

Jane's condition deteriorates over the coming months, and she is admitted as her pain is not well controlled. She regularly needs two PRN doses. It is decided to give her pain relief SC as she is struggling to take the medication orally.

9. Convert between equivalent doses of PO and SC morphine
   - Calculate daily oral morphine requirement = regular morphine (2 x 45mg) + PRN (2 x 15 mg) = **120 mg daily oral morphine requirement**
   - Convert to SC equivalent dose (10 mg PO = 5 mg SC therefore divide 2) = **60 mg daily SC morphine**
   - Give total requirement over 24 hours in a syringe driver.
   - Calculate as required dose = 1/6 of total daily morphine requirements = 60 mg ÷ 6 = **10 mg SC morphine PRN**
   - Prescribe antiemetic and ensure laxative is prescribed.

Jane's pain management is optimised, and she is well enough to go home with a syringe driver and the nursing care she needs.

For further information, see the Palliative Care and Oncology chapter.

READING LIST: PRESCRIBING APPENDIX

AAGBI. (2010). *AAGBI safety guideline. Pre-operative assessment and patient preparation.* www.rcoa.ac.uk.

Baker, E., Burrage, D., Hitchings, A., & Lonsdale, D. (2019). *The top 100 drugs: Clinical pharmacology and practical prescribing.* Elsevier

BNF. (2020). https://bnf.nice.org.uk/ [Accessed April 21]

Clunie, G. P. R., Wilkinson, N., Nikiphorou, E., & Jadon, D. (2018). *Oxford handbook of rheumatology.* Oxford University Press

Elkins, M., Davenport, R., & Mintz, P. (2022). Chapter 37 transfusion medicine. In *Henry's Clinical Diagnosis and Management by Laboratory Methods.* Elsevier. https://www.clinicalkey.com/#!/browse/book/3-s2.0-C20180017521.

HEE e-LFH. (2020). *Anaesthesia eLA, core training, preoperative assessment and management.* https://portal.e-lfh.org.uk.

Jones, M., & Tomson, C. (2018). Acute kidney injury and 'nephrotoxins': Mind your language. *Clinical Medicine (London), 18*(5), 384–386.

Kidneys, Think (2016). *Guidelines for medicines optimisation in patients with acute kidney injury.* https://www.think-kidneys.nhs.uk/aki/wp-content/uploads/sites/2/2016/03/Guidelines-for-Medicines-optimisation-in-patients-with-AKI-final.pdf [Accessed April 2021]

NICE. (2019). *NG148: Acute kidney injury: Prevention, detection and management.* https://www.nice.org.uk/guidance/NG148. [Accessed April 2021]

NICE guideline. (2022). *NG125: Surgical site infections: Prevention and treatment.* www.nice.org.uk/guidance/ng125/. [Accessed April 2021]

Note: Page numbers followed by "f" indicate figures and "t" indicate tables.